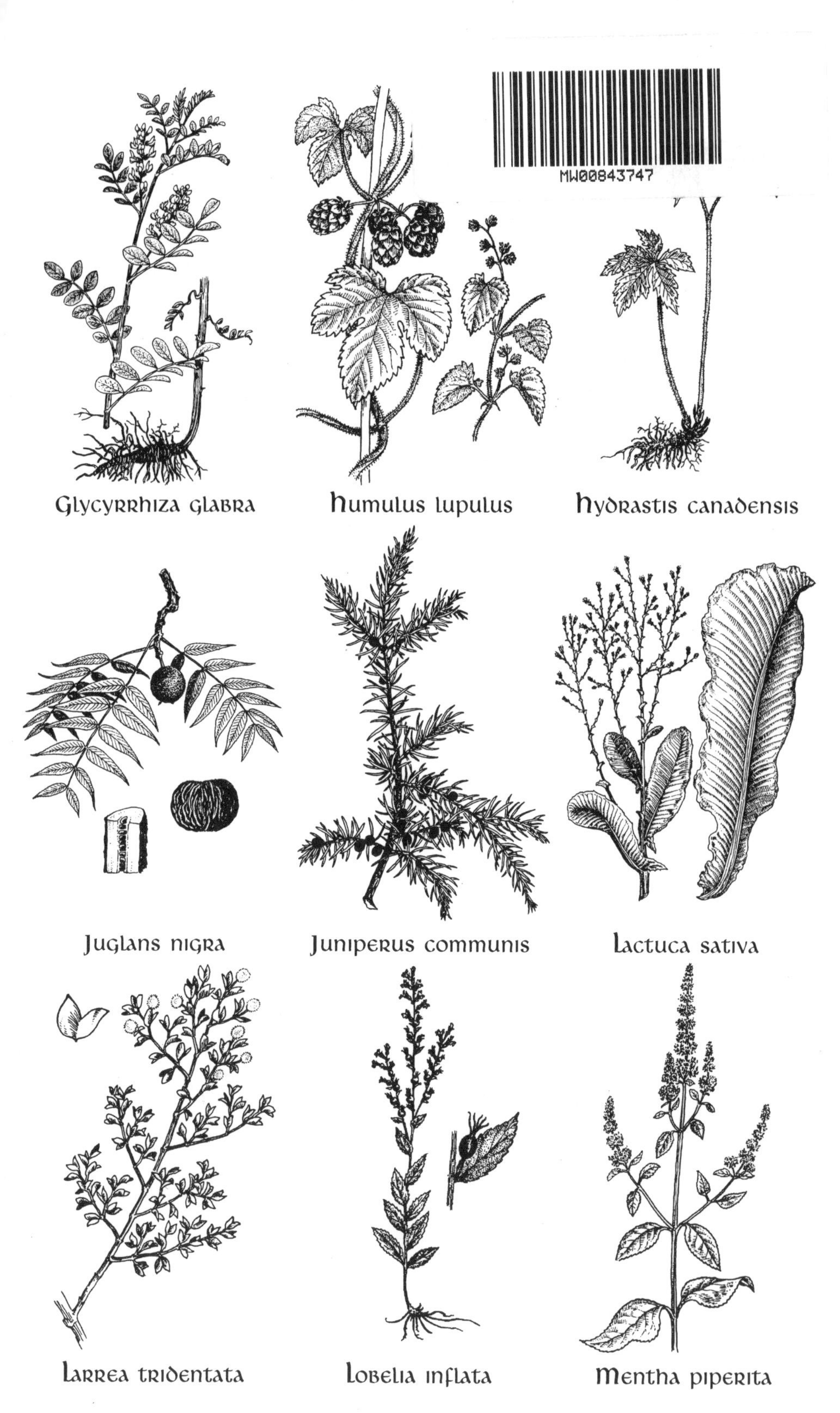
MW00843747
Glycyrrhiza glabra
Humulus lupulus
Hydrastis canadensis
Juglans nigra
Juniperus communis
Lactuca sativa
Larrea tridentata
Lobelia inflata
Mentha piperita

SCHOOL OF NATURAL HEALING

Dr. John R. Christopher

SCHOOL OF NATURAL HEALING

THE REFERENCE VOLUME ON HERBAL THERAPY
FOR THE TEACHER, STUDENT
OR PRACTITIONER

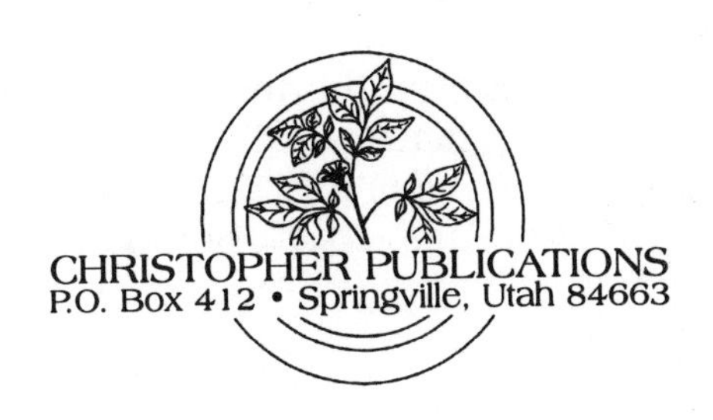

Published by Christopher Publications, Inc.
P. O. Box 412
Springville, Utah 84663

ISBN 1-879436-01-9
Library of Congress #90-205323

First Printing
September 1976

Third Printing
July 1978

Fifth Printing
September 1979

Seventh Printing
July 1986

Ninth Printing
March 1991

Eleventh Printing
January 1996
Revised and Expanded
20th Anniversary Edition

FOREWORD

The contents of this volume were originally presented as a series of lectures given by Dr. John Raymond Christopher to groups interested in natural healing. When audiences heard the principles of diet and the use of herbs contained in the lectures, they asked for a reference book.

The first edition appeared as a correspondence course of twenty lessons taken directly from the lectures. In 1976, as the demand increased for the valuable information contained herein, Dr. Christopher decided to publish the course in book form so everyone who wished could learn about his successful approach to healing with herbs.

A mastery of the concepts in this book can change a person's life to a fuller enjoyment of health and vigor. Dr. Christopher's personal experiences and his refreshing attitude of faith can become a source of lasting joy to the serious student.

FOREWORD TO THE 20TH ANNIVERSARY EDITION

Changes in the political health climate, the current resurgance of interest in herbal healing, advances in word processing technology, and the concentrated, scrutinizing labors of the entire staff of Christopher Publications over the past year have made this expanded, revised edition the most valuable resource of herbal therapeutics and formulation since Dr. Christopher himself presented the lectures. For the first time since the original mimeograph version, Dr. Christopher's famous formulations are included.

Other improvements found in this edition include:

The bi-nomial nomenclature of the herbs has been updated to the current standard usage.

All formulas have been reviewed for accuracy and, where necessary, have been corrected and simplified.

Herbal references and medicinal categories are posted at the top of each page for accessibility.

Measurements have been updated to current standards in millegrams, teaspoons, and ounces.

David Christopher, M.H. -project director
Dean G. Morris, M.H. -editing director

TABLE OF CONTENTS

TABLE OF CONTENTS
HERBS IN ALPHABETICAL ORDER

INTRODUCTION

Last summer my family went camping with some friends in the arid regions of southern Utah. One morning, our friend asked me for help with her daughter who had diarrhea. Miriam, the little daughter, had ignored the delicious herbs, berries and seeds we were foraging and the salads we prepared and instead stuck to hot dogs, chips, and candy, and thus earned some real discomfort. We knew she needed to cleanse and nourish, but with the heat we also recognized the risk of dehydration and the need to stem the flow of fluids escaping her small body. Being an Herbalist graduate of The School of Natural Healing founded by Dr. John R. Christopher, I recognized right away the root cause of her condition. Her bowel was malnourished and had become loose in the effort to remove waste. We needed to provide herbs that would give tone, or contract the tissue, as well as nourish the system. Because of this book, *School of Natural Healing*, I was able to determine the proper therapeutic category of astringent/tonic herbs that would help Miriam. My mind rummaged through the powders, extracts, and ointments I had stocked in my herbal first-aid kit. I couldn't come up with just the right remedy from my preparations, so I turned to the surrounding medicine chest of Nature for her answers.

I looked around for an herb from the astringent category and quickly spotted a grove of gambel oak (Quercus gambelii) next to Miriam's tent. Here was nature's answer to her needs. With gratitude we broke off some small branches, picked off the leaves, and had Miriam chew on the twigs while we prepared a warm infusion of the leaves. From the twigs and herbal tea, natural relief came quickly. Recently, her mother informed me that the oak has now become "her" herb. Whenever she feels a tummy ache or intestinal discomfort, she climbs the nearest oak tree to find her medicine.

I thank God for oak trees and the ability to teach people how to use them to help themselves. I thank Dr. Christopher for his text's contribution to the art of natural healing. Within these pages you will find herbs categorized by their therapeutic action. The study of these categories gives us freedom from memorizing the countless specific medicinal applications of each herb. Instead we choose an available herb whose therapeutic action will heal the root cause of the condition.

School of Natural Healing continues to be the primary resource for the herbalist training offered by The School of Natural Healing. This text has been a valuable aid to me from the beginning of my study to my current work as a professional herbalist. This text provides a compilation of many areas of study requisite for a natural healer.

For the novice, the chapter on general disease gives the symptoms, useful herbs and therapies for diseases, and also instructs on the root cause of the condition. The botanist will find the emphasis on botanical names and detailed identifying characteristics of the herbs thorough and precise. The horticulturist will find helpful information on growing your own herbs. For the commercial herbal provider, Dr. Christopher gives personal experience in determining herb quality. For the nutritionist, Dr. Christopher provides unique and simple instruction on proper diet and cleansing for a strong foundation to support the healing power of herbs. Herbal practitioners will find the chapters on therapeutic categories inspiring. Herbal pharmacists will find an unequaled resource of pages filled with proven formulas, preparation instruction, and congenial combinations. Only a Master Herbalist with years of successful clinical application and remarkable teaching skills could combine each of these essential studies into one masterful work. Whatever your healing interest may be, I commend this book to you with all my heart.

Dean G. Morris, M. H.

BIOGRAPHY OF
DR. JOHN RAYMOND CHRISTOPHER

Adapted from *An Herbal Legacy of Courage*
David Christopher, M.H.

The quality that I remember most when thinking of my famous father, Dr. John R. Christopher, was his extraordinary positive attitude. This positive outlook was reflected in a cheerfulness that never quit. Even when he suffered physically or even through endless persecution from the medical establishment, because of his herbal treatments, he maintained his love of life and deep concern for those in need.

Living in an era when natural remedies are much the fashion, we may often forget what a pioneer Dr. Christopher was, and what he sacrificed and suffered to help bring about the renaissance of herbal healing in North America. Appreciation for his singular struggle comes when you see his life's path in the following biography.

He was born November 25, 1909 in Salt Lake City, Utah, to Jean Ramone and Lorena Roth Raymond. Both were emigrants to the United States, and for some unknown reason, they left their infant son and an older sister at the Salt Lake City Orphanage. When prospective parents came to that orphanage, the children would be lined up so the couple could make their choice. On one such day, Leander and Melissa Ann Craig Christopher visited the orphanage, looking for a son. Suddenly, without invitation, a baby, dressed only in a diaper and thin undershirt, toddled up, crawled into Melissa's lap, and snuggled into her shoulder. She exclaimed softly, "This is our son!"

The original parents had stipulated that both children remain together, so now Raymond (often called "Ray") and his sister Ruby had a new family. They lived in Salt Lake City in the Avenues district, which was then a semi-rural neighborhood. The first glimpse the Christophers had of Raymond's unusual future came one winter's night when young Ray lay critically ill with croup. The parents were pacing the floor with him, distressed because of the high fever and labored breathing, wondering if he would have the strength to catch another breath. Suddenly a knock came at the door. Leander, startled because of the late hour, answered.

Standing on the porch was a bearded man in short sleeves, with no coat in the bitter cold. He announced to Leander that their young child was ill but would not die; that he had an important mission to perform. Leander listened to the stranger give explicit directions on how to cut the phlegm and stop the croup.

Leander started into the house to follow these instructions, but then turned to thank the visitor and invite him into the house to get warm. But the man was gone without a trace. There were no footprints in the deep snow. Ray's parents followed the man's instructions, and he recovered. The Christophers never forgot this experience, and Ray always remembered that his life had an important purpose because of it.

That Ray became a healer is appropriate and also ironic, because he had been born with advanced rheumatoid arthritis, walking with a cane even as a child, or often confined to a wheelchair. Along with the arthritis, he developed hardening of the arteries. Despite the constant pain and suffering, young Ray was cheerful and optimistic. Doctors at the time predicted that he would never reach the age of thirty.

Raymond's adopted mother suffered from a lifetime affliction of diabetes and dropsy, which left her exhausted and debilitated. As Ray, just a little boy, observed her suffering from his own wheelchair, he resolved one day to be a doctor. His mother laughed a little, commenting that he couldn't even stand the sight of blood, that he couldn't bear to see chickens or other animals killed for the evening meal. What kind of doctor could such a person be?

Raymond answered, "Mother, I will be able to heal people without cutting them up. There will be natural ways of doing it." This answer from a young child became a charter for his life's mission. When Raymond was sixteen years old, such a doctor visited the Christopher home: an Iridologist who could ascertain a person's condition from examining the iris of the eye. This doctor, seeing in her irises the very conditions she had been treated for over the years, recommended dietary changes and gave Mrs. Christopher some herbs. As the doctor left, Ray said, "That's the kind of doctor I'm going to be when I grow up." Several months later, Raymond tried to locate the doctor, but he had been arrested for practicing medicine without a license, and put into jail—a foreshadowing of Ray's own future.

After he graduated from high school, he heard of another natural doctor in Canada, who massaged people's feet to heal them. He was in such demand that people lined up to see him, even pitching tents for weeks at a time as they waited. Ray wanted to see this man, not only to have his rheumatoid arthritis healed, but to study under him. He prepared to make the trip. His parents tried to discourage him, since they had no money at that time in the middle of the Depression. Nevertheless, Ray continued to prepare for the trip, till he heard that this man, too, had been arrested.

Ray worked during the days at his father's lumber mill, and at night he played with a dance band to save for college. He graduated with honors from Henager's Business College in Salt Lake City. Because he had a photographic memory and a way with words, he wanted to go to law school. He was accepted at the University of Utah School of Law.

The day before classes began, Ray was riding in the car of a friend and they were hit by another vehicle. Ray was pronounced dead at the scene. His grief-stricken parents arrived at the morgue to identify the body—when his mother suddenly screamed! She had seen the faintest flicker of an eyelash! The mortician bent over Ray, and he too saw the slightest motion of life in him. He was rushed to the hospital, where he lay in a coma for several days, and then, after drifting into consciousness, lay helpless only able to speak. Nurses had to feed him, shave him, and carry him to the bathroom.

One afternoon, a driver from the lumber company came to visit him. He tried to cajole him into coming back to work. Ray just laughed, knowing he couldn't even move his hand. The driver suggested a chiropractor. But when Ray mentioned this possibility to the four doctors who were treating him, they scoffed at him. Nevertheless, this driver convinced Ray's parents to take him to a chiropractor. Ray resisted with all he had, but they carried him out, and to the chiropractor they went.

Several days after his chiropractic treatment, Ray was working again at the office. He was still bandaged about the head, but he regained his strength and could work as he used to. However, his injuries had damaged his photographic memory and given him trouble with his short-term memory. One day he went to the bank to deposit company funds, and his mind went completely blank. He located some police officers, asking them for help. They found his identification and took him back to the office, and his memory finally returned.

During this recuperation period, he would suffer periodic pain in the head and back from the injuries of his accident. At times the pain was so severe he couldn't sleep. And at the same time he was helplessly watching his mother die from complications of diabetes and Bright's Disease. Her condition stopped responding to even the highest doses of insulin, and her arms were purple from constant needles. She began to die, slowly poisoned with gangrene. As Ray watched her painful death, helpless to do anything for her, he prayed that he could learn how to stop such suffering.

His own pain caused him to experience many sleepless nights. To help pass through these he would study and read. In addition to many good books, he chose to read from the scriptures. One night, confined to a chair with arthritis, he picked up *The Doctrine and Covenants,* a book of scripture from The Church of Jesus Christ of Latter-day Saints. It fell open to Section 89, commonly known as "The Word of Wisdom," a health code for the church. Ray had read this many times before, but this time he gained some unique impressions. The words *sparingly*—referring to meats—and *wholesome*—referring to grains and vegetables—deeply moved him. He vowed to follow the health code strictly, and developed for himself a diet of fruits, vegetables, grains, nuts, and seeds.

He was astonished to see his health improve immediately and dramatically. Within a few months, he gained weight, began sleeping soundly at night, and had enough energy for a full day's work. In 1939 he wrote *Just What is the Word of Wisdom?,* a booklet that described this experience and outlined his ideas about diet and health. Not long after, Dr. John A. Widtsoe, an authority in the Mormon church and author who had also written on the Word of Wisdom, called Ray on the phone, praising his booklet as being "well ahead of its time." He urged Ray to distribute it to as many people as he could.

Ray began to do so, talking to as many people as would listen about his ideas on health. Many of them responded with derision and ridicule. With typical good humor, he often retold one particular story. He was still working at the lumber mill, and at lunchtime, one of the workers told him he was wanted at his office. There lay a sumptuous meal, set with a fine tablecloth and beautiful china: fresh green alfalfa ("common cow hay," as he later described it), dried wheat and rolled oats, and an elegant decanter of apple juice. The workers waited to see what he would do. With characteristic good grace, he pulled out his chair and plucked up the fancy cloth napkin. "How nice of you! This is really wonderful!" he exclaimed, and ate every bite. They never kidded him again, but he lived lonely among his peers, since vegetarianism was not understood at the time.

Ray married Irene Short in 1935, and had two daughters, Sandra Joy and Carol Ann, but this marriage did not work out, and they were divorced in 1943. He later met Wendella Walker, fell immediately in love, and they were married on August 14, 1944, in the Salt Lake Temple of The Church of Jesus Christ of Latter-day Saints. She always supported his ideas about health and his work, and together they had five children: John Rulon, Ruth Ellen, David Wendell, Janet Lorene, and Steven Craig.

A PRESCRIPTION FOR THE MESS SERGEANT

When World War II broke out, and just a few months after the Christophers were married, Ray received a draft notice on his doorstep summoning him to active duty. A 35-year-old man, divorced and newly married, with two families to support, he reported for service but requested status as a conscientious objector, presenting his Word of Wisdom booklet as evidence of his firm beliefs.

"I'll serve my country with pride on the front lines," he said, "I'll carry stretchers that can save people. But I will not carry a gun. I cannot kill another human being." During basic training, he was told to carry a gun on night watch, but he refused. The officer thrust a night stick at him, but he shook his head, and refused to carry a night stick, too, because you could kill people with a night stick. The officer ordered Ray to be confined to quarters under guard till next morning, when he was tried for his rebellion. The officer hearing the case slapped his palm sharply on the table and shouted, "This is ridiculous! A conscientious objector that won't carry a nightstick? What if everyone in the world felt as you do?"

"Then there would be no war," Ray answered.

"That's the answer I needed," the officer responded. "Take this card. It shows that you are a conscientious objector, and no one will challenge you again."

From Fort Douglas, Utah, Ray travelled to North Fort at Washington's Fort Lewis, where he was assigned to supervise a medical dispensary. Here was more irony—Raymond Christopher, a buck private, gave orders to pharmacists and therapists, all of whom outranked him. Even the cleaning boy outranked him. Ray, in charge of the entire operation, served under a Major Shumate.

At first Ray felt frustrated and angry. Having learned and seen so much healing using natural methods and nutrition (he had all ready helped many people), here he was confined to use standard medical treatments. He knew that there are better ways. He saw cases among the soldiers that he knew would quickly respond to natural treatments. However, Major Shumate was firmly against any such treatments. So he spent his time observing the effects of orthodox medications, seeing firsthand the futility of the treatment. He saw that standard medicine only treats symptoms instead of the cause of disease. But one day a soldier came to the dispensary with a supposedly incurable condition, and this changed the course of his life.

At a staff meeting, composed of the heads of eight dispensaries, Major Shumate, a private dermatologist in civilian life, said he had never seen a case of contagious impetigo so severe. The soldier had been hospitalized nine times, where his case had cleared up temporarily, but it always flared up when he was released. Specialists from the eastern U.S. had been called in, but nothing had worked.

Major Shumate brought the soldier in, and, except for Ray, they all gasped with horror. The soldier's head had been shaved as much as possible, but wherever the stubble of hair grew, the scalp was covered with a crusty scab nearly an inch thick.

"What a beautiful case of impetigo!" exclaimed Ray (who had never seen one quite that bad).

"You must be a born doctor," said Shumate, slapping him on the shoulder, "It's one of the most amazing things I have ever seen, too. But unfortunately, we have to release this man from the army."

"I object to that!" cried the soldier, "I came into this army a clean man. I caught this thing while I was here, and now you're asking me to take this filth home to my wife and children. I won't do it."

"I'm sorry, but there's nothing more we can do," responded Shumate, "We've done everything possible. We've used every cure medical science has to offer, and nothing has worked. We have to give you a release, and it will be an honorable discharge."

"Wait," Ray said. "That man can be healed."

Shumate whirled to face him. "None of your blasted herbs!" The other officers rolled their eyes and guffawed.

The soldier spoke up. "I should have something to say about this. I don't care if he puts horse manure on my head, as long as he heals me."

Shumate paused, and then said, "All right. If you sign papers releasing the government and the army from any liability, you can try this treatment."

The papers were signed, and the soldier was placed under twenty-four hour military police surveillance to prevent escape. As the meeting broke up, one of the officers jeered, "When will the big unveiling be?"

"Monday morning!" Ray snapped back, without really thinking. Then he realized—he just had one week. Here, far from home without the herbs that he generally used, he had to treat the worst case of impetigo he had ever seen. Immediately he called a Salt Lake friend who had a black walnut tree in his backyard. He explained his dilemma, and his friend agreed to gather the black walnut husks, even though the ground was covered with snow. They were transported overnight to Fort Lewis. Ray picked them up in the morning—sopping wet, which could weaken their potency. Not only that, but Ray only had rubbing alcohol, not grain alcohol, which was not available through the army medical system. And instead of fourteen days to macerate the tincture, he figured he could take only two days. He carried the tincture with him, shaking it vigorously all the time.

At last he strained the tincture and made a compress to fit over the soldier's head like a football helmet. He left instructions that the compress should be kept wet with the tincture for the rest of the week. He also wrote a prescription to the mess sergeant, for wholesome foods for the soldier to eat.

All too soon Monday morning arrived, and the dispensary heads all met, ready to ridicule Ray for his herbal treatments. "Everybody ready?" asked Shumate in a mocking tone. "Private Christopher, are you ready to show us your miracle?"

"I'm ready," responded Ray, feeling nervous but determined. "I haven't seen him yet, but we'll take a look."

The guards ushered the soldier in, and Ray skillfully cut away the adhesive tape. As he lifted the compress off, the scab came off with it, and the soldier's scalp was as clean and pure as a baby's. The impetigo was gone, with no scarring.

The officers all gasped. Shumate shouted; "I've never seen anything like this in all my medical practice!" He took Ray aside. "I've misjudged you, Private Christopher," he admitted. "From this day on you have full permission to practice with herbs. Set yourself up a laboratory here. Do whatever you like as long as you're under my jurisdiction at Fort Lewis."

And with that Ray became the only practicing herbalist in the United States Army during World War II. His black walnut tincture became famous, not only to cure impetigo, but for fungus infection and jungle rot. When soldiers learned that Private Christopher could cure jungle rot, his patient load multiplied tenfold. Eventually this tincture was successful in curing scrofula, eczema, ringworm, shingles, and chronic boils.

BPE, THE BLOOD PRESSURE FORMULA

During his time at the dispensary, Ray started his personal search for an herb that could relieve his own serious health problem, high blood pressure and hardening of the arteries, which he had suffered since adolescence. He began working with cayenne, which is high in calcium and vitamin C. He found that cayenne is one of the best remedies for the heart. He saw that it restores and retains the elasticity of the blood vessels, correcting or preventing hardening of the arteries and preserving the health of the circulatory system. Ray also found that cayenne equalized blood circulation and brought blood pressure to normal. He even found that cayenne was powerful enough to stop a heart attack in progress. In later years, carrying cayenne in his herbal doctor's bag, he never lost a person to a heart attack. He remembered one woman who had suffered from heart problems for eighteen years. She had taken powerful heart medication for more than seven years. After starting cayenne, she was able to stop this medication within months. Her varicose veins also completely cleared.

Soon Ray added ginger, parsley, golden seal, garlic and Siberian ginseng root to cayenne to create a formula called BPE, which equalizes blood pressure and builds the health of the circulatory system. This formula, along with a healthy diet and lifestyle, prolonged Ray's own life many years after the doctors' predictions. At age 45, ten years after the doctors predicted he would die, Ray had a full physical examination. The doctors were astounded to see that he had the blood pressure of a healthy teenager. Just before his death, Ray's blood pressure at seventy years was that of a young man in his twenties.

During World War II, racial prejudice was still rampant. Ray began to understand and feel the distress of the black soldiers who were treated so negatively at the dispensaries. Black soldiers often suffered physical agony in silence rather than go there. But soon word spread that the dispensary head at Fort Lewis was different; within months he was seeing dozens of black soldiers every day. They received kindness as well as the superior care from herbal treatments.

At Fort Lewis dispensary, Ray had the chance to experiment with different herbs that he had only studied about previously. There he began to develop his own herbal formulas, which remain to this day a singular contribution to herbal medicine.

HARVESTING WEEDS AT DAWN

When Ray's military obligation was over, Major Shumate invited him to spend another tour of duty in the dispensary and let the Army pay for his medical education. But Ray preferred to go home to Olympia, Washington, home to his wife. Now he was ready to become a natural doctor, his childhood dream. Coming home with the knowledge and first-hand experience of using herbs in the army, he wanted to expand his skills and help others.

He and his wife agreed that he should travel to Canada to study under Dr. H. Nowell at Dominion Herbal College. There he earned his Master Herbalist Degree. He returned home to Olympia to set up his first practice. But during those final war years and their aftermath, Ray found it difficult to practice as an herbalist.

First of all, it was hard to build enough of a practice to support his small family. In those post-war years, jobs were scarce, and most people had little money to pay for treatment. And unlike today, it was impossible to order herbs through wholesale houses. There were few enough of these businesses, and most of these were forced to close their doors in those lean years. But Ray figured out what to do and did it with typical vigor: he secured a job weeding gardens each morning for ready cash, and then took the medicinal varieties home in large burlap bags

He would spread his morning's harvest across the counter tops of their small kitchen. Then he would wash each weed, rinsing out the soil carefully. He sorted them carefully into categories and then prepared them to use for his patients that afternoon. Ray turned a difficulty into a blessing: he had cash to sustain his family, and also had the freshest herbs one could desire. But he never withheld any knowledge to line his wallet; he taught his patients to harvest their own herbs from their own backyards and treat themselves.

One of the most successful "weeds" he used was plantain. Ray knew that Galen and Pliny, ancient herbalists, had used it as a powerful blood purifier to kill infection rapidly. He also knew that it would relieve blood poisoning that can result from cuts, slivers, bites, and stings. In one astonishing case, Ray treated a man who had slipped at work and drove a chisel deep into his palm. The man couldn't afford to take time off, nor to pay any doctors' fees, so he wrapped the hand with a dirty rag and finished his day's work. He even worked for a few additional days.

By the time he arrived at Ray's office, his hand was swollen and hot and a red streak ran from the badly infected hand up the arm. A painful lump the size of a baseball in his armpit prevented the man from dropping his arm to his side. The man was frantic with pain and fear. Ray asked him why he hadn't sought medical treatment when the condition became so severe, but the man was afraid that his arm would have been amputated. Ray taught him how to dig up plantain plants, wash and crush them, put them on the wound and bandage them in place. He was to add fresh herb to the poultice every time it dried out. He was also to drink at least three cups a day of the tea. The man wanted to come back for a checkup, but Ray assured him that he would be healed completely by the next day.

The man did return in three days, but only to report what seemed to him a miracle. On the first day, the red streak had disappeared within a few hours and the swelling in the armpit had reduced. By evening, the wound was much better, and within a day or two, the condition was completely healed. The man had full use of his hand and arm and was able to earn a living for his family.

In a similar case, a young girl had cut her foot on a shell while clam hunting at the beach. She had continued to run and play for the afternoon, but by the next morning her foot and leg were swollen and feverish. She also had a red streak forming toward her groin. Ray gave her similar instructions as he had for the man with the chisel wound. The wound healed quickly, and the next day the child skipped into Ray's office to pay him. He protested that the pay was too much, but the child said, "Mama told me to bring you this much because my foot healed so quickly." As it turned out, the Christophers were paid many times over for this assistance, because this girl's family owned a smorgasbord in Spokane, and were some of the few people in the area who were able to get butter and fresh produce because of wartime rationing. Throughout the remainder of the war, they saw to it that the Christophers had a little butter and some fresh fruits and vegetables as a token of their appreciation.

Because plantain and other herbs are only available during the summer, Ray began to concoct concentrates, tinctures, and ointments to use year-round. Once a mother called Ray about her ten-year-old son who had been stung by a wasp. His hand was severely swollen and he had passed out from the pain.

Ray tucked a jar of plantain ointment into his bag and went on the house call. When he arrived, the child was still unconscious and his hand swollen to twice its size. Ray quickly spread a thick layer of plantain ointment over the bite about the size of a silver dollar, covered the ointment with gauze, and used a gauze bandage to hold the patch in place.

"Is that all you're going to do?" the mother asked. "That's all that needs to be done," Ray smiled and told her that the ointment would draw the poison from the sting and relieve the pain and swelling. The boy soon regained consciousness and sat up. Within a half hour, the pain was much relieved, and by next day he was out playing baseball with his friends.

BONE, FLESH AND CARTILAGE (BF&C)

Building on his early experiences with black walnut tincture, Dr. Christopher developed the Bone, Flesh and Cartilage formula for skin trouble. The additional herbs made a wonderfully effective remedy for minor burns, infection, cuts, abrasions, bruises, hemorrhages, sore gums, bunions and corns. It also removes calcium deposits that exacerbate arthritis. A nurse in California used it to dissolve a bone spur on her heel. It has healed skin cancers. And it works, as the black walnut tincture does, for eczema, psoriasis, and other chronic skin conditions.

The beloved story of how Dr. Christopher came by the BF&C formula begins when a woman came to his office early one morning, panicky and desperate. Hours earlier, her fourteen-year-old daughter had attempted suicide. She left the daughter in the care of several neighbors to find help from Dr. Christopher. The girl had developed, almost three years before, a severe case of dermatitis, with heavy scales on her face, neck, arms and hands, legs and feet. No physician or specialist had been able to identify her condition, much less find a cure. She began to gorge herself, became extremely overweight, and eventually decided to end her life. As Ray listened to this desperate mother, he offered a silent prayer for help and "a formula came immediately to my mind," as he related it. He jotted the herbs down and gave the mother complete instructions on how to make and apply the fomentations and tea, and sent her to an herb shop to get them.

Four days after this mother had come to his office, she called to report that the scabs and scales were gone, and the girl's skin began to show what the mother termed, "a healing glow." Six months later she was a cheerleader at school and enjoying all the social activities of girls of her age.

BF&C has been known to heal wounds, even surgical incisions that have failed to heal. One California woman had an abdominal surgical wound that had been draining for more than three years. She applied the ointment to the wound and took the capsules internally. Within seven days, the wound was entirely healed.

BF&C has even been known to regenerate tissue. Ray's nephew was a passenger in a car accident, and although relatives held onto him so that he wasn't thrown from the car, he was dragged for some distance along the hot asphalt, and his small fingers were scraped to stubs as far as his first knuckles. Ray gave the child capsules of BF&C and told the parents to mix the powder with honey and wheat germ oil. Within two months, the fingers had healed, complete with perfectly formed fingernails. When Ray next saw his nephew, the child ran toward him and threw his arms around him. "Look, Uncle Ray!" he shouted. "My fingers grew back!"

In a similar story, a young woman came to Ray and said, "How do you like my fingers?" He said he thought they were beautiful, clean, and well manicured. "Can you tell which finger was cut off?" she asked him. He couldn't tell, even when he looked close. She told him her story: her finger had been amputated below the knuckle. She had used BF&C, and the knuckle had regenerated. Gradually, all the bone and flesh filled in, and even the fingernail grew back perfectly formed.

BURN PASTE

One of Dr. Christopher's most dramatic cases of skin regeneration involved two ten-year-old boys who were playing with matches and gasoline, when the gas burst into flame. Both boys were severely burned. The surgeon at the hospital said that the hands would either have to be amputated at the wrist and iron claws attached to both arms, or the boys could endure several years of painful skin graft surgeries. After years of such surgery, the boys would have nothing better than mummified claws which could never move like fingers.

One set of parents told the surgeon to begin operations; the other set of parents took their child to Dr. Christopher. He cringed at the badly scarred skin, tendons, muscles and nerves. He gave the parents a salve made of comfrey, honey, and wheat germ oil. He told the parents to keep a thick layer of this burn ointment on the area.

Within a week, the parents took their son to see the surgeon, who was dumfounded. The burns had healed from third-degree to first-degree. "What on earth have you been using?" he asked. The parents just said, "An old-fashioned remedy." "Whatever it is, keep on using it. I don't think there's need for surgery now. I can't believe it. But these hands are going to heal without scar tissue."

A year after the burn, the first boy remained in the hospital. The parents had invested hundreds of thousands of dollars on the surgery and skin grafting, but the boy ended up with stiff, unbending claws that the boy hid with gloves.

The other boy, whose parents had applied the herbal salve, healed completely. The tendons, nerves, muscles and flesh were all renewed, with no scar tissue. Even the fingernails grew back. The family's total investment was less than twenty dollars for the herbal salve.

INF FORMULA

From his experiences with plantain, Ray developed INF, a formula to kill infection. He began with plantain; then added black walnut hulls, which kill infection, destroy worms and parasites, and relieve infection of poisonous snakebite or rabid animal bites. He added calendula flowers, marshmallow root, golden seal root, and bugleweed, herbs that kill infection and clear toxins from the lymphatic system.

RED CLOVER COMBINATION

Soon Ray hoped to team INF with a formula to purify the bloodstream and remove infection that circulated throughout the body. He came up with the famed

Red Clover Combination, a purifying formula of red clover blossoms, chaparral, licorice root, peach bark, Oregon grape or barberry root bark, poke, and stillingia or echinacea, cascara sagrada bark, sarsaparilla root, prickly ash bark, burdock root, and buckthorn bark. Ray chose each ingredient carefully, after much herbal study about each herb's characteristics.

He began with red clover blossoms, an alterative herb which gradually purifies and cleanses the bloodstream and corrects any deficiencies in the circulatory system. It also removes obstructions in this system while it nourishes and builds the tissues, reducing any spasms or irritability in the blood vessels.

He added chaparral for its ability to clear up all infections, even stubborn ones. He had seen it heal boils, abscesses, carbuncles and other sever infections by purifying the bloodstream. He had used it to clear up several severe cases of acne within six weeks because of its power to purify the bloodstream.

He chose echinacea because in those days it was famous for clearing blood poisoning. It is now know also for its supreme action to enhance the immune response. Dr. Christopher used echinacea with success in clearing up infection associated with gangrene, ulcers and cancers. He saw it clear staph infections in the bloodstream. To complete the formula, Dr. Christopher added two of nature's most powerful blood purifiers, burdock root and buckthorn bark.

Ray began trying out the Red Clover Combination, and it worked fast and well. One of the most dramatic cases was a forty-five-year-old man who had developed severe sepsis throughout his system. He had lost his hair and fingernails. His eyes were ulcerated and he had even developed some of the symptoms of leprosy. He had lost so much weight that he looked like a skeleton. Ray gave him the Red Clover Combination, together with nutritional guidelines, and within six weeks he had regained weight and had no signs of infection.

A middle-aged woman had been diagnosed with cancer so advanced that her doctor had sent her home, with no further treatment, to die. Ray started her on the Red Clover Combination, as well as a diet of fresh fruits, vegetables, grains, seeds and nuts, and he also advised her to avoid hard water, processed foods, sugars, and cholesterol-containing foods. He also started her on the three-day cleanse once a month. Several months later, after following these directions, she had a checkup with her doctor, and the cancer was gone. She was cured.

As Ray used the Red Clover Combination for various conditions, he was amazed at its powers. A baby was born to an Rh-negative mother and an Rh-positive father which usually necessitates draining the baby's blood followed by total blood transfusion. Sometimes the treatment is successful, but sometimes the baby develops complications or even dies. The mother had previously borne three children who had to have the transfusion. When she had to have open-heart surgery a few years later, the doctor warned her not to get pregnant again, or she and the baby could lose their lives. However, she wanted a large family and went to Ray for help. He put her on the three-day cleanse, the Red Clover Combination, and the mucusless diet, including at least a gallon of distilled water and a quart of red raspberry tea each day. She followed the program and eventually became pregnant. She maintained the program throughout the pregnancy, and when the baby was born, he had no Rh factor. The family eventually had two more Rh-free babies.

CSK PLUS FOR WEIGHT CONTROL

During his practice in Olympia, Ray developed many of his formulas in response to particular needs. One woman had come to him in despair, having gained a hundred pounds in the years since she had married. Ray put her on the mucusless diet, as well as the three-day cleanse once a month. He promised her that if she would follow the program, she would lose the weight naturally and permanently. Several months later, she called him and invited him to a celebration—she had lost all the weight! After a wonderful vegetarian dinner, she led Ray and the family to the back yard. He was puzzled as he sat in one of the chairs surrounding a freshly-dug grave which was scattered with bright wildflowers. He thought they must be planning to bury a well-beloved pet.

Then the children began carrying from the house aluminum pots and pans, putting them inside the grave. They marched to the outside cellar, hauling up slabs of bacon and large smoked hams, adding them to the aluminum pans. At a time of rationing and severe economic depression, Ray saw this as a significant sacrifice—and an inspiration for another of his formulas.

He put together CSK Plus, to be used in weight loss. He combined chickweed, safflower flowers, burdock root, parsley, Norwegian kelp, licorice root, fennel seed, echinacea, black walnut hulls, papaya leaves, and hawthorn berries. Throughout the years, he saw people experience astonishing results with the formula. The licorice root and fennel seed curb the appetite and relieve cravings. Historically, the ancient Greeks nibbled on fennel seeds to control hunger during fasting. Knowing that the body holds on to fat reserves if it is missing essential trace elements, he included the powerful nutritional herbs such as kelp and parsley. He added the papaya leaves to help with metabolism and absorption. The other herbs help cleanse the blood and regulate the adrenal and thyroid glands.

THE NERVINE FORMULAS—B&B, MEM AND RELAXEZE

Ray, or as he was coming to be known by this time, Dr. Christopher, developed other formulas for those who were suffering. A family brought in a fifteen-year-old boy who had constant epileptic seizures, as many as twenty-five in one day! He could not be left unattended, and the family had hired nurses to watch him day and night. The epilepsy created roaring noise inside his head, and in an attempt to stop it, the boy pounded his head against the walls until blood poured from his ears, nose, and mouth. No doctors throughout the state could help in the condition. The boy could not talk and had never attended school. He was diagnosed as severely retarded and doctors recommended institutionalization. Instead, the family came to Dr. Christopher in a last attempt for help.

Ray recommended the mucusless diet and therapeutic massage. Then he came up with two herbal combinations to build and strengthen the nervous system. He showed the parents how to make the teas and give them to the boy. Within six months, this boy, who had been thought retarded, was speaking, and had tutors brought in twice a week to keep up with him in his learning! Instead of being handicapped, he was actually brilliant! Within a few months, he was at the normal level for his age. He enrolled in school, seizure-free from then on.

Dr. Christopher developed and used formulas that came to be known as B&B, MEM, and Relax-Eze. MEM heals the nervous system tissue, restores memory, and strengthens thought processes. Relax-Eze also feeds and rebuilds the nerves and reduces irritation of the nervous system, soothes spasms and tics, and relieves pain.

Relax-Eze is based on skullcap, a nervine herb without the side effects of pharmaceutical nerve medications. It is naturally calming for those who are troubled by worry or emotional distress. Dr. Christopher often used it to help with insomnia. One woman who had been troubled throughout her life with chronic insomnia had never slept more than thirty minutes at a time. After one cup of Relax-Eze tea, she slept soundly throughout the night.

During his practice in Olympia, Dr. Christopher developed two career trademarks: his famous house calls and his success with incurable diseases. He would sometimes travel more than fifty miles one way in the middle of the night to patients he had never even met. On one of these house calls, he found a man who was in the throes of pain and paralysis of arthritis. From his wheelchair, he said, "Please, help me. No one has been able to help me yet. I have tried every doctor, but nothing has worked. My money is gone. I have nothing left."

"Don't worry," said Ray, stroking the man's gnarled hand. "You don't need money to pay me. Let's see what we can do for you." From his bag, Ray took his morning's harvest of burdock root, firm and fresh. He chopped the roots and brewed burdock tea, telling the man to drink as many cups a day as he could tolerate. Then he made poultices from the tender burdock leaves, placing them over the painful joints. He taught the man how to make his own poultices, how to eat properly and take quarts of fresh juices.

Within weeks, the man's joints began to loosen, and he could stand for the first time in years. Soon he could walk—and then run! Eventually he was completely healed. Only a few months after he first saw Dr. Christopher, he was back on the job as a night watchman, without pain or difficulty.

Dr. Christopher had special understanding and empathy for arthritic conditions since he had suffered from the same ailment early in his life. His knowledge came first-hand: if he stayed on the mucusless diet, with olive oil or wheat germ oil, he scarcely noticed his arthritis. But if he ate breads or pastries, he needed a cane to walk. If he ate sugar, he became crippled. And if he ate red meat, he was back to his wheelchair within two days.

AR-1

He knew first-hand the healing benefits of burdock root, which works a chemical reaction on calcified joints of arthritis. He used it as the basis of AR-1, his arthritis and rheumatism formula. He added yucca stalk, wild yam root, hydrangea, Brigham tea, chaparral, black walnut hulls, black cohosh root, wild lettuce leaves, sarsaparilla root, valerian root, and cayenne; herbs that detoxify and cleanse the condition, remove calcium deposits, relieve pain and kill infection. He saw this formula work miracles in even the most advanced cases. He always warned patients not to expect healing to take place all at once. In arthritis there is much rebuilding and healing to do. To the AR-1 formula, he added hot fomentations over extremely painful joints, a quart or two of kidney bean pod tea daily, the mucusless diet, and daily use of the BF&C formula.

FEN-LB

Dr. Christopher usually found that people with incurable conditions were willing to try herbs, even if they had disdained them before. One veterinarian doctor had contracted undulant fever fourteen years earlier in the packing houses where he had inspected meats for the federal government. No matter what advanced treatments were tried, his condition worsened. By the time Ray arrived at the house, the man was completely helpless. Attendants had to roll him over to prevent bedsores, and he couldn't even feed himself. He said, "I've never tried herbs, but I'm at the end of my rope! They only give me a few days to live—I want to live!"

Ray knew that the man needed a thorough cleansing, and quickly. He gave blood cleansing herbs and juices. And then he prescribed what became one of his most famous formulas, to clean the bowels and colon. Dr. Christopher knew that more than ninety percent of all disease is caused by congestion in the colon. Processed foods weaken the bowel, creating pockets and balloons filled with old fecal matter, a perfect place for germs to proliferate. And the hard material absorbs moisture, spreading the toxins back into the body.

Fen-LB works not only as a laxative to clean the bowel, but as a food to tone, rebuild and strengthen the colon at the same time. He began with barberry bark, which stimulates the flow of bile and acts as a non-habit-forming laxative. He added cascara sagrada bark, a famed laxative herb that strengthens the peristaltic muscle. Then he included cayenne to stimulate the cells of the bowel and stop bleeding; ginger to relive gas and stop cramping and pain; lobelia which acts as a catalyst as well as stopping pain and cramping; red rhubarb root, a laxative that also relieves nausea; turkey rhubarb, another gentle, pure laxative; fennel which relieves gas; and golden seal to heal, rebuild and prevent infection. This formula works on both the small and large intestine.

Within six weeks, the veterinarian, who had been so near to death, was out mowing the lawn. Passing neighbors were astonished: "I thought you were dead!" they called out to him. "No sir! I've turned to herbs. And if you want to feel this great, you should see Dr. Christopher yourself!" Cases like this eventually filled the waiting room of Dr. Christopher's office each morning.

One case in particular was a woman who came because of severe pain in her shoulders, so intense that she could not even lift her arms. After examining her briefly, Ray determined she had a large pocket of fecal matter trapped at the ascending transverse junction of her colon. Toxic waste had drained through her bloodstream, irritating the nerves of her shoulder and eventually causing this excruciating pain. Ray began by massaging the reflexology point on her foot that corresponded to the point of congestion. She screamed with pain as he kneaded the spot. This eased the pain in her shoulders. By taking the Fen-LB formula, she had no more pain again.

Though his practice continued to flourish, Ray and his family were becoming homesick for their former mountain home and for their friends and relatives in Utah. They decided to close his practice in Olympia, Washington and return to Salt Lake City.

HOME TO UTAH

In the early days of Utah history, herbalism had been well-accepted; the early church leaders had been committed to herbal healing. But things had changed in Utah, it was now a center of orthodox medical healing, unready for natural healing. During this time, he completed a naturopathy degree from Iowa's Institute of Drugless Therapy and an herbal pharmacist degree from the Los Angeles Herbal Institute.

Ray couldn't make enough in his practice to make ends meet, so he started work as a salesman, often travelling out of state. As he travelled, he seemed drawn to people who needed his help, and he always offered it freely. He recalled the phone call he had from a family with eight children in a tiny frame house in Great Falls, Montana; people he had met selling encyclopedias. The mother was frantic. An intestinal flu was running through the community, and two of her eight had come home with it. Dr. Christopher knew that the family only had one bathroom—a disaster if all should come down sick with intestinal flu! Remembering a thick patch of red raspberries along the family's back fence, he told her to gather the leaves, only stripping a third from any one bush. She was to brew a tea of the leaves.

"Give the sick children nothing but raspberry tea," he advised. "Give them all they can drink, and nothing else. Give the others tea, too. That's all they should eat or drink till the flu has cleared up." He told her that the family should be fine by morning if they followed these instructions.

A few days later, she called to tell him that the children were indeed fine by morning, instead of suffering for weeks, as had their classmates. No one else in the family got the flu. The mother had borne and raised sixteen children, and later graduated from Brigham Young University as a registered nurse. At graduation, she was honored by the university president and her classmates with a standing ovation. Over the years, as she practiced nursing, she also helped patients with herbal remedies.

GARLIC, ROSEHIPS AND PARSLEY FOR COLDS AND FLU

Dr. Christopher knew that raspberry leaves could cure a viral infection of a cold or the flu. He knew other herbs worked as well, and combined some of these remedies in a formula for colds and flu. He started with garlic, proven to kill both bacteria and viruses. He added rose hips, parsley, watercress and rosemary leaves. He made this into tablets and capsules and advised patients to take these with a cup of steam-distilled water. For faster action, the capsules could be opened and made into tea.

SHA FOR HAY FEVER

Just as medical doctors could not do much for colds and flu, hay fever presented a similar problem. Wanting to avoid chemical remedies, Dr. Christopher developed SHA, a combination based on a natural plant extract of pseudoephedrine, with Brigham tea, marshmallow root, burdock root, parsley, cayenne, chaparral, golden seal root, and lobelia. Used together with the mucusless diet, it feeds and strengthen the pulmonary organs to ease nasal and respiratory congestion, working as a natural decongestant and antihistamine. For stubborn hay fever, Dr. Christopher advised patients to thoroughly chew and swallow a thick pulp of grated horseradish root and apple cider vinegar three times a day.

ADRENETONE

Often Dr. Christopher was called upon to help patients whose bodies were worn out by stress. He developed Adrenetone to rebuild the adrenal glands, which are always exhausted when there is stress. He began with mullein leaves, the perfect "gland food." He added licorice root, famed for directly supplying the adrenal glands with needed nutrients. He added gotu kola to relieve fatigue and stimulate the adrenal glands; cayenne which brings oxygen and other nutrients to the glands, and ginger which flushes out congested capillaries. He finished with Siberian ginseng, famed for easing stress and boosting endurance among Soviet athletes, and hawthorn berries which tone the heart and reduce its load during stress.

PROSPALLATE

In response to a patient's distress, Dr. Christopher developed Prospallate, to dissolve kidney stones, kill infection, and clear sedimentation in the prostate gland. Dr. Christopher discovered that this was also an effective formula for gonorrhea. The formula consisted of cayenne, uva-ursi, parsley, golden seal root, gravel root, juniper berries, marshmallow root, ginger root and Siberian ginseng, to be taken with parsley tea.

JUNI-PARS

To help patients with incontinence, bed wetting, kidney stones, or bladder/urinary infection, Dr. Christopher developed Juni-pars for the kidneys and bladder. As a base he used two of the most effective and fastest-acting natural diuretics—juniper berries and parsley. Juniper also corrects problems in voiding urine, and parsley is one of the best-known herbs for rebuilding urinary tissues. One woman in Chicago lay dying with edema. After only four days of parsley tea and parsley fomentations, she was healed. To those two herbs, he added ginger root, to help the herbs work together; uva ursi leaves which dissolve kidney stones and other inorganic calcification; marshmallow root which acts as a soothing and healing emollient to ease the flow of urine; cramp bark which relives spasms; and golden seal root which kills infection and heals tissues. Numerous patients who took this formula were able to overcome incontinence and chronic urinary tract conditions.

Despite his success in developing these formulas, and his family's joy in being together with extended family in Utah, Ray was becoming increasingly frustrated. He could not be licensed in the state of Utah. One of the city's naturopaths, suggested that he become licensed in Wyoming and then return to Utah. Dr. Christopher decided to follow his advice. On the trip out, the family realized how hard their financial situation had actually been. They ran out of gas twenty miles out of Evanston. With no money to buy more, Ray walked to the nearest farmhouse. The farmer gave Ray gasoline from the tank of his tractor. On borrowed fuel, the Christophers arrived in Evanston.

EVANSTON

The family found a place to live with a spacious office in front for Ray. With nothing to live on but a few boxes of food they'd packed in the car, they hung out a sign announcing their arrival and waited for patients. Local people had a hard time with this new arrival—many of them didn't even know what a naturopath was. All they had experience with was orthodox physicians.

Just when Ray was afraid they'd have to starve, a few patients started trickling in, most for minor ailments like athlete's foot or a sprained ankle. These few didn't provide enough of a living for the Christopher family to pay their bills and put food on the table. When circumstances were the worst, the Christophers received a phone call from Della's sister Jane. She told them she wanted to serve a mission for the Church of Jesus Christ of Latter-day Saints. She knew that her father couldn't afford to support her financially, and she hoped to find someone who could. Ray offered to support her on a mission for the two full years.

When he hung up the phone, he and his wife looked at each other. What had he done? Sometimes there was hardly enough food; the adults would scant themselves so the children could have their fill. But they shared a faith in the Lord and gratitude for what they had. As Jane prepared to enter the mission home, she asked Ray where he might like to see her serve as a missionary. He said, "My father was from Paris, and my mother was from Switzerland. I would love to see you serve in the French-Swiss mission! But tell them to send you where they need you the most."

The Christophers borrowed money against their naturopathic equipment in the Evanston office to supply her with clothing and other necessities for the mission. With the last of their funds, they boarded the train with her for Salt Lake City.

The line of missionaries was long, waiting to enter the mission home where they receive and prepare for their assignments to some corner of the globe. When Jane reached the front of the line, the receptionist paused. "Where would you like to go?" he asked.

"I want to go where you need me the most," she replied.

"The place you are needed most is the French-Swiss Mission."

The Christophers were delighted. But then they boarded the train back to Evanston and reflected on what they had done. With the last few dollars in his pocket, Ray and Della had a meal in the dining car and prayed for the family's future.

When he entered his office waiting room the morning of his return, he was astonished. It was filled. Patients sat in every available space, waiting for appointments to see the new naturopath in town. There was money to keep Jane on her mission. There was money to feed his family again! The patients were the best advertisements Dr. Christopher could hope for. Word-of-mouth recommendations came from people who had suffered for years, unable to get help from the orthodox medical community. There was the woman whose arthritic joints were at last freed, the asthmatic whose airways were finally opened, and the polio victim who at last walked.

In one dramatic case, a man arrived in his wheelchair, hoping for some relief from the pain of his affliction, but resigned to the doctor's pronouncement that he would never walk again. "I know I can relieve your pain," Ray told him," and if you'd like to walk again, I think I can help you do that, too." With the mucusless diet and herbal remedies, the man left the office with new hope. Within a few months, he was walking around town, telling others about Dr. Christopher.

Although their business flourished, the Christophers had a hard time adjusting to the cold climate of Evanston. One of their favorite jokes was: "We missed that one day of summer—we were in Salt Lake that day!"

SANCTITY OF LIFE

Throughout his practice, Dr. Christopher opposed birth control and refused to assist in abortion. He remembered one belligerent young women who came to him seeking an abortion. Although his patient schedule was full, he counseled her for almost an hour about the sanctity of life. "Let this baby come; give it life; take care of it and love it."

"I hate you!" she screamed, jumping from her seat. "If I had a gun, I would kill you! I'm going to get rid of this baby, and if you won't do it, I'll find another doctor who will!" As she ran from the office, he pleaded with her to remember the things he had said.

About a year later, the woman came into his office, with a sweet baby in her arms. "I just want to thank you," she said, stroking the baby's head. "I told you I hated you, that I wanted to kill you, but you made me think. I went to three other doctors for an abortion. Each time as I sat in their waiting rooms, I heard your voice. I couldn't go through with it. This baby has changed my life; she is the most beautiful thing I could ever have been given."

Another day, the phone rang, with a woman on the line who was hemorrhaging rapidly, about to lose her baby. She'd had miscarriages before and wanted to save this one. He told her to stay in bed till he arrived. Just then the phone rang with another woman, on the opposite end of town, in the same precarious situation: hemorrhage, losing a baby. He told her to stay in bed. He stuffed more herbs in his bag and raced off.

Dr. Christopher directed each woman to take half a cup of false unicorn tea every half hour till the bleeding stopped, stay in bed and take plenty of fresh juices. Within months, each came to Dr. Christopher's office to show him their beautiful, fully formed babies.

NU-FEM

Dr. Christopher's experience with false unicorn led him to develop two formulas for women. The first, Nu-Fem, was formulated to rebuild a malfunctioning reproductive system. Along with false unicorn, it contains golden seal root, blessed thistle, cayenne, uva ursi leaves, cramp bark, false unicorn root, red raspberry leaves, squaw vine, and ginger root. Nu-Fem was effective for menstrual cramping and flooding, for infertility. With its natural source of estrogen, Nu-Fem corrects an estrogen imbalance, which is often the source of many female problems.

In one particular case, Dr. Christopher treated a seventeen-year-old girl from Texas whose cycle was so exhausting that she was hospitalized each month for dehydration and excessive vomiting. When she took Nu-Fem, her problems disappeared. Another woman in Evanston had suffered from terrific pain during menstruation for ten years. She had invested thousands of dollars on specialists, without receiving any relief. After using Nu-Fem for only ninety days, she had a regular, pain-free cycle.

Nu-Fem also rebuilds the feminine organs, particularly the uterus. An Ohio woman had suffered severe pain from a badly tipped uterus. After taking Nu-Fem for five days, the pain cease, and within several weeks, the doctor was astonished to see that the uterus was no longer tipped.

Nu-Fem also aids in conception and makes normal pregnancies possible. One couple who for fourteen years were unable to conceive, came for instruction. They took Nu-Fem, distilled water, the mucusless diet, and wheat germ oil and received the child they had longed for. Nu-Fem also helped a forty-one year old woman from Portland who had suffered nine miscarriages, all within the second or third month of pregnancy. Nu-Fem restored her reproductive system, and she too was able to bear a child.

Nu-Fem is wonderful to use during pregnancy as well. It can relieve the nausea of morning sickness, quiet false labor, help bring good contractions once labor has started, check hemorrhage, aid in a rapid and safe delivery, relieve after-pains, and enrich the mother's milk. Cramp bark aids in proper positioning of the fetus and prevents painful leg cramps during pregnancy. Squaw vine is a traditional Native American herb for easy delivery. Cayenne improves strength and endurance during pregnancy and helps stop hemorrhage after delivery.

CHANGEASE

Dr. Christopher's second female formula based on false unicorn is known as Changease. He recommended it for puberty, pregnancy, nursing, and menopause, including "male menopause." The herbs in Changease provide precursors to hormones, which the body can easily convert to the hormones that it requires. Synthetic hormones, on the other hand, cannot be completely assimilated by the body. They may be stored in the body tissues, with potentially serious side effects. Changease can help with the changes associated with puberty, can be an outstanding pregnancy supplement, and can relieve hot flashes and other symptoms associated with menopause. Because both men and women require varying amounts of female hormones, it can be used for hormonal imbalance in men as well.

Blessed thistle is one of the important herbs in both formulas. This wonder herb, which can bring up the milk supply in a nursing mother. Dr. Christopher remembered one mother who lost her milk for almost two months. Her baby could not digest formula, soy formulas, or animal's milk. He was almost dead from starvation and dehydration. Blessed thistle brought this mother's milk back, and saved the baby's life. Another mother was ordered by a doctor to wean her three-month-old infant. Her milk was insufficient, he said. Blessed thistle gave her a good supply of rich milk. Still another mother of a large family grew fatigued and began to lose her milk, and just two capsules of blessed thistle each night restored so much milk that her nightclothes were wet with it.

But perhaps the most dramatic story about blessed thistle was the family where the mother was killed in an automobile accident. The seventeen-year-old sister brought the baby to Dr. Christopher; the infant had been thrown clear of the car and was uninjured. But it could not digest formula or animal's milk. The young woman began to take blessed thistle tea, and soon she had a good, rich milk supply. She nursed the baby till it was weaned.

Similarly, a woman came to Dr. Christopher, intending to adopt a baby and wanting to breast feed. It was their fourth adoption, but she hadn't been able to nurse any of them. Dr. Christopher helped her get onto a good diet, plenty of fresh juice, lots of distilled water each day, and at least three cups of blessed thistle tea a day. A few months later, she came to see him, and, throwing back her robe, showed him a chubby Navajo baby, nursing from her stark white breast. She said, "I love my four children so much, but I feel so close to this one. He is blood of my blood."

With such success, Dr. Christopher's practice in Evanston grew steadily. Each day the small waiting room was filled to capacity, all day long. Some cases were simple, some complex, and some involved mental illness.

One such woman came into the office with her sixteen-year-old daughter. The girl had Down's Syndrome, and had been institutionalized in Lander, Wyoming. The girl could not speak. The woman wanted to keep her daughter home with her. Dr. Christopher recommended a complete program, and within three months, the girl was quicker and brighter, more responsive, and was even speaking simple sentences! The officials were so amazed that they allowed the child to stay at home with her family.

One night there came a pounding at the door; when Dr. Christopher opened it, there were two young men, supporting a wizened old man who was struggling for every breath of air. Dr. Christopher recognized the wheezing sounds of asthma. "Please!" cried one of the young men. "Our regular doctor is out of town and we can't find his assistant. Can you help keep Pap alive?" Dr. Christopher settled the old man in a chair and gave him a cup of peppermint tea. The man had been sick with asthma for twenty-six years. For twenty of those it had been so severe that he could not hold a job. He could not lie down in bed because he choked up so much that he risked death. His sons built him a special chair to sleep in at night. The sons both worked to support the family's needs, including the high medical bills from this condition. The man required shots, respiratory therapy, and oxygen treatments, often more than twice a week.

Dr. Christopher helped the man sip the peppermint tea. Ten minutes later, he gave him a teaspoonful of lobelia tincture. Ten minutes later, as the four of them talked, Dr. Christopher spooned in another dose, and ten minutes later, another. Dr. Christopher began to quietly gather pots, pans and buckets. Suddenly the man began vomiting. From two till five in the morning he vomited the thick, sticky, blackened phlegm that had choked his airways. Because of the peppermint tea, his muscles were relaxed and he suffered no soreness from the hours of heaving.

Just after five o'clock, well before dawn, Dr. Christopher said, "You can take your father home now; he is finished with the treatment. He is fine now." The two rushed to their father's side to take him home, but he said, "You don't have to help me, boys. I'll walk." Dr. Christopher settled into bed for an hour's rest before starting the next day's work. The boys took the man home to his chair but he said, "Put me to bed, boys. I'm going to sleep in a bed tonight."

"You can't, Pap. It will kill you!"

But the father insisted and went to bed. He fell into a heavy sleep for thirty hours. When he woke up, after sleeping soundly for the first time in twenty years, he said, "I'm healed. I'm going out to get a job." He got a job as a gardener, and he never lost a day's work. He slept in a bed every night thereafter.

RESP-FREE

For all respiratory complaints, Dr. Christopher developed Resp-Free, a natural plant extract of ephedrine in an herbal base of chickweed, marshmallow root, mullein leaves, comfrey leaves and lobelia. This formula would expel thick mucus secretion and rebuild the lungs. It would also soothe inflammation, relieve pain, and heal hemorrhage in the lungs. This would be used in addition to the mucusless diet, distilled water, oil massage, and BF&C applied externally.

HERBAL EYEBRIGHT

Formulated around the herb eyebright, this formula feeds the cell structures around the eyes. Dr. Christopher used it in many instances to help restore sight. It would be brewed into a tea for use as an eyewash, as well as taken internally. It could relieve the pressure of glaucoma, remove scar tissue on the cornea caused by infection, and remove cataracts. An elderly man in Fort Worth, Texas, suffered from both glaucoma and cataracts—and was healed completely with the formula. A Michigan woman used it for ten days and removed cataracts on both eyes. A woman in Kentucky, who had lost 80 percent of her sight due to a subretinal hemorrhage, had her sight completely restored. A California woman had the beginnings of cataracts when the gel broke in both her eyes. Her vision failed, and her eyes were so dry that she had to lift her eyelids with her fingers each morning. With Herbal Eyebright, both eyes healed and the cataracts dissolved.

And, most dramatically, an elderly woman had lived in blindness for many years; with the formula, her sight was restored. A young man who had suffered an eye injury and had gone without sight for ten years was able to see again. Two young adults, blind since birth, used the formula and were able to see!

One Missouri baby had been born with Coloboma; one eye was smaller than the other. Three leading specialists proclaimed the blindness to be permanent. The mother began patiently using Herbal Eyebright with a dropper in each of his eyes. Within three months, this supposedly blind baby was reaching for objects. By the age of three, he ran freely, his vision perfect.

Another couple had a baby born without optic nerves. Dr. Christopher knew that giving sight to such a child was almost impossible. But he knew that the formula could cause no harm, so he recommended Herbal Eyebright in the eyes and given internally, and B&B tincture dropped in the ears and given internally. Six months later, the same couple brought the child to a lecture. He chased balls across the room and picked them up; he had normal sight.

Dr. Christopher often laughed about an experience he had in Evanston. He was called to a farmhouse forty miles away in Woodruff, Utah. The rancher and his whole family were very sick from an undiagnosed sickness. The farm work and housework were all close to a standstill, because the family was so weak. "What are you eating?" Ray asked.

"Oh, we eat well," said the rancher. "I just stored up a thousand pounds of white flour, and we have plenty of canned goods to see us through the winter."

"Have you ever considered whole wheat?" Ray asked

"You could never force *that* down me," the rancher jeered. "I don't believe in it. There's no sense in it at all."

"Now, you're a rancher," said Ray, "and you've got some prize horses and cattle out there. Do you feed them carrots?"

"You bet," the rancher smiled, "I've got about half a ton of carrots out there."

"Do you ever eat them?"

"Naw. . .they're just for the horses—you know, to keep them in good condition."

"What about grains?"

"I've got coarse-ground grains in the shed for the cattle."

"You bring in from the shed a thousand pounds of those coarse-ground grains. Prepare it over low heat till it is soft and chewy, stir in a little honey or some fresh-diced fruit. You eat that. And take your thousand pounds of white flour, and give it to the cattle."

"What?" the man said angrily, "That would kill my prize cattle!" Then the man's face reddened as he realized what he had said. "You caught me," he admitted. "All right. I'll do it your way."

Within a few weeks, the family had received good health and vitality once again.

HOME TO SALT LAKE—AND TROUBLE

The Christophers finally prepared to return to Utah, to family, friends and a familiar setting. Once they returned, he set up an office similar to the one he'd had in Evanston. But even though he had been licensed in Wyoming, he could not receive similar licensing in Utah. Some of the people in the area were adamant against herbs and vowed to prosecute anyone who prescribed their use. Even the few patients that made their way to Dr. Christopher were considered suspect.

One day, a young man and his sister called Dr. Christopher to their home. Lying in bed was their mother, in terrible pain, almost at death's door. The children explained that she was riddled with cancer and had been given only hours to live. They wanted to fulfill her wish of dying at home and wanted something to ease her pain during her last hours. Ray had been warned against visiting the woman because of legal ramifications. But he could not turn his back when there was pain. He leaned close to her and said, "I don't know how long you'll be with us, but if you will follow this program for a few days, you will be free of pain. And I believe you will enjoy ease until your time comes." She nodded weakly, with a smile. He left the family with dietary instructions and a handful of herbal formulas.

As he left the house, he noticed neighbors peering from behind heavy lace curtains. He visited her several times, and soon she was able to get out of bed, to talk walks among her beloved gardens, to smile, to associate with her children. One morning a few months later, she gathered her children around her and bid them goodbye, telling each how she loved them. She closed her eyes and died, without pain. The children phoned Ray with the news, expressing their gratitude for her final few months of joy and companionship.

A few days later, the police came to Ray's house, handcuffed him, and arrested him for murder, and took him to jail. The neighbors had noted his license plate and filed charges against him when the woman died. She had been sentenced to die within a few hours and Dr. Christopher had prolonged her life by a few weeks, and eased her pain. Yet he paid the price, because he was, in the words of the prosecuting attorney, an "unorthodox physician." Ray's defense wasn't sure that they could avoid a prison term.

The children of the deceased offered Ray's greatest defense. The young son passionately told how Ray's treatments had taken away his mother's pain and allowed her to live much longer than expected. He told how she got out of bed, walked around, and was happy. The judge rapped his gavel, saying, "Case dismissed." Ray always believed that the Lord was in court with him that day.

Unfortunately, there were many more times that Dr. Christopher felt handcuffs slapped around his wrists, when his family had to post bail to free him from unfair imprisonment. His wife always supported him through arrests, trials, and imprisonments. As he'd leave the house each day to attend the sick, he'd called back over his shoulder, "I'll phone you when I get to jail tonight!" and they'd both smile and wave goodbye.

Unfortunately, this prediction often proved true. There were so many arrests and trials—although, at his funeral, National Health Federation official Clinton Miller pointed out that Ray never showed bitterness or retaliation, with "no anguish in his face, no concern, no bitterness, just beauty." Eventually legislation was passed aimed specifically against Dr. Christopher, so that he could not practice natural healing anymore. But as distressing as this was, it opened a door to Dr. Christopher.

When he could no longer treat patients, he began to lecture and teach. At his peak, he lectured in more than 120 cities a year. The halls were filled to capacity; eager students stood in the aisles and lined the walls in an effort to learn from him. In 1979, he began a newsletter, which, together with his books, reached tens of thousands of more people than his practice could ever have done.

His work did not stop there, however. Starting from his service at Fort Lewis, continuing in Evanston, and then on through Salt Lake, many of his patients became herbalists. Even the rancher in Woodruff who refused to feed his prize cattle white flour bought a fruit farm, learned reflexology and works as a full-time herbalist.

Dr. Christopher practiced open-heartedly, without guile, with selfless concern for his patients and later for all his students. He never held back information on his formulas to gain more money; he freely shared any information he thought could help someone else. He took people into their yards and taught them to use the "weeds," when he could have easily bottled them himself for profit. He shared the ingredients of his formulas freely.

Throughout his life, Dr. Christopher maintained a wonderful sense of humor. He loved to tell the story about a man who was hospitalized, with doctor's orders for an enema. A nurse administered it, and then was called away on an emergency before recording the treatment. Soon a second nurse appeared, and gave him a second enema. But she, too, failed to record the treatment. Then a third nurse did the same. When the man heard a knock on his door, he called out, "Who goes there? Friend or enema?"

The press was sympathetic to Dr. Christopher's troubles. *The San Francisco Recorder* published an editorial commenting on Ray's arrests and the accompanying $50,000 bond, saying, "Where hardened criminals, guilty of crimes of violence and threats to society, are given low bail, some members of the legal profession are requesting that an investigation be made to determine what prompted such an excessive bail in this case. Could this be a ploy to take the heat off the doctors in the current malpractice mess by making it unpleasant for acupuncturists, herbal, and natural healers? Just asking!"

Dr. Christopher continued to teach until the last of his life, when in 1983, he had slipped on the treacherous ice outside his home in Covered Bridge Canyon, Utah, and suffered what became a fatal accident. He was seventy-three years old, and through trials and suffering through his long life, he blazed the path to a way of life we take for granted today, with natural foods, healthy lifestyles, and healing with herbs. This volume remains a landmark in herbal healing, and as you read it, remember the man who sacrificed to make it possible.

CHAPTER 1

GENERAL DISEASE

This chapter describes common afflictions, diagnoses the cause of the problem, locates the afflicted areas and suggests the dietary remedy and the herbs used to speed recovery. Specific directions for herbal preparations for certain ailments may be located either in the general chapters or in the index.

Although the names of these listed afflictions may be different in common medical terminology and medical science may break down the ailments into further subcategories, the causes and cures of the conditions are simple and recognizable. The most effective herbs are typed in *italics*.

ABSCESS

Symptoms:
A collection of pus within a body cavity. According to Thomas Duskier, "The brighter the redness, the smaller will be the abscess. The softer the feeling and the darker the appearance the more extensive will be the destruction of the tissue. Thick yellow pus is termed 'healthy', thin watery and greenish pus is always bad, indicating prostration and difficulty in healing."

Cause:
An abscess is nature's way of purifying the body, bringing waste materials into a deposit that can be easily drawn out. Pus is formed by the loss of organic sulphur from cell, so that the cells decay. Herbs containing organic sulphur, such as garlic, rebuild and prevent this deficiency condition.

Herbal aids:
Poultices will bring an abscess to a head and clear it out. A poultice of slippery elm, wild sage, and lobelia (equal parts) is good; another poultice that will draw very rapidly and will relieve pain at the same time is mullein (three parts) and lobelia (one part). Others are flaxseed, lobelia, and golden seal; leek boiled in milk; sour dock, hyssop and green fennel; ground ivy and yarrow; carrot; potato.

Useful herbs:
Bayberry bark, cayenne, cloves, garlic, ginger, hemlock bark, herb Robert, *lobelia,* mugwort, *mullein,* sassafras, *slippery elm,* stinging nettle leaves.

AGUE

Symptoms:
A malarial fever which is attended by paroxysmal and recurrent chills.

Cause:
This is a condition of malnutrition and poor blood circulation.

Herbal aids:
Moist heat and profuse perspiration or sweating with diaphoretics are needed, (yarrow is one of the best). Tonic or alterative herbs (Brigham tea, burdock, ginseng) must be used to build up the body, with special attention to a proper, healthful diet.

Useful herbs:
Avens, *bayberry bark,* broom, butternut bark, *camomile,* common holly, dogwood bark, *gentian root, Irish moss, Jesuit's bark, oak bark, Peruvian bark, prickly ash bark,* smartweed, sorrel, sumach (bark or root), tansy, *tormentil root,* tulip tree bark, *vervain,* willow, wormwood, yellow bearsfoot root.

APOPLEXY

Symptoms:
The sudden loss of consciousness, sensation, and voluntary motion, caused by the rupture or obstruction of an artery of the brain, very often resulting in death; also gross hemorrhage into any organ, such as the lungs, spleen, etc.

Cause:
This is a serious catarrhal condition of the body, wherein the normal excreting channels are blocked and the denser glutinous and fibrinous matters overload the bloodstream.

Herbal aids:
The suddenness of apoplexy requires the fastest therapeutic action. Cayenne pepper (one teaspoon to the cup) may be administered quickly; tincture of lobelia (three drops to one-half teaspoon, according to the size and age of the individual) should be given regularly; the antispasmodic tincture is excellent.

Useful herbs:
Bibernell, bittersweet, *black cohosh,* black hellebore, blue cohosh, *burdock, catnip,* coriander seeds, couch grass, cowslip, crow foot, *burdock,* hedge hyssop, lavender, *lily of the valley,* masterwort, peony (seeds and root), pepper cress seed, rosemary, skullcap, soapwort, *vervain,* white mustard seed.

ARTHRITIS

Symptoms:
Inflammation of the joints. Arthritis is an ailment of the body that is an old chronic condition. There are many forms: such as gout or rheumatoid arthritis which are different from the common variety of arthritis. The joints become enlarged and painful, being very tender to any movement or pressure (the pain may be con-

stant or intermittent). Often the hands draw back or to one side, and in chronic conditions the muscles shrink and will eventually wither away. This affliction may have a decided effect on childbirth both to the mother and the newborn child.

Cause:
Arthritis is caused by acids and waste matter in the body, which eventually become solidified and lock the joint. This condition is caused and aggravated by improper diet. Some of the worst intakes are eggs, bread, milk, meat, salt, sugar, etc., because they cause arthritic calcification. The use of extremely hard water (generally of twelve or more grains in hardness) will often accentuate an arthritic condition where softer water will help relieve it. Sometimes an individual with a good inherent structure can throw off the hardest water without arthritic effect. The weaker person may drink water that is not very hard and absorb from it relatively larger quantities of the inorganic minerals.

Herbal aids:
For eliminating toxic substances from the bowels, one may use a high enema of slippery elm or white oak bark tea. The system should be cleansed by a daily sweat bath with pleurisy root; massage (except the inflamed joints) with angelica, black cohosh, buckthorn bark, columbo, gentian root, skullcap, or valerian root. One may use poultices such as cayenne, lobelia, mullein, slippery elm for relieving pain of the swollen joints; liniments of oils, such as cayenne, coconut, lobelia, origanum are also good.

Useful herbs:
Bearsfoot, bitter root, blackberry, black cohosh, buckthorn bark, burdock, *hydrangea, Irish moss*, saw palmetto berries, skullcap, winter green, yellow dock.

ASTHMA

Symptoms:
The system is filled with waste matter and mucus. Asthma is characterized by labored breathing (dyspnea), wheezing with dry and painful coughing which is often due to an extreme irritation of the mucus membranes in the nasal passages or bronchial tubes. The symptoms are accompanied by constriction of the chest (bronchial spasm) and expectoration of mucus (mucoid sputum). Asthma may result in an excessive development (hypertrophy) of the glandular elements. This affliction is commonly believed to be due to hypersensitivity to inhaled or ingested substances such as odors, pollen, dust, smoke, etc.

Cause:
Asthma is caused by malnutrition. Only by diligent and consistent effort to change embedded habits will one get permanent relief. The cough is a result of nature's effort to expectorate mucus from the lungs, after which breathing becomes easier. Often times the cause of asthma is basically a nervous condition because the nerves are irritated.

Herbal aids:
When a person is in a convulsion there are certain herbs that will give very fast relief. One of these is tincture of lobelia, and a valerian decoction with a little cayenne added to relieve spasms. If such an attack comes after a meal one should use an emetic, such as a large dose of lobelia or use the Yoga finger method.

Drink several cups of warm water, then place the middle finger deep down the throat and press the tongue until regurgitation starts. Mustard is also good to clean the stomach and lungs. Prior to the emetic, a peppermint or spearmint tea should be used to soothe the area and alleviate the discomfort of continual vomiting.

Hot fomentation of castor oil, comfrey, lobelia, mullein, etc., may be placed over the stomach, liver, spleen and lung areas. Frequent hydrotherapy baths or lengthy sweat baths are beneficial, followed by a cold shower or sponging.

Another helpful method is to take a vapor bath twice a week, inhaling steam from a decoction of cudweed, ragwort, wormwood, or a decoction of the following herbs, taken warm, (equal parts) will prove very beneficial: elecampane root, horehounds, hyssop, skunk cabbage root, vervain, wild cherry bark (and to this preparation add tincture of lobelia or antispasmodic tincture). Clear the bowels with an injection of catnip or barberry bark.

This affliction also calls for plenty of outdoor exercise, deep breathing, and good ventilation while sleeping. The whole body system should be built up with tonic herbs such as chickweed, comfrey, marshmallow, mullein, etc. Diet should be mostly fruits and vegetables, avoiding all processed devitalized foods.

Useful herbs:
Agrimony, anemone pulsatilla, angelica, anise seed, asarabacca, *asthma wood,* balm of Gilead, balsam of Tolu, beet root juice, *belladonna leaves, Bethroot, bitter candy tuft, black cohosh,* blue cohosh, *blood root, boneset,* cajeput oil, catawba tree, *cayenne,* cherry laurel, *cleavers* (small), coltsfoot, comfrey root, coral bloom, coughwort, cramp bark, cubeb berries, cypripedium, daisy, dragon root, dragon turnip, *elder berries, elecampane root,* ephedra herb, flaxseed, *garlic, ginger, grindelia, ground ivy, henbane leaves, hickory bark, honeysuckle, horehounds,* hyssop, Indian poke, *Indian hemp,* Indian turnip, Irish moss, *licorice root,* lady's slipper root, *lobelia,* lungwort, maiden hair, masterwort, milkweed, mullein, myrrh, nettle, plantain, *pleurisy root,* prickly ash, *red clover tops,* red root, red sage, ribwort, river weed, *rosin weed leaves,* sage, saw palmetto berries, senna, *skunk cabbage, slippery elm bark,* snake weed, spinet root, spikenard, storax, succory, sunflower seeds, thorn apple plant, thoroughwort, *thyme,* wall germander, *walnut leaves,* water ash, wild plum bark, *yerba santa leaves,* vervain, wild cherry.

ASTHMATIC ASPHYXIA

Symptoms:
Suffocation or coma from asthmatic bronchiolar spasm resulting in a deprivation of oxygen.

Cause:
See "Asthma."

Herbal aids:
Tincture of lobelia, or an antispasmodic tincture taken internally is excellent. One can also massage the outside of the body rubbing the tincture thoroughly between the shoulder blades, across the upper rib-cage area, through the chest and bronchial areas.

Useful herbs:
See "Asthma."

BLEEDING

Symptoms:
The escaping of blood internally or externally. Blood coughed from the lungs is generally of a bright red color and is usually mixed with sputum. The problem is often preceded by nausea and stomach disorder with blood passing through the bowels.

Cause:
Bleeding, unless it is by injury, is caused by a calcium deficiency in the body. Bleeding from the nose (epistaxis) is generally caused by the rupture of a small vessel in the nose due to pressure in the head (with a rupture occurring at the weakest point). Diet is very important in this case.

Herbal aids:
Cayenne will take care of most bleeding problems, external or internal by the time you can count to ten. For bleeding of the lower bowel (commonly called dysentery) use mullein (preferably in milk). In the urinary tract, marshmallow (preferably in milk) is generally faster. Other excellent herbs; comfrey root, *European Goldenrod,* self-heal, *shavegrass,* shepherd's purse, and wild alum root may be used.

In bleeding of the nose, raise the arms above the head and administer cayenne dissolved in hot water, or the extract of witch hazel may be sniffed in the nostrils. A decoction of equal parts of bistort root, cranesbill root, avens or raspberry taken internally works well.

Useful herbs:
Bleeding of the nose (epistaxis): *Alum root* (snuffed), Bethroot, calamine, cancer root, cayenne, forget-me-not leaves, gall oak powder (on cotton), globe thistle, groundsel, *nettle leaves* (snuffed), onion juice in vinegar (snuffed in the nose), *shavegrass,* walnut leaves, willow bark and sprouts. The bark is to be used on the nose and the sprouts in the nose.

Bleeding of the lungs: Bethroot, black cohosh, blood root, *bugleweed, comfrey root, cranesbill root,* cypress tree, hounds tongue, kidney liver leaf, lungwort, mullein, nettle leaves, oak bark, shavegrass, *shepherd's purse,* St. John's wort, succory, *witch hazel, whortleberry, yarrow.*

Bleeding of the stomach: Bethroot, *cayenne* (one of the fastest healers of bleeding ulcers), *geranium root,* groundsel, ladies mantle, mullein, oak bark, *shavegrass, shepherd's purse,* tormentil, whortleberry, *witch hazel, yarrow.*

Bleeding of the bowels: Adder's tongue (expressed juices), Bethroot, geranium root, groundsel, ladies mantle, mullein, oak, red root, *shavegrass, shepherd's purse, tormentil, witch hazel, whortleberry, yarrow.*

Bleeding of the urinary tract: *Bethroot, buchu,* calendula (tincture), chervil, clown woundwort, *comfrey,* European goldenrod, false sweet flag, garden daisy, garlic, ground ivy, groundsel, herb Robert, lungwort, *marshmallow, mayflower,* nettle leaves, oak bark, peach leaves, plantain, pyrola, sanicle, *shavegrass,* veronica, *vervain,* yarrow.

BLOOD PRESSURE

Symptoms:
The pressure exerted by blood upon the walls of the arteries, depending upon the force of the heart beat, the elasticity of the vessel walls, the resistance of the capillary network and the volume and viscosity of the blood. In *Back to Eden,* revised and expanded second edition p.365, says the following:

> Blood pressure reflects the contractile powers of the heart and the resistance of the blood vessels. The blood pressure increases slowly during life so that the normal blood pressure at age thirty is approximately 125 and at age sixty it is about 140 mm/Hg. Persons who are weak physically have a slightly lower pressure. The blood pressure rises to some degree during exercise.

The old accepted routine of taking the blood pressure count has been 100 systolic plus the age, wherein a person of thirty years, it was felt, should have a normal blood pressure of 130, and a person of forty a blood pressure of 140, etc. But this is very erroneous, because at any age heavy meat eaters will have a higher blood pressure than vegetarians. There is actually no hard and fast rule on blood pressure.

Cause:
(See "HIGH BLOOD PRESSURE" or "LOW BLOOD PRESSURE")

Herbal aids:
(See "HIGH BLOOD PRESSURE" or "LOW BLOOD PRESSURE")

Useful herbs:
(See "HIGH BLOOD PRESSURE" or "LOW BLOOD PRESSURE")

BRONCHITIS

Symptoms:
An acute or chronic inflammation of the mucous membrane of the bronchial tubes.

Cause:
This is a condition from improper diet and results in bowel problems. Relieving the effects of the condition will not heal it. Bronchitis usually develops from a cold which settles in the lungs and develops into a chronic condition if not healed, eventually going into consumption or tuberculosis.

Herbal aids:
Comfrey and almond are specifics for bronchitis. Since constipation is one of the chief causes of the problem, the bowels must be cleared and kept open with the lower bowel tonic or herbal laxatives. If one has shortness of breath and needs the throat cleared of mucus, use an emetic.

Cayenne is very effective for cutting the phlegm, as are fruit juices such as grapefruit, lemon, orange, or pineapple. Chickweed, comfrey, marshmallow or mullein are the greatest cleansers to get the mucus out of the body. One can relax the throat, stomach, and bronchi rapidly with a very small amount of lobelia.

Other useful aids for relief are a hot vapor or steam bath followed by a cold shower or sponging; also hot fomentation of pleurisy root or mullein (with lobelia in it) on the chest and spine. If you want to speed up any fomentation, add cayenne as a counterirritant.

Useful herbs:
Abscess root, Acadia (mucilage), anise seed, asthma weed, aya pana (Eupatorium ayapana), balsam of copaiba, balsam of fir, balsam of tolu, Bethroot, bitter candy tuft, *blood root,* blue violet, calamus, *cascarilla bark,* cayenne, chickweed, cleavers (small), coltsfoot, *comfrey root,* copaiba, cubeb berries, *elecampane root,* fennel, flaxseed, *garlic,* ginger, *golden seal, grindelia squarrosa, gum Arabic, hickory bark, horehounds, hyssop herb, Irish moss,* Indian turnip, *Iceland moss,*

Ivy (American), jaborandi, *licorice,* lungwort, *marshmallow, mullein leaves,* myrrh, old fashioned balsam, onion, Peruvian balsam, *pleurisy root,* red root, red sage, sanicle, saw palmetto berries, Senegal, senna, skunk cabbage, *slippery elm bark,* snake weed, spikenard, stillingia, sumbul, sunflower seeds, thoroughwort, wahoo bark, wake robin, *walnut leaves,* water fennel seed, white pine, white pond lily, *wild cherry bark, yerba santa leaves.*

BURSITIS

Symptoms:
Inflammation of the bursa, or small sac interposed between parts that move upon one another. This causes a rheumatic or arthritic tendency that affects different parts of the body, often the shoulders.

Cause:
The cause of bursitis is the same as arthritis and rheumatism: malnutrition and poor circulation. Generally, the problem of most bursitis in the shoulder and neck areas comes from a congested condition in the transverse colon. A toxic acid condition irritates a specific area causing the specific inflammation.

Herbal aids:
Fomentations and liniments will give very quick relief but this is just giving relief and not healing. A fomentation, poultice or tea of burdock leaves (three parts) and lobelia (one part) is good. Wormwood oil in combination with other oils is one of the fastest and most effective pain relievers. Cleanse the inflamed tissue of the toxic accumulations with the cleansing program and change to a mucusless diet.

Useful herbs:
Apple cider vinegar and honey, chaparral, lobelia and mullein (poultice), sassafras.

CATARRH

Symptoms:
Chronic inflammation of the mucus membrane of the air passages of the nose and throat with an exudation containing mucin and epithelial cells. This is an excessive and often morbid mucus discharge from the nose, throat, larynx, bronchi, stomach, duodenum, etc. Catarrh can go through the entire body from the head to the feet. Catarrh in the lungs is similar to colds, flu and pneumonia. When it becomes chronic the person has tuberculosis or consumption.

Cause:
Catarrh is caused by eating devitalized or processed foods; by eating excess starches and glutinous foods; by poor circulation, lack of sunshine, fresh air, exercise; by eating wrong food combinations; by eating many soft and cooked foods; by drinking with meals; and by poor elimination.

When foods are not digested, fermentation takes place in the digestive tract, alcohol and acetic acid are formed, and various forms of catarrh clog the membranes. When this thickened mucoid matter is dispatched to the skin, the skin glands become obstructed, resulting in colds and fevers. The fibrinous and glutinous substances (excess starches and carbohydrates, especially those rendered inorganic in cooking) overload the blood and tissues and cannot be passed off fast enough through the intestinal tract. The eliminative system becomes clogged and the mucus is forced into the various mucus glands or membranes.

Although there is only one basic cause, the manifest symptoms are varied according to the form and location. The problem induces such diseases as arthritis, asthma, biliousness, Bright's disease, bronchitis, cystitis, diphtheria, dysuria, gravel, jaundice, laryngitis, pleurisy, rheumatism, tonsillitis, etc. If catarrh collects in the blood stream and congest circulation, it becomes high blood pressure and finally apoplexy.

Herbal aids:
One should keep away from the mucus forming foods, and the diet should consist entirely of leafy and juicy vegetables and fresh fruits. As catarrh is a general mucoid complaint, one must thoroughly cleanse the stomach, liver and intestines. One must keep the mucous membrane in the nasal passage clean.

The "musts" for catarrh are proper diet, outdoor exercise and good elimination. If one doesn't get enough fresh air and exercise, the catarrh will develop into hay fever, asthma, or tuberculosis. Take vinegar and honey copiously, especially for children (here you may add some glycerine).

Useful herbs:
African tea plant, angelica, *anise seed, asthma weed, avens root, bayberry bark, bistort root (intestines), black mallow flowers, blood root, borage, buchu, burdock root, cascarilla bark, cayenne, coltsfoot, comfrey,* coriander seed, couch grass, coughwort, cubeb berries, *elder flowers* and *berries, elecampane,* fennel seed, fringetree, *garlic* (Mucous membranes), golden seal, hyssop, *Iceland moss,* Indian hemp, Indian turnip, *Irish moss,* jaborandi, juniper berries, lemon balm, *licorice root,* lobelia, lungwort, *marshmallow,* meadow anemone, milfoil, mullein leaves, parsley, Peruvian bark, pichi tops (vessels), *princes pine* (bladder), Seneca snake root, Senegal, *skunk cabbage,* raisins, storax, sumac sun dew, swamp cabbage, sweet gum bark, tormentil, turtle bloom, *uva ursi* (bladder), watercress, water plantain, *white oak bark,* white pine, *wild cherry bark,* witch hazel, yarrow, *yerba santa* (bladder).

CHOLERA MORBUS

Symptoms:
An acute, infectious affliction characterized by profuse, purging evacuations, vomiting, prostrating collapse, muscular cramps and suppression of the urine.

Symptoms develop rapidly and become dangerous in six to twelve hours. Children may be restless and go into stupor or have convulsions.

Cause:
Cholera is a deficiency condition from improper diet, unsanitary conditions, and often occurs in hot weather. As future foreboding problem conditions continue to afflict our society there will be more epidemics, so we must be prepared to handle cholera. The only way to avoid this deadly killer is to build up the body so that the cholera organisms will not affect the system.

Herbal aids:
Rice water will check the diarrhea as will peach leaves, raspberry leaves, and sunflower leaves. A warm bayberry and catnip enema is very soothing. Antispasmodic tincture is soothing and relaxing and the slippery elm tea is nutritional and cleansing.

Useful herbs:
Uva Ursi, prickly ash, *queen of the meadow, raspberry leaves,* red clover, rhubarb, smartweed, *tormentil root,* wild alum root, *wild yam.*

CHOLESTEROL

Symptoms:
A monohydric alcohol found in the body as a glistening white, crystalline substance. It is insoluble in water and found in bile, gall stones, and nerve tissue.

Cause:
This is a mucus condition stemming from improper foods.

Herbal aids:
The diet must be changed. Herbs that reduce cholesterol will help but not correct the condition. Apple cider vinegar and honey, cayenne, or any of the cleansing herbs are good.

Useful herbs:
Bayberry bark, Brigham tea, buckthorn bark, burdock root, chaparral, ginseng, *prickly ash bark, red clover blossoms, sassafras bark,* stillingia, *white oak bark* (see chapter two on "The Alterative Herbs").

COLD
(Also known as common cold, coryza, rhinitis.)

Symptoms:
This is a disorder in the respiratory tract caused by exposure and resulting in catarrh and the invasion of microbial cleansers. The affliction is usually mild and short, and is characterized by a chilly sensation followed by sneezing, watering of

the eyes, congestion and discharges from the nose and throat, coughing, earache, and often fever.

Causes:
A cold always signals a congestion of catarrh and faulty elimination affecting the circulatory as well as the excretory organs.

Herbal aids:
Often all that is needed is copious amounts of raspberry leaf tea and some bowel cleaning. A very powerful remedy is the infusion of dried elderberry flowers and dried peppermint leaves taken internally as hot as possible. The diaphoretic herbs will open the pores and discharge waste obstructions.

When a cold occurs the whole system is involved. At the first sign of a cold, one should clean the nose and mouth of the toxic accumulations (through snuffing and gargling); and after the cold is broken with the sweating aids, the patient should be sponged with equal parts cold water and vinegar to close the pores, put to bed, and given fruits or fruit juices.

Useful herbs:
Ammoniac gum, angelica, bayberry bark, black cohosh, blood root, *blue vervain,* blue violet, *boneset*, butternut bark, button bush, *catnip, cayenne,* chestnut leaves, cloves, coltsfoot, dittany, elder flowers and *berries, feverfew, flaxseed, gentian, ginger,* ginseng, *golden seal, grindelia, ground ivy,* hemlock bark, hops, horehounds, hyssop, Indian hemp, Irish moss, *licorice, lobelia,* lungwort, malabar nut, marshmallow, masterwort, mouse ear, *mullein leaves*, nettle, pennyroyal, peppermint, pleurisy root, prickly ash, *motherwort,* rosemary, saffron, *sage, sarsaparillas, saw palmetto berries, smartweed, tansy, valerian, vervain,* walewort (alternate for elder), water pepper, white pine, *wild cherry, wintergreen, wood betony, wood sage, yarrow, yerba santa.*

COLIC

Symptoms:
Paroxysmal abdominal pain due to smooth-muscle spasm, obstruction by calculi, nervous indigestion, or distention or enlargement of any of the hollow viscera.

Cause:
In all cases, this is due to improper diet, digestive disorder, and poor elimination.

Herbal aids:
Wild yam, cramp bark, some nervines and antispasmodic tinctures relieve cramping. The bowels should be cleansed with a catnip injection. Hot bran fomentation over the stomach-abdominal area will give ease and comfort.

For gassy colic, the following decoction is excellent; dandelion root, fennel seeds, marshmallow root, sweet flag root (with cayenne and ginger added as stimulant carriers).

For bilious colic, use a decoction in equal parts of agrimony, barberry bark, centaury, dandelion root, or an infusion of a handful of fresh parsley will do the job.

Useful herbs:
Angelica, anise, balm leaves, balsam of Tolu, *bayberries, black walnuts, blessed thistle,* blue cohosh, bog bean, boneset, buckthorn bark, calamus, *camomile,* camphor gum, caraway seed, carrot seed, cascarilla, *catnip, cayenne,* celandine, centaury (European), cinnamon, galangal, gentian root, ginseng, *ground nutmeg,* guaiac wood, gum guaiacum, gum hemlock, *gum myrrh,* Indian turnip, Ipecac, juniper berries, *licorice root,* linden flowers, masterwort, *motherwort, nutmeg flowers,* orange peel, origanum, Peruvian bark, pimpernel, pleurisy root, prickly ash, raisins (seedless), *rosemary, rue, sassafras, senna, silverweed (cinquefoil), spearmint, star anise, stone root, summer savory, sweet flag, tansy, thyme,* tormentil, valerian, *wild yam, wintergreen, wood betony,* wormwood.

COLITIS (Colon trouble)

Symptoms:
Inflammation of the colon or large intestine, especially its mucous membrane. This is characterized either by runny or constipated bowels, mucoid discharge from the bowel, weakness felt in the abdomen, often headache, pain, dizziness, etc.

Cause:
This is caused by faulty diet, too many food mixtures irritating the stomach and bowels, hasty eating (insufficient mastication and saliva), taking liquids while eating, excessive use of cathartics, and foods cooked in aluminum.

Herbal aids:
Any of the following herbs used as a high enema are very beneficial and soothing: alum root, bayberry, burdock, golden seal, myrrh, or yellow dock. This irritation can be soothed by drinking teas of cayenne, comfrey, marshmallow root, mullein leaves, or slippery elm. The lower bowel tonic is excellent. Alleviate irritation of the bowels by pureeing foods until some healing takes place and normal food roughage can be handled.

Useful herbs:
Aloes, *anise seed, bayberry bark,* blackberry root, columbo, fire weed, fleabane, golden seal, myrrh, peppermint, sassafras, slippery elm, sweet gum bark, vervain, wahoo bark, white oak bark, wild cherry bark.

CONGESTION

Symptoms:
An abnormal collection or over accumulation of blood in an organ. This is due to insufficient dilation of the blood vessels.

Cause:
See: "CATARRH."

Herbal aids:
Use cayenne or another stimulant externally or internally. A very good external application for breaking up bronchial congestion is the use of mullein (three parts) and lobelia (one part) with cayenne added as a counter-irritant.

Useful herbs:
Aloe, anise, *apple cider vinegar, blessed thistle, camomile,* caraway, *cayenne,* fennel, fringetree (liver), lavender flower, linden, *mandrake* (liver), *peppermint, rue, sage, veronica, yarrow.*

CONSTIPATION

Symptoms:
A condition of peristaltic malfunction in the bowels wherein the fecal matter becomes condensed and compressed and the evacuations are infrequent and difficult. This condition is produced by our modern way of life—the eating of highly refined and demineralized foods instead of a plain and coarse diet, the strain and stress of rapid living, hastily eaten meals, and lack of exercise.

When toxic waste matter is left to stagnate in the lower bowel tract, the system becomes polluted with poisonous gases which congest and irritate the surrounding organs, causing adhesions, and other ailments. A person should have bowel movements as often as regular meals are eaten.

Herbal aids:
You may get quick, temporary relief by using an herbal laxative to clear the lower bowel tract, but only the lower bowel tonics will get at the cause. With the lower bowel tonic, we feed the eliminative organs and allow them to work on their own and eventually eliminate the use of enemas, colonics, and laxatives. The proper procedure is to build up the body, to cleanse it, and see that the bowels work freely.

Often prune juice or fruits will give relief and start the peristaltic motion coming again with ease. The afflicted person can assist in restoring natural bowel action by drinking copious amounts of water between meals (one-half hour before and two hours after eating) and by eating proper foods at regular intervals, especially bulky foods. Avoid any inorganic or concentrated foods.

If one needs a quick herbal laxative, any of the following herbs may be used: agar, or seaweed, boneset, *bran,* butternut bark, *California bark berry root,* and *Chinese Rhubarb root, culver's root, Indian senna leaves, mandrake root,* psyllium seed, *sacred bark, senna, turtle bloom leaves, Virginia snake root.*

One should be wary of an incorrect use of laxatives and purgatives, because liquefied fecal matter is immediately absorbed by the intestinal villi into the bloodstream, and if there is excess toxic matter, it will be thrown out of the bloodstream into the lungs, skin, kidneys, or other organs, producing a chronic toxemia thus laying the foundation for chronic disease.

Useful herbs:
Aloe leaf, American black alder berries, anise, asafetida, *balmony leaves*, benzoin gum, bitter root, European black alder bark, *black root, blackthorn flowers,* blue flag, *buckthorn bark, butternut bark,* caraway, cascaras bark, cayenne, celery seed, *chickweed,* cinnamon, colic root, coriander, couch grass, culverts root, dandelion root, elder, elecampane, fennel, fringetree, ginger, Indian senna fruit, *licorice, mandrake root, may apple root, Oregon grape root,* origanum, papaw seeds, peppermint, podophyllum root, *poke root, quaker button seeds* (powder), psyllium, *rhubarb* (herb and root), *sacred bark* (cascaras sagrada), *sassafras,* scammony, senna leaves, sweet weed, *Turkey rhubarb,* Virginia poke root, *wahoo bark, walnut bark,* white ash, wild Oregon grape.

CONVULSIONS

Symptoms:
Violent and involuntary muscular contractions.

Cause:
Some irritation of the nervous system, such as afflictions of the spinal cord or brain; head injury; a toxic condition of the blood; teething, worms, hysteria, intense pain, griping of the bowels, fear, etc.

Herbal aids:
Know the cause before administering any herbal remedy. If convulsions are caused by poisons taken into the body through the stomach, then emetics must be used quickly. If they are from fright or fear, an antispasmodic tincture with cayenne will usually stop the attack at once. If the convulsions are caused from an impacted bowel, catnip injection will relieve the constipation and soothe the nervous system.

Often the individual is in no condition to take oral aids. In such cases give an enema or an injection of antispasmodic, nervine or catnip, which will ease and soothe the convulsive condition.

Useful herbs:
All-heal, *antispasmodic,* asafetida, betony, black cohosh, blue cohosh, bull nettle, calamine, *catnip, cayenne,* cedron, *camomile,* dwarf elder, *fennel,* fit root, *garlic, gentian, German camomile* (infant), honeysuckle, Indian poke, *ladies slipper, lobelia,* masterwort, motherwort, pennyroyal, peppermint, red clover, red root, rue, *sassafras, skullcap, skunk cabbage root,* spearmint, twin leaf, *valerian,* wild yam.

COUGH

Symptoms:
The sudden involuntary and violent expulsion of air after deep respiration due to irritation.

Cause:
This is often caused by a stomach disorder that comes from overloading the system with food, wherein fermentation occurs causing phlegm. It may also be induced by inflammation in the bronchial tubes due to a neglected cold. Worms may be the cause. Many coughs are from a nervous condition, where coughing may eventually become habitual.

Coughs are highly misunderstood. Usually a sore throat and coughing are caused by the sinuses draining the eustachian tubes, which is like pouring acid down the throat. A cough usually comes from a lowered vitality in the system from improper diet, loss of sleep, lack of exercise, and fresh air, improper breathing, poor elimination, or improper night clothing and bedding.

Herbal aids:
Acute coughs can often be relieved with a little honey and onion syrup. When it is the result of an old acute condition, clear out the morbid condition as rapidly as possible without causing irritation. In old cough conditions, comfrey with vervain or mullein are very good.

The antispasmodic tincture is also excellent, and it is good to massage the chest area across the back with an antispasmodic tincture during attacks of spasms. Antispasmodic tincture may be used both internally and externally as a liniment on the throat.

If cough is due to a neglected cold, any of the diaphoretic herbs are excellent. To relieve the coughing spasms, use horehounds, comfrey, or a small amount of lobelia. High enemas of herbal laxatives will relieve congestion of the bowels, and if the cough is severe (asthma, whooping cough) load the stomach with liquids and induce vomiting.

Useful herbs:
Althea, anise, arbor vitae, balm of Gilead buds, balsam of fir, balsam of Peru, bal-

sam of Tolu, Bethroot, *black cohosh,* blood root, boneset, bugleweed, button bush, cascaras sagrada, catechu, *cayenne, cherry bark,* chestnut leaves, coltsfoot leaves and root and flowers, comfrey, elder flowers, elecampane root, European centaury, fennel, field scabious flowers, figs, *garlic, ginger,* great laurel, grindelia squarrosa, ground ivy, hickory bark, *honey, horehounds leaves* and *flowers,* hyssop, ipecac, *lobelia,* lungwort, maidenhair, malabar nut, *Irish moss,* Island moss, Jamaica dogwood, *licorice root,* linden, liverwort, mandrake, *marshmallow root,* meadow anemone, *Mimosa gum, mullein leaves,* nutmeg, pimpernel root, plantain, *pleurisy root,* poplar bark, poppy capsules, raisins, *raspberry leaves,* rock candy, rue, sacred bark, sage, sassafras, saw palmetto, Seneca snake root, Senegal, *slippery elm bark,* snake weed, soapwort, *spearmint,* spikenard roots, squills, storax, strawberry leaves, sundew, sunflowers, swamp cabbage, sweet gum bark, tamarack bark, veronica, violet, wahoo bark and root, white pine, white root, *wild cherry bark,* wild marjoram, wild potato, *wood betony,* wood root, yerba santa.

CRAMPS

Symptoms:
Painful, spasmodic, and involuntary contractions of the muscles; in the stomach, in a muscle, in the uterus or genital organs, in the bladder, or in the kidneys.

Cause:
Panic and fear, food, or a congested condition in the stomach and the bowel.

Herbal aids:
The first thing to do is to locate the condition and then cleanse the bowel, if that is what is needed. Use an antispasmodic or cramp bark. For stomach cramps take a little tincture of rhubarb in water. For uterine cramping, use cramp bark, squaw vine, or wild yam. Many times when a cramp comes on, all that is needed is one-half teaspoon of ginger in a cup of hot water.

Useful herbs:
All-heal, anise, balm, *black cohosh, blessed thistle, blue cohosh,* cajeput (oil), calamine, *camomile,* caraway, cardamon seed, *cayenne, chickweed, cloves,* coral, cowslip, *cramp bark,* daffodil, dill, fennel, goose grass, juniper berries, *ladies slipper,* linden flowers, *lobelia,* masterwort, motherwort, nettle, *nutmeg* (oil), *parsley, pennyroyal, peppermint* (herb and oil), pleurisy root, prairie hyssop, *rue, sage, skullcap, silverweed, skunk cabbage,* Stone root, *thyme,* twin leaf, *valerian*, whortleberry, *wood betony*, yarrow.

CYST

Symptoms:
A pouch or sac without an opening, having a distinct membrane enclosure, and containing fluid or semi-fluid morbid matter. This usually develops within an organ or a body cavity.

Causes:
Cysts are unwanted material in the body that can be dissolved and cleared with the proper use of herbs. Cysts are often caused by a rundown condition of the body where the malfunction is so intense in a specific area that the cell structure gets out of hand and grows additional unneeded lumps or polyps.

Herbal aids:
In breaking up a cyst, the use of walnut herbs (leaves, bark, or the green hull or dried pulp around the shell of the nut) are excellent. The use of chaparral may be used internally or externally.

Useful herbs:
Apple cider vinegar, Brigham tea, burdock root, cayenne, chaparral, honey, mullein, plantain, sarsaparilla, yellow dock (ovarian or genital areas).

DEBILITY

Symptoms:
Weakness, absence or loss of strength (asthenia), loss of vital strength or muscular power (adynamia).

Cause:
In debility, the condition is generally caused by a rundown body as a result of an improper diet. Do not overfeed since the body is already overworked, and the heart is already overburdened, and the organs are tired from trying to digest heavy foods. The kind "angels of mercy" that bring in cakes, pies, and the little "goodies" to the invalid and say; "Now you must eat to get your strength--you must eat to get your strength built up," are not really "angels of mercy" since they only aggravate the problem.

Herbal aids:
In some cases the whole digestion must be rebuilt. A speedy recovery may be had with juice therapy alone or with slippery elm gruel. Other nutritional herbs such as Irish moss or comfrey may be used successfully.

Useful herbs:
Alder, almond (sweet), angelica, anise seed, avens root, balmony bark, barberry, Bethroot, bittersweet, black alder bark, boneset, camomile, canella, cardamon seed, *cayenne,* celandine, *cloves, comfrey,* common birthwort, *elecampane, gentian root, ginseng, golden seal,* gold thread, guaiac, *Iceland moss,* Indian cup plant, magnolia tree, myrrh, oak leaves, peach (pits), Peruvian bark, *poplar bark,* prickly ash, *quaker button,* quassia, queen of the meadow, ragged cup, *rhubarb, Salem root, sorrel, star grass, raisins, tansy, tormentil, wafer ash, wake robin, white ash, white poplar, yarrow.*

DIABETES (Or diabetes mellitus)

Symptoms:
This is a constitutional disease where carbohydrates are not used properly due to failure in the pancreas to secrete sufficient insulin. The body tissue cannot oxidize carbohydrates at a normal rate. This is characterized by excessive discharge of urine, sugar in the urine, excessive thirst and hunger, and progressive emaciation.

Cause:
Malnutrition and malfunction in connection with a bad pancreatic condition cause diabetes. Stay away from sugars and starches which will go into diabetes very quickly due to a weakened pancreas. Baking soda and aluminum cookery greatly aggravate diabetes.

Herbal aids:
Diabetes is a forerunner for Bright's disease. Heavy users of insulin have been able to cut their intake rapidly by a number of herbal remedies such as verde cactus and ginger, cedar berries, and chaparral. Clean the colon area with a high enema of burdock root, yellow dock root, or bayberry bark. Assist nature in its elimination of sugars and body poisons through the skin by taking long hot baths. Accompany the baths by taking internally diaphoretic teas. Finish off with a cold shower or by sponging with cold water and vinegar.

Use the lower bowel tonic herbs to regulate elimination. Hot fomentation of castor oil, etc., may be used on the spine, stomach, and pancreas areas to obtain relief. The patient should avoid all processed denatured foods and "secondary" foods such as animal by-products—meat, milk, eggs, fish, etc. Herbs such as Irish moss and slippery elm are nutritive mucilages that soothe while they feed the irritated digestive areas.

In general, the diet for diabetes should consist of the fresh fruits and tender greens and vegetables "in the season thereof" from the garden, preferably raw or cooked at low heat. Deep breathing and plenty of vigorous outdoor exercise are also vital.

Useful herbs:
Alum root, beech, bilberry leaves, bistort, *blueberry leaves, blue cohosh,* buchu, bugleweed, butter weed, Canada flea bane, cedar berries, cheese plant, *dandelion root,* devil's club, dog grass, flaxseed, German cheese plant, globe flower root, *golden seal,* huckleberry leaves, Indian hemp, ivy leaved toad flax, jaborandi, jambul seed, knotgrass, *marshmallow root, milfoil,* mistletoe, nettle leaves, cranesbill root, unicorn root, hemlock spruce, *malva root, pinus canadensis, poplar bark, queen of the meadow, raspberry leaves, red root, rhus aromatica, saw palmetto berries, slippery elm, sumac berries,* sweet fern, *sweet sumac,* thyme, tormentil, *unicorn, uva ursi,* white pine needles, wild alum root, wintergreen, wormwood, yarrow, yellow dock.

DIARRHEA

Symptoms:
A common symptom of gastrointestinal affliction, either from acute infection, inflammation of the mucous membrane, or psychogenic causes. It is characterized by frequent, morbid and profuse bowel evacuations.

Cause:
Diarrhea is the most severe form of constipation caused by a complete blockage in the lower intestine. Liquids only will come through while solids are retained. The body must be cleansed as quickly as possible or diarrhea will go into dysentery.

Herbal aids:
The use of peach leaf tea or ripe peaches themselves will often stop common diarrhea. Sunflower leaf tea is one of the most potent but must be used in very small amounts.

Useful herbs:
Alum root, amaranth, angelica, avens root, balm mint, barberry, *bayberry bark, blackberry* (root and berries), black haw, *black root, bugleweed, camomile,* catechu, *cayenne,* chocolate root, cinnamon, cloves, columbo, *comfrey,* copaiva, cranesbill, elder, gentian root, ginger root, gum myrrh, hardhack, hearts-tongue, *Iceland moss, Irish moss,* Judas tree, kino, knotgrass, ladies mantle, lady slipper, *mace, marshmallow, mimosa gum, mullein,* nettle, nutgall, nutmeg, oak bark, peppermint, Peruvians bark, pilewort (celandine), plantain, poplar, prince's feather, *raspberry leaves,* red oak bark, rhatany root, rhubarb, ribwort, rock rose, rosemary, sage, sheep laurel, shepherd's purse, silverweed, *slippery elm,* sloe, smartweed, spearmint, *squaw vine,* St. John's-wort, strawberry, *sunflower leaves, sweet sumac, thyme, tormentil root, uva ursi, walnut leaves,* white pond lily, white poplar, whortleberry, *wild alum root,* willow bark, *witch hazel,* wormwood, yarrow, *yellow dock.*

DIPHTHERIA

Symptoms:
An acute febrile and contagious affliction common with children, characterized by the formation of a fibrous, inflammatory membrane (yellowish or greenish) on the mucous membrane of the air passages, usually the pharynx, larynx, and trachea. The tonsils become inflamed and are dark red, but the uneven swelling gives the appearance of white patches. This is further characterized by pain, swelling and obstruction, fever, prostration, and often cardiac damage, which sometimes results in paralysis and death.

Cause:
Diphtheria is caused by impure blood, improper diet or contaminated foods, and

unsanitary conditions. A deficiency of organic calcium and vitamin C is the basis for diseases of this type.

Herbal aids:
With diphtheria the throat area should be cleared of the false mucous membrane, with a bayberry and raspberry combination, garlic, or a purified type of turpentine as a fomentation. Take a few drops in a tea. Quick relief is given through antispasmodic and cayenne fomentation on the chest and the lung area. Antispasmodic tincture and cayenne can be taken internally (this will also ward off the danger of paralysis).

One should always give an emetic before allowing the patient to go to sleep, and the bowels should be cleaned of the poisons with high enemas accompanied with stimulant herbs. Any of the following may be used as enemas: bayberry bark, raspberry leaves, catnip, chickweed, white oak bark, shepherd's purse, wild alum root, echinacea, strawberry leaves, raspberry leaves. A hot vapor bath is beneficial as is a hot foot bath of mustard and water. Also apply fomentation of mullein and ragwort to the throat. Decoctions of raspberry leaves, mullein, agrimony, bayberry bark or lemon juice will relieve the soreness in the throat. Ample fresh pineapple juice is also very good.

Useful herbs:
Agrimony, bayberry bark, cayenne, echinacea, eucalyptus, *golden seal,* Indian hemp, jaborandi, *lemon Juice, lobelia, mullein leaves,* myrrh, *oak bark, persimmon bark, quince seed and fruit, raspberry leaves,* red sage, wild indigo.

DIZZINESS (Vertigo)

Symptoms:
A swimming or swirling sensation of the head; a sensation of lack of equilibrium.

Cause:
Dizziness can be caused by constipation when pressure causes the nerves to become impinged. There are many other reasons for dizziness such as the menstrual period, an injury or a fall on the head, compacted sinuses, or blood pressure problems.

Herbal aids:
Cayenne will give relief.

Useful herbs:
Basil, black alder, black horehounds, benzoin, buckbean, calendula, caraway, cardamon, *catnip, centaury (European), cloves, coltsfoot, coriander, cowslip, cubeb, dandelion,* galangal, *garlic,* lavender, mastic, mountain flax, mullein, roman leopard's bane, rose leaves, rosemary, *rue, sage,* savory, senna, single peony, storax, sweet flag, tansy, *valerian, veronica, wild plum bark, wood betony.*

DROPSY (Generalized edema or anasarca)

Symptoms:
Abnormal and excessive accumulation or infiltration of diluted lymph serum in the interfibrillar spaces of the subcutaneous connective tissue or in the serious (peritoneal or pleural) cavities of the body which do not drain. This condition is accompanied by swelling, scanty urine, poor appetite, sluggishness, and debility. The swelling usually begins in the feet and ankles and proceeds up the legs towards the abdomen.

Cause:
Heavy salt users often have dropsy as do diabetics. We do not pinpoint the symptoms as to locality (hydrocephalus, hydrothorax, ascites, etc.), as does orthodox medicine, but the general problem is that fluid does not eliminate properly through the kidneys and skin.

Dr. Edward Shook had the following to say about dropsy:

> When sulfuric acid is generated within the organism, it immediately unites with water and swells up. This action produces heat, which expands the capillaries. The osmotic pressure forces the serum through the walls of the blood vessels, producing inflammation and dropsy. Hence the using of inorganic matter is always poisonous to the human organism in spite of all the apparent evidence to the contrary. (*Advanced Treatise in Herbology,* lesson 8 page 101)

Herbal aids:
Exceptional results have been attained with dropsy by the use of parsley, parsley root, juniper berries, verde cactus, ginger, and chaparral. Diet is the key to eliminating the cause. Meats, pastries, salt, etc. should be avoided. Eat fruits (grapes and coconut especially), sprouts, leafy and green vegetables (do not mix fruits and vegetables). Use vapor baths and diaphoretics to open the pores, stimulants to increase and regulate circulation, diuretics for kidneys, and be sure to treat the whole digestive system with tonics. Also rub the body with vinegar and cold water and be sure to keep the bowels cleaned.

Useful herbs:
Adders tongue, agrimony, angelica, *anise,* arbor vitae, asarabacca, ash leaves, *asparagus,* balm leaves, balmony, bitter candy tuft, bitter root, *black alder bark, black cohosh,* black hellebore, black root (with cream of tartar), *blessed thistle,* blooming spurge, blue cohosh, *blue flag,* broom, buchu, buckthorn bark, *burdock root, butternut bark,* button snake root, *camomile,* Canada fleabane, caper bush, *carrot,* celandine, *celery,* cleavers, colocynth, coriander seed, *couch grass, cucumber* (single seeded), currants, *dandelion root,* elder (dwarf) or *wild bark, elecampane root, fennel, flaxseed, garden daisy, golden seal, haircap moss, hawthorn,*

hearts tongue, hedge agrimony, hedge hyssop, *horseradish, Hydrangea,* hyssop, Indian hemp, Indian physic, iris, *Irish moss, ivy* (American), *jalap, juniper berries,* kidneywort, knotgrass, larkspur, *lily of the valley, lobelia, mandrake root,* marjoram, masterwort, meadow lily, meadow sweet, milkweed, mugwort, mulberry (French), mullein, nettle leaves, origanum, *parsley herb, parsley root, pennyroyal, Peruvian bark,* plantain, pimpernel, *pipsissewa,* poplar buds, *prickly ash berries, quassia,* queen of the meadow, *quince seed* and *fruit,* raisins, red chickweed, rosemary, sandalwood, *sassafras, shavegrass,* skunk cabbage, sloe tree, sourbush, sow fennel, spearmint, squills, succory, sundew, *tansy,* twin leaf, uva ursi, wahoo, wall pellitory, wall rue, *walnut leaves,* water starwort, white ash, *white mustard herb* and *seeds, white pond lily,* wild carrot seed, wintergreen, wolfsbohne, wood betony, *yellow dock.*

DYSENTERY (Summer complaint)

Symptoms:
An affliction characterized by inflammation of the large intestine or colon. The symptoms are griping pains, constant strain to evacuate the bowels (tenesmus), intense diarrhea, and frequent discharge of mucus and blood. These are symptoms of impure blood, fever, sleeplessness, lack of appetite, and sometimes a swollen abdomen. In advanced cases, there is pallidness, rapid breathing, slow pulse, and hot urine.

Bleeding from the bowels is quickly healed by mullein in milk. Give a warm, very high enema with an astringent such as white oak bark, bayberry bark, wild alum root, etc. Use fomentation of lobelia, castor oil, etc. placed on the abdomen and spine, followed by a liniment application of wormwood oil. The patient should be nurtured with a diet of light alkaline foods and mucilage herbs, such as slippery elm and Irish moss, barley or oatmeal water.

Cause:
The cause is improper diet, liquids with meals, overeating, wrong food combinations, impure water, use of liquor, tobacco, coffee, tea, eating fruits or vegetables that have begun to decompose or chronic constipation.

Useful herbs:
Acacia powder, alum root, asarabacca, balm, balsam of copaiba, balsam of Peru, bamboo, barberry, *bayberry bark, bethroot,* birth bark, bistort, *blackberries, black root,* blood root, buckthorn brake, *bugleweed, burdock, camomile, cascarilla,* chocolate root, cinnamon, calumba, *comfrey,* copaiba, cow parsley, cudweed, dandelion, dragons blood, fever bush, fire weed, fleabane, geranium, ginger, Goldenrod (European), groundsel, hearts-tongue, house leek, *Iceland moss, Irish moss, joint weed,* Judas tree, kino, knotgrass, *lady's slipper* (enema), leptandra, logwood, magnolia, *marshmallow,* masterwort, *mimosa gum,* mountain ebony, mullein, nettle, peach (pits), *peppermint,* periwinkle (small), pilewort, plantain, pleurisy root, prince's feather, *quince seed* and *fruit,* ragweed, raspberry leaves,

red sandalwood, ribwort, saffron, sanicle, *sheep laurel, shepherd's purse, silverweed, simaruba bark, skunk cabbage, slippery elm,* sloe tree, Solomon's seal, *squaw vine,* St. John's wort, St. Thomas tree, *strawberry leaves* and *root, tormentil root, Turkey rhubarb, uva ursi* (decoction or syrup), *valerian* (enema), wall pellitory, wallwort, whortleberry, *wild cherry bark,* willow (bark of root), *witch hazel, yarrow.*

DYSMENORRHEA

Symptoms:
Difficult or painful menstruation. There may be intense congestion of the pelvic viscera, pain between menses, inflammation, mechanical obstruction to the menstrual fluid, uterine mucosa, problems with the ovaries, pain of mental or psychic origin, problems in the pelvic region, sudden and severe spasmodic uterine contraction, problems of the oviduct, and other problems of the uterus and vagina.

Cause:
Weakness in the generative organs, colds, or a general body weakness.

Herbal aids:
Pain may be quickly relieved with squaw vine or bark, or any emmenagogue. Stimulants should be given to equalize circulation, and ginger is excellent. Pennyroyal and vapor baths will relieve the colds and congestions. Use the corrective tonics.

Useful herbs:
Balm, *black cohosh,* black haw, blue cohosh, Bethroot, *camomile, cramp bark, devil's bit, dogwood (Jamaica), false unicorn root,* figwort, *ginger, golden seal, ironweed, lily root, partridge berry, pimento berries, poke root, raspberry leaves,* rue (German), spearmint, squaw mint, *squaw vine,* star grass, sumbul, thyme, unicorn root, uva ursi, white ash bark, *white poplar bark.*

DYSPEPSIA

Symptoms:
Disturbed or deranged digestion, sour stomach, acid stomach, indigestion, poor assimilation.

Causes:
Dyspepsia is a hyperacidity condition in the body, where certain cooked and secondary substances cannot be digested. The problem may also be with the liver, or the gall bladder. This is caused by eating processed and devitalized foods.

Herbal aids:
Instead of using those aids which are highly advertised and are high in aluminum, which cause aluminum poisoning, use the herbs for the nerves, stomach and bow-

els. Carminatives will assist the stomach herbs to improve elimination. Alteratives will cleanse the blood and tone up other excretory organs. Stimulant-diuretics will help eliminate waste matter that may be causing the problem. Demulcents or emollients will soothe the irritated stomach lining.

Useful herbs:
Adrue (*Cyperus articulatus*), *aloes, angelica, anise, balmony, bayberry bark,* bay leaves, beech, bitter root, *black alder bark, blood root, blue vervain, boneset, buchu,* calamus, *camomile,* caraway, cardamon seed, cascaras sagrada, *cascarilla, cayenne,* chocolate root, *cloves,* calumba, cow parsnip, devils bit, dogwood; *dwarf elder, elecampane root,* galangal, gentian root, ginger, ginseng, golden seal, gold thread, horehounds, *Hydrastis, Iceland moss, ipecac, ironwood, lever wood, life everlasting, magnolia tree, milkweed root, nutmeg,* orange peel, *origanum, papaw seed, peach leaves, peppermint, Peruvian bark, pichi tops* (fabiana), *plantain,* pleurisy root, prickly ash, *quaker button,* quassia, *raspberry leaves, rhubarb,* rose pink, rush, sage *spearmint,* star grass, sundew, tag alder, *tansy, thyme,* unicorn, Virginia snake root, wahoo, white ash, *white poplar, wild cherry,* witch hazel, yarrow, yellow dock.

DYSPNEA

Symptoms:
Difficult breathing.

Cause:
This usually arises from mucus in the air passages in the trachea, the nostrils, lungs, etc.

Herbal aids:
Take a cup of cayenne tea and antispasmodic tincture internally and massaged on the chest area. With a breast-fed baby, the mother should take a tea of balm, hyssop, or pennyroyal. For the baby, where the problem is largely in the nose (sometimes referred to as snuffles), a mixture of milk and olive oil in the nose is good. The bowels may need to be relieved with a small injection of lobelia.

Useful herbs:
Almond (sweet), *blue vervain, comfrey root,* coriander, *dandelion, hawthorn,* imperial masterwort, *garlic, lobelia, sarsaparillas* (German), soapwort, veronica.

FATIGUE

Symptoms:
Exhaustion of strength, weariness from exertion or any condition involving over-activity diminishes the vital energy.

Cause:
Fatigue is usually caused by insufficient oxygen in the body either through diet, wearing synthetic clothes, or through improper breathing. It may be caused by being in congested areas where there is insufficient good air for breathing. The oxygen supply to the body is very important because waste matter accumulates if there is a lack of oxygen to every cell. Overeating also robs the body of the oxygen that should be distributed to various other places. Not only should one use proper herbs and proper foods to rebuild the body, but it is also necessary to take steps to avoid overtiring the body and learn the science of breathing properly.

Herbal aids:
Brigham tea, carrot juice, cayenne, ginseng, grape juice, lobelia, sarsaparillas.

Useful herbs:
Same as above.

FEVER

Symptoms:
The elevation of the body temperature above normal (98.6° F., 37° C). It is characterized by increased heat, accelerated pulse, general functional derangement, and usually is accompanied with thirst and loss of appetite.

Cause:
Fever is not a disease but a condition in the body wherein the balance of circulation has become disturbed. This is nature's way of trying to burn out the toxic poisons. When the body becomes exposed to excessive chilling or dampness, the capillaries near the surface contract and the pores close by becoming obstructed with body waste matter. This results in a containment of body heat and a sudden rise of body temperature. In fever the natural body function is to increase the heat to a point wherein the thick glutinous and fibrinous matters loading and congesting the system are made liquid enough to pass through the fine and delicate excretory membranes and tubules.

Herbal aids:
If the fever is from cold or flu, eliminate the mucoid condition and you will eliminate the problem. Raspberry and other sweetening herbs are very beneficial. Raise the body heat with moisture, a stimulant and diaphoretic herbs so the restricted blood vessels relax, the obstructed pores open, and the morbid material washes out in the subsequent profuse perspiration.

Useful herbs:
Aconite root, apple tree bark, bitter root, *blood root, blue vervain* (hot), boneset, borage, buckbean, buckthorn bark, butternut, calamus, *camomile, cascarilla, catnip, centaury, cinchona bark, cleavers,* calumba, coral, culverts root, dandelion, dogwood bark, European black alder bark, fenugreek, *feverwort, fireweed, fit root,*

friar's cap root, gentian root, hyssop, Indian hemp, *lobelia,* magnolia, *mandrake,* masterwort, *nettle, parsley, pennyroyal, peppermint, Peruvian bark, pleurisy root, poplar, quassia bark, raspberry leaves, roman motherwort, sage,* shepherd's purse, sumac berries, sweet balm, *tansy, thyme, valerian, vervain, Virginia snake root, wahoo, water avens root,* wild cherry, willow, wintergreen, *wood sage, wormwood, yarrow, Yerba buena herb.*

FLATULENCE

Symptoms:
Gassy condition in the alimentary canal, especially the gastrointestinal tract.

Cause:
Flatus (which is gas or air in the gastrointestinal canal) is the result of poor digestion. The food becomes fermented and sour in the stomach due to an acid condition. This is caused by wrong food combinations, drinking with meals, hasty eating, or poor mastication.

Herbal aids:
There are a number of herbs that will help relieve gas. Some of the best are *wild yam, celery seed tea,* and peppermint or spearmint teas. Carminative teas are specifics for the stomach area to soothe the flatulent condition and to correct the digestive functions. Golden seal with myrrh is an excellent stomach tonic.

Useful herbs:
Angelica root and *seed, anise seed,* balsam of Tolu, barberry, *bayberries,* bishop's root, *calamus root, camomile flowers,* camphor, Canada snake root, caraway seed, cardamon seed, catnip, cloves, calumba, *coriander seeds,* cow parsnip, *cumin seed, dill, fennel seed,* fever bush, galangal, gentian root, *ginger,* Goldenrod (oil), guaiacum (gum), hemlock (gum and oil), *lemon balm, lovage root,* mace, melissa, milfoil, mint, *myrrh* (gum), *nutmeg,* orange peel, origanum, *parsley root, peppermint, rue,* sage, sarsaparillas, sassafras, senna, spearmint, *sweet flag, thyme,* unicorn, *valerian, water mint, wild yam, wintergreen* (oil and herb), wood betony, yarrow, yerba buena, zedoary root.

FLU (Or influenza or gripe)

Symptoms:
An epidemic affliction, characterized by catarrhal inflammation of the mucous membranes of the throat and bronchi, accompanied by mucopurulent discharge, fever, vascular prostration, and severe neuralgia pains. Complications of pleurisy and neuritis may appear. This condition is characterized by chilling, stuffy head, dizziness, sneezing, loss of appetite, fever, coughing sore throat, etc.

Cause:
Flu is an advanced cold condition. A body catches flu when it is full of waste mat-

ter and toxins through lowered vitality and by body exposure to cold and dampness. This is due to mucus in a weak spot in the body—in this case, the respiratory tract. The contributing factors to this weakness are shallow breathing and a lack of oxygen to that particular area.

Herbal aids:
The fastest way in eliminating this body condition is by proper diet and rest, and by flushing the body system with diaphoretics. Take a ginger bath (using up to a pound of ginger to a tub of water), or a mustard-cayenne bath with cold sheeting. The antispasmodic agents relax the constringed cell structure, loosen and discharge the mucoid matter. Fruit juices (especially hot lemon juice) should be taken alternately with the herbal teas. After the cleansing crisis, the body system should be built up with tonic herbs and with nutritious, non-mucous forming foods.

Useful herbs:
Agrimony, angelica, bay leaves, bayberry bark, black cohosh, black root, bethroot, *blood root,* blue cohosh, boneset, butternut bark, calamus, cayenne pods, *chickweed, cinnamon bark,* cloves, coltsfoot, *comfrey, culverts root, elder flowers,* European filbert, *fennel, feverfew, flaxseed, ginger, ginseng, golden seal, holy thistle,* hyssop, juniper berries, Indian hemp, lady's slipper, *lobelia, lungwort, marshwort, mullein, mustard, myrrh,* nettle, orange peel, pennyroyal, peppermint, pimpernel, *pleurisy,* poplar, red sage, *sacred bark,* saffron, slippery elm, sweet balm, *tansy, thyme,* valerian, *vervain,* wahoo, *wild cherry bark,* white pine, willow bark, witch hazel, wood betony, wood sanicle, yarrow, *yerba santa.*

GANGRENE (Mortification)

Symptoms:
Mortification or death to a part of the body due to interference with and failure of the local blood supply. The moist type gangrene begins with inflammation, with the dying or dead tissues becoming bluish or black. The dry gangrene results from contracted arterioles where circulation is poor, and it begins with yellow or black spotting in the tissue.

Cause:
Gangrene is the advanced condition of blood poisoning.

Herbal aids:
This condition will never happen to a person who has good blood circulation and whose blood has been cleansed. Soak the afflicted area with marshmallow root tea, covering the area with tea as hot as the patient can take and leave it there for long periods of time. Soaking works faster than the poultice or the tea, but drinking the tea along with the soaking will speed the action. Plantain used as a poultice is also excellent. Pain in the infected part can be relieved by adding a small amount of lobelia. Be sure that the bowels move properly by cleansing them with

the lower bowel tonic.

Useful herbs:
Black alder bark, black willow bark, bryony, *bugleweed,* calamus, *camomile* (poultice), camphor, carlina thistle, cayenne, calumba, *comfrey root,* echinacea, *geranium root, golden seal,* hemlock, *linden, charcoal, marshmallow root, myrrh,* nettle, *oak bark,* Peruvian bark, *pleurisy root, poplar, smartweed, vervain, walnut leaves,* willow bark.

GOUT

Symptoms:
A metabolic affliction due to excessive uric acid in the blood which deposits uriate of sodium in and around the joints. This is associated with the high blood level and decreased urinary excretion of uric acid, and is often accompanied with fever and excessive increase in leukocytes. There may be intermittent and sudden attacks of acute, painful arthritis that last from a few days to a few weeks. These attacks come at night and usually affect only one joint. The first joint involved is usually the bigtoe, and the afflicted joint may be hot, red, tender, with the adjacent skin being very shiny. When there are repeated attacks, degeneration of the joints may occur, resulting in deformity. This is accompanied with indigestion, flatulence, constipation, heart trouble, and scanty urine (sometimes red). The ankles and knees may swell as the problem progresses.

Cause:
This condition is caused from overloading the system with improper foods. If the general living habit is not changed, the condition that starts on the big toe will go into various parts of the foot and ankle and sometimes into other parts of the body. Babies may be born with gout or rheumatoid arthritis, although it is usually caused by improper diet. The author himself was gout with rheumatoid arthritis from the time he was able to walk. Gout is always rheumatoid arthritis, but rheumatoid arthritis is not always recognized as being gout because at times it comes to different parts of the body instead of just the foot.

Herbal aids:
The eliminative organs must be improved. Drink apple cider vinegar with honey and bathe the area in hot apple cider vinegar. To speed healing, take MCP pectin (one teaspoonful three times a day). Herbal teas work well to relieve pain. Tincture of lobelia with apple cider vinegar baths on the afflicted parts is very good. A good herb combination is equal parts of skullcap, valerian, and yarrow taken in tea form to assist in freeing the toxic waste from the tissues and to eliminate the waste through the various excretory organs.

Useful herbs:
Angelica, *arbor vitae,* balm of Gilead, birch leaves, bitter candy tuft, *blackberry,* black ramsthorn, *blue violet,* broom, buckthorn bark, *burdock root,* cajeput oil,

calamus, *cayenne,* cherry tree wood, common ash, cough grass, dwarf elder leaves, English cowslip, European ash leaves, garden daisy, gentian, *German rue, ginger, gout wood, gravel root, Hydrangea root, juniper berries,* kidneywort, *lily of the valley, marshmallow root,* meadow saffron, Mt. Laurel, mugwort, nettle leaves, pennyroyal, plantain, *queen of the meadow* (gravel root), rest harrow, rhubarb, rue, sarsaparillas, shavegrass, succory, tacamahaca, violet flowers, wood betony, yarrow, yellow parilla.

GRIPING

Symptoms:
An intense spasmodic pain in the lower bowels.

Cause:
Overloading the stomach or bowel may cause the peristaltic area to cease functioning. This can be very painful and is generally caused by malnutrition, poor assimilation, or by gorging, and by improper types of food. The overuse of corn which is not chewed properly or eating too many green apples are good examples of causes of bowel griping. Do not permit such unhealthful self-indulgence.

Herbal aids:
Use hot packs of mullein or slippery elm with one-fourth part lobelia on the afflicted area; or, if tincture of lobelia is used, rub it into the specific area and over the spine area controlling the affected part. Taking a few drops of tincture of lobelia in warm water will stop the griping immediately. The use of a hot castor oil pack with a hot water bottle over it on the area will often stop the pain. If the griping is low in the bowel, use a catnip tea enema.

Useful herbs:
Anise seed, balm, bay leaves, caraway seed, *catnip, coriander, ginger, pennyroyal, nutmeg, thyme.*

HEADACHE (Cephalalgia)

Symptoms:
Pain in or around the head.

Cause:
This is often the result of a disturbance in some other part of the body, such as digestive disorders in the stomach, liver or bowel; problems in the abdominal area; menstrual irregularities, impingements in the cervical; concussion, eye strain, nervous excitement, fatigue, etc. The headache is a mechanism which signals some serious problem elsewhere. The common headache is due to faulty elimination, and the waste matter causes problems until the toxic wastes reach the stomach nerves and affects them. Sometimes headaches are caused from panic, fear, or worrying about the unknown. Headaches of this type are the hardest to relieve,

generally requiring something strong like a heavy nervine tea with lobelia in it to diminish the nervous excitement. A nerve tea such as valerian or skullcap with a few drops of tincture of lobelia to a cup will give relief.

Herbal aids:
Improve elimination with the lower bowel tonic (use the cathartics and enemas only in case of emergency). If the problem is in the stomach area, use any of the following stomach herbs: angelica, balmony, black alder, elecampane, gentian root, raspberry leaves, rhubarb, strawberry leaves, wild cherry, wormwood. Use ginger for a menstrual problem. To relieve the local headache pain, two or three drops of tincture of lobelia in a little water three times a day or up to every hour if required will often give temporary relief. If the contents of the stomach causes the problem, empty that area with an emetic. Where the nerves are raw, the following herbs are excellent: catnip, peppermint (hot), rosemary herb, skullcap, spearmint, wood betony, and since plenty of rest is needed, any of the foregoing herbs along with hops tea is very soothing and will produce sleep.

Useful herbs:
Angelica, anise seed, bitter root, *blessed thistle,* blood root, blue violet, box tree leaves, buckthorn bark, calamine (external), calendula, *camomile, cascaras amarga, catnip, cayenne,* celery seed, coltsfoot, coriander, cudweed, dandelion, dittany, elder flowers, feverfew, fringetree, *ground ivy* (fresh juice as snuff), guarana, horehounds, ivy tree, *lady's slipper* (nervous), lavender flowers, licorice, *marjoram, millet,* mother of thyme, mountain balm, oak balm, oak bark, peach tree, pennyroyal peppermint, pimpernel, prickly ash, *red root,* rhubarb, rose flowers, *rosemary, rue, skullcap, senna, saw fennel, stone root, succory, sweet balm, thyme, tansy, valerian,* violet, virgin's bower, *wild marjoram, wood betony, yerba santa.*

HEARTBURN (Cardialgia)

Symptoms:
A burning sensation or gnawing pain in the area of the chest over the heart (precordium) or beneath the sternum and near the heart, usually a symptom of indigestion or esophageal spasm. Generally this comes from gastric pyrosis, a stomach problem characterized by belching (eructation) an acid, irritating fluid.

Cause:
As heartburn is an acid condition of the system, it is necessary to go on a complete cleansing program to clean out the system. Proper foods, proper eating habits, and effective elimination are very important. A cure is effected only with a complete change of living habits.

Herbal aids:
Prompt and temporary relief may be given for heartburn with cramp bark, ginger, wild yam, etc. Massaging tincture of lobelia externally into the area and taking two or three drops regularly internally is often sufficient.

Useful herbs:
Angelica, anise, burnet, calamus, caraway seed, *catnip, dill, fennel ginger,* mint, nutmeg, *origanum, peppermint, sage, sarsaparilla, sassafras,* spearmint, *thyme,* valerian, *wild yam,* willow, wintergreen, wood betony, yarrow.

HEART TROUBLE

Symptoms:
An abnormal, unhealthy and morbid condition of the heart.

Cause:
The principle cause of heart trouble is wrong diet which causes the system to become sluggish with waste products which collect in the blood stream. Because of lack of exercise, the circulation becomes poor and the blood supply to the extremities becomes congested and overburdens the digestive organs and the heart. Sometimes the heart valves become tired and weak from malnutrition and poor tone. Often the heart is slowed down because of cholesterol which restricts the walls and makes it difficult for the life giving fluid to flow without causing high blood pressure which is very tiring to the heart muscles and eventually stops the heart completely. If the blood is not in good condition, a clot may form in the heart. A recent and excellent article on the dietary aspects of heart disease which is a good warning to offenders is: Ray G. Rowley, M.D., "An 1833 Guide for the Prevention of Heart Disease," *The Improvement Era,* 72:3 (August 1969), pp. 60-63.

Herbal aids:
Refrain from harmful mucus-forming food and drink. Take cayenne regularly. The best herb for the heart is hawthorn berries (for syrup see page 582). The heart valves can be toned up with the use of cayenne, heart tonics, and wheat germ oil. For irregular beating, a tea of black cohosh, lobelia, skullcap, and valerian (with a little cayenne added) is excellent, and lily of the valley is especially good to quiet the heart.

Useful herbs:
Almond (sweet), angelica, anise seed, annatto tree seed, avens (European), *balm,* blackberry, *black cohosh, blessed thistle, blood root,* borage, bugleweed, cactus grandiflora, candy tuft (enlarged heart), *cayenne,* cinnamon, cloves, coriander, cubeb, day lily, *elecampane,* galangal, *garlic, ginger, golden seal, grape juice,* guaiacum wood, *hawthorn berries, horehounds, knot grass, licorice, lily of the valley, mistletoe, motherwort,* nutmeg, peppermint, *prince's pine, raisins,* rhubarb, roman motherwort, sage, skullcap, sheep laurel, snow berry, *sorrel, tansy, valerian, vervain, wintergreen, wood betony.*

HEMORRHAGE

Symptoms:
A discharge or escape of blood from the blood vessels, either by passage of blood cells through the intact and unruptured walls (diapedesis) or by flow through the ruptured walls.

Cause:
This problem is caused by severing or rupturing a blood vessel. If the rupture is from an artery, the blood (usually bright red) spurts and flows fast. If it is a vein, the blood is dark and flows more slowly and constantly.

Herbal aids:
Hemorrhage throws many people into shock and can bring on death very rapidly. If the wound is small, the blood usually coagulates and the area seals itself, but if the rupture is large, some herbal aid is needed. The first thing one should think about is cayenne as quickly as possible. Using one teaspoon to the cup, as hot as can be taken without scalding. This will stop any hemorrhage, internal or external, by the time a person can count to ten. If the rupture is external and cayenne is not available, comfrey placed over the wound will stop bleeding quickly.

Useful herbs:
Bayberry bark, Bethroot, blackberry (uterus), *black pepper, bugleweed,* Canada burnet, *cayenne,* chocolate root, comfrey root, *dandelion,* dwarf nettle, *European goldenrod, fleabane* (bowels and uterus), garden burnet, gentian root (uterus), *geranium root, golden seal* (rectum), great burnet, ipecac, kino (gum), lady's mantle, laurel, *lemon juice* (cold), life everlasting, *marshmallow,* milfoil, mullein, nettle, *oak bark,* Paul's betony, pilewort, *pomegranate,* ramie plant, rock brake, *sheep laurel, shepherd's purse,* sloe tree, sorrel, *St. John's wort,* tag alder (cones), *tormentil root, walnut leaves, watercress, white oak bark,* wild alum root, witch hazel, *yellow dock.*

HICCOUGH

Symptoms:
This is a sudden inspiration of air caused by spasmodic contractions of the diaphragm. An irritation of the phrenic nerve causes the contraction of the diaphragm.

Cause:
This is generally caused by overloading food or drink into the stomach. Relaxation is the most important thing. Often hiccoughs can be stopped merely be bending over with the head downward and tipping a glass of liquid to drink it while upside-down. A few drops of antispasmodic tincture taken internally and rubbed on the chest area will often bring relief, as will a teaspoon of onion juice, a cayenne poultice on the chest area, black cohosh tea, blue cohosh, or wild car-

rot flowers or seeds.

Useful herbs:
Adders tongue, *antispasmodic tincture, black cohosh, blue cohosh, dill,* fennel, hearts tongue, Indian hemp, mint, onion juice, orange juice, *wild carrot seed.*

HIGH BLOOD PRESSURE

Symptoms:
Excessive pressure is exerted on the valves and the pumping muscles of the heart. A pressure is also exerted on the functioning lifelines in the body—the arteries, the capillaries, etc. This condition is characterized by a red or flushed complexion, excess weight, discomfort, and sometimes skin pallor. High blood pressure is the result of improper living habits which cause a rundown condition in the body.

Cause:
A thickening of the blood from catarrhal and excess glutinous and fibrinous matters loading the circulatory system. Generally there is a clogging of the bowel with putrid body waste, making it necessary to cleanse the excretory systems in order to purify the blood.

Herbal aids:
With high blood pressure, cholesterol and mucus form a sludge within the body. Avoid the mucus-forming foods and take herbs that act as a solvent by liquefying impurities such as cayenne, garlic or sassafras. Take cayenne, working up to a teaspoon three times a day. This increases the power of the heart and corrects the circulation problems. Garlic in copious amounts will bring down high blood pressure. Pure tomato juice is very good as a nutritional and medicinal herb. Wheat germ oil is excellent for feeding the heart and helps cut the cholesterol and facilitate its removal from the area. Avoid the use of liquor and tobacco, do not keep late hours, and avoid over-tiredness and worry. There is an intricate inter-relationship between one's living habits and their body condition.

Useful herbs:
Black cohosh, blue cohosh, boneset, broom, buckthorn bark, cassia bark, cayenne, culver's root, European black alder bark, fruit, linden flowers, myrrh, peppermint, *poke root, red clover, rue,* sanicle, *sassafras bark, skullcap, sweetwood root, valerian,* vervain, *water shamrock, wild cherry bark.*

HIVES (Urticaria, or nettle rash)

Symptoms:
An eruption on the skin resembling the condition produced by the stinging of nettles, characterized by the appearance of intense itching, elevated welts and a surrounding redness of skin in patches (erythema). The inflammation may appear in

patches or may be widely distributed over the entire body. It can last a few hours to a day or two.

Cause:
A person will never get hives if the body is in good condition and the blood stream is clear, free and clean. Hives can come from the sting of an insect. This irritates the system and causes it to throw off poisons rapidly in the form of large welts. Sometimes hives will be as large as the palm of the hand and swell up with considerable puffiness. In some cases, a person will eat certain combinations of food and come down with hives after exercise. This cuts the poison loose from the body and brings it to the surface. Hives can be so intense that the eyes will close and swell the tissue over the entire body. This is caused by an acid condition.

Herbal aids:
Rubbing wheat germ oil onto the area is a great help. Use elder leaf tea or chickweed as a wash, and chickweed or elder ointment to heal the condition. Quick relief can be obtained by drinking celery seed, comfrey, chickweed, burdock root or seed, etc. Burdock seed is one of the most potent to relieve the skin and lymph areas rapidly. A half-pound to a pound of ginger in a tub of hot water will help give relief. The bowels must be cleared since the worse cases of hives can come from constipation. The mucusless diet is the most important thing for rashes and hives.

Useful herbs:
American hellebore, *asafetida,* black cohosh, *burdock seed,* coca, *German camomile, queen of the meadow,* hops, *Indian poke, lady's slipper, lever-wood, lobelia,* motherwort, mullein, nettle, origanum, peppermint, *poplar bark, quaker button, skullcap,* sheep laurel, smilax, Solomon's seal, twin leaf, *valerian, wood betony.*

HYSTERIA

Symptoms:
A psychoneurotic disorder characterized by emotional excitability, extreme emotionalism involving motor and vasomotor, sensory and visceral functions. This is a condition that varies from mild excitement to laughing and crying with extreme nervous tension, accompanied by fits, convulsions, loss of sensibility and mania.

Cause:
Hysteria is considered to be due to mental causes, such as autosuggestion, dissociation or repressed emotion. This condition only occurs while a person is awake and is therefore a willed emotional release to obtain sympathy, to frighten, etc., if another person is involved. This type of person suffers much anxiety and fear.

Herbal aids:
For immediate relief, give a nervine tea such as an infusion of lady's slipper, skull-

cap, ginger, raspberry leaves, poplar bark, balmony, calumba root, cayenne, or antispasmodic herbs to relax the nerve tension. Add a little tincture of lobelia to the nervine as an antispasmodic. If it is impossible to administer these aids orally, the same tea in the form of an enema will ease the condition very quickly. Rest and cheerful surroundings are needed. The digestive system needs to be toned up properly.

Useful herbs:
Antispasmodic tincture, black cohosh, blue cohosh, catnip, *cayenne, celery seeds, linden flowers, mistletoe, motherwort, pennyroyal, peppermint, rue,* saffron, skullcap, skunk cabbage, *tansy, valerian, vervain.*

INDIGESTION

Symptoms:
Poor, incomplete or difficult digestion.

Cause:
Indigestion is poor assimilation or difficulty in processing the food correctly in order to get the proper value from it. The whole body must be toned up and the diet changed. The use of aluminum-based digestive tablets sold on the market give only temporary relief and aluminum poisoning is a side-effect. Eat proper foods and use the Lower Bowel Tonic which is prescribed in the cleansing program.

Herbal aids:
A good digestive tonic such as sarsaparillas or ginseng may be taken fifteen or twenty minutes before eating. Apple cider vinegar sweetened with honey may be taken before meals.

Useful herbs:
Agrimony, ammonia (gum), angelica, anise seed, balm, balmony, *barberry bark, bay leaves,* beech bitter root, *black root, black strap molasses, blessed thistle, blood root, buckbean, cascaras sagrada,* cascarilla bark, *cayenne, cherry bark,* chicory, cinnamon, *cloves, coltsfoot, couch grass, cow parsley, Culver's root, damiana, European centaury, fennel, garden balsam, gentian root, German camomile, ginger, ginseng,* gold thread, *golden seal,* ground ivy, *hops,* hyssop, knot grass, *juniper berries, lavender, linden flowers, lobelia,* madder root, *marjoram, melissa, nutmeg,* orange peel, *parsley seed, peppermint* (herb and oil), *Peruvian bark, quaker button, red root,* rhubarb, rosemary, sage, shavegrass, stone root, *tansy, thyme, Turkey rhubarb,* wahoo, *white poplar,* wild basil, *wild cherry bark,* wood betony, wormwood.

INFLAMMATION

Symptoms:
A local response to cellular injury or an affliction characterized by capillary constriction, then dilation, white corpuscle or leukocytic infiltration, redness, local heat and swelling from congestion, the exudation of noxious wastes in fluids, and the deposition of fibrin to replace the damaged tissue. Serum or white corpuscles are pushed and cause expansion or an elevation of the temperature which carries through the walls of the capillaries into the surrounding tissues or interstices.

Cause:
Inflammation is often caused by an abrasion of the clothing, bites of poisonous insects, bumping, shingles, welts, by an acid condition of the body affecting the nervous system, or from an internal acid condition of the urine or the orifice of the genital area.

Herbal aids:
This condition must be aided instead of inhibited. If the process is stopped it can be compared to putting the cork on the poison bottle. When inflammation is accompanied by blood poisoning use plantain to purge the poisons from the body. If inflammation is caused by a rheumatoid or arthritic condition, either burdock leaves or mullein in combination with lobelia will facilitate cleansing.

Useful herbs:
Chickweed, cayenne, fenugreek, flaxseed oil, golden seal, gum Arabic, hops, hyssop, lobelia, *marshmallow root,* mugwort, mullein, sarsaparillas, *slippery elm, smartweed, Solomon's seal, sorrel, tansy, white pond lily, witch hazel.*

JAUNDICE (Icterus, or hepatitis)

Symptoms:
A morbid affliction characterized by yellowness of the skin, eyes, mucus membranes, and urine, due to bile pigments in the blood and tissues. This is the result of the malfunction of hepatic cells which hold back the bile or obstruct the bile ducts, wherein the bile diffuses into the body fluids and impregnates the system and tissues.

Cause:
The problem arises due to improper diet resulting in a derangement of the function of stomach, liver, and bowels. The liver is the main seat of the problem. The bile does not excrete properly and is passed off into the blood stream and the body tissues, causing a toxic condition (called cholemia) causing indigestion, sluggishness, fatigue, constipation, upset stomach, chills, vomiting, and fever. The stools become a light clay or chalky color, the skin takes on a gold cast, yellow shows in the whites of the eyes, and bile deposits in the skin cause itching.

Herbal aids:
Carrot juice will bring the skin from clear to yellow (as the liver clears) and then back to normal, which is a sign that the bile is now cleared and flowing properly into the intestinal tract. Tonics for the liver are helpful, such as barberry, carrot juice, blueberry bark, cranesbill (crow foot) root, red raspberry root, and white oak bark. Proceed with caution since rapid unloading of toxic bile may upset the body and induce vomiting as well as turn the skin extremely yellow. Take golden seal and drink fruit juice to help cleanse. Other excellent herbs for this liver problem are agrimony, dandelion, mandrake root, self-heal and yarrow. Unsweetened fresh lemonade is good.

Useful herbs:
Agrimony, ale hoof, alkanet, ash leaves, balmony, *barberry, bayberry bark, betony, bistort, bitter root, black alder bark,* bittersweet, black strap molasses, *blessed thistle, blood root, boneset,* borage, broom, calamine, *camomile, cascaras sagrada,* celandine, *chicory,* cleavers, *columbine seeds,* couch grass, dandelion, *dwarf elder, elecampane, European vervain, fennel, fringetree bark, fumitory, gentian root, ginger,* golden seal, ground ivy, groundsel, *henna leaves, herb Robert, hollyhock,* hops, horehounds, hyssop, *madder root,* master of the wood, marjoram, *nettle leaves, origanum, parsley, peach tree* (leaves and pits), pennyroyal, Peruvian bark, pichi tops (fabiana), *plantain, poplar,* prickly ash, rue, *self-heal, sheep laurel, silverweed, sorrel, spearmint* (oil), St. John's wort, succory, *tansy, Turkey rhubarb, vervain,* wahoo, water plantain, *wild cherry bark,* wood betony, wormwood, yarrow.

KIDNEY TROUBLE

Symptoms:
An unhealthy, morbid condition of the kidneys.

Cause:
Kidney trouble is caused by a local infection.

Herbal aids:
The greatest aids for this problem are juniper berries, marshmallow root, parsley, and watermelon seeds.

Useful herbs:
Black birch leaves, black Indian hemp root, birch leaves, *broom tops, buchu leaves, button snake root, celery seed, cleavers,* corn silk, *couch grass root, cubeb berries, European goldenrod* (Solidago virgaurea), goldenrod (S. odora), *gravel plant, gravel root, Irish moss, juniper berries, kava kava root, lovage root, marshmallow root,* meadow sweet, *mountain cranberry* (berries and leaves), *mountain mahogany leaves, parsley herb and root, partridge berry, pichi tops* and *leaves* (fabiana), prince's feather leaves, *prince's pine,* purple foxglove leaves, shavegrass, squill root, *trailing arbutus, uva ursi leaves, wild cherry bark, whortleberry*

leaves.

LOW BLOOD PRESSURE

Symptoms:
Insufficient blood pressure for normal circulatory and nutritive activity.

Cause:
Low blood and high blood pressure are both due to malfunction of the circulatory system. High blood pressure in many cases works just like low blood pressure. Cholesterol must be eliminated from the system in order to get the blood flowing more freely. The condition is brought about by improper diet, insufficient rest and exercise and a lack of vitality within the system.

Herbal aids:
More oxygen is needed to correct this condition. Garlic is a good oxygen carrier. One of the greatest aids for low or high blood pressure due to oxygen starvation is deep breathing, which serves as a catalyst and helps the herbs react more rapidly. An immediate increase in circulation may be obtained by the use of cayenne and non mucus-forming foods. Grape juice as well as other juices rebuild and give endurance to the system.

Useful herbs:
Blue cohosh, burnet, *cayenne, gentian, golden seal,* hyssop, *prickly ash,* red pepper, *sassafras, skullcap, vervain,* wood betony.

LUMBAGO

Symptoms:
A backache or rheumatic pain in the loins or lower back (the lumbar of the lumbosacral regions) with extreme pain and tenderness.

Cause:
Lumbago is an inflammation of the lumbar muscles and is considered by many to be rheumatism of the lumbar muscles.

Herbal aids:
Lumbago is one of the most painful conditions. The use of vapor baths and the cold sheet treatment will bring relief. A massage with a tincture of cayenne and prickly ash liniment with antispasmodic tincture will work very well. The eliminative functions should be corrected, especially the bowels which need to be cleaned during attacks. Garlic and lobelia enemas work well.

Useful herbs:
Black cohosh, burdock root, chaparral (creosote), gravel root, shepherd's purse,

uva ursi, vervain.

MEASLES

Symptoms:
This is mainly a child's disease, although adults may contract it. It is an infectious febrile affliction, characterized by round red eruptions on the skin, and catarrhal inflammation of the mucous membrane passages. It begins after two weeks incubation with the common cold (coryza), cough, inflammation of the conjunctive (referred to as conjunctivitis), and the appearance of small red spots surrounded by white areas. On the third or fourth day of chills and fever, dark rose-red maculopapular eruptions appear (concentric and confluent groups) on the face or behind the ears. In three or four days the eruption fades, and the skin sheds or peels (including the mucous membranes). Measles begin with sneezing and dry coughing, redness of the eyes and sensitivity to light. The red rash appears on the fourth day. The fever subsides on the sixth day, and peeling continues until the ninth to eleventh days.

Cause:
Measles is evidence that the body is loaded with toxic poison and is trying to expel it with the assistance of nature. Microorganisms are brought into activity by nature as the cleansing scavengers.

Herbal aids:
This disease must be brought to the surface through the skin as rapidly as possible. Diaphoretic herbs such as yarrow and raspberry leaf are excellent. Use vapor baths (such as ginger, mustard and cayenne) which quickly bring the toxic wastes to a head. Moisture is required or the organic calcium will turn into inorganic calcium because of the feverish dry body heat, which causes further tissue damage. Rheumatic fever is often the aftermath of diseases such as chicken pox and measles. Take care of the bronchi and the eyes. Avoid bright light, since the eyes are weak at this time. The bowels should be kept open with the lower bowel tonic. A catnip enema is soothing and beneficial. Ripe fruits will assist in the cleansing process.

Useful herbs:
Alkanet, bistort root, *camomile, catnip, cleavers,* ginger, *lady's slipper,* licorice, linden flowers, lovage, *peppermint, pleurisy root, raspberry leaves,* red sage, saffron, *sage,* tormentil, *valerian,* vervain, yarrow.

MUCUS

Symptoms:
A viscid, slippery secretion is produced by the mucous membranes which moistens and protects their surfaces. This consists of water, mucin, inorganic salts,

epithelial cells, and leukocytes, etc., held in suspension.

Cause:
Mucus must not be confused with the mucous membrane, the latter being part of the body. Mucus accumulates excessively on top of the membrane. This mucoid filth is caused by improper diet.

Herbal aids:
Apple cider vinegar and honey are highly recommended. Tomato juice, onion and garlic will cut mucus rapidly. Many anti-catarrhal herbs are available which will do the job.

Useful herbs:
*Bayberry, **bistort,*** bitter root, coltsfoot, cranesbill root, fire weed, golden seal, gum Arabic, hyssop, *red raspberry, white pond lily, yarrow.*

NAUSEA

Symptoms:
Any feeling of discomfort in the stomach region, with aversion to food and a tendency to vomit.

Cause:
The problem has a number of origins, such as bilious attacks, pregnancy, undigested food, etc.

Herbal aids:
With some people, the discomfort can be cleared up quickly by chewing hard, common cloves. With others, it takes something a little more potent such as catnip, peach leaves, peppermint, raspberry leaves, spearmint or sweet balm. A few drops of tincture of lobelia or antispasmodic tincture is very good. A combination of cinnamon, cloves, spearmint, and Turkey rhubarb will bring good results when used as prescribed later in the book.

Useful herbs:
Anise seed, cinnamon bark, cloves, European avens, giant Solomon seal, *ginger, golden seal* (pregnancy and other), *lavender, mint, origanum, peach leaves, pennyroyal* (not for pregnancy), *peppermint, raspberry leaves, spearmint, sweet balm,* whortleberry, *wild yam.*

NEURALGIA

Symptoms:
A severe, intermittent pain lasting a short time. The pain radiates along the course of a nerve and its branches, but is not associated with any manifest changes in the nerve structure. The tender spots are often where the nerves exit and paroxysm

can be produced by contact with a certain area (the trigger zones). Often there are sharp, stabbing attacks of pain in the eye, brow, temples, or back of the neck. There are also various forms of neuralgia along the spinal column, and the various internal organs (viscera), along the sciatica nerve, or in a joint.

Cause:
Neuralgia is caused by irritation of the nervous system and by heavy mucus throughout the body. An acid condition is also a factor.

Herbal aids:
The sharp, excruciating pains can generally be relieved by placing a poultice or fomentation of mullein and cayenne over the area. Relief may also be obtained by applying a liniment of equal parts cayenne and prickly ash tincture. To remove the cause, rebuild the body with tonics, change the diet and improve the person's general health.

Useful herbs:
Same as for neuritis.

NEURITIS

Symptoms:
Injury or lesions of one or more nerves accompanied with hypersensitivity, loss of sensation (anesthesia), sensation of tingling, crawling or burning of the skin (paresthesia), paralysis, reduction in muscle size (muscular atrophy), and loss of reflexes in a body part.

Cause:
Mucus in the system. Mucus causes an upset in a specific area conducting nerves into the spinal column and throws out a vertebrae which causes even more irritation. The nerves and the worn sheath around the nerves must be rebuilt, and the acid condition of the nerves removed by taking nervines. Besides using the cleansing program, rebuild the entire nervous system.

Herbal aids:
Neuritis is frightening because of the pain. Use nervines and antispasmodic to correct the cause. Ease the pain with fomentation, poultices and the green drinks.

Useful herbs:
Apple cider vinegar fomentations (hot), *black cohosh, burdock root* and seed, *celery juice* and *celery seed tea, comfrey drink, hops, lady's slipper, lobelia, mistletoe, Peruvian bark, skullcap, valerian, wood betony.*

PALPITATION

Symptoms:
An abnormal and rapid fluttering, pulsation, or beating of the heart.

Cause:
Weak heart valves having poor tone may be the cause. Fever and excitement from panic can add to the problem. The fluttering of the heart is due to weakness within the entire body system, but more specifically in the heart area. High cholesterol and dense mucoid stoppage can cause sluggishness of the blood flow.

Herbal aids:
Take cayenne, wheat germ oil, and hawthorn berry tonic. Motherwort is another specific

Useful herbs:
Angelica, arnica, asafetida, balm leaves, balsam of Tolu, black cohosh, black haw, blue cohosh, borage, buckthorn root, burnet cahinca, *cayenne, cherry laurel,* cleavers, cuckold, gentian, greater pimpernel root, gum of guaiacum, *gum of hemlock, hawthorn, kola* (heart failure), lavender, *lily of the valley,* meadow anemone, meadow saffron, *Mexican fever plant, motherwort,* oil of hemlock, *oil of wintergreen, pheasant's eye* (valves), pink root, *rue, silverweed spurge* (hard breathing), swamp beggars tick, *tree of heaven.*

PARALYSIS

Symptoms:
A rapid, complete or partial loss of muscle function and motion or merely a loss of sensation because of nerve injury or neuron destruction. A slight loss of function is called "palsy."

Cause:
Most cases of paralysis are caused by calcium deficiency. Paralysis is generally classified as incurable but no disease is incurable. The problem is due to toxic wastes in the body and it becomes essential to cleanse the body and give it tone and a positive regeneration in order to correct the paralysis.

Herbal aids:
Paralysis can be cleared with cayenne alone. Correct the cause with a cleansing program and the regenerative diet. Use nerve tonics and antispasmodic.

Useful herbs:
Black cohosh, catnip, cayenne, dandelion root, ginger, golden seal, Hydrangea, *lady's slipper, poke root* (bowels), *poplar bark, prickly ash berries, red clover,* red pepper, *rosemary, skullcap, valerian root, vervain, wild cherry bark, yellow dock.*

Paralysis of throat: As an aid, chew ginger root often.

PERITONITIS

Symptoms:
Inflammation of the peritoneum, or the smooth, transparent, serious membrane lining the interior of the abdominal cavity and surrounding the digestive organs and other internal organs (viscera) such as the heart, liver, intestines, etc.

Cause:
This is another mucus-derived problem.

Herbal aids:
Use lobelia in either tea or tincture form. Also use garlic (enema, tea, or tincture) and a diet of liquids and juices. Castor oil fomentation over the abdominal area will give relief.

Useful herbs:
Apple cider vinegar and honey, garlic, onion, blood purifiers of a powerful nature (chaparral, Brigham tea, burdock root and seed in equal parts, sassafras), the lower bowel tonic, lobelia.

PLEURISY (Pleuritis)

Symptoms:
Inflammation of the pleura (membrane covering the lungs), usually accompanied by fever, painful and difficult respiration, cough, and mucoid exudation into the pleural cavity.

Cause:
The cause of pleurisy is mucus forming in a weak area caused by the failure to breath deeply. It is common where there is general debility of the body, especially in the lung area.

Herbal aids:
Use of pleurisy root (a specific), slippery elm, comfrey root, hyssop, and vervain.

Useful herbs:
Agrimony, angelica, boneset, borage, buckthorn bark, bugloss, *caraway* (oil of), *calamus, cayenne, chickweed,* colocynth, coral, *cough grass, crawler, dandelion, elder,* European bitter polygala, flaxseed, gamboge, *gum Arabic,* heart's ease, *Indian hemp, lady's slipper, lobelia,* maidenhair, mandrake root, marshmallow, mullein, nettle, pleurisy root, skullcap, skunk cabbage, slippery elm, sour dock, strawberry leaves, succory, *valerian, yarrow.*

QUINSY

Symptoms:
A severe acute inflammation of the tonsil and peritonsillar tissue with swelling, fever, and generation of pus (peritonsillar abscess) accompanied by chills, fever, painful swallowing, swollen throat and tongue, and dry mouth. It may induce panic if the tightening in the throat area makes breathing difficult.

Cause:
The cause is frequent sinus drainage with mucus coming down the eustachian tubes and causing irritation. The basic cause is a dirty transverse colon, which causes poison in the sinus and head areas and then drains down into the throat.

Herbal aids:
Use an antispasmodic (such as lobelia) both internally and externally (wrapping the throat with a soaked fomentation). This can also be aided quickly by the use of a bayberry gargle (drinking several tablespoons every hour or so) or using mullein (three parts) and lobelia (one part). This should draw off the toxic poison into the blood stream and disperse it quickly. Use a hot water bottle and either a poultice or a fomentation.

Useful herbs:
Agrimony, black currant, blood root, cayenne, house leek juice, clary, cudweed, Culver's root, *glycerine, guaiac tincture, hyssop, Jews ear, ipecac, lovage, mandrake root, marshmallow, old field balsam,* quince, quinsywort, ragwort, *raspberry leaves, red sage, sage, sanicle, slippery elm bark,* violet, *walnut, wormwood.*

RHEUMATISM

Symptoms:
Afflictions of muscle tendon, joint, bone or nerve, resulting in discomfort and disability due to stiffness of the joints or muscles, pain on motion, etc. In this category, often included are rheumatoid arthritis, degenerative joint diseases, spondylitis, bursitis, fibrositis, myositis, neuritis, lumbago, sciatica, and gout.

Cause:
Poor elimination causes rheumatism due to toxic matter becoming stagnated in various parts of the body. Thomas Deschauer explains:

> Urea should be daily expelled from our body, an ounce every day. Urea, as you might know, is completely changed waste matter, and as such easily expelled. Now if the process of turning the dead tissues into urea is incomplete—it forms uric acid. Certain foods and drinks cause the urea to be left unfinished. Or if the urea is hindered or stopped to be expelled, it also returns into the system and forms uric acid. This can

be done by stopping perspiration, by cooling off quickly, by neglect of proper bathing, changing of underclothing, inhaling urea at night while sleeping in ill-ventilated room, etc. Avoid all these things if you want to get well. Some persons have what is known as the uric acid habit, that is, the waste matter does not break down completely. This tendency is due to an extremely abnormal and diseased condition of the blood.

Herbal aids:
Rheumatism can be relieved rapidly by a cleansing program and by the use of burdock root tea, with the burdock root and leaf fomentation (on the painful areas). Use apple cider vinegar and honey to cut the toxic wastes loose and expel them from the body. Use MCP pectin (1 teaspoon three times a day) in water (it tastes like weak lemonade), or chaparral tea (three times a day, a teaspoon to the cup). The bowels and urethral tract should be kept open. A stimulant diuretic for the kidneys will aid in waste elimination and a diaphoretic should be used to assist in eliminating through the skin.

Useful herbs:
Angelica, *ash,* balm of Gilead, *balsam of Tolu, belladonna, birch, bitter root, bittersweet twigs, black alder bark, black cohosh root, black willow bark, blessed thistle,* blue cohosh, blue flag, blood root, boneset, buchu, buckbean (herb), buckthorn bark, burdock root, candy tuft, *cayenne, celery, centaury, colchicum seed,* calumba, coltsfoot, *Culver's root,* dogwood bark, elder flowers and *berries,* European avens, germander, *glycerine, gravel root, guaiac wood* and *gum, gum Arabic* (mucilage), *gravel root, Hydrangea, hyssop* (muscular), *Indian hemp,* Indian physic, *Irish moss, kava kava root, lobelia, melissa, mezereon bark, mother of thyme, mugwort, mullein, mustard, myrrh, nettle, Oregon grape root,* origanum, pareira brava, *peppermint,* pipsissewa, *pleurisy root, poke root* and *berries, poplar, prickly ash bark, quassia, rest harrow, rheumatism weed herb, rosemary, sarsaparillas,* skullcap, silverweed root, skunk cabbage, snow berry, soapwort, spikenard bark, sumac berries, swamp hellebore, toothache bark, *tormentil, Turkey rhubarb, twin leaf root, Virginia snake root, wahoo* (bark of root), wake robin, watercress, white ash bark, *white pine,* wild blackberry roots, *wild cherry bark, wild yam,* willow, wintergreen, wood betony, *wormwood, yellow dock root,* yellow parilla, yellow poplar bark.

RHEUMATOID

Symptoms:
A chronic arthritis affecting multiple joints and resulting in debility, weakness and loss of weight. There is painful limitation of motion, often with deformity, and sometimes a complete fusion of a joint (bony ankylosis). Rheumatism, arthritis and gout are very similar, although the basic cause may be the same.

Cause:
Improper diet consisting of unwholesome, denatured, and processed foods.

Herbal aids:
Taper off of the "secondary" and inorganic-type foods such as eggs, starches and carbohydrates. Eat the regenerative organic foods as much as possible. Chaparral (creosote bush) is one of the best herbal remedies. Another fine remedy which is excellent internally as a decoction and externally as a liniment is the following combination of herbs: black cohosh, cayenne, lobelia, mullein and prickly ash. The daily use of apple cider vinegar and honey will do wonders. There are many aids for the rheumatic-type problems such as arthritis, neuritis, sciatica, neuralgia, etc., and more formulas are given in the sections of the individual herbs.

Useful herbs:
Same as "gout" and "arthritis." See "rheumatism."

SCIATICA

Symptoms:
Neuralgic pain along the course of the sciatica nerve which runs down the back of the thigh. It is supposed to be due to inflammation or injury to the nerve, resulting in pain, numbness, tingling and tenderness along the course of the nerve, and eventual wasting away of the muscles that are enervated by the malady. With inflammation of the sciatica nerve, there is extreme pain around the hip region and in the lumbar muscles.

Cause:
Crippling pain of the lower extremities has long been blamed on the sciatica nerve, but actually it is not a nerve problem at all. It is due to toxic poison from the sigmoid section of the bowel, the area going from the descending colon over to the rectal area. This important small section of the intestines is subject to kinks or pockets which cause toxic poisons in the area and in the leg area, which in turn irritate the sciatica nerve, dislocating the sacroiliac. When the affected part of the bowel is cleaned out with the lower bowel tonic and cleansing program, the poisons no longer affect the nerve area.

Herbal aids:
The best remedy is to empty the bowel and cleanse the sigmoid, then give organic aid as fast as possible. The greatest herb for this problem is chaparral supplemented by burdock root tea. Sassafras and Brigham tea may also be added. This combination makes a delicious drink when sweetened with honey. Do not drink it with chaparral (creosote bush) tea. Bathing the feet in hot apple-cider vinegar will help, and if you wish faster action, place the right foot into a pan of chopped garlic (with the bare foot on the garlic), and the left foot in hot apple-cider vinegar. This will start a circulatory movement which will give quick relief. The internal use of apple-cider vinegar and honey (a tablespoonful of each, three times a day), or MCP pectin (a teaspoonful three times a day) will speed the cleansing. For external fomentation or poultices, use burdock root or crushed burdock leaves, with one-fourth part lobelia added, or a hot apple-cider vinegar fomentation.

Useful herbs:
Apple-cider vinegar, chaparral, MCP pectin, broom, *burdock,* rue, sassafras, tansy, wintergreen.

SCROFULA

Symptoms:
Tuberculosis of the cervical lymph nodes, particularly with enlargement and cheesy degeneration of the lymphatic glands of the neck.

Cause:
Scrofula is caused from mucus accumulating into large lumps in specific areas of the lymphatic glands. This is basically a diet problem. The mucusless diet will decrease the mucus in the area. Poultices and cleansing will complete the process.

Herbal aids:
Use three parts mullein and one part lobelia as a fomentation or poultice over the area to reduce swelling. The entire blood stream must be purified and the whole body cleansed to affect a cure.

Useful herbs:
Abscess root, adders tongue, *adders violet, agrimony,* American ivy bark, American sarsaparillas, *bayberry bark, bearsfoot, bittersweet bark, black walnut,* bladderwrack, blood root, *blue flag,* blue vervain, *burdock root,* button snake root, *camomile, coltsfoot, comfrey root,* dandelion root, echinacea, elder flowers, fig-wort, frost wort, gentian, guaiac, *Irish moss,* iron weed, *juniper berries, lavender, lever-wood, quince seed* and *fruit, red clover,* rock rose, *rosemary, wild sage,* sassafras, soapwort, stillingia, sumac, sweet gum, tag alder, turkey corn, *valerian, wormwood,* yellow dock, yellow parilla.

SHOCK

Symptoms:
A state of profound depression of the vital processes due to various causes from emotional trauma to injury which reduces the blood pressure and venous return, thus impairing circulation which may cause irreversible circulatory failure and eventually death.

Cause:
Bad news or an automobile accident will bring on shock sufficient to weaken the body and bring on the problem. With perfect body function, a shock would not have this effect. It could cause a disquieting moment, but the body system would not undergo the extreme shock. The shock is greater when the person is not well.

Herbal aids:
When a person goes into shock, the administration of medicinal aids orally will

often be difficult or impossible. In this case an anus injection (or enema) which will cause relaxation is applicable. Use one cup (to a pint maximum) of catnip, peppermint, skullcap, spearmint, or valerian. Massage the abdomen and parts of the spine with lobelia externally and make sure that the patient gets undisturbed rest. Cayenne should be taken internally to equalize the blood pressure and insure that the internal functions will remain stabilized during the intense systemic distress.

Useful herbs:
Catnip, cayenne, hops, lady's slipper, lobelia, mistletoe, peppermint, skullcap, spearmint, valerian.

SORE

Symptoms:
A place where the skin and flesh are ruptured or bruised and are therefore tender and painful, such as an ulcer, boil, wound, etc.

Cause:
Sores can be caused from problems internal or external, from abrasion, from running into an object, irritation of shoes on the foot. The hands can become sore from a specific type of tool or some excessive use of a piece of equipment. Internal sores can come from pimples that have been picked, from boils or from an acid condition of the body. There are many possible causes which can be aggravated by poor diet.

Herbal aids:
Most skin sores can be aided by the use of comfrey. Use three parts comfrey with one part lobelia to relieve pain and restore the skin. For ulcers, boils or wounds, see the index.

Useful herbs:
Aloes, *bayberry bark, bistort root, bittersweet, blood root, blue violet,* borage, *burdock root, calamus, camomile, elecampane root, elder leaves, flaxseed, golden seal,* hemlock, masterwort, mullein, *myrrh, peach,* pimpernel, *plantain, poke root,* poplar, *prickly ash, sage, sanicle, self-heal, skunk cabbage,* Solomon's seal, St. John's wort, sumac berries, valerian, vervain, virgin's bower, *walnut husks* (green), *white clover, witch hazel,* wood sage, *yellow dock.*

SPASMS

Symptoms:
A sudden, involuntary, and unnatural muscular contraction.

Cause:
Spasms may arise from calcium deficiency, panic, fear or overeating.

Herbal aids:
If the spasm is in a muscle and easy to reach, a good nervine (especially wormwood oil) as a liniment massaged into the problem area will give quick relief. For internal spasms (such as in the stomach area) give a few drops of lobelia tincture each half hour.

Useful herbs:
Antispasmodic tincture, Bethroot, block cohosh root, black hawk bark, blue cohosh, Brigham tea, *camomile flowers,* cassia bark, *catnip, cayenne,* cedron, *cramp bark,* dragon turnip root, *female regulator herb, fennel, fit root, horse nettle berries, lady's slipper root,* linden flowers, *lobelia,* peony root, *pomegranate bark, quaking aspen bark, red clover, red root, rosemary leaves,* rue, *sassafras, skullcap, skunk cabbage,* spearmint, *squaw bush root,* squaw mint herb, *squaw root, twin leaf, valerian, water mint herb, wild yam root.*

STROKE

Symptoms:
A sudden, severe seizure or attack often termed apoplexy. Apoplexy is generally accompanied by a stroke. A stroke does not necessarily mean apoplexy because a stroke can come without heat prostration which occurs in apoplexy.

Cause:
A calcium deficiency in the body, where the organic calcium has been burned out by a former fever or by an inheritance to an inorganic calcium, which is devoid of life and does not sustain the muscle, nerve, and bone structure. This causes weakness and inability to use the organ involved.

Herbal aids:
Cayenne should be used generously. Cayenne is known to have relieved paralyzed condition of strokes, even though the person has been in a wheelchair for years. Through the use of cayenne and the cleansing herbs many have been able to walk again.

Useful herbs:
Brigham tea, burdock root and *seed, cayenne, chaparral, comfrey* (green drink) *fomentation* or *poultice, ginger* (bath or tea, especially for throat), *sassafras.*

TUMOR

Symptoms:
A swelling. An abnormal formation of parasitic, non-inflammatory cells or tissue arising from the cells of the host, yet progressive and independent in their growth. Tumors can be malignant or non-malignant; they can be fast-growing or slow-growing, and they can be in many parts of the body, such as the lymphatic glands or nodes, the urinary and genital areas, or the abdominal structure.

Cause:
The inability to eliminate unhealthy material.

Herbal aids:
Rebuild tissue so the body can slough off the tumor accumulation. This is done by toning the body generally with alteratives.

Useful herbs:
Bayberry, blue flag, blue violet, *burdock root,* celandine, *chickweed, coltsfoot, coral, elder flowers, flaxseed,* hops, *Irish moss,* marigold flowers, mullein, mugwort, myrtle, *red foot,* rock rose, *sage, sanicle, tansy, skunk cabbage, slippery elm,* sorrel, *St. John's wort, walnut leaves and husks* (green), white pond lily, *wild yam,* witch hazel, wood sage, *yellow dock.*

TYPHOID FEVER

Symptoms:
An infectious affliction characterized by an enlargement of the spleen and the mesenteric lymph nodes and catarrhal inflammation of the intestinal mucous membrane. After two or three weeks incubation, there is weakness, headache, vague pains, tendency to diarrhea and nosebleed, and pronounced stupor. The stools have a peculiar pea-soup color. At times there is constipation, and usually there is slight congestion of the lung accompanied by a cough. On the seventh to ninth day, peculiar eruptions of small, slightly elevated, rose-colored spots appear on the chest and abdomen. Frequently there is a complication of intestinal hemorrhoids, peritonitis, pneumonia, nephritis and perforation of the bowel.

Cause:
The basic cause is contagious cleansing-organisms that are introduced through contaminated foods.

Herbal aids:
With fevers, use moist heat to facilitate the cleansing and eliminate the toxic backlog in the system. Induce profuse perspiration by the use of hot yarrow or raspberry leaf tea and by soaking in a tub of hot water with up to a pound of ginger, and a teaspoon each of mustard and cayenne. Follow with the cold sheet treatment.

Useful herbs:
Bitter root, blood root, *camomile, cranesbill root, golden seal, mimosa gum, myrrh, Peruvian bark, pleurisy root, quince seed and fruit, red raspberry leaves,* red sage, *white oak bark, wild cherry bark, yarrow.*

ULCER

Symptoms:
An interrupted surface or superficial sore having an inflamed base which discharges pus. It is distinguished from abscess, which is a localized collection of pus in any part of the body, and has its origin deep in the tissues.

Cause:
An ulcer is a large accumulation of dead cells that have decayed and formed pus.

Herbal aids:
An ulcer is similar to a tumor. It is an accumulation of foreign material in the body, but with an ulcer, a drawing agent must be used. Use a poultice of powdered slippery elm or mullein (three parts) and lobelia (one part), or wild sage. Cayenne will speed the process.

Useful herbs:
Agrimony, angelica, bayberry bark, beech, bistort root, bittersweet, *blue violet, bog bean, borage, bugleweed, burdock root, calamus, carrot* (poultice), *cayenne,* celandine, *chickweed, comfrey root, cranesbill root, elder flowers* and *leaves,* fenugreek, *garlic, golden seal,* gold thread, mullein, myrrh, pennyroyal, pilewort, *poke root,* poplar, prickly ash, psyllium, *quince seed and fruit, ragwort, raspberry leaves,* rock rose, *sage,* sanicle, shavegrass (urinary), *slippery elm, sorrel, St. John's wort,* twin leaf, *valerian,* virgin's bower, *water* pepper, *white clover, white pond lily, wintergreen,* wood *sage, wood sanicle, yarrow.*

VOMITING (Or emesis)

Symptoms:
The forcible ejection or spewing of the stomach contents through the mouth.

Cause:
This may be either a voluntary body activity or it may be induced when it is necessary to cleanse the stomach of undigested food poison, and excess body waste. Enemas, fasting, the use of the lower bowel tonic, or mild herbal laxatives, will cleanse the stomach. The nerve action of fear or panic sometimes induces vomiting.

Herbal aids:
Use some type of herb to calm the stomach area. This may be done simply by taking teas of peach, peppermint, or raspberry leaves, or by simply chewing cloves. For the more difficult advanced cases, turkey rhubarb will do a thorough job.

Useful herbs:
Adder's tongue, angostura, *antispasmodic tincture,* camphor water, *catnip,* cinnamon bark, *clover, cloves,* calumba, European avens, gentian root, knot grass,

lobelia, oil of walnut, origanum, *peach leaves, peppermint, mullein, mustard* (poultice), *raspberry leaves,* spearmint, *sweet almond,* sweet balm, *sweet basil, white poplar bark,* white swallow wort, *whortleberry.*

WHEEZING

Symptoms:
A lightly audible sibilant, whistling or sighing sound produced in labored breathing, signaling an obstruction of air passages due to a spasm, edema, inflammation, a foreign body, tumor, or external pressure.

Cause:
When there is wheezing, there could be serious trouble in the body which signals a need for immediate cleansing.

Herbal aids:
Lobelia and nervines are generally used most effectively. Whenever there is heavy congestion in the lungs or bronchi, use chickweed, lobelia, or mullein.

Useful herbs:
Antispasmodics, apple cider vinegar and *honey, black walnut, catnip, chickweed, comfrey* (preferably fresh, chewed or used as a vegetable), *lobelia, marshmallow, mullein,* etc.

WHOOPING COUGH

Symptoms:
An infectious catarrhal inflammation of the air passage with violent convulsive coughs (paroxysms), consisting of several expirations followed by a loud, sonorous whooping inspiration. This is generally a children's disease and begins with spasmodic coughing spells. The face reddens, and the eyes bulge. Sore throat, and often vomiting may occur. Advanced cases develop into bronchopneumonia.

Cause:
Whooping cough is a rapid accumulation of mucus in the throat, which causes choking and will cause death if not cleared. Eliminate the mucus as fast as possible.

Herbal aids:
Lobelia herb or tincture used in fomentation, as well as a few drops internally every few minutes works well. To cut the phlegm, use a bayberry tea as a gargle (swallow after gargling). Use crushed garlic with cayenne and honey every few minutes to help clear the throat.

Useful herbs:
Anemone, *antispasmodic tincture, black cohosh,* blood root, blue cohosh, *blue violet, boneset,* chestnut (American), coltsfoot, cubeb berries, daisy, *elecampane root, flaxseed, garlic, lobelia, mistletoe, onion, peach leaves,* poets narcissus, *poke root, red clover, red raspberry, red root,* saw palmetto berries, *skunk cabbage, slippery elm, thyme, tormentil root,* trumpet moss, *vervain,* wake robin, *wild cherry bark.*

WOUND

Symptoms:
A cut or breach of the skin or other membrane (internal or external), either by violence or surgery.

Cause:
Wounds are caused in many ways, such as battle, falling, tears, etc.

Herbal aids:
The best herb is comfrey (which is also called "knit bone"), or you may use all-heal, chickweed, golden seal, or mullein without recourse to the orthodox method of need-le and stitches. Walnut combinations assist in healing, but comfrey is probably the most effective because it possesses a powerful cell proliferative.

Useful herbs:
Aloes, arnica flowers, balm of Gilead buds, bayberry bark, beech, bistort root, bladderwrack, *burdock root, calendula flowers, camomile, carrot* (poultice), *chickweed, comfrey root, cranesbill root,* echinacea, *elder leaves,* fenugreek, *figwort herb, garlic* (oil), *golden seal, Irish moss, marigold flowers, marshmallow root, marsh rosemary root, mullein leaves, myrrh,* pilewort, pimpernel, *plantain leaves, poke root,* poplar, prickly ash, *red oak bark, rosemary leaves,* sage, *self-heal, slippery elm,* Solomon's seal, *St. John's wort, sweet clover, tormentil root, walnut husks* (green), *white oak bark, white pond lily, wild sage leaves, witch hazel leaves,* wood sage, *wood sanicle, yarrow.*

YELLOW FEVER

Symptoms:
An acute, infectious, often fatal, febrile affliction of the tropical and sub-tropical regions of America, characterized by jaundice, hemorrhages, vomiting, etc. The affliction begins with a chill and pain in the head, sudden onset of fever (103-105° F.), vomiting, constipation, scanty and albuminous urine. A period of diminution (remission) occurs, another fever attack, jaundice develops, and the vomit becomes darkened from the presence of blood. The disease is often fatal, occurring in the typhoid state or from uremia.

Cause:
A thick and sluggish blood stream. Mucus clogs the body to the point that a fever takes over without which the body cannot clear itself. Yellow fever or other forms of fever do not occur when the body is in a healthy condition. The clogged condition is triggered by an organism carried by a mosquito.

Herbal aids:
Work the fever out through the skin by the use of diaphoretics, vapor baths, heat baths and cold sheeting and change the diet.

Useful herbs:
The same herbs previously mentioned with other fever conditions such as colds, flu or pneumonia may be used.

CHAPTER 2

THE ALTERATIVE HERBS

Among the alteratives there are upwards of 100 specialized plants which clean the blood and the eliminative tissues and organs. Being skilled in using alteratives will greatly help you in helping people heal from disease. Dr. Nowell wrote:

> Alteratives, or, as they are sometimes called, Antiscorbutics, are remedies which gradually alter and correct impure conditions of the blood. It is because of this that many of these agents are commonly called "Blood Purifiers" or "Blood Sweeteners."
>
> They alter the character of the blood stream because of being possessed of certain properties which the Vital Force can use in stimulating or strengthening the organs of nutrition and secretion, building up so that waste material may be carried and a supply of helpful pabulum may be provided for the organism.

Blood impurities occur because of the improper functioning of one or more organs—most frequently the secretory organs—which fail to carry out impurities of the blood. Toxicity may also come from improper food or impure air. As you work to clean the blood, also find out the cause of the disease in order to cure that as well.

Many herbs may be classed as alteratives, as they promote the elimination of impurities. Some herbs work fast on a given organ to relieve engorgement, but such an agent should scarcely be called an alterative. The true alterative slowly but surely cleans and purifies the bloodstream and, at the same time, steadily tones up the organ or organs which may not be able to secrete impurities from the blood.

The liver, kidneys, and skin are the chief organs for carrying off impurities and waste matter. If the liver is torpid and bile retained in the system, we may find in one case the retained bile has affected the digestion, and in another case, caused a skin eruption. An acne type skin eruption is one of the first signs of failure to maintain an open avenue of elimination through the liver and bowels. If the kidneys fail to secrete as they should or are not furnished with the proper amount of clean water, the bloodstream can remain toxic. The skin may not be eliminating well, or the lungs may be unable to oxygenize the blood due to impure air being breathed.

So you can see that you need to know what organ is involved when prescribing alteratives. In addition, you need to know the specific qualities of each herb. For example, there are stimulating and toning alteratives and there are relaxing alteratives. Food, air, emotional stress, and other essential factors must be improved in addition to using herbs, or the bloodstream may remain toxic.

PLANTAIN or RIBWORT
(Plantago major; P. lanceolata; PLANTAGINACEAE)

***Common names*:**
Plantain, ribwort, waybread, ripple grass, broad-leaved plantain, ribbed grass, snakeweed, white manfoot, Englishman's foot, cuckoo's bread, common plantain, lance-leaf plantain; Plantain lanceole (Fr.) Spitzwegeric (Ger.); Llanten (Span.). The broad-leaf plantain is Plantago major and the lance-leaf is Plantago lanceolata, which are treated in this text as medicinal equivalents.

Identifying characteristics:

Stem Stiff, channeled, smooth, six to eighteen inches high.

Leaves Broad-leaf: Ovate, blunt, abruptly contracted at the base long and channeled petiole, blade is four to eight inches long, three to four inches broad, five to eleven strong fibrous ribs, entire or coarse and unequally dentate-serrate margins, dark green.
Lance-leaf: Lanceolate, sharp-pointed, on long and tough stems, strongly ribbed length-wise, dark green.

Flower Broad-leaf: Inflorescence or dense spike of four-parted flowers, purplish-brown, about five inches long.
Lance-leaf: Short head, studded with tiny, dull-white, four-parted flowers, long, slender stamens.

Fruit Cells containing two to four seeds (in the spike).

Taste Mildly astringent.

Odor None.

Part used:
Root, leaves, flower spikes, seeds.

Therapeutic action:
Cooling alterative, depurant, diuretic, emollient, mildly astringent, refrigerant, deobstruent, antiseptic, vulnerary, antivenomous, styptic, antisyphilitic, anthelmintic (vermicide).

Both the roots and leaves have moderately diffuse and stimulating alterative effects for the circulatory system. They also assist the glandular system, healing the lymph and epidermal areas in scrofulous and skin diseases. Plantain is an excellent remedy for kidney and bladder troubles. It is an effective remedy for poisonous bites and stings, since the poison of fresh stings is extracted rapidly, often within an hour's time.

It is the best herb for blood poisoning: reducing the swelling and completely healing a limb where poisoning has made amputation imminent. Finally, it is very useful for easing pain and healing problems in the lower intestinal tract. This valuable "weed" is often found in soils close to most habitations, in parks, sports fields, etc.

Medicinal uses:
Poisonous bites and stings, boils, carbuncles, tumors, inflammation, scrofula, eczema, frog or thrush, blood poisoning, malignant and bleeding ulcers, bleeding of minor wounds, diarrhea, piles, cuts and scratches, erysipelas, burns, scalds, leucorrhea, lumbago, bed-wetting, syphilis, dropsy, toothache, worms, running sores, itch, ringworm, mastitis, poison ivy, bruises.

Preparations:
Fluid extract, infusion, powder, tincture. Glycerine may be used as a preservative.

Dosage:

Fluid extract	1/2-1 teaspoon
Infusion	2 fluid ounces 3 to 4 times daily
Powder	1-3 grams
Tincture	1/2-1 fluid teaspoon

ADMINISTRATION

Anal

Diarrhea, hemorrhoids, piles: Use a strong tea (steep one ounce of the granulated herb for twenty to thirty minutes in one pint boiled hot water), let cool, inject one tablespoonful three of four times daily (or more frequently in bad cases), and especially after each bowel movement.

Piles (ointment): Make an ointment by simmering two ounces of the granulated or powdered herb (double this for fresh) in one pint of oil (olive, soybean, safflower, peanut), add beeswax to thicken, apply on soft cotton or gauze and use a band or belt to hold it in place.

Oral

Blood poisoning: Use internally and externally (see "skin").

Diarrhea, kidney and bladder trouble, lumbago, scanty urine, bed-wetting: Drink one teacupful of the tea four to five times daily until relieved.

Dropsy: Drink the tea from the seeds.

Scrofula, syphilis: Use as a tea and an external application.

Thrush or frog: Make a decoction, simmering one ounce of seeds in one and one-half pints of water and reducing to one pint; sweeten with honey and give one tablespoonful three or four times daily.

Skin

Stings and bites of poisonous insects, plants, animals, boils, carbuncles, tumors: Bruise the fresh leaves and apply to the affected area, cover and keep moist with the juice of plantain leaf; change poultice before it dries.

Bleeding of minor wounds; cuts, scratches, bruises, etc: Apply a poultice of the fresh, bruised or mashed leaves; drink the tea internally.

Malignant or bleeding ulcers: Apply the infusion with glycerine on well-saturated cotton or lint, cover, and change as often as necessary.

Toothache: Apply the fine powder of the roots to the affected area.

Burns, scalds, erysipelas: Use the strong tea as a frequent wash, and drink the infusion internally.

Inflamed eyes: Use a finely-strained tea made in distilled water as a wash.

Itch, ringworm, running sores, old wounds: Make a strong tea of equal parts of plantain and yellow dock (Rumex crispus), and bathe the affected area frequently as a wash.

Blood-poisoning: Use plantain as a fomentation or poultice and increase the normal internal dosage.

Vaginal

Leucorrhea, menorrhagia: Use a strong tea as an injection or douche, and drink the tea internally.

FORMULAS

Diarrhea

3 parts	Plantain (Plantago major; P. lanceolata)
4 parts	Silver weed (Potentilla anserina)
2 parts	Knotgrass (Polygonum periscaria)

Preparation: Steep 1 ounce of the mixture for 20 minutes in 1 pint of water, cover; strain and allow to cool until blood-warm.

Administration: Inject 1 tablespoonful or more three or four times daily and after each bowel movement.

Scrofulous tumor, glandular swellings, etc. (ointment)

3 ounces	Plantain leaves (Plantago major; P. lanceolata)
6 ounces	Fumitory herb (Fumaria officinalis)
3 ounces	Yellow dock root (Rumex crispus)
12 ounces	White resin
12 ounces	Olive oil
12 ounces	Beeswax

Preparation: Simmer the ingredients slowly together for one hour; strain and stir while cooling; when cool place in jars and keep in a cool place.

Administration: Apply to the affected parts as needed.

CASE HISTORY

The greatest herb for blood poisoning.
Dr. Christopher had a man come for help with blood poisoning. Red streaks were running up his arm, he had a large lump under the arm pit and was in extreme pain. His fingers were swollen so large that his hands were spread wide. Dr. Christopher simply bruised some leaves of the plantain herb, made them into a poultice and applied it over the entire arm. Within twenty-four hours the fingers were normal, the lump was gone, and the tell-tale red line had entirely disappeared. The herb had drawn the poison completely out.

In another case, a girl cut her foot on a poisonous seashell, and her leg swelled up with the usual red streaks and a knot as large as a baseball formed in the groin. A plantain poultice was put on her leg, and within one hour the pain was gone. The poultices were renewed every hour, and she was completely healed in a very short time.

Plantain is also useful for poisonous stings, bites, plants. A 2-year-old was stung on the neck, and the part swelled to enormous size. Again, the remedy was simple, yet wonderfully effective: four plantain leaves were bruised and bound around the neck, and within one hour there was no sign that anything had been wrong with the child.

Growth characteristics:
Perennial root: one of the most common flowering "weeds" spread with European colonization found about door yards, in lawns in meadows, along the borders of fields, and in the hedgerows.

Collection:
The fresh, mature leaves may be used anytime.

Sister plants:
Hoary Plantain (Plantago media; PLANTAGINACEAE): (seeds) similar therapeutic properties and uses to P. major; specific for blight on fruit trees (rub green leaves on affected part); broad elliptical leaves spread horizontally close to the grouped fragrant flowers on short spike (long stalk) with conspicuous light purple anthers.

RED CLOVER, WILD CLOVER or TREFOIL
(Trifolium pratense; LEGUMINOSAE)

Common names:
Red clover, wild clover, trefoil, purple clover, meadow clover, honeysuckle clover, cleaver grass, marl grass, cow grass.

Identifying characteristics:

Stem — Erect or reclining, more or less hairy, branching, six to twenty-four inches high.

Leaves — Usually compounded of three growing on alternate sides of stem; leaflets are oval or oblong, marked with a white crescent and often dark-spotted near the center.

Flower — Terminal ovoid head, consisting of many small magenta, purplish-pink sweet-scented tubular corollas crowded together, one-half to one inch long and broad, and egg-shaped stipples at base, shriveled and purplish-brown on drying. Powder is greenish-brown.

Taste — Sweetish and slightly bitter.

Odor — Faintly aromatic and tea-like.

Part used:
Flowering tops.

Therapeutic action:
Alterative, mildly stimulant, sedative, deobstruent, nutritive, somewhat antispasmodic, depurative, detergent.

Red clover is wonderful for scrofulous and skin diseases, as an antidote to cancer, and for bronchitis and spasmodic affections. It is excellent to add to alterative compounds. You will find this an effective and reliable remedy in wasting disease and for weak and delicate children. The warm infusion is soothing to the nerves.

Medicinal uses:
Spasmodic and bronchial coughs, whooping cough, cancer, indolent ulcers (red clover is highly recommended for any part of the body), scrofula, scaly skin (red clover has an old and persisting reputation for this), rickets, bronchitis, wheezing, chest weakness, St. Vitus' dance, leprosy, pellagra, fresh wounds, syphilis, old

sores.

Preparations:
Fluid extract, infusion, powder, tincture. The strength of the preparation may be made twice as strong with safety and the same dosage given.

Dosage:

Fluid extract	1/2-1 fluid teaspoon
Infusion	2 to 3 fluid ounces 3-4 times daily, between meals
Powder	1-3 grams (2-6 #0 capsules at 500 mg each)
Tincture	20 drops or 2/3 teaspoonful

ADMINISTRATION

Anal

Cancer: Inject a strong infusion of the tea five or six times daily and also drink internally.

Oral

Alterative: Red clover is usually combined with other alterative agents, such as stillingia or queen's delight (Stillingia sylvatica), burdock root (Arctium lappa), yellow dock (Rumex crispus), prickly ash (Zanthoxylum americanum), blue flag (Iris versicolor), etc. to better bring out its alterative properties.

Bronchitis, bronchial and spasmodic coughs, whooping cough: Drink the infusion freely.

Lack of vitality and nervous energy: Drink the infusion.

Cancer: Drink four or more times daily on an empty stomach.

Skin

Scaly skin: Use a strong tea as a wash, or apply an ointment.

Indolent ulcers, cancer: Apply the extract or bathe freely with a strong tea, and drink internally; or see "FORMULAS."

Vaginal

Cancer: Inject a strong tea with a bulb syringe (holding the vagina closed after insertion to force the tea around the head of the womb), retain several minutes before expelling, five or six times daily.

FORMULAS

Alterative compound

1 ounce   Red clover (Trifolium pratense)
1 ounce   Burdock root (Arctium lappa)
1 ounce   Yellow parilla (Menispermum canadense)
1/2 ounce   Mullein (Verbascum thapsus)

Preparation: Simmer the ingredients in 2 quarts of water down to 1 quart; strain, sweeten with honey, allow to cool; bottle and keep in a cool place.

Dosage: 2 fluid ounces, 3-4 times daily.

Dr. Thompson's famous Cancer Plaster

> Take the heads of red clover, and fill a brass kettle, and boil them in water for one hour; then take them out and fill the kettle again with fresh ones, and boil them as before in the same liquor. Strain it off and press the heads to get out all the juice, then simmer it over a low fire, till it is about the consistency of tar, when it will be fit for use. Be careful not to let it burn. When used it should be spread on a piece of bladder, split and made soft. It is good to cure cancers, sore lips and old sores.

Note: It is not necessary to make as large an amount as indicated. Be sure to use a stainless steel pan. Dr. Nowell recommends that the foregoing preparation be mixed with dandelion extract (Taraxacum officinale) to alleviate the severe smarting that red clover may cause after being applied, and to accentuate the therapeutic value. Apply the plaster on clean gauze.

Anti-cancer remedy

1 part   Red clover blossoms (Trifolium pratense)
1 part   Poke root (Phytolacca americana)
1 part   Licorice root (Glycyrrhiza glabra)
1 part   Cascara sagrada bark (Rhamnus purshiana)
1 part   Sarsaparilla root (Smilax officinalis; S. ornata)
1 part   Prickly ash bark (Zanthoxylum americanum)
1 part   Burdock root (Arctium lappa)
1 part   Buckthorn bark (Rhamnus Frangula)
1 part   Stillingia root (Stillingia sylvatica)
1 part   Oregon grape root (Berberis aquifolium)
1 part   Peach bark (Prunus Persica; Amygdalus Persica)
1 part   Chaparral leaves and small stems (Larrea tridentata)

Preparation: 1 teaspoon to the cup; infuse with boiling water.

Dosage: 1/3 cupful 3 times a day, increase 1/3 cup each 3 weeks up to a cupful 3 times a day.

**Cancerous growths,
leprosy affections, pellagra**

1 part	Red clover (Trifolium pratense)
1 part	Violet (Viola odorata)
1 part	Burdock root (Arctium lappa)
1 part	Yellow dock (Rumex crispus)
1 part	Dandelion root (Taraxacum officinale)
1 part	Rock rose (Helianthemum Canadense)
1 part	Golden seal root (Hydrastis Canadensis)

Preparation: Infuse mixed herbs in boiling hot water; let set covered until cool enough to drink.

Dosage: 2 fluid ounces 3 times daily.

Syphilis

1 ounce	Red clover (Trifolium pratense)
1 ounce	Burdock seed (Arctium lappa)
2 ounces	Oregon grape root (Berberis aquifolium)
1/2 ounce	Blood root (Sanguinaria canadensis)

Preparation: Using the granulated or powdered herbs, pour over 1 pint of boiling hot water and 1 pint of hot apple-cider vinegar; cover and steep for 2 hours; strain and keep in a cool place.

Dosage: 2 fluid ounces 4 times daily.

Congenial combinations:
The alterative properties in red clover are best brought out in combination with other alterative herbs.

Growth characteristics:
Perennial root, annual stem; common throughout Canada and the United States, Europe, Central and Northern Asia; grows in fields and meadows, and along the roadside; flowers April to November.

Collection:
Gather the flowers while in perfect bloom.

Sister plants:
White Clover or Dutch Clover (Trifolium repens; LEGUMINOSAE); blossoms:

boils, ulcers, skin diseases; equal parts white clover and yellow dock (Rumex crispus) makes an excellent salve; solitary round heads of white pinkish flowers on leafless stems.

Melilot or King's Clover (Melilotus alba; LEGUMINOSAE); Flowers: similar uses to melilot; tiny white flowers or slender racemes; small, narrow or oblong trifoliate leaf; entire plant has a sweet, vanilla-like scent when dried, and is used for flavoring.

POKE ROOT, POKEWEED or SKOKE
(Phytolacca americana; P. vulgaris; P. decandra; PHYTOLACCACEAE)

Common names:
Poke root, pokeweed, scoke, pigeon berry, garget, ink-berry, red ink plant, American spinach, crow berry, jalap, cancer-root, cancer jalap, American nightshade, cokan, pokan bush, Virginia poke, poke berry, branching phytolacca; Mechoacan du Canada, Raisin d'Amerique, Morelle a Grappes, Herb de la Laque (French); Amerikanische Scharlachbeere, Kermesberro (German).

Identifying characteristics:
Stem Round, smooth, stout, pithy, erect, branching, green when young and red or purple toward the end of summer. Four to ten feet high, about one or two inches in diameter.
Leaves Scattered, alternate, oblong to lanceolate and tapering at both ends, five or more inches long and about three inches broad, smooth on both sides, rich-green, entire, petiolate.
Flower Numerous and small in racemes, white with a green center pink tinted outside, about one-fourth inch across, bracted racemes two to eight inches long, calyx of four to five rounded persistent sepals simulating petals, no corolla, conspicuous green ovary, curved styles.
Fruit Round berry, very juicy, dark purplish, one-third inch thick, hanging in long clusters from reddened foot stalks, ten-seeded (glossy, black- purple) purplish-red juice.
Root Large, cylindrical, one to three inches thick, frequently fleshy and fibrous, easily cut or broken, annulate (ringed), longitudinally wrinkled, covered with a thin yellowish-brown or brownish-gray bark, internally whitish, fibrous fracture. Powder: Brownish-yellow.
Taste Sweetish, acrid.
Odor Slight.

Parts used:
Fresh root (most potent); berries, also leaves.

Therapeutic action:

relaxant, alterative, cathartic, emetic, resolvent, deobstruent, detergent, antisyphilitic, antiscorbutic, nutritive; leaves: anodyne, cardiac-depressant. Poke root is one of the most powerful botanical alteratives, especially beneficial where the glands (especially the thyroid and spleen) are hard, swollen or enlarged. Poke root is excellent for all skin problems, and especially useful for hardened liver and scanty flow of bile. It works almost magically on new abnormal growths, as well as bony enlargements from direct injury, even chronic conditions. It is healing to inflamed kidneys and enlarged lymphatic glands and is an effective and rapid anti-cancer agent. Both the root (boiled in two changes of water) and the tender leaves make an excellent spring tonic, and the tender leaves may be used as greens for the dinner table. Poke root has a slow, but persistently powerful, action.

Dyspepsia: Poke root has been considered as a valuable remedy for this problem.

Rheumatism: Poke root has been used very successfully in treating the various forms of this problem.

Cancer: Poke root is a valuable remedy for treating cancer.

Medicinal uses:

Chronic rheumatism, skin diseases, syphilis, ulcers, scabies, eczema, tonsillitis, diphtheria, feverish conditions (babies), goiter, cancer, mammary abscesses or gatherings, enlarged lymphatic glands, malignant tumors, granular conjunctivitis, dysmenorrhea, leucorrhea, paralysis of the bowels, headaches (of many sources), felons, hard liver, biliousness, nephritis, scrofula, itch, chronic pharyngitis, obesity (adipose tissue), hemorrhoids.

Preparations:

Fluid extract, infusion, tincture.

Dosage:

USE ONLY THE PRESCRIBED DOSAGES: the herb is potent.

Fluid extract	(root) 1/4-1/2 fluid teaspoon
Fluid extract	(berries)1/2-1 fluid teaspoon
Infusion	1 teaspoonful to 1 tablespoonful 3 times daily, before or after meals; children 1/2-1 teaspoonful according to age.
Tincture	3-10 drops

ADMINISTRATION

Caution: Don't use large doses of poke root as an emetic, as the action on the system is too potent.

Anal

Hemorrhoids: Use the fluid extract as a wash and injection.

Oral

Goiter, mammary abscesses or gatherings (mastitis), enlarged lymphatic glands (especially of the neck): Use 1/2-1 teaspoonful of the fluid extract in 1 glassful of water, give 1 teaspoonful of the mixture every 2-3 hours; or 10 drops of the tincture every 4 hours.

Feverish condition (babies): Give 1 drop of the tincture in 1 teaspoonful of water every 3 hours.

Chronic rheumatism: Use the infusion in teaspoonful dose alone or the extract as indicated; or the infusion in compound with black cohosh (Cimicifuga racemosa) and wintergreen (Gaultheria procumbens).

Obesity (adipose tissue): Use an infusion of the berries.

Cancer of the breast: See “FORMULAS.”

Goiter: Use the fluid extract externally as a liniment, and drink internally in very small doses (as indicated in “Dosage”).

Felons: Use the fluid extract as a poultice for rapid suppuration.

Tumors, glandular enlargements, etc.: See “Formulas.”

Skin diseases, syphilis, scrofula, eczema: Use the liniment or the infusion as a wash, and drink internally.

Gathering of the breasts (caked breasts, mastitis): Take the fluid extract internally, and apply the liniment or solid extract to the area of the inflammation.

FORMULAS

Infusion of poke root

1/2 ounce	Poke root, cut or finely ground (Phytolacca americana)
1½ pints	D-cell or distilled water

Preparation: Bring the water to a boil and pour boiling hot over the herb, steep for 3-4 minutes; strain, allow to cool, bottle, and keep in a cool place.

Dosage: 1 teaspoonful to 1 tablespoonful 3 times daily, before or after meals.

Children: 1/2-1 teaspoonful according to age.

Fluid extract of poke root

1 pound	Poke root (Phytolacca americana), cut into thin sections and bruised thoroughly into a pulp
6 ounces	70% alcohol
12 ounces	D-cell or distilled water.

Preparation: Pour the menstruum of alcohol and water over the herb, cover closely and let stand for 5 days; press off the liquid under the heaviest pressure possible, strain, place in a tinted bottle and keep in a cool place.

Dosage: 3-10 drops, well diluted with warm or cold water (best given alone).

Tincture of poke root

1 pound	Poke root (Phytolacca americana), fresh and coarsely ground.
1/2 gallon	40% alcohol.

Preparation: Macerate the herb in the alcohol solution for 2 weeks; filter.

Dosage: 10 drops every 4 hours (adult); this can be increased somewhat until the patient becomes relaxed.

Compound poke root liniment

3 ounces	Poke root, fluid extract (Phytolacca americana)
1 teaspoon	Bayberry, powder (Myrica cerifera)
1 teaspoon	Sassafras, oil (Sassafras, oil) (Sassafras albidum)
1/2 teaspoon	Bay or laurel (Laurus nobilis)
2 ounces	Tragacanth, thick mucilage of gum (Astragalus gummifer)

Preparation: Mix the first four herbs well, then add the mucilage (this makes 6 ounces); shake well together.

Administration: Apply to affected parts 4-5 times daily. For non-malignant tumors and enlargements, use plenty of friction or kneading.

Cancer compound

2 ounces	Poke root, fluid extract (Phytolacca americana)
1 ounce	Gentian root, fluid extract (Gentiana lutea)
1 ounce	Dandelion root, fluid extract (Taraxacum officinale)
Sufficient	Honey water or simple syrup

Preparation: Mix the fluid extracts together and add sufficient honey water or simple syrup to make 1 pint.

Dosage: 1 teaspoonful after each meal.

Cancer of the breast
(poultice)

Sufficient	Poke root, fresh and ground fine (Phytolacca americana)
Sufficient	Poke root, fluid extract (diluted to 1/16 strength); or use infusion of the fresh root
Sufficient	Bayberry powder (Myrica cerifera)

Preparation: Use the fresh root each time and grind sufficient only for one use; roll this on a piece of muslin, cheesecloth or other thin material, large enough to cover the breast entirely (cut a hole large enough for the nipple).

Administration: Apply the poultice to the breast, moisten once daily with the fluid extract, and cover with plastic to help retain moisture; leave on three days, then apply fresh poultice. In two weeks, the surface of the breast will break out in pustular sores; in about four weeks from the beginning of treatment, all hardness will be gone from the breast area, leaving it soft. Then wash carefully with diluted apple-cider vinegar and cover with bayberry powder and allow the entire breast surface to dry; in 7-10 days thereafter the entire surface will be healed.

Cancerous sores (liniment)

1 part	Poke root, fluid extract (Phytolacca americana)
1 part	Yellow dock, fluid extract (Rumex crispus)
1 part	Blood root, fluid extract (Sanguinaria Canadensis)

Administration: Apply the ointment 3 times daily, and before each fresh application wash affected area with a good brandy. Note: As an excellent internal alterative tea for this condition, drink 3 teacupfuls of walnut leaf tea (Juglans nigra).

Chronic rheumatism

4 ounces	Poke berries (Phytolacca americana)
4 ounces	Dwarf Elder berries (Sambucus Ebulus)
4 ounces	Sumac berries (Rhus glabra)
4 ounces	Blackberry or bramble root (Rubus villosus)

Preparation: Simmer the herbs for 20 minutes in 2 quarts of water; add sufficient sugar or honey to make a syrup.

Dosage: 1 teaspoonful 3 times daily.

Growth characteristics:
Perennial root; found widely in the eastern part of the United States, also in Europe and northern parts of Africa; grows in dry, waste soils (especially in burnt-over districts), roadsides, thickets, field borders, hillsides; flowers June-October. Dr. Nowell commented that "the physician will be well advised to grow his own roots and make his own preparation. It grows very quickly; seed sown in the fall will come up in the spring and will produce in the summer a root one foot long and some two inches thick. The berries on the ground will, if gathered, provide seed for the sowing of another crop."

Collection:
Probably no other medicinal herb deteriorates as rapidly and completely with age as poke root; therefore, the *fresh* root should be dug and used for each preparation, or make the fresh root into a fluid extract or tincture promptly after gathering and cleaning. The young and tender shoots gathered in spring may be prepared and eaten similar to spinach, asparagus, etc. The leaves should be gathered just prior to the maturing of the berries, and the berries are collected when fully mature or ripe, August-October.

Drying and preservation:
Poke root is best preserved as a fluid extract or tincture. The fluid extract sold by pharmaceutical concerns is improperly prepared from old and dried roots and is not a reliable agent, so the herbalist should prepare his or her own.

Sister plants:
-(Phytolacca octandra; CHENOPODIACEAE); root: similar medicinal characteristics and uses to poke root; the young and tender shoots may be used as vegetable greens in the springtime; found in Central and South America.
-(Phytolacca acinosa; CHENOPODIACEAE); root: similar medicinal characteristics and uses to poke root; the young and tender shoots may be used as vegetable greens in springtime; found in northern India.

BURDOCK ROOT
(Arctium Lappa; Lappa minor; COMPOSITAE)

Common names:
Burdock root, Lappa, clothburr, thorny burr, fox's cloth, beggars buttons, hardock, hareburr, burrburr, turkey burr, bardana.

Identifying characteristics:

Stem	Stout, wide spreading branches, 2-6 feet high, coarse.
Leaves	Heart-shaped (cordate-oblong and rhubarb-like), large and wavy, rough, fleshy, dentate, petiolate, alternate, whitish beneath.
Flowers	Purple, globular heads, with a calyx of imbricated scale (burs or

	bracts) with hooked extremities for adhering lightly to objects.
Fruits	Achene, globoidal, 1/2-1 inch broad, imbricated scale with hooked (burs) extremities that adhere to anything. The seed is obovate-oblong, angular, slightly curved, one-fourth inch long, brownish-grey, wrinkled.
Root	Nearly simple, fusiform or spindle-shaped, 1/5-4/5 inch thick, 10-30 inches long, brownish-grey externally, longitudinally wrinkled, annulate crown (often with a woolly tuft of leaf remains), somewhat horny fracture, dark cambium separates the thick outer bark from the yellowish or whitish porous, and radiate wood, hollow center or contains white pith-like tissue. Powder: light brown.
Taste	Roots and seeds: mucilaginous, sweetish, slightly bitter. Leaves and stems: bitter.
Odor	Slight.

Parts used:
Roots (first year's growth), leaves; seeds; stalk (nutritive). The root has the most powerful alterative characteristics.

Therapeutic action:
alterative, tonic, diuretic, diaphoretic, stomachic, aperient, depurative, antiscorbutic, demulcent.

It is one of the best blood-cleansers in nature but does not nauseate. Burdock root benefits the skin, soothes the kidneys, and relieves congestion of the lymphatic system. It increases the flow of urine and is useful for weight loss. The stalk, when cut before the flower opens and stripped of the bitter rind, can be boiled or used in salads (eat raw with oil and apple-cider vinegar); it has a delicate flavor of asparagus.

Medicinal uses:
Skin troubles, rashes, pimples, boils, scurvy, eczema psoriasis, itch, rheumatism, scrofula, syphilis, leprosy, cancer, gout, pulmonary affections, catarrh, urinary deposits, swellings, hemorrhoids, burns, wounds, eruptions, canker sores, sciatica, gonorrhea, kidney and bladder troubles, colds, fevers, etc.

Preparations:
Decoction (roots), fluid extract, infusion (leaves), powder, solid extract, tincture.

Dosage:

Decoction (root)	2 fluid ounces 3 to 4 times daily.
Fluid extract	1/2-1 fluid teaspoon
Infusion	(leaves) 1 teacupful 3 to 4 times daily
Powder	2-4 grams (2-8 #0 capsules at 500 mg each)
Solid extract	325 mg-1 gram
Tincture	30-60 drops (1/2-1 fluid teaspoon) 3 to 4 times daily

ADMINISTRATION

Oral

Promote perspiration (diaphoresis) in colds and fevers: Double the dose in hot water, adding 1/8-1/4 teaspoon of ginger (Zingiber officinalis) to each teacupful.

Pain: Drink an infusion of the tops.

Skin diseases, boils, carbuncles, pulmonary catarrh, scrofula, leprosy, syphilis, rheumatism, etc.: Drink the decoction regularly.

Skin

Large sores, skin diseases, inflammation, swelling: Apply a hot fomentation of the tea to the affected part, cover with plastic or oiled silk to prevent evaporation, and bandage; leave on until almost dry, then cleanse the area and make another application; repeat until healed.

Skin eruptions, burn wounds, swellings, hemorrhoids: Apply the burdock ointment; see "FORMULAS."

Rashes, pimples, boils, scurvy, eczema: Use a decoction of equal parts burdock root and yellow dock (Rumex crispus) as a wash, and drink the combination as a tea.

Goiters: Mix burdock root powder with olive oil and apply externally over the affected gland and inflamed area.

Locked joints: Apply a poultice of the root over the affected parts.

FORMULAS

Decoction of burdock root

4 ounces	Burdock root, cut or powdered (Arctium lappa)
3 pints	Distilled or d-cell water
8 ounces	Glycerine (for longer preservation)

Preparation: Simmer the herb in the water for 30 minutes; strain, sweeten with honey, allow to cool, bottle and keep in a cool place. For longer preservation simmer the herb in the water for 30 minutes, strain, return the liquid to the cleansed vessel, and reduce by simmering to 1 pint; strain, allow to cool, add the glycerine and shake well together; keep in a cool place; do not sweeten until using.

Dosage: 2 fluid ounces 3 to 4 times daily. 1-2 tablespoonfuls for the stronger decoction with glycerine, (diluted in some water); stronger doses may be used in severe and difficult cases, when the stomach is not nauseated thereby.

Strong decoction of burdock root

4 ounces	Burdock root, cut (Arctium lappa)
2 quarts	Distilled or d-cell water
1/4 pint	Glycerine

Preparation: Soak the herb for 1 hour in the water; bring to a boil and reduce by simmering to 1 quart; strain; return the liquid to the clean vessel and reduce by simmering to 3/4 pint; add the glycerine and mix well, allow to cool, bottle and keep in a cool place.

Dosage: 1 teaspoonful to 1 tablespoonful in water (3 times as strong as the infusion). Large doses may purge the bowels, so regulate the dosage accordingly.

Glycerin extract of burdock root and walnut leaves

8 ounces	Burdock root, cut (Arctium lappa)
8 ounces	Walnut leaves (Juglans nigra)
1/2 pint	Glycerine

Preparation: Place the herbs in 1 gallon of Distilled or d-cell water; reduce by simmering to 1/2 gallon; strain the liquid and set aside; cover the herbs again with water in the clean vessel and simmer another 10 minutes; strain and mix in the glycerine; allow to stand until cool, bottle and keep in a cool place.

Dosage: 2 teaspoons to 1 tablespoonful in water 3 to 4 times daily between meals.

Uses: Relaxed and a tonic conditions of the alimentary tract, tumors, cancers, ulcerations, kills worms and parasites (vermicide), syphilis, scrofula, tuberculosis, hardening of the arteries, fibroid growths, mucoid deposits, bronchial catarrh, dryness of mucous membranes, dysentery, diarrhea, prolapsed uterus, prolapsus and hemorrhoids, enlarged prostate, hernia, croup (paint on glottis while tongue is pressed down and forward), skin diseases (apply on lint or cotton), etc.

For injections and douches, dilute in water according to the condition of the patient and the amount of astringency or stimulation desired (in dilution, the action is more demulcent and soothing, and less arousing and stimulating).

Acne

1 ounce	Burdock root (Arctium lappa)
1 ounce	Sarsaparilla (Smilax officinalis; S. ornata)

1 ounce Yellow dock (Rumex crispus)
1 ounce Sassafras (Sassafras albidum)
1/2 ounce Dandelion root (Taraxacum officinale)
1/2 ounce Prickly ash bark (Zanthoxylum americanum)
1/2 ounce Stillingia (Stillingia sylvatica)
1/4 ounce Camomile flowers (Chamaemelum nobile; Anthemis nobilis)

Preparation: Simmer the first 7 herbs for 10 minutes in 1 quart of water, pour hot liquid over the camomile flowers, cover, steep for 10 minutes, strain, and cool; sweeten with honey, bottle and keep in a cool place.

Dosage: 1 tablespoonful 3 to 4 times daily before meals and at bedtime.

Blood Purifier

4 tablespoons Burdock root (Arctium lappa)
4 tablespoons Yellow dock (Rumex crispus)
1 tablespoon Blood root (Sanguinaria canadensis)
1 pint Glycerine

Preparation: Place the herbs in 1½ quarts of boiling water and reduce by slow simmer down to 1 quart; strain, sweeten with honey and the glycerine, mix well; when cool, bottle and keep in a cool place.

Dosage: 2 fluid ounces 3 to 4 times daily.

Boils (poultice)

1 part Burdock root (Arctium lappa)
1 part Sarsaparilla (Smilax officinalis; S. ornata)
1 part Yellow dock (Rumex crispus)
1 part Black alder (Prinos Verticillatus)

Preparation: Mix with hot water to poultice consistency.

Administration: Apply over area hot until relieved.

Skin affections, eczema, etc. (wash)

1 ounce Burdock root (Arctium lappa)
1 ounce Yellow dock root (Rumex crispus)
1 ounce Yarrow (Achillea millefolium)
1 ounce Marshmallow root (Althaea officinalis)

Preparation: Simmer the herbs in 2 quarts of water and reduce to 2½ pints; strain.

Administration: Bathe the affected parts frequently with warm decoction (at least 2 times daily).

Skin affections, eczema, etc. (decoction)

1 ounce	Burdock root (Arctium lappa)
1 ounce	Centaury herb (Erythraea centaurium)
1/2 ounce	Fumitory leaves (Fumaria officinalis)
1/2 ounce	Yellow dock root (Rumex crispus)
1 teaspoon	Cayenne (Capsicum frutescens; C. minimum)

Preparation: Simmer the first 4 herbs for 15 minutes in 3 pints of water; strain hot over the cayenne; cover until cool; sweeten with honey, bottle and keep in a cool place.

Dosage: 2 fluid ounces 4 times daily.

Itch ointment

1 pound	Burdock root, freshly grated (Arctium lappa)
8 ounces	Olive oil
1 ounce	Beeswax

Preparation: Simmer the ingredients slowly for 2 hours; strain through coarse cloth or fine wire sieve; stir until solidified; place into jars.

Administration: Apply to affected parts night and morning; at the same time, drink the decoction of the root internally.

Rheumatism

1 ounce	Burdock root (Arctium lappa)
1 ounce	Yarrow (Achillea millefolium)
1 ounce	Buckbean or bogbean (Menyanthes trifoliata)
1/2 ounce	Meadowsweet or steeplebush (Spiraea tomentosa)
1/2 ounce	Raspberry leaves (Rubus idaeus)
1/2 ounce	Barberry bark (Berberis vulgaris)
1 ounce	Licorice (Glycyrrhiza glabra)
1 teaspoon	Cayenne (Capsicum frutescens; C. minimum)

Preparation: Simmer the first 6 herbs for 20 minutes in 3 pints of water, add the licorice just a few minutes before removing from the heat; strain hot over the cayenne; cover until cool; sweeten with honey, bottle and keep in a cool place.

Administration: Use the vapor bath at first daily, gradually reducing to once a week; get the patient to perspire, keep up the circulation, and clear the bowels.

Dosage: 2 fluid ounces 4 times daily.

Sciatica, rheumatism

1/2 ounce	Burdock root (Arctium lappa)
1/2 ounce	Yarrow (Achillea millefolium)
1/2 ounce	Cleavers (Galium aparine)
1/2 ounce	Figwort (Scrophularia nodosa)
1/2 ounce	Angelica (Angelica atropurpurea)
1/4 ounce	Ginger (Zingiber officinalis)

Preparation: Infuse the herbs in 1 quart of boiling-hot, distilled water and steep well-covered for 2 hours; strain, sweeten to taste with honey, bottle and keep in a cool place.

Dosage: 2 fluid ounces 4 times daily.

Spring tonic

1 part	Burdock root (Arctium lappa)
1 part	Yellow dock (Achillea millefolium)
1 part	Sarsaparilla (Smilax officinalis; S. ornata)
1 part	Dandelion root (Taraxacum officinale)
1 part	Celandine (Chelidonium majus)
1 part	Senna (Cassia angustifolia)
1 part	Uva ursi (Arctostaphylos uva-ursi)
1 part	Juniper berries (Juniperus communis)
1 part	Spikenard (Aralia racemosa)

Preparation: Infuse the herbs in 1 quart of boiling-hot, distilled water and steep well-covered for 1/2 hour; strain, sweeten to taste with honey, bottle and keep in a cool place.

Dosage: 6-8 fluid ounces 3 to 4 times daily.

Ulcers in any part

4 ounces	Burdock root (Arctium lappa)
1 pint	Comfrey mucilage (Symphytum officinale)

Preparation: Boil the burdock root briskly for 15 minutes; strain and return the liquid to the clean vessel, reduce to 1 pint; when cool, add the comfrey mucilage (see page 339), shake well together until mixed, sweeten with honey, keep in a cool place.

Administration: Apply saturated on lint or cotton, keep moist and change often (do not allow to dry before removing).

Dosage: 2 fluid ounces-1/2 teacupful 3 to 4 times daily.

Uses: This remedy has also cured many cancers, bad cases of syphilis, and skin diseases.

CASE HISTORY

Feeding his own skin problems
While Dr. Christopher served in the army during World War II, a soldier come to him with a bad case of boils under both arms. Dr. Christopher lanced and treated them as usual, but in a week the soldier was back with another crop. He said that he had been plagued with the problem all his life. Dr. Christopher asked him if he wanted to rid his body of the boils, and he said he did. So Dr. Christopher gave him a prescription, for the mess sergeant (not for the druggist): no fried foods, no milk, no meat, no potatoes, no soft drinks, but all fresh fruits and vegetables. Needless to say, the boils promptly cleared up and there was no recurrence. These diseases must be treated by clearing up the bloodstream and keeping it clean.

Growth characteristics:
Biennial, found in the northern parts of the United States, also in Europe and northern Asia. Grows along roadsides and in rich waste places (wherever there is nettles, there also will be found burdock); flowers July-September.

Collection:
The roots of the seedling or one-year-old plant should be dug in the fall or early spring.

CHAPARRAL or CREOSOTE BUSH or GREASEWOOD
(Larrea tridentata; L. divaricata; ZYGOPHYLLACEAE)

Common names:
Creosote bush, greasewood, black bush, grease bush; Gobernadora (Span.).

Identifying characteristics:

Stem	Evergreen shrub, erect, 2-9 feet high, tangle-branched, brittle, leafy.
Leaves	Small, olive-green, resinous, appear divergently.
Flowers	Bright yellow, 1/2 inch across, terminal.
Fruit	Small, white, densely woolly, globose seed capsule.
Taste	Extremely bitter and disagreeable.
Odor	Strong-smelling, tarry.

Parts used:
Leaves and small stems.

Therapeutic action:
alterative, diuretic (lithotription), tonic, depurative, astringent, anti-arthritic, anti-rheumatic, anti-scrofulous, emetic (large doses), anti-venomous.

Chaparral or creosote bush is especially known for its use in cancer and arthritis. It was considered to be a cure-all by many native Americans. It is a potent healer to the urethral tract and to the lymphatic system. It tones up the system and rebuilds the tissue. It cleanses the lower bowel and tones peristaltic muscles. It is very bitter, but for the needy and courageous, it works fast for difficult conditions.

Medicinal uses:
Cancer, arthritis, rheumatism, stony deposits, stomach disorders, bladder problems, kidney troubles, hemorrhoids, leucorrhea, amenorrhea, dysmenorrhea, prolapsed uterus, pains, aches, bruises, cuts, inflammation of minor wounds, chicken pox, snake bites, venereal disease, sores, tetanus.

Preparations:
Infusion, powder.

Infusion: Use 1 teaspoonful of the herb to each cupful of water; put the appropriate quantity of the herb into a glass or stainless steel thermos bottle, fill it with boiling hot water, and immediately cork or cap; infuse for 24 hours, strain, and sweeten with honey; bottle and keep in a cool place. See also "FORMULAS."

Dosage:
Infusion 1 teacupful (6 to 8 ounces) 3 times daily
Powder 2-3 grams (4-6 #0 capsules at 500 mg each) 3 times daily.

ADMINISTRATION

Anal

Piles, hemorrhoids: Use externally as a sitz bath.

Oral

Cancer, arthritis, rheumatism, etc.: Drink the tea for 3 weeks, after which the capsules or tablets may be used.

Skin

Old sores, inflammation: Apply a hot fomentation of the infusion.

Bruises, cuts, minor wounds: Use the infusion as a wash.

Vaginal

Leucorrhea, amenorrhea, dysmenorrhea, prolapsed uterus: Use the infusion as a douche.

FORMULAS

Chaparral tea (not bitter)

2 tablespoons Chaparral or Creosote bush (Larrea tridentata; L. divaricata)
4 teaspoons Elder flowers (Sambucus canadensis; S. ebulus)
2 teaspoons Peppermint (Mentha piperita)

Preparation: Place the chaparral herb and 1¾ pints (28 oz.) of distilled or d-cell water into a 1-quart Mason jar, cap, and place in the oven for 5-6 hours at 180-200 F. (or make the tea in a thermos bottle, see "***Preparations***" above), strain, and clean the bottle, place the last 2 herbs in the bottom, pour in the chaparral tea, and seal; allow to stand all day or 2 hours, shaking the bottle occasionally. Strain through muslin and pour the tea back through the strainer over the herbs several times; sweeten with honey, bottle, and keep in a cool place.

Dosage: 1 teacupful (6 ounces) 3 times daily

Chaparral ointment

1 ounce Chaparral or Creosote bush (Larrea tridentata; L. divaricata)
1/2 cup Olive oil
1/2 ounce Beeswax (to add firmness)

Preparation: Place the ingredients in the oven for 1 hour at 180 F.; strain through a wire sieve and stir until solidified; place into a jar.

Administration: Apply to the affected part as needed.

Growth characteristics:
Perennial; this plant is native characteristic to the sparse scrubby vegetation of dry desert plains in the southwestern United States and northern Mexico (covering wide areas to the exclusion of most other woody plants); it grows in low altitudes and sometimes up to 3000 feet and forms a characteristic zone of vegetation in the Gila, Colorado, Mohave and similar deserts, but is also cultivated in desert gardens as ornamental; its flowers appear in early spring, and the seeds follow shortly after and make good food for desert rodents and other wild life.

Collection:
The best time to gather is when the seeds are matured in the springtime or in the fall, but do not hesitate to gather at other times.

Drying and preservation:
Take care to preserve the valuable volatile oils.

OREGON GRAPE or MOUNTAIN GRAPE
(Berberis aquifolium; Mahonia aquifolium; BERBERIDACEAE)

Common names:
Oregon grape, mountain grape, wild Oregon grape, rocky mountain grape, holly-leaved barberry, California barberry, trailing mahonia, mahonia.

Identifying characteristics:

Stem	Low-trailing shrub, glabrous (smooth, without hairs or projectiles).
Leaves	Holly-like, shining, evergreen, coriaceous (tough, leather-like), thick, ovate, acute, petiolate, dentate with spin-bearing teeth.
Flowers	Small, numerous, yellowish-green, on racemes.
Fruit	Bluish-purple berry, globular, acid pulp, resembles whortleberry.
Root	Long cylindrical rhizome, branching roots, knotty, tough, hard, yellowish wood, brownish bark, 1 inch thick, bark 1/25 inch thick and separable into layers, radiate wood with small pith, splits on drying, wrinkled, hard fracture. Powder: Yellowish-brown.
Taste	Distinctive and bitter, yellow saliva on chewing.
Odor	Slight.

Part used:
Rhizome and roots.

Therapeutic action:
Alterative, depurant, tonic, slight stimulant, hepatic, tonic laxative, diuretic, antiscorbutic, antisyphilitic, antiscrofulous, antiperiodic, nerve tonic.

Oregon grape is one of the best blood purifiers and liver stimulants. It creates appetite, promotes digestion, improves absorption, and increases strength and vitality. It also helps heal the bowel as a gentle tonic-cathartic, and the genito-urinary tract, and is very healing to the lymphatic system and skin tissues.

Medicinal uses:
Chronic skin diseases, psoriasis, chronic eczema, scrofulous, and syphilitic cachexia (condition of general ill health), atonic dyspepsia, chronic constipation, weak digestion, flatulence, jaundice, kidney and liver troubles, rheumatism, chronic uterine diseases, leucorrhea.

Preparations:
Decoction, fluid extract, powder, tincture.

Dosage:

Decoction	2 fluid ounces 3 times daily, 1 hour before meals.
Fluid extract	1/2-1 fluid teaspoon.
Powder	1-3 grams.
Tincture	30-60 drops (1/2-1 teaspoonful).

ADMINISTRATION

Oral

Chronic constipation: Combine Oregon grape root (2 parts) with cascara sagrada (Rhamnus purshiana) (1/2 part). Take in doses of 2 fluid ounces, but if this relaxes the bowels too much, reduce the dose; take regularly.

Scrofula, jaundice, kidney and liver troubles, rheumatism, leucorrhea, weak digestion, etc.: Use the strong decoction.

Skin

Skin diseases: Drink the decoction or strong decoction internally, and use externally as a fomentation or wash.

FORMULAS

Decoction of Oregon grape root

2 ounces	Oregon grape root, cut or powder (Berberis aquifolium)
1 quart	Distilled or d-cell water

Preparation: Boil the herb slowly for 20 minutes in an appropriate and covered vessel; strain through cloth; sweeten to taste with honey; when cool, bottle and keep in a cool place.

Dosage: 2 fluid ounces 3 times daily, 1 hour before meals.

Strong glycerine decoction of Oregon grape root

8 ounces	Oregon grape root, cut (Berberis aquifolium)
1/2 gallon	3 pints distilled or d-cell water
1/2 pint	Glycerine

Preparation: Simmer the herb until the root is barely covered with water; strain and set the liquid aside; retain the herb in the pot, add 3 more pints of water, and reduce by simmering until the root is again just covered with water; strain and mix the two quantities of liquid together; return to the clean pot and reduce by simmering down to 1 pint, add the glycerine and mix; allow to cool, bottle and keep in a cool place.

Dosage: 1 teaspoonful, well diluted in water, 3 to 4 times daily. Children 10 to 20 drops, according to age, condition, etc.

Syphilis

2 teaspoons	Oregon grape root, cut or powdered (Berberis aquifolium)
1¼ teaspoons	Red clover (Trifolium pratense)
1 teaspoon	Burdock seeds (Arctium lappa)
1 teaspoon	Cascara sagrada (Rhamnus purshiana)
4/5 teaspoon	Blue flag (Iris versicolor)
2/3 teaspoon	Prickly ash berries (Zanthoxylum americanum)
2/3 teaspoon	Blood root (Sanguinaria canadensis)

Preparation: Simmer 15 minutes after soaking in water for one hour.

Dosage: 2 tablespoonfuls or more 3 or 4 times a day.

Congenial combinations:
Cathartics: Oregon grape root is beneficially combined with cascara sagrada (Rhamnus purshiana) for cases of atonic dyspepsia with chronic constipation.

Tonics: Oregon grape root may at times be substituted for golden seal (Hydrastis Canadensis).

Growth characteristics:
Perennial; found in North America, western Nebraska, the Rocky Mountain region and extending to Arizona, Oregon, Washington and British Columbia (Canada); cultivated in England after 1923.

Collection:
The best time to gather the roots is in the late fall or early springtime.

Sister plants:
-Holly grape or mountain grape (Mahonia repens; BERBERIDACEAE); rootbark, berry: identical in the therapeutic action. This species grows in shaded woodland throughout the west and looks very much like M. aquifolium though it generally grows closer to the ground.
-Barberry (Berberis vulgaris; BERBERIDACEAE); bark, rootbark, berry: almost identical in the therapeutic action.

BLUE FLAG, FLAG LILY or WATER FLAG
(Iris versicolor; IRIDACEA)

Common names:
Blue flag, flag lily, water flag, iris, liver lily, snake lily, poison flag, larger blue flag, blue iris, vegetable mercury plant, dragon flower, kings evil herb, flower-de-luce, dagger flower.

Identifying characteristics:

Stem	Stout, straight, almost circular (angled on one side), sometimes branching above 2-3 feet high.
Leaves	Sword-shaped, erect, narrow, equitant (folded and overlapped in a flat compact cluster at base), somewhat whitish, 1/2 inch wide 2½ feet long (shorter than stem).
Flowers	Lily-like, large, beautiful, violet-blue with yellowish, grayish or whitish markings at base of sepals, and purple-veined six divisions of the perianth all united into a short tube, outer segments above 2½ inches long.
Fruit	Oblong capsule, not prominently 3-lobed, 2 rows of flat seeds packed closely in each cell.
Root	Cylindrical rhizome, horizontal, creeping, fleshy, annulate joints (2 or more inches long, 3/4 inch in diameter), often branched, 2-8 inches long, compressed towards larger end where there is a cup-shaped scar and numerous rings of scars above, grayish-brown, root-scars and remnants below short fracture, internally yellowish, central stele with vascular bundles scattered through the central column, distinct endodermis and cortex. Powder: brownish.
Taste	Acrid and nauseous.
Odor	Slight, but not distinctive.

Parts used:
Dried rhizome and roots.

Therapeutic action:
Positive alterative, cathartic, diuretic, stimulant, cholagogue, emetic, antisyphilitic, resolvent, sialogogue, anthelmintic (vermifuge), hepatic, purgative (fresh).

Blue flag is a powerful liver stimulant, claimed to be a therapeutic equal to mandrake root (Podophyllum peltatum), though less irritating. It clears the bile-ducts of mucus and restores the normal flow of bile. It benefits the secretive glands of the intestines, stimulates the flow of saliva, and is healing to the lymphatic system. It is mild and effective, especially in chronic and torpid conditions. Blue flag is most effective for cleansing impurities from the blood and for correcting skin diseases. It helps resolve inflammations and lesions.

***Medicinal uses*:**
Rheumatism, dropsy, cancer, impurity of blood, constipation, malarial jaundice, bilious remittent fever, chronic liver troubles, duodenal troubles, catarrh, skin diseases, syphilis, scrofula, fluor albus, venereal affections.

Preparations:
Decoction, fluid extract, powder, solid extract, tincture. The fresh root is somewhat acrid and purgative but drying removes these negative characteristics, while retaining the healing qualities.

Dosage:

Decoction	2 fluid ounces 3 to 4 times daily.
Fluid extract	1/2-1 fluid teaspoon.
Powder	650 milligrams (1300 milligrams as a cathartic).
Solid extract	650 milligrams to 1 gram.
Tincture	1/2-2 fluid teaspoons.

ADMINISTRATION

Oral

Cathartic: Give in small doses; often the fluid extract used for this purpose, or 1 #00 capsule of the powdered root.

Emetic: Give a large dose (4-5 capsules).

FORMULAS

Dr. Fox's cancer liniment

2 ounces	Blue flag, tincture (Iris versicolor)
1 ounce	Red clover, tincture (Trifolium pratense)
1 ounce	Blood root, tincture (Sanguinaria canadensis)

Preparation: Mix thoroughly (for the above tinctures use 90 proof grain alcohol or ethanol as the solvent).

Administration: Saturate a cloth and apply to the affected area twice daily; cover with plastic to retain moisture.

Ward's blood purifier

1/2 ounce	Blue flag (Iris versicolor)
1/2 ounce	Burdock root (Arctium lappa)
1/2 ounce	Red clover (Trifolium pratense)
1/2 ounce	Yellow dock (Rumex crispus)

3/4 ounce Sarsaparilla (Smilax officinalis; S. ornata)
1 teaspoon Wild ginger or Canada snake root (Asarum canadense)

Preparation: Simmer the herbs in 3 pints of water and reduce down to 2 pints; strain, sweeten to taste with honey; allow to cool, bottle and keep in a cool place.

Dosage: 3 tablespoonfuls 3 times daily.

Felon

1 part Blue flag (Iris versicolor)
1 part American hellebore (Veratrum viride)

Preparation: Boil the roots for 20 minutes in equal parts of milk and water.

Administration: Soak the felon for 20 minutes as hot as can be tolerated; then bind on the roots for 1 hour.

Growth characteristics:
Perennial, found in North and Central America; grows in rich, moist, marshy places, but it will also grow in an average-moist, shady spot in a garden; flowers May-July. About every 3 years dig up the plants and cut or divide the rhizomes so that each piece has at least 1 good bud; in cooler climates this should be done directly after blooming.

Drying and preservation:
Slice transversely and dry; seal in an airtight container and store in a dark place; this will preserve the virtues for quite a long period of time.

Sister plants:
-Orris or Florentine Iris or White Flag (Iris Florentine; I. germanica; I. pallida; IRIDACEA); dried rhizome or root: due to its violet fragrance it is used in various powders (such as tooth, dusting, etc.); and because of its spicy flavor it is often used for flavoring foods; masticator for perfuming breath (breath-sweetener for garlic, etc.); it is also used for diarrhea, bronchitis, dropsy, and teething infants; sword-shapes leaves, stem rises 1-2 feet high and bears 2 large white or bluish flowers; grown near Florence in N. Italy, Germany, France, Morocco.
-Yellow Flag or European Wild Flag or Fleur-de-lis (Iris pseudacorus; I. lutea; I. aquatica; IRIDACEAE); rhizome or root: dysmenorrhea, leucorrhea, astringent lotion; also useful for making ink and yellow dye; small, bright yellow flower veined with brown; should be grown by a natural pool or along a water course; very acrid taste.
-Gladwyn (Iris foetidissima; IRIDACEAE); rhizome or root: cramps, convulsions, stomach disorders, rheumatism; has a characteristic stinking odor.

SASSAFRAS

(Sassafras albidum; S. officinale; S. varifolium;
Laurus sassafras; LAURACEAE)

Common names:
Sassafrax, saxifrax, knutze, sassafras, saloop, ague tree, cinnamon wood; Sassafras Cortex Radix (Br.); Ecorce de Sassafras (Fr.); Sassafrasrinde (Ger.); Sassafras (Span.).

Identifying characteristics:

Stem	Varies from a shrub in the North to a very tall tree in the South; 10-18 feet high, 1-2 inches thick, many slender branches, wood is light, strong, durable, aromatic, whitish and reddish; the young end twigs are smooth and green, bases of stems and large branches are grayish, rough, deeply furrowed, and divisible into layers.
Leaves	Varying shape, 4-6 inches long, bright green, alternate petiolate, glabrous or smooth above and downy beneath.
Flowers	Small, greenish-yellow racemes that appear before the leaves, fragrant.
Fruit	Oval drupe, succulent, size of a pea, deep blue.
Root	Bark: Bright orange-brown with reddish-brown inner surface, irregular curved or quilled pieces (dried), nearly smooth, irregular ridges, soft and brittle, short fracture (cork layer). Inner bark: yellowish-white, numerous oil cells, 1 inch thick. Powder: reddish-brown. Root Chips: Brownish-white tint, distinct concentric rings marked off by 3 rows of porous vessels and slender medullary rays, has distinct taste of sassafras.
Taste	Sweetish, aromatic, slightly mucilaginous, astringent.
Odor	Agreeably aromatic.

Parts used:
Rootbark, root pith, root chips (root), bark, stem pith, oil.

Therapeutic action:
Rootbark: alterative, aromatic, diuretic, diaphoretic, stimulant, emmenagogue, anti-rheumatic, arterial depressant (when taken in large doses over a long period).

Pith: mucilaginous, demulcent, emollient, anti-poison.

Oil: anodyne, stimulant to neuralgia, anti-poison, cleanses the blood of narcotic effects of tobacco, henbane, etc., anti-emetic.

Sassafras is a blood purifier and destroys certain micro-organisms, such as protozoa. It makes a good diaphoretic when drunk hot and in quantity. It heals the alimentary and eliminative systems and effectively cleanses the whole body.

Sassafras is often used to cover the disagreeable taste of herbal bitters, which are often the alterative herbs. The pith makes an excellent demulcent and healing drink for the stomach and intestines. It is also an antidote for poisoning by acid or alkaline corrosives.

***Medicinal uses*:**
Skin diseases, rheumatism, scrofula, impure blood, syphilis, poison-ivy, poison oak, tobacco poisoning, cold, amenorrhea, ophthalmia (inflamed eyes), toothache, varicose ulcers, spasms and pains in the heart region, diarrhea, colic, flatulence, spasms, problems of the kidneys, bladder, chest and throat, tonic after childbirth.

Preparations:
Fluid extract, infusion, mucilage, oil (distill from the root bark with water or steam; soluble in 90% alcohol), poultice, tincture.

Dosage:
DO NOT TAKE DURING PREGNANCY.

Fluid Extract	1/2-1 fluid teaspoon.
Infusion	1 tablespoonful-2 fluid ounces 3 to 4 times daily.
Mucilage	4 teaspoons.
Oil	1/2-1 teaspoonful (1 part oil of sassafras in 4 parts of olive oil; do not give to children under 10, always use the oil diluted unless directed otherwise (externally used).
Powder	1/2-1 gram.
Tincture	1/4-1/2 fluid teaspoon.

ADMINISTRATION

Don't overdo sassafras by giving unlimited doses or for more than 3-4 weeks consecutively; the oil especially should not be given in overdose or taken over an extended period of time.

Oral

Diaphoretic; recent cold: Drink 2 fluid ounces of the infusion in equal parts of very hot water upon retiring.

Emmenagogue; amenorrhea: Drink 1 teacupful of the infusion without dilution; heat until blood-warm, then sip slowly 1 mouthful at a time over 1/2 hour, keep the lower area warm by wrapping in a blanket, and place feet in a mustard and water bath during the 1/2 hour period.

Skin disorders, rheumatism, syphilis: Drink an infusion of equal parts sassafras and sarsaparilla (Smilax officinalis; S. ornata) and 1/2 part Guaiacum officinale.

Counteract effects of poison of henbane or black henbane (Hyoscyamus niger), tobacco poisoning, blood purifier, diarrhea, colic: Use the oil, but do not give to children under 10 and do not give an overdose.

Children's blood troubles, colic: Give 1-2 teaspoonfuls of the infusion sweetened with honey 2 times daily (morning and evening).

Poison ivy, poison oak: Give the infusion internally and use it often externally as a wash.

Inflammation of the stomach and bowels, diarrhea, dysentery, inflamed throat, poisoning by acid or alkali corrosives: Give the mucilage of sassafras pith.

Pains and spasms in the region of the heart, flatulence: Give the warm infusion.

Varicose ulcers: Give the infusion and also use externally as a wash.

Skin

Warts, corns, hard bony growths: Mix the undiluted oil with a thick sugar syrup and apply to the affected part.

Toothache: Apply the oil onto the affected area (dilute slightly with olive oil).

Ophthalmia, inflamed eyes, conjunctivitis: Use the mucilage of pith as an eye-wash or lotion.

Poison oak, poison ivy: Apply the infusion on saturated cotton to the affected area, cover with plastic and bandage, or use as a wash; also drink the infusion internally.

FORMULAS

Infusion of sassafras bark

1 ounce Sassafras bark, cut or powdered (Sassafras albidum)
2 ounces Glycerine 1-1/4 pints distilled or d-cell water

Preparation: Pour the boiling-hot water over the herb, cover and allow to steep for 15 minutes; strain and mix in the glycerine; allow to cool, bottle and keep in a cool place.

Dosage: 1 tablespoonful to 2 fluid ounces 3 to 4 times daily.

Mucilage of sassafras pith

1 teaspoon	Sassafras pith, powdered (Sassafras albidum)
1½ pints	Distilled or d-cell water

Preparation: Place the ingredients in a quart jar (do not heat the water) cover and shake well; let stand for 4 hours, shaking several times during the period until obtaining a uniform mixture, strain through unbleached muslin or cheesecloth; bottle, keep in a cool place.

Dosage: 2 tablespoonfuls.

Oil of sassafras and olive oil compound

2 teaspoons	Sassafras oil (Oleum sassafras; Sassafras albidum)
8 ounces	Olive oil (Oleum olivae; Olea Europaea)
2 ounces	Honey

Preparation: Warm the olive oil (not hot); place the olive oil into a quart jar and add the sassafras oil; close and shake until dissolved or thoroughly mixed; add the honey and shake well; keep well-capped and in a cool place.

Dosage: 1 teaspoonful to 1 tablespoon 3 times daily.

Dr. Shook's High Blood Pressure Formula (hardening of the arteries, etc.)

1½ teaspoons	Sassafras bark (Sassafras albidum), a blood cleanser.
1½ teaspoons	European goldenrod (Solidago virgaurea), relieves congestion, also a diuretic.
1½ teaspoons	Buckbean or bogbean or water shamrock (Menyanthes trifoliata), stimulates digestion.
1½ teaspoons	Black cohosh or black rattlesnake root (Cimicifuga racemosa), relieves nervous tension, reduces arterial action.
1½ teaspoons	Poke root or pigeon berry (Phytolacca americana), stimulates glandular action.
6 teaspoons	Indian senna fruit (Cassia angustifolia), activates the bowels.
15 teaspoons	Buckthorn or European black alder bark (Rhamnus Frangula), cleans and regulates the system.
1½ teaspoons	Cassia bark or Chinese cinnamon (Cinnamomum cassia), stimulates the circulatory system.

Preparation: Mix well and use 1 teaspoonful of the mixture to each cup of boiling hot water; simmer for 2-3 minutes, then steep for 10 minutes (or steep in hot water for 1/2 hour); strain, sweeten to taste with honey, allow to cool, bottle and leave in a cool place.

Dosage: 1 teacupful 3 times daily, before of after meals; OR, take 1 #00 capsule or 1/2 teaspoonful of the powder mixed into honey 3 times daily, before or after meals.

Deafness

5 drops	Sassafras oil (Oleum sassafras; Sassafras albidum)
1/2 ounce	Olive oil (Oleum olivae; Olea europaea)

Preparation: Mix well together.

Administration: Place 2-3 drops into the ear, 1 to 2 times daily.

Rheumatic liniment

1 ounce	Sassafras, tincture (Sassafras albidum)
1 ounce	Prickly ash, tincture (Zanthoxylum americanum)
1 ounce	Cayenne, tincture (Capsicum frutescens; C. minimum)
1 ounce	Myrrh, tincture (Commiphora myrrha, var. molmol)
1 ounce	Camphor, tincture (Cinnamomum camphora)
8 ounces	Distilled or d-cell water

Preparation: Shake the ingredients well together.

Administration: Apply to the affected parts.

Sciatica, inward inflammation

1 ounce	Oil of sassafras (Oleum sassafras; Sassafras albidum)
1 ounce	Oil of rosemary (Oleum rosemary; Rosmarinus officinalis)
1 ounce	Oil of oregano from marjoram (Oleum origani; Origanum vulgare)
1 ounce	Cayenne, tincture (Capsicum frutescens; C. minimum)
1 ounce	Gum camphor (Cinnamomum camphora)
12 ounces	Grain alcohol (50 to 95%) or ethanol

Preparation: Mix well together.

Administration: Massage well into the sore places on the body.

Spring tonic
(purifying and thinning the blood)

1 part	Sassafras (Sassafras albidum)
1 part	Sarsaparilla (Smilax officinalis; S. ornata)
1/2 part	Mezereon bark (Daphne mezereum; D. gnidium; D. laureola)
1/2 part	Guaiac (Guaiacum officinale)

Preparation: Decoction; simmer for 10 minutes.

Dosage: 1/2 cupful or more, 3 to 4 times a day.

Relaxing and stimulating liniment

1 ounce	Oil of sassafras (Oleum sassafras; Sassafras albidum)
4 ounces	Lobelia, fluid extract (Lobelia inflata)
4 ounces	Ladies slipper, fluid extract (Cypripedium calceolus)

Preparation: Mix well together.

Administration: Massage well into the affected area.

Stimulating liniment

1 part	Oil of sassafras (Oleum sassafras; Sassafras albidum)
1 part	Oil of cloves (Oleum caryophulli; Syzygium aromaticum)
1 part	Oil of cinnamon (Oleum cinnamomi; Cinnamomum zeylanicum)

Preparation: Mix together well.

Administration: Massage well into the affected areas.

Growth characteristics:
Perennial; common to the woods from Canada to Florida to Texas and Mexico, cultivated in Maryland, Virginia and Louisiana; grows best in light, sandy soil and in the open; flowers March-May.

Collection:
Gather the root bark from recently-felled trees only; the oil made from the roots of old stumps is reddish (instead of yellowish) and should be avoided.

Drying and preservation:
The oil gets darker and thicker with age, so it should be kept well-capped in brown bottles, and in a cool dark place.

SARSAPARILLA
(Smilax officinalis; S. ornata; S. medica; S. papyracea; LILIACEAE or SMILACEAE)

Common names:
Honduras sarsaparilla, Jamaica or Central American sarsaparilla, Mexican or Vera

Cruz sarsaparilla, Guayaquil sarsaparilla, Paraguyian or Brazilian sarsaparilla, red sarsaparilla; Salsepareille (Fr.); Sarsaparille (Ger); Zarzaparilla (Span.).

Identifying characteristics:

Stem — Large thorny climber, many stiff, woody, angular, ridged thorns or prickles or nodes.

Leaves — Quadrangular, cordate, glabrous, leathery, dark glossy green, 4-12 inches long, 3-6 inches wide, entire, round lobes at base.

Flowers — Small, petiolate umbels of 10-20 together, dioicous.

Fruit — Small red berry, 1/3 inch thick, 2-3 seeded.

Roots — Honduras (S. officinalis): Dark orange-brown, 6-8 feet long, 1/12-1/5 inch thick, spreading, longitudinally wrinkled or finely furrowed, shipped usually without earth, and only occasional fibrous rootlets attached, light gray fibrous central cylinder, internally reddish-brown, light-yellow porous woody zone, whitish pith.

Jamaica (S. ornata): Grayish or reddish brown, 6-8 feet long, 1/12-1/5 inch thick, spreading, longitudinally wrinkled, nearly smooth, and rarely furrowed, shipped without earth and with numerous coarse fibrous rootlets, short fracture or tough and fibrous in central cylinder, porous wood zone, yellow or white pith; resembles the Honduras variety, but redder, less wrinkled, more starchy and yields more extract.

Mexican (S. medica): Grayish-brown or dark brown, finely hairy and nearly devoid of branches or fibrous rootlets, 1/8-1/4 inch thick, shrunken when dried and forming sharp longitudinal ridges and broad furrows (often containing a blackish earth), bark or cortex is brittle, mealy whitish-brownish, horny, touch and fibrous fracture of the central cylinder, yellow and porous woody zone, distinct whitish pith. Stem branches are slender and often without prickles.

Guayaquil (S. officinalis): Dark, much fiber, thick, furry bark, somewhat starchy (amylaceous), internally pale yellow rhizome and stem portions are often included in shipping.

Paraguyian, Brazilian, Rio Negro, Lisbon (S. papyracea); considered to be a variety of S. officinalis: Dark, few rootlets, starchy and acrid, resembling Honduras; older stems and branches remain square, angles with flattened thorns or prickles, leaves much more membranous. Powder: Grayish-brown.

Taste — Sweetish, mucilaginous, slightly acrid.

Odor — Nearly odorless.

Part used:

Root.

Therapeutic action:
Alterative, diuretic, tonic, stimulant, relaxant, demulcent, diaphoretic, cathartic, anti-arthritic, anti-syphilitic, depurant, deobstruent, anti-scorbutic, carminative.

Sarsaparilla is a wonderful tonic blood-purifier. It contains organic sulphur (anti-putrefaction), a small amount of magnesium sulphate (equals Epsom salts as a laxative), iron (oxidizer and vitalizer of the blood), calcium oxalate (high in oxygen and absorption of carbon dioxide), potassium chloride (fibrin solvent), and magnesium (bitter tonic). It will promote profuse perspiration when taken hot, it will increase the flow of urine, and it is a powerful agent to expel gas from the stomach and intestines. Recent research has found that the root contains valuable plant hormones: testosterone, progesterone, and cortin.

Medicinal uses:
Scrofula, rheumatism, gout, syphilis, skin eruptions, pimples, arthritis, tetters, ringworm, poison antidote, internal inflammations, colds, catarrh, fever, ophthalmia, flatulence (stomach and bowels), venereal disease, sores, chronic abscesses, necrosis, old ulcers, psoriasis, physical debility, weakness, sexual impotence, infant venereal disease.

Preparations:
Decoction, fluid extract, powder, solid extract, tincture. Sarsaparilla is generally compounded with other alterative agents.

Dosage:

Decoction	2-8 fluid ounces.
Fluid Extract	2-4 fluid teaspoons.
Powder	1/2-1 teaspoonful.
Solid Extract	1/2-1 gram.
Tincture	1-2 fluid teaspoons.

ADMINISTRATION

Oral

Deadly poison: Cleanse the stomach thoroughly with lobelia emetic (Lobelia inflata); then drink the sarsaparilla decoction copiously.

Diaphoretic, colds, fever: Drink the decoction or compound decoction hot.

Skin

Arthritis, gout joints, etc.: Drink the decoction as given in "FORMULAS"; dilute this same decoction with equal parts of hot distilled water, and apply hot fomentation of this solution to the affected part; cover with a heavy towel to retain heat; change as often as necessary until relief is obtained.

Sty: Apply a hot fomentation of strong tea over the eye.

Venereal disease (infant): Use the decoction as a local wash; mix the powdered root into the food.

FORMULAS

Sarsaparilla-yellow parilla compound
(arthritis, gout, etc.)

5 ounces	Sarsaparilla root, cut (Smilax officinalis; S. ornata; S.medica)
3 ounces	Yellow parilla root, cut (Menispermum canadense)
1/2 gallon	Distilled or d-cell water
6 ounces	Glycerine

Preparation: Boil the herbs briskly in the water until the water is 1 inch above the herbs (towards the last simmer slowly to allow the roots to settle); strain and set the liquid aside, return the roots to the vessel, cover the herbs with fresh water, simmer for 10 minutes; strain and mix the two quantities into a liquid together; return this liquor to the cleaned vessel and reduce by simmering to 3/4 pint; strain through cheesecloth and add the glycerine; allow to cool, bottle, keep in a cool place.

Dosage: 1 tablespoonful 3 to 4 times daily (regulate the dose according to the bowel movements).

Blood Purifier

1 ounce	Sarsaparilla root (Smilax officinalis, S. ornata; S. medica)
1 ounce	Burdock root (Arctium lappa)
1 ounce	Guaiac chips (Guaiacum officinale)
1 ounce	Cleavers (Galium aparine)
1 ounce	Fumitory (Fumaria officinalis)
1 ounce	Licorice root (Glycyrrhiza glabra)

Preparation: Pour 3½ quarts of boiling-hot water over the herbs and simmer down to 2 quarts; strain, sweeten to taste with honey, allow to cool, bottle and keep in a cool place.

Dosage: 1/2 teacupful 3 to 4 times daily before meals.

Rheumatism

Add the following herbs to the finished product of the above "Blood Purifier" formula when cool:
1 ounce Prickly ash, tincture (Zanthoxylum americanum)

1/2 ounce	Stillingia or queen's delight (Stillingia sylvatica)

Dosage: 2 fluid ounces 3 to 4 times daily.

Compound decoction of sarsaparilla

4 ounces	Sarsaparilla root (Smilax officinalis; S. ornata; S. medica)
2 ounces	Sassafras bark (Sassafras albidum)
2 ounces	Guaiac chips (Guaiacum officinale)
2 ounces	Licorice root (Glycyrrhiza glabra)
1 ounce	Mezereon (Daphne mezereum)

Preparation: Boil the herbs in 2 quarts of water and reduce down to a quart; strain and set the liquor aside; return the herb to the vessel, add 2 more quarts of water and reduce by simmering down to 1 quart; strain, mix the two quantities of liquid together; sweeten to taste, allow to cool, bottle and keep in a cool place.

Dosage: 2 fluid ounces 4 times daily.

Coffin's sarsaparilla compound

1 ounce	Sarsaparilla root, cut (Smilax officinalis, S. ornata; S. medica)
1 ounce	Sassafras root bark or chips (Sassafras albidum)
1/2 ounce	Virginia snake root, bruised (Aristolochia serpentaria)
1/2 ounce	Licorice root, sliced (Glycyrrhiza glabra)

Preparation: Macerate the herbs for 10 minutes in 1 quart of water; take out the sarsaparilla root and bruise it, then return it to the liquid; boil gently for 10 minutes and allow it to stand until cool, strain, sweeten to taste, bottle and keep in cool place.

Dosage: 2 fluid ounces 3 to 4 times daily.

Sarsaparilla root beer

2 ounces	Sarsaparilla root (Smilax officinalis, S. ornata; S. medica)
2 ounces	Sassafras root bark (Sassafras albidum)
1½ ounces	Wintergreen herb (Gaultheria procumbens)
1/2 ounce	Tansy (Tanacetum vulgare)
1/4 teaspoon	Brewing yeast (or regular baking yeast can be used)
1 pint	Molasses

Preparation: Cover the herbs in water and simmer until all the strength is extracted (30 to 45 minutes); strain, add the molasses; when cool, add the brewer's yeast; after 2 hours, add 2½ gallons of lukewarm water; it will be "worked" in 5-6 hours, then should be bottled, well-stoppered or capped, and kept in cool place.

Dosage: Drink at will as a refreshing, cooling and healthful beverage.

Spring tonic

8 ounces	Sarsaparilla root (Smilax officinalis S. ornata; S. medica)
2 ounces	Licorice root (Glycyrrhiza glabra)
1 ounce	Burdock root (Arctium lappa)
3 teaspoons	Senna leaves (Cassia angustifolia)
1 ounce	Cascara or sacred bark, fluid extract (Rhamnus purshiana)
5 ounces	Glycerine

Preparation: Simmer the first 4 herbs gently in 1 quart of water for 30 minutes; strain hot over the cascara and glycerine, cover and allow to stand until cool; sweeten to taste with honey; bottle and keep in a cool place.

Dosage: 1 teaspoonful 3 times daily before meals.

Skin diseases

1 part	Sarsaparilla root (Smilax officinalis; S. ornata, S. medica)
1 part	Quassia (Quassia amara; Picraena excelsa)
1 part	Sassafras rootbark (Sassafras albidum)
1 part	Licorice root (Glycyrrhiza glabra)
1 part	Juniper berries (Juniperus communis)
1 part	Bittersweet (Solanum dulcamara)
1 part	Dandelion root (Taraxacum officinale)
1 part	Burdock root (Arctium lappa)

Preparation: Simmer herbs for 15-20 minutes.

Dosage: 2 fluid ounces to 1/2 cup 3 times a day between meals.

Stomach weakness

6 teaspoonfuls	Sarsaparilla root (Smilax officinalis, S. ornata; S. medica)
6 teaspoonfuls	Yellow dock root (Rumex crispus)
6 teaspoonfuls	Cascara sagrada bark (Rhamnus purshiana)
5 teaspoonfuls	Virginia snake root (Aristolochia serpentaria)
5 teaspoonfuls	Indian turnip or Jack-in-the-pulpit (Arisaema triphyllum)
4 teaspoonfuls	Boneset tops and leaves (Eupatorium perfoliatum)
4 teaspoonfuls	Gentian root (Gentiana lutea)
3 teaspoonfuls	Mandrake root or Mayapple (Podophyllum peltatum)

Preparation: Decoction, soak one hour in 2 gallons of water. Simmer down to 2 quarts then add 1 pint of glycerine.

Dosage: 1 teaspoonful to 1 tablespoonful in water 3 times a day.

Growth characteristics:
Perennial; found in Tropical America, Mexico to Brazil to Peru; grows best in swampy forests. Honduras: grown in Honduras, Guatemala, Peru, Colombia, Central America. Jamaica: grown chiefly in Costa Rica, some in the Amazon Valley. Mexican: grown in the Mexican Andes, around Orizaba, Vera Cruz, etc. Guayaquil: grown in West Andes Valleys. Para, Brazilian, etc.: grown in northern Brazil, Guiana, (Para, Marannam).

Collection:
Gathering is quite troublesome as the plants occur in thick undergrowth. Fully grown plants often yield 30-60 pounds at first cut and every 2 years thereafter, they will yield smaller quantities of more slender and less starchy roots. Care must be taken in selecting sarsaparilla, as age may render its medicinal value nearly or entirely inert, or the species may be inferior. The best quality has many roots from the stem, persistent acrid taste (a decidedly acrid impression should be left in the mouth after having chewed a piece of the root for a short time), and closely set prickles or thorns and leaves.

***Sister plants*:**
-Smilax glauca (Mex.), S. syphilitica (Brazil), S. utilis; commercial varieties.
-China Root (Smilax china; SMILACEAE); rhizome: native to China and Japan, similar therapeutic characteristics to sarsaparillas.
-German Sarsaparilla (Carex arenaria): similar therapeutic characteristics.
-Other plants having similar therapeutic characteristics to sarsaparillas: Smilax pseudo-china, S. tamnoides, S. aspera, S. papyracea.
-Aralia nudicaulis; ARALIACEAE; American or wild sarsaparilla; similar but weaker properties and therefore used more as a tonic.

ECHINACEA, BLACK SAM(P)SON or CONEFLOWER
(Echinacea angustifolia; Brauneria angustifolia; B. pallida; COMPOSITAE)

Common names:
Echinacea, Sampson root, black Samson, coneflower, pale purple coneflower, angustifolia, rudbeckia.

Identifying characteristics:

Stem	Simple, stout, bristly hairy, naked above.
Leaves	Alternate, strongly 3-nerved, rough, hairy, thick, 3-8 inches long, lanceolate, acuminate, entire.
Flower	Single large head, color varies according to species; deep purple, pale purple, purple-red, rose-pink, whitish.
Root	Rhizome, nearly entire cylindrical, tapering, spiral, grayish-brown, 4-

	8 inches long, 1/6-3/5 inches thick, annulate (ringed), longitudinally furrowed, wrinkled, occasional stem-scars, thin brown bark, yellowish porous wood in narrow wedges with numerous slender black fibers (which give a grayish appearance to the broken surface), circular or angular pith, short and fibrous fracture. Powder: Grayish.
Taste	Sweetish, then bitterish with a tingling sensation (no benumbing effect).
Odor	Faintly aromatic.

Parts used:
Root (rhizome).

Therapeutic action:
Alterative, antiseptic, stimulant, tonic, antiscrofulous, diaphoretic, sialogogue, aphrodisiac, depurant, anti-venomous, anti-putrefactive, deodorant.

Echinacea is a very effective blood-purifier, and it is a powerful and stimulating antiseptic and antiputrefactive agent. It is very valuable for correcting autoinfection, where a person has not been eliminating toxins well, and the tissues and fluids have become septic or putrefactive, with resultant weakness. It heals infected skin wounds and provides pain relief; and it eliminates the disagreeable odors of pus formation and fetid discharges from infected wounds.

It is excellent wherever tissue decay is imminent or taking place, repair power is poor, and where there are unhealthy or bloody-tinged discharges. Echinacea is a good appetizer and greatly improves digestion and is useful in goitrous or scrofulous conditions. It relieves non-venomous bites and stings, and the Sioux Native American Indians used the freshly-scraped root as a successful antidote for snake bites and hydrophobia.

Medicinal uses:
Blood poisoning, tuberculosis, fermentative dyspepsia, carbuncles, boils, eczema, chronic ulcers, syphilis, scrofula, goiter, peritonitis, poisonous bites or stings, gangrene, typhoid fever, diphtheria, pus formation, tonsillitis, chilblains, bleeding gums, halitosis, enlargement and weakness of prostate gland, inflammations, abscess, septicemia, sores, infections, wounds, cancer, erysipelas, sexual impotence.

Preparations:
Decoction, fluid extract, infusion, powder tincture.

Dosage:

Decoction	1 tablespoonful 6 times daily
Fluid Extract	1/2-1 teaspoon
Infusion	2 fluid ounces 3 to 4 times daily
Powder	1-2 grams

Tincture 1/2-1 fluid teaspoon

ADMINISTRATION

Oral

Tuberculosis: Fine results have been obtained by using echinacea alone or in combination with elecampane root.

Ulceration, purulent skin diseases: See "FORMULAS."

Fever, typhoid fever: Drink the hot tea until sweating occurs, and administer hourly thereafter until the system is relieved of toxic buildup.

Fermentative dyspepsia: Use echinacea in combination with other stomachic tonics, such as golden seal (Hydrastis Canadensis).

Skin

Boils, carbuncles: Make an external application of equal parts of echinacea and ground pine or club moss (Lycopodium clavatum), while taking the echinacea tea or syrup internally; another effective poultice is to use flaxseed (Linum usitatissimum), lobelia (Lobelia inflata), slippery elm powder (Ulmus rubra; U. fulva), and cayenne (Capsicum frutescens; C. minimum) with echinacea tea and apply fresh 2 times daily for 4 days.

Snake bites, mad dog bites, etc: Apply the freshly scraped root upon the wound.

FORMULAS

Ulceration, purulent skin diseases, etc

3 ounces Echinacea root, cut (Echinacea angustifolia)
3 ounces Marshmallow root, cut (Symphytum officinale)
1 ounce Blue flag root, cut (Iris versicolor)
1 ounce Cloves, powder (Syzygium aromaticum; Eugenia aromatica)
1 ounce Golden seal root, cut (Hydrastis Canadensis)
4 ounces Vegetable Glycerine
1/2 ounce Myrrh, tincture (Commiphora myrrha, var. molmol)

Preparation: Mix the first 5 herbs together and place into 1/2 gallon of distilled or d-cell water and let stand for 12 hours; bring to a boil and simmer for 1 hour, stirring frequently, strain and press all liquor from the herbs; return the liquor to the cleansed vessel and reduce by simmering to 1 quart; stir in the glycerine and myrrh, cover and allow to cool; bottle in brown actinic bottles, keep in a cool, dark place.

Dosage: 1-2 tablespoons with lemon or orange juice 3 times daily before meals.

Growing characteristics:
Perennial; found in central and eastern Kansas, and west of Ohio in the United States; cultivated in Great Britain; flowers July-October.

Sister plants:
(Echinacea purpurea and Echinacea pallida; COMPOSITAE); fresh root: possesses similar therapeutic properties and uses.

PURPLE LOOSESTRIFE
(Lythrum salicaria; LYTHRACEAE)

Common names:
Purple loosestrife, loosestrife, spiked loosestrife, flowering sally, sage willow, rainbow weed, purple grass, purple willow herb, willow strife, blooming sally; Salicaire, Lysimaque rouge (Fr.); Braune (Rothe); Weiderich (Ger.)

Identifying characteristics:

Stem	Square or quadrangular, 2-4 feet high. Somewhat reddish simple and branching toward top.
Leaves	Pairs, nearly sessile, broadly lanceolate, often cordate (heart- shaped) base, 2-5 inches long, entire margins.
Flowers	Terminal spike with numerous large, showy flowers, reddish purple, 6-8 in rings around the stalk, each with 6 line petals.
Root	Woody, branching at the crown, throws out fibers.
Taste	Soothing, astringent.

Parts used:
Herb.

Therapeutic action:
Alterative, antispasmodic, diuretic, diaphoretic, astringent, febrifuge, tonic, demulcent, cholagogue. Purple loosestrife is one of the most useful alterative and astringent herbs for the mucous, secretory, vascular, and nervous systems. Its astringent action is potent but not drying as it promotes secretions of the mucous membranes and leaves them moist. It has special affinity for the liver, kidneys, bladder, and the biliary systems. Its astringent and tonic properties are valuable for intestinal problems, because it promotes secretions of the mucous membranes and strengthens the muscles.

Medicinal uses:
Cholera morbus, cholera infantum, fever, constipation, hepatic troubles, diarrhea, dysentery, hemorrhages (passive bleeding), leucorrhea, wounds, sores, ulcers,

restore eyesight and clouded vision, blindness, bladder problems, sore throat, quinsy, typhoid fever.

Preparations:
Decoction, fluid extract, powder, tincture.

Dosage:

Decoction	2 fluid ounces 3 to 4 times daily.
Fluid Extract	1/2-1 teaspoon.
Powder	1-3 grams (4-6 #0 capsules at 500 mg each).
Tincture	1/2-1 fluid teaspoon.

ADMINISTRATION

Purple loosestrife is an excellent agent to be used alone or in combination with other compatible herbs.

Oral

Cholera, fevers: See "FORMULAS."

Diarrhea, dysentery: Give in doses of 2 fluid ounces as required.

Leucorrhea, hemorrhages, passive bleeding: See "FORMULAS."

Skin

Clouded vision, inflamed or injured eyes, blindness: Make the tea in distilled water, strain well and use as an eyewash several times daily.

Wounds, ulcers, sores: Use the tea as a wash, or apply in ointment form.

Quinsy, sore throat: Use the warm decoction as a gargle; drink the decoction internally as an herbal tea.

FORMULAS

Leucorrhea, hemorrhages, passive bleeding

2 parts	Purple loosestrife (Lythrum salicaria)
1 part	White pond lily root (Nymphaea odorata)
1 part	Bayberry bark (Myrica cerifera)
1 part	Bur marigold or water agrimony herb (Bidens tripartita)
1/2 part	Ginger root (Zingiber officinalis)

Preparation: 1 teaspoonful to the cup of boiling water; steep till cool.

Dosage: 1/2 cup 3 or 4 times a day.

Cholera, fevers

5 ounces	Purple loosestrife, fresh herb, (Lythrum salicaria)
1 ounce	Ginger, crushed (Zingiber officinalis)

Preparation: Simmer the ingredients in 3 pints of water and reduce to 1½ pints; strain, sweeten to taste, allow to cool, bottle and keep in a cool place.

Dosage: 2 fluid ounces-1 teacupful every 1/2 hour until the patient feels easier; then regulate as the case indicates.

Growth characteristics:
Perennial; found in many places in the United States, Europe, and Central Asia; has an affinity for water; grows by waterways, luxuriantly on river islands and banks, in swamps and on marshy borders; flowers July-September.

Sister plants:
(Lythrum hyssopifolia; LYTHRACEAE): has similar therapeutic properties.

Allied plants:
Yellow Loosestrife or Wild European Loosestrife herb (Lysimachia vulgaris; PRIMULACEAE); passive bleeding, wounds, epistaxis (nosebleed), menorrhagia (profuse menstruation), relaxed throat, etc.; rather stout, downy species with auxiliary and terminal clusters of good-sized yellow flowers.

YELLOW DOCK, CURLED DOCK or SOUR DOCK
(Rumex crispus; R. obtusiolius; POLYGONACEAE)

Common names:
Yellow dock, curled dock, sour dock, curly dock, narrow dock, garden patience.

Identifying characteristics:

Stem	Coarsely angled, 1-4 feet high, erect, simple.
Leaves	Narrow and lanceolate-oblong, crisped and wavy at the margin, 6-14 inches long, decreasing in size toward the summit, acute, dark green.
Flowers	Numerous on terminal and auxiliary panicles, pale green, drooping and interspersed with the leaves below.
Fruit	Flower panicles turn into a dense mass of rusty-brown 3 winged capsules.
Root	Spindle-shaped, nearly simple with few rootlets, somewhat twisted, up to 12 inches long and 3 inches thick, yellowish-brown, annulate or ringed above longitudinally wrinkled, indented root-scars, stem scars

	or hollow remains, short fracture, internally dusty and fibrous, woody center with concentric rings and a radiate structure, rather thick barked. Powder: brownish.
Taste	Astringent, mucilaginous, bitterish.
Odor	Slight.

Part used:
Root.

Therapeutic action:
Alterative, tonic, depurative, astringent, cathartic, antiscorbutic, anti-syphilitic, detergent, antiscrofulous, nutritive (leaves).

Yellow dock is considered to be the most medicinal variety of the dock family. The roots of yellow dock have been found to contain as much as 40 percent iron compounds, making yellow dock one of the best blood builders in nature. It is very effective as a blood-purifier, and excellent for the lymphatic system. It is very valuable for all skin disorders and has therapeutic characteristics that are similar to sarsaparilla (Smilax officinalis) and turkey rhubarb (Rheum palmatum).

Medicinal uses:
Skin disorders and eruptions, scorbutic diseases, scrofula, glandular tumors, swellings, leprosy, itch, syphilis, liver congestion, biliousness, cancer, running ears, ulcerated eyelids, sour stomach, lack of pep or vitality, intermittent fevers, food (leaves), sores, anemia, cough, laryngeal irritation and catarrh, arsenic poisoning, hemorrhage, diarrhea.

Preparations:
Decoction, fluid extract, infusion, powder, solid extract, tincture.

Ointment: Mix the freshly-bruised root with leaf-lard, butter, or olive oil and beeswax.

Dosage:

Decoction	2 teaspoons -1 tablespoon in 1 cup of water 3 times daily (strong)
Fluid Extract	1/2-1 fluid teaspoon
Infusion	2 fluid ounces 3 to 4 times daily between meals
Powder	1-4 grams
Solid Extract	325 milligrams-1 gram
Tincture	1/2-1 teaspoonful

ADMINISTRATION

Be sure that the patient abstains from black or Chinese tea and coffee, as these are incompatible with iron tonics, such as yellow dock, and will produce toxic results.

Oral

Children: As the root is somewhat astringent, it is best to use the infusion in a diluted form, preferably in honey water.

Delicate stomachs: Give the infusion in smaller doses, gradually increasing them.

Iron tonic (blood maker, blood builder) general tonic: Drink the strong decoctions; see "FORMULAS."

Skin

Cough, laryngeal irritation and catarrh: Use the decoction as a gargle, and drink the tea internally.

Itch, sores: Apply the ointment as needed, or use the tea as a wash.

Glandular tumors, inflammation: Make a strong decoction of hot tea; saturate a natural fiber cloth in the tea; wring out excess and apply a fomentation over the affected part.

Vaginal

Douche: Inject into the vagina.

FORMULAS

Infusion of yellow dock

1 ounce	Yellow dock root, cut (Rumex crispus)
1½ pints	Distilled or d-cell water

Preparation: Bring the water to a boil and immediately pour over the herbs, cover tightly, and allow to steep for 30 minutes; strain, allow to cool, bottle and keep in a cool place.

Dosage: 2 fluid ounces 3 to 4 times daily between meals. Children: 1 teaspoonful to 1 tablespoonful in honey water.

Strong decoction of Yellow dock
(iron tonic)

4 ounces	Yellow dock root, cut (Rumex crispus)
3 pints	Distilled or d-cell water
3 ounces	Glycerine

Preparation: Boil the root slowly for 15 minutes in 2 pints of water, strain with 1 pint of water and simmer for 10 minutes, strain, place the two quantities of the liquid in a clean pot and reduce by simmering to 3/4 pint; remove from the heat, add the glycerine (which will make the quantity 1 pint total), allow to cool, bottle and keep in a cool place.

Dosage: 1 teaspoonful to 1 tablespoonful in 1/2 glass or 1 cupful of water 3 times daily. Do not drink tea or coffee while drinking these organic iron preparations.

Anemia #1

2 ounces	Yellow dock root, powder (Rumex crispus)
4 ounces	Sarsaparilla root, powder (Smilax officinalis)
1 ounce	Yellow parilla root, powder (Menispermum canadense)
1/2 ounce	Sassafras bark (Sassafras albidum)

Preparation: Simmer the ingredients in 2 quarts of water and reduce to 1 quart; strain, dissolve sufficient honey to make into a syrup, allow to cool, bottle and keep in a cool place.

Dosage: 2 teaspoonfuls-1 tablespoonful after each meal.

Anemia #2

1 ounce	Yellow dock root (Rumex crispus)
1 ounce	Buckbean or bogbean root (Menyanthes trifoliata)
1 ounce	Comfrey root (Symphytum officinale)

Preparation: Simmer slowly for 20 minutes in 1 quart of water; strain, sweeten to taste with honey, allow to cool, bottle and keep in a cool place.

Dosage: 2 fluid ounces every 4 hours.

Blood purifier

1 part	Yellow dock root (Rumex crispus)
1 part	Red clover tops (Trifolium pratense)
1 part	Brigham tea or Ephedra or Ma-Huang (Ephedra sinica)
1 part	Burdock root (Arctium lappa)
1 part	Figwort root (Scrophularia nodosa)

Preparation: Simmer the herbs 20 minutes in distilled water.

Dosage: 2 fluid ounces 3 times a day. Use this also as a wash.

Gonorrhea, gleet

1 part	Yellow dock root (Rumex crispus)
1 part	Red clover tops (Trifolium pratense)
1 part	Burdock root (Arctium lappa)
1 part	Slippery elm inner bark (Ulmus rubra; U. fulva)
1/2 part	Myrrh gum (Commiphora myrrha, var. molmol)

Preparation: Take 1 teaspoonful of the cut or powdered herbs and place in a teacup; pour over and fill with boiling hot water (or measure accordingly for larger amounts); cover and steep, strain and sweeten.

Dosage: 1 teacupful (6 to 8 ounces) 3 times daily.

Scrofula

2 ounces	Yellow dock root (Rumex crispus)
2 ounces	Dandelion root (Taraxacum officinale)
2 ounces	Stillingia root (Stillingia sylvatica)
2 ounces	Bittersweet twigs (Solanum dulcamara)
1 ounce	Sassafras root bark (Sassafras albidum)
1 ounce	Figwort root (Scrophularia nodosa)
1 ounce	American ivy or Virginia creeper bark or twigs (Ampolopsis quinquefolia (Mich.); Vitis Hederacea (WILLD.)

Preparation: Simmer the ingredients in 3 quarts of water and reduce to 2 quarts; strain, sweeten to taste with honey, allow to cool, bottle and keep in a cool place.

Dosage: 1 tablespoonful 3 times daily.

Special iron compound
(good for arsenic poisoning)

3 ounces	Yellow dock root, cut (Rumex crispus)
3 ounces	Bugle weed herb, cut (Lycopus americanus)

Preparation: Simmer the herbs for 10 minutes in 1 pint of water; strain; sweeten to taste with honey; allow to stand until cool.

Dosage: 2-3 fluid ounces every hour until the whole amount is consumed.

Growth characteristics:
Perennial root, native to Europe and now common to the United States; grows in waste ground, cultivated soil, along roadsides, about rubbish, etc., thriving wherever there is iron present; flowers June-July.

***Sister plants*:**

-Great Water Dock or Red Dock (Rumex aquaticus; POLYGONACEAE) root: Skin diseases, sluggish liver (use in combination with mild laxative), ulcers of the mouth, medicinal cleanser and first-rate tooth powder; medicinally similar to yellow dock, largest of all the docks, reaching 6-7 feet tall; stem erect, thick, striated, hollow, branching; leaves very large, some 2 feet long, pale green turning to reddish-brown, broad and sharp-pointed; flowers, small greenish yellow with white threads that turn brown; root large, reddish-brown, porous bark, large pith with honeycombed cells.

-Water Dock (Rumex Britannica; POLYGONACEAE); root: medicinally similar to yellow dock but more astringent (often mistaken for and collected indiscriminately with yellow dock); grows 5-6 feet high; leaves 1-2 feet long, lanceolate, acute transversely-veined, slightly crisped.

-Blunt-Leaved Dock (Rumex abtusifolius; POLYGONACEAE); root: similar but less-valued medicinal properties to yellow dock.

-Red-Veined Dock (Rumex sanguineus; POLYGONACEAE); root: distinguished by red leaf veins and stems; similar but less medicinal value than yellow dock.

-Herb Patience or Spinach Dock or Monk's Rhubarb or Patience Dock (Rumex alpinus: R. patio; POLYGONACEAE); herb: blood purifier, liver complaints, skin diseases, dysentery; native of the Alps, but common to various parts of Great Britain in the vicinity of ancient monasteries; foreign names: Patience, Parelle, Oseille Spinard (Fr.); Winter pinat (Ger.); Lapazio, Paxienza, (Ital.).

Note: Several species of Rumex have sour leaves, and are popularly called *Sorrel* to distinguish them from the others which are called *Dock.*

-Sorrel or Red Top Sorrel or Garden Sorrel (Rumex acetosa; POLYGONACEAE); leaves, flowers and root: fevers, kills putrefaction in the blood, expels worms, menorrhagia, stomach hemorrhages, gravel in the kidneys, jaundice, scurvy, scrofula, skin diseases, cancer (especially as a poultice), boils, tumors; leaves eaten as salad in the springtime have potent antiscorbutic properties, and the leaves used similar to spinach as greens and high in nutritive value; leaves, oblong, arrow-shaped below, rather firm, with a broad-toothed, membranous, stipular sheath around the stem base.

-Sheep Sorrel or Field Sorrel (Rumex acetosella; POLYGONACEAE); fresh herb or juice: urinary and renal diseases, fevers, scurvy, etc; highly nutritive when used green in salads; leaves, arrow-shaped, 1½ inches long and 1/2-3/4 inch broad, sour taste; flowers small, greenish, becoming red when in fruit; root yellowish, shallow and running.

-Turkey Rhubarb or Chinese Rhubarb (Rheum palmatum; R. officinale; POLYGONACEAE).

Allied Plants:

Sarsaparilla (Smilax officinalis; S. ornata; S. medica; SMILACEAE).

GARLIC
(Allium sativum; LILIACEAE)

Common names:
Garlic, poor man's treacle; Rhoblauch (Ger.); Ajo (Span.)

Identifying characteristics:

Stem	Stalk simple, erect, grows directly from bulb, sheathed leaves below, leafless and terminal flower umbel above.
Leaves	Long, narrow, flat, grass-like.
Flowers	Globular terminal umbel, containing small and whitish flowers grouped together with swathes (membranous bract surrounding them).
Bulb	Subglobular, 1-2 inches broad; compound of 8-15 bulblets (cloves) held together by whitish membranaceous scales or skin (as a sac) and attached to flattened circular base having numerous yellowish-white roots; each clove is covered by the whitish membranaceous scale-like leaves, with an underlying pinkish epidermal layer which coheres but is easily separable from the solid portion.
Taste	Warm and persistently acrid; onion-like but much stronger.
Odor	Intensely pungent and disagreeable.

Parts used:
Bulb, preferably fresh.

Therapeutic action:
Alterative, stimulant, diaphoretic, sudorific, diuretic, expectorant, antiseptic, antispasmodic, disinfectant, tonic, nervine, cathartic, emmenagogue, carminative, anthelmintic (vermicide), rubefacient, vulnerary, antivenomous, antisyphilitic, condiment, anti-catarrhal, digestant.

Garlic's medicinal value is largely in its highly volatile essential oil, so be careful in its preparation. Anciently it was used in both healing and nutrition, as it was known to build physical strength and energy. It is a valuable nervine tonic and is especially useful in lowering hypertension; laboratory tests have proven this. It equalizes blood circulation, and it is a useful expectorant for all respiratory affections and infections.

It has a special affinity for the respiratory tract, beneficially influencing bronchial secretions, though it rapidly diffuses throughout the whole system. The odor is so readily diffusible that when the juice, oil, or other form is applied to the soles of the feet, in seconds it is exhaled by the lungs and detected on the breath.

Garlic stimulates the gastric juices and has active carminative properties to correct any fermentative and gaseous conditions in the stomach. It arrests intestinal putrefaction and infection, while stimulating the healthful growth of the "friendly bacteria." The garlic oil is reportedly so popular in Russian medicine that it is referred to as "Russian penicillin," and the hospitals and clinics have used the volatile garlic extracts almost exclusively in the form of vapors and inhalants.

The use of garlic as an antiseptic and vulnerary during World War I was sensational; wherever there is pus, it is a safe and certain remedy. Its anthelmintic properties and action is deadly to round-and pin-worms. It also appears to be a powerful agent against tumor formation. Laboratory experiments have shown that it kills both harmful bacteria and viruses as well.

Unfortunately, it is the fragrant element in the garlic, called "allicin," which contains its antibacterial properties, so it is difficult to avoid the unpleasant smell. Some products claim to offer garlic's medicine without the smell, but we like to use the raw garlic or home-prepared garlic so that we know its vital.

Medicinal uses:
Tuberculosis, asthma, bronchitis, skin diseases, stomach ulcers, leg ulcers, athletes foot, boils, abscesses, epilepsy, worms, high blood pressure, low blood pressure, pimples, carbuncles, tumors, kidney disease, poisonous bites and stings, indigestion, catarrh, pneumonia, earache, infantile convulsions, leprosy, psoriasis, smallpox, intestinal disorders (chronic colitis), respiratory affections and infections, dropsy, sounds, aging, insect repellent, fevers, nervous and spasmodic coughs, hoarseness, whooping cough, typhus, cholera, hypertension, headaches, backache, dizziness, vomiting, nausea, diarrhea, dysentery, dyspepsia, heart palpitation, chills, loss of weight, restlessness, diphtheria, colds, colic, pleurisy, intercostal neuralgia, dyspnea, pharyngitis, cramps, heartburn, sore throat, rhinitis (clogged and running nose), nicotine poisoning, lip and mouth diseases (ulcers, fissures, etc.), diabetes, ague, pulmonary phthisis, sciatica, hysteria, ringworm, scrofulous sores, rheumatism, inflamed eyes, eye catarrh, chapped and chafed hands, flatulence, paralysis, neuralgia pains, retention of urine (bladder weakness), heart weakness, eczema, pityriasis, cancers, swollen glands, tubercular joints, necrosis.

Preparations:
Fresh bulb, juices, oil, syrup, tincture. Do not boil garlic juice; this will reduce its active virtues considerably. The freshly prepared juice is medicinally more effective than other diluted and preserved forms.

Dosage:

Fresh Bulb	1/2-2 teaspoons (1-2 cloves)
Juice	1/2-1 fluid teaspoon.
Oil	Several drops to 2 teaspoons.
Syrup	1-2 teaspoonful.
Tincture	1 tablespoonful.

ADMINISTRATION

Garlic treatment generally should be continued over a period of time. When using garlic oil, be sure to shake well before using so that the preparation is thoroughly mixed.

Nasal

Rhinitis (clogged and running nose): Apply the garlic into the nostrils and take the garlic internally.

Tuberculosis, whooping cough: Inhale the vapors of the freshly expressed juice that has been diluted with equal quantities of water.

Oral

Nervous and spasmodic cough, hoarseness, etc.: Take the freshly expressed juice mixed with syrup, honey, or other appropriate vehicle.

Chronic colitis, ulcerated stomach, etc.: Take the garlic oil internally over a period of time, 2 teaspoons 3 to 4 times daily.

Worms: Give 10-30 drops of the fresh juice or 1 teaspoon of garlic syrup.

Colds: At the onset, place a clove of garlic on each side of the mouth between the teeth and cheek. The cold will disappear within a few hours or within a day.

Chronic diseases of the upper respiratory tract (inflamed tonsils, salivary glands, neighboring lymph glands, pharyngitis, laryngitis, bronchitis, etc.: Keep garlic in the mouth constantly during waking hours, renewing morning and evening after the cloves have absorbed the poisons; or use another appropriate garlic preparation such as a mixture of fresh minced garlic, cayenne pepper and honey.

Asthma, whooping cough, cough, pneumonia, smallpox, bronchitis, dyspnea, etc.: When there is spasm, give 1 teaspoonful of the syrup with or without water every 15 minutes until the spasm is controlled, then give 1 teaspoonful every 2 to 3 hours for the rest of the day; thereafter give 1 teaspoonful of the syrup 3 to 4 times daily. Use the foot poultice. Mix the freshly expressed juice with leaf lard and rub on chest, throat, and between the shoulder blades.

Tuberculosis, cardiac asthma, dyspnea: Give 2 teaspoons to 1 tablespoonful of the syrup 3 to 4 times daily between meals.

Dropsy, heart disease: See "FORMULAS."

Hysteria, flatulence, sciatica: Give an infusion of garlic in hot soymilk (tofu-milk) and water.

Skin

Rheumatic pains: Rub the affected areas with cut garlic; or massage in garlic oil.

Chapped and chafed hands or other parts: Massage garlic oil well into the affected parts.

Earache, inflammation of the middle ear, ear disease: Pack a small clove of garlic in gauze and place into the external ear passage; or drop 4-5 drops of oil into the ear channel, put over this a piece of cotton, and keep warm. You may add a few drops of warm B&B Tincture (see "Herbal Combinations", page 594).

Pimples: Rub several times daily with garlic; the visible eruptions will disappear without leaving a scar, but this does not remove the cause. Purify the skin by cleansing the blood; see "FORMULAS."

Wounds: Garlic placed on the lip of unclean wounds will cleanse them in 4 to 5 days; grated garlic placed near the most virulent bacteria will kill them in 5 minutes.

Skin diseases, septic wounds: Apply the garlic tincture on gauze and cover.

Eczema, pityriasis, psoriasis, ulcers, cancers, swollen glands, tubercular joints, necrosis, etc.: See "FORMULAS."

Lip and mouth diseases (ulcers, fissures, etc.): Apply a paste of garlic (made by rubbing garlic in a mortar) to the affected part on a sterile gauze and retain 8 to 12 hours.

Indolent tumors, ulcerated surfaces, wounds: Apply the freshly expressed juice.

Scrofulous sores, ringworm: Apply a poultice of freshly-grated garlic.

Sciatica, paralysis, neuralgia pains: Massage garlic oil over the affected area.

Retention of urine (due to bladder weakness): Apply a garlic poultice on the abdominal and pubic regions.

Athlete's foot: Wash the parts in hot, soapy water; rinse and dry well; massage in the garlic oil 2 to 3 times daily. Apply once a week to prevent recurrence.

Foot Poultice: Remove the outer membranes of the cloves of garlic; chop it up finely and mix 1 part garlic to 1 part Vaseline, enough to cover the bottom of each foot with a thickness of about 1/4 inch (for children use 1 part garlic to 3 parts petroleum jelly). Apply olive oil to the feet first then spread on the preparation; bandage each foot with soft cloth, place in plastic bags, then cover the feet with old socks to prevent the poultice from being kicked off during the night. Remove the poultice in the morning, or retain it longer if desired. Do not use where the skin is irritated or extremely delicate, as it can cause blistering. This poultice is used to heal the entire body.

FORMULAS

Oil of Garlic

8 ounces	Garlic, peeled and minced (Allium sativum)
Sufficient	Warm olive oil

Preparation: Place the garlic in a large jar and use sufficient olive oil to completely cover the garlic; shake and allow to stand in a moderately warm place for 2 to 3 days; strain through unbleached muslin or cotton; bottle and keep in a cool place.

Dosage: A few drops to 2 teaspoonfuls 3 to 4 times daily.

Tincture-syrup of Garlic

1 pound	Garlic cloves, peeled and minced (Allium sativum)
Equal parts	Apple cider vinegar and distilled water (sufficient to cover the minced garlic)
Equal part	Hot syrup of yellow D sugar (see "*Syrup*" page 544)

Preparation: Place the minced garlic into a large jar, cover with the apple cider vinegar and distilled water, shake well and allow to stand for 4 hours; strain and add an equal quantity of syrup, stir and shake together; cap and keep in a cool place.

Dosage: 1 tablespoonful 3 to 4 times daily. Children: 1 teaspoonful or more according to age.

Tincture-syrup (glycerite) of garlic

1 pound	Garlic cloves, peeled and minced (Allium sativum)
Equal parts	Apple cider vinegar and distilled water (sufficient to cover the minced garlic)
1 pint	Glycerine
3 pounds	Pure honey

Preparation: Place the garlic into a wide mouth jar, cover with the vinegar and water; close, shake well together; allow to stand in a cool place for 4 days, macerating (shaking thoroughly) 1 to 2 times daily; add the glycerine, shake and allow to stand another day; strain with pressure and filter through muslin or thin linen cloth; add the honey and stir until thoroughly mixed; seal the jar tightly and keep in a cool place.

Dosage: 1 teaspoon to 1 tablespoonful 3 to 4 times daily between meals.

Uses: Asthma, bronchitis, catarrhal conditions, phthisis, tuberculosis, coughs, dyspnea, heart weakness, internal ulcerations, etc.

Aromatic vinegar
(to cover the pungent odor and taste of garlic, aid in flatulence)

3 ounces	Caraway or kummell seed, powdered (Carum carvi)
3 ounces	Fennel seed (Foeniculum vulgare)
1 quart	Apple cider vinegar
1 pint	Glycerine

Preparation: Simmer the 2 herbs slowly in the apple cider vinegar, covered, for 15 minutes; strain and allow to cool; when cool, add the glycerine and mix in well.

Uses: This should be used in place of the vinegar and water and glycerine. It is much more acceptable to those who can't stand the taste and smell of garlic.

Dropsy, heart disease

8 ounces	Parsley seeds, powdered (Petroselinum crispum)
2 ounces	Lily-of-the-valley root, cut or granulated (Convallaria majalis)
8 ounces	Garlic, expressed juice (Allium sativum)
8 ounces	Yellow D or brown cane sugar
1 pint	Glycerine

Preparation: Boil the first 2 herbs slowly for 20 minutes in 3 pints of distilled or D-cell water; strain, return to the clean pot and reduce by simmering to 1 pint; set aside to cool and when warm but not hot, add the remaining ingredients and stir in well; when cool, bottle and keep in a cool place.

Dosage: 1-2 teaspoonfuls in water as required; give the larger dosage to bring about diuresis, and to slow the heart's action and increase the tone of its contraction, then give the smaller dosage 3 to 4 times daily.

Eczema, pityriasis, psoriasis,
ulcers, cancers, swollen glands, tubercular joints,
necrosis, etc.

8 ounces	Garlic, expressed juice (Allium sativum)
8 ounces	Glycerine

1 pint Burdock seeds, strong decoction (Arctium lappa)

Preparation: Mix the ingredients thoroughly together.

Administration: Saturate lint or cotton and apply over the area; cover with plastic or wax paper, and secure with adhesive tape; change 2 to 3 times daily.

Dosage: Internal: 1 teaspoonful 3 to 4 times daily, until the affections disappear.

CASE HISTORY

Famous "Four Thieves Vinegar":
During the Dark Ages in Europe when plagues were rampant, those who ate garlic daily were not infected. The famous "Four Thieves" garlic preparation was credited with saving many lives when a plague struck the city of Marseilles in 1722. This preparation is supposed to have originated with four thieves who plundered the dead bodies of plague victims while being protected by the liberal use of aromatic garlic vinegar during the plague. Recent research corroborates this protection (a word to the wise with an eye toward possible future conditions).

Congenial combinations:
Aromatics: Garlic odor and taste can be covered effectively by adding a few drops of oil of anise (Oleum anisi-Pimpinella anisum; Illicium verum), oil of caraway (Oleum cari-Carum carvi), oil of cinnamon (Oleum cinnamomum-Cinnamomum zeylanicum; C. loureirii), or any other aromatic oil.

Growth characteristics:
Native of central Asia, cultivated in southern Europe, and America; grows best in rich, sandy and moderately moist soil with ample sunlight; propagated by seed or bulb division; cloves are planted in the fall about 2 inches deep and 6 inches apart in drills or rows like onions; keep free from weeds and hoe up soil around plants.

Collection:
The bulbs are dug in the late summer after the leaves die down.

Drying and preservation:
The bulbs should be free of foreign matter, then placed in netted bags, and hung in a cool, dry place where there is ample circulation of air.

Sister plants:
-Onion (Allium cepa; LILIACEAE); herb bulb: cough, colds, gravel, dropsy, digestive disorders, nervousness, etc.; onion has similar but weaker medicinal characteristics than garlic.
-Leek (Allium porrum; LILIACEAE); bulb: similar medicinal characteristics and uses as onion.

For a listing of alternative herbs which may be used when the foregoing are not available, please see chapter 17.

CHAPTER 3

THE ANTHELMINTIC HERBS

The Helpful Role of anthelmintics:
The three most common types of worms found in the body are: the thread or seat worms (Oxyuris vermicularis), the round worms (Ascaris lumbricoides-lumbrici), and the tape worms (Taeince-Taenia solium, bothriocephalus latus). There are also other less-common worm types that enter the body, such as hook worms (Ancylostoma duodenale, Nectar americanus) for which thymol and oil of Chenopodium (American wormseed) are specifics and those of unclean pork (Trichinella spiralis), etc., which thrive on toxic conditions in the body.

The thread or seat worm is rather easily destroyed or expelled because it is usually found in the lower bowel and does not adhere to the intestinal wall. Herbs such as cathartics, astringents, aloes, quassia, calumba, apple cider vinegar, etc., are effective against these intestinal vermin.

The roundworm is most likely to be found in and often clinging to the intestinal wall, and can cause considerable harm and physical discomfort, especially to children. If roundworms are not checked, they may increase to the point that they enter the stomach, and even travel up the esophagus in the pharynx, with most unpleasant and upsetting results. You can see roundworms in the stools, and you can also know you have them because they greatly disturb the balance of the stomach. The anthelmintic herbs are particularly useful and beneficial to eliminate roundworms and tapeworms. The anthelmintic agents are classed as to their action against the worm parasites:

VERMIFUGES cause the expulsion of worms from the body.
VERMICIDES destroy worms in the body.
TAENIAFUGES cause the expulsion of tapeworms from the body.
TAENIACIDES kill tapeworms in the body.

The difference in the action of a worm medicine often depends on the medicinal dosage given and how soon after administration the bowels are moved—thus, a large dose of an anthelmintic, if it remains in the intestine, will destroy, while a smaller dose will merely expel the worm. Almost all anthelmintics are potent and must be respected as such; and concentrated preparations must always be used in wisdom. Generally, in the case of thread or seat worms, an enema is sufficient; and, in case of round worms, follow the following procedure:

1. Go on a three day cleanse/fast drinking only one type of juice and distilled water and take the anthelmintic morning and night, preferably with wormwood.
2. On the morning of the 4th day, drink 6-8 ounces of senna (Cassia acutifolia; C. angustifolia) tea alone to cleanse and purge the bowel of the parasites (other suitable cathartics are also acceptable; see below).

The tapeworm is somewhat more obstinate, but the foregoing procedure will also work, using male fern or pomegranate as the anthelmintic. Continue taking the remedy a few days after the worm sections have ceased to pass, and use lobelia along with an antibilious cathartic. Dr. Shook gives some good advice:

> Doctors generally have the patient fast for a day or two before taking tapeworm remedies, but this is unnecessary, because the worm, being a parasite, cannot be starved. This only makes the patient feel weak and nauseated, and when he finally takes the medicine on a starved stomach, he may throw it up. A far better way, from our experience, is to advise the patient to eat, for a day or so, foods the tapeworm dislikes, such as onions, garlic, pickles and salted fish. This weakens the worm and tends to loosen its grip, so that when the medicine is taken, the tapeworm can be expelled more easily.

WORMWOOD or ABSINTHIUM
(Artemisia absinthium; COMPOSITAE)

Common names:
Wormwood, absinthium, absinthe, old woman, green ginger, common wormwood; absinthe (Fr.); Wermut (Ger); Ajenjo (Span.).

Identifying characteristics:

Stem	Numerous, bushy (branched and leafy), firm, flowering, 2-3 feet high, whitish, closely covered with fine silky hairs; lower part is perennial and almost woody from which new shoots spring forth each year. Powder (herb): Brownish, yellowish-green.
Leaves	Hoary from the fine silky hairs on both sides, grayish-green, 1-3 inches long, 1½ inches broad, three times pinnatifid (pinnately- cleft lobes), lobes linear and obtuse, alternate, broadish, blunted, leafstalks with slightly winged margins, lower leaves on longer petioles.
Flowers	Small and nearly globular flower heads, racemose, pendulous, greenish-yellow tint, hairy and convex receptacle arranged on an erect leafy pinnacle (the leaves thereon are reduced to 1-3 linear segments).
Fruit	Achene, abovoid, without pappus (the tuft of hairs that crowns the fruit of the majority of the composite family).
Root	Woody, branched at crown, numerous fibers below.
Taste	Leaves and flowers extremely bitter. Root warm and aromatic.
Odor	Characteristic (dried herb with flowers has strong and aromatic odor).

Part used:
Herb; oil (external only).

Therapeutic action:
Tonic, anthelmintic, (vermifuge) stomachic, stimulant, febrifuge, hepatic, aromatic, antiseptic, nervine, antivenomous, antibilious, carminative.

Wormwood is an extremely bitter remedy (next to rue, the most bitter herb known); it is rarely given to children. But it is valuable to the digestive system: it stimulates appetite, promotes digestion, and corrects stomach disorders. It is especially useful for atonic and debilitated conditions. It is an excellent nervine tonic, and it will expel intestinal gas. The leaves are antiseptic and correct putrefaction, as well as counteracting the effects of poisonous plants such as hemlock, toadstool, etc. The leaves and flowers expel roundworms, and they are excellent for correcting and toning the liver and gall bladder. The oil is valuable for external use as a very stimulating liniment.

Medicinal uses:
Roundworms (lumbrici), atonic dyspepsia, diarrhea, bilious and liver troubles, epilepsy, flatulence, debility, nervous conditions, melancholia, jaundice, nausea, morning sickness, intermittent fevers, gout, rheumatism, swelling, sprains.

Preparations:
Fluid extract, infusion, oil, powder, tincture.

Dosage:
Wormwood should be given in small and repeated doses.

Fluid Extract	1/2-1 fluid teaspoon
Infusion	2 fluid ounces
Oil	Use externally only
Powder	650-1300 milligrams
Tincture	5-30 drops

ADMINISTRATION

Oral

Round worms (vermifuge): Take 2 fluid ounces to 1 teacup of the infusion night and morning, or take the dosage night and morning and an active cathartic every 2nd or 3rd morning; or take 1/2-2 grams of powder night and morning, followed by an appropriate cathartic as indicated; or see "FORMULAS" (especially for children). This will clean the worms from the stomach and leave it toned up.

Dyspepsia, melancholic, jaundice, debility, etc: Take 2 fluid ounces of the infusion 3 to 4 times daily.

Skin

Rheumatism, sprains fomentations, neuralgia, etc: Apply fomentation of the herb; or, use the oil as a liniment.

FORMULAS

Dr. Shook's anthelmintic vermifuge

1/2 ounce	Wormwood herb (Artemisia absinthium)
1/2 ounce	Tansy herb (Tanacetum vulgare)
1/2 ounce	Santonica buds (Artemisia santonica, A. pauciflora)
1/2 ounce	German camomile flowers (Matricaria chamomilla)

Preparation: Boil 1 quart of water and, when boiling, pour over the herbs; allow to simmer 2 to 3 minutes (cover well); allow to cool, strain, bottle and keep in a cool place.

Dosage: 1 tablespoonful to 2 fluid ounces 2 times daily. Children: 1 teaspoonful to 1 tablespoonful 2 times daily.

Cystitis (inflammation of the bladder)

2 ounces Wormwood herb (Artemisia absinthium)
2 ounces Life root or golden ragwort root or herb (Senecio aureus)
2 ounces Camomile flowers (Chamaemelum nobile; Anthemis nobilis)

Preparation: Simmer the herbs 15 minutes in 5 pints of water.

Administration: Foment over the affected parts as hot as convenient: give composition tea freely (see page 147-148) and continue to foment until the patient sweats; follow this with the cystitis formula found on page 241.

Indigestion, dyspepsia

3 parts Wormwood herb (Artemisia absinthium)
2 parts Shavegrass herb (Equisetum hyemale; E. arvense)
2 parts Aniseed (Pimpinella anisum)
2 parts Thyme herb (Thymes vulgaris)

Preparation: Infuse 1 teaspoonful of the mixed herbs into 1 pint of boiling hot water; cover well and steep 20 minutes, strain, sweeten to taste, and keep cool.

Dosage: 2 fluid ounces 3 to 4 times daily.

Migraine Headache

1 teaspoonful Wormwood herb (Artemisia absinthium)
1 teaspoonful Culver's root (Veronicastrum virginicum)
1/4 teaspoon Cayenne (Capsicum frutescens; C. minimum)

Preparation: Steep the first 2 herbs for 20 minutes in 1 pint of boiling hot water (cover); strain, stir in the cayenne, bottle and keep in a cool place.

Dosage: 2 fluid ounces as needed (regulate to suit bowels).

Round worms (vermifuge)

1 ounce Wormwood herb (Artemisia absinthium)
1 ounce Rue herb (Ruta graveolens)
1 ounce Peach leaves (Prunus Persica; Amygdalus Persica)

Preparation: Pour 1 quart of boiling hot water over the herbs and steep for 1 hour (cover well); strain, sweeten well, bottle and keep in a cool place. Children: 1/2 teacupful (3 ounces) 3 to 4 times daily on an empty stomach.

Growth characteristics:
Perennial; found nearly all over the world from United States to Siberia; grows best in shady conditions; flowers June-September. It is easily propagated in the autumn by root division or cutting, or the seed may be sown in autumn soon after they are ripe (they are slow to germinate); plant 2 feet apart.

Collection:
Gather the herb when it is in flower, June-September.

Drying and preservation:
The herb should be dried with care so that its aromatic and volatile properties are not lost. Immediately after drying, the herb should be placed in an air-tight container, as otherwise it will absorb about 12% moisture from the air.

Sister plants:
-Beach Wormwood or Dusty Miller (Artemisia Stellerana; COMPOSITAE); creeping stems 2 feet long, leaves are whitish, broad, deeply cut; spreads rapidly.
-Sea Wormwood or Old Woman (Artemisia maritima; COMPOSITAE); herb: has similar, but less potent therapeutic properties and medicinal uses as wormwood, which it resembles but is smaller; stem rises 12-18 inches, leaves are similar but twice pinnatifid, small and oblong flower-heads (3-6 tubular florets, yellowish or brownish tint).

MALE FERN or FILIX MAS or BEAR'S PAW ROOT
(Dryopteris Filix-mas; D. marginalis; Aspidium Filix-mas; POLYPODIACEAE)

Common names:
Male fern, filix mas, bear's paw root, male shield fern, sweet brake, knotty brake, shield root; felix mas, Radix Filicis maris (Br.); Fougere male (Fr.); Rhizome Filicis, Farnwurzel, Wurmfarn, Waldfarn, Johanniswurzel (Ger.).

Identifying characteristics:

Stem	No true stem (fronds).
Leaves	Fronds, several, 2-4 feet high or long, wide and spreading, bipinnate, stiff, erect, broadly lanceolate, bright green, oval, acute, leafy nearly to bottom, stalk covered with brown scaly hairs; PINNAE (leaflets are arranged alternately on the mid-rib which is also hairy), the lower ones decreasing in size and each pinna divided again almost to its own mid-rib, the pinnules being oblong and rounded, with their edges slightly notched and their surface somewhat furrowed. The sort or clusters of spore cases are on the upper half of the frond, at the back of the pinnules, in round masses towards the base of the segments, covered with a conspicuous, roundish heart-shaped indusium or membrane.

Flowers	None, asexual fructification.
Fruit	Spores (dust-like, almost invisible seeds), contained in little roundish membrane or indusium (resembling the shields of ancient days), appearing as small dots situated on the veins near the mid-rib.
Rhizome	Horizontal, stumpy and creeping, 6-12 inches long, 2-3 inches thick, lies on the surface or just below the surface of the ground, covered with a stipes bases or "fingers", cylindrical, nearly straight, or brownish black, light brown when peeled; somewhat greenish internally, short fracture, spongy, 6-12 small wood or vascular bundles forming an irregular circle; matted roots (black, wiry, branched) spring from under surface, crown is brown, tangled mass (hairy bases of the leaves, undeveloped and rolled fronds). Powder: Greenish, brownish.
Taste	Bitterish, nauseous sweet, acrid, astringent.
Odor	Unpleasant, slight.

Parts used:
Root (rhizome and stipes).

Therapeutic action:
Anthelmintic (taeniafuge, vermifuge), astringent, tonic, vulnerary. Many species of the genus "Polypodium" have been sold as "American Aspidium," with disappointing results, but the European Aspidium will almost always eliminate worms.

Medicinal uses:
Expel worms (tape, round, seat or pin), wounds, rickets.

Preparations:
Fluid extract, infusion, oil, oleo-resin, powder, tincture. The fluid extract is prepared freshly as the root deteriorates rapidly, usually becoming greatly reduced in potency within 1-2 years.

Dosage:

Fluid extract	1-4 fluid teaspoons
Infusion	1 teacupful night and morning
Oil	5-30 drops
Oleo-resin	(extract) 3/4-1½ teaspoons
Powder	1/2-3 teaspoons
Tincture	1-1½ fluid teaspoons

ADMINISTRATION

Oral

Worms: Follow the procedure given on page 117 or take 1/2-1 teaspoonful of powder in the morning on an empty stomach (this can be administered in a capsule, mixed in honey, as an infusion, or in an emulsion—thick mucilage of gum Arabic and water), followed by a brisk purge of senna and ginger or butternut bark; or take 30 drops of oil (emulsion, capsule, warm water) night and morning, followed by a cathartic herb; or use the fluid extract, etc.

Worms (children): Mix equal parts of fluid extract and glycerine (shake well together). For ages 4 to 7 years, give 6 drops in jam; 7 to 12 years, give 12 drops in jam, over 12 years, give 1-2 teaspoonfuls in 1/2 teacupful (3 oz.) of cold water; follow with a cathartic tea (2 ounces of senna, 1/2 ounce of mountain flax, 1 large sliced lemon, steep for 30 minutes in 2 pints of boiling hot water). Administer the anthelmintic at 6 a.m. on an empty stomach, give the cathartic tea (to children over 12 years) at 8 a.m., serve breakfast at 9 a.m.

Skin

Wounds: Make into an ointment with olive oil and beeswax and apply to area.

FORMULAS

Male fern electuary

4 ounces Male fern, powder (Dryopteris Filix-mas)
Sufficient Honey

Preparation: Mix with sufficient honey to form a paste.

Dosage: 1 teaspoonful to 1 tablespoonful at night; follow in the morning with a senna or butternut laxative.

Worm powder (all types of worms)

2 ounces Male fern, powder (Dryopteris Filix-mas)
1/2 ounce Senna, powder (Cassia acutifolia, C. angustifolia)
1/4 ounce Jalap, powder (Ipomoea purga; I. jalapa)

Preparation: Mix thoroughly.

Dosage: 1/2 level teaspoonful in syrup or honey.

Dr. Shook's tapeworm remedy

4 grams Male fern root, powder (Dryopteris Filix-mas)
100 milligrams Mandrake root or Mayapple, powder (Podophyllum peltatum)
260 milligrams Jalap root, powder (Ipomoea purga; I. jalapa)
12 drops Broom pine oil (Pinus palustris)

Preparation: Mix well and fill into 6 capsules, equally divided.

Dosage: Take 1 capsule every 10 minutes until all are taken.

Note: Examine stools closely and do not forget the *thinnest* part of the worm bears the head. This must be eliminated or a new worm may grow.

Congenial combinations:
Male fern combines well with gum Arabic or acacia (Acacia Senegal), especially as an emulsion.

Growth characteristics:
Perennial; found in North America (Canada, westward to Rocky Mountains, Mexico), Andes Mountains of South America; Himalaya Mountains of North India, Europe, North Asia, Polynesian Islands; North Africa, South Africa; grows best for medicinal uses in temperate climates and on strata of volcanic origin, luxuriant in woods and shady situations, along moist banks and hedgerows. Germany was the chief supplier of European male fern.

Collection:
Dig and gather the older rhizomes in late autumn after the fronds die down.

Drying and preservation:
The potency in the root (rhizome) deteriorates rapidly in 1-2 years, so the fluid extract and tincture forms are best for preservation.

Sister plant:
Polypody Root or Female Fern or Rock Brake (Polypodium vulgare)

POMEGRANATE
(Punica Granatum; P. legrellei; P. sempervirehs; PUNICACEAE)

Common names:
Pomegranate, pomegranate bark, grenadier, punic apple, garnet apple, carthiginian apple; Granati Cortex (Br.); Ecorce do Grenadier, Ecore do Balaustier (Fr.); Granatwurzelrinde, Granatrinde (Ger.); Corteza de Granada (Span.); Melogranato, Malicorio, Scorzo del Melogranati (Ital.).

Identifying characteristics:
Stem — Shrub or small tree, up to 15 feet high, angular branches with spiny ends, young shoots and buds red, tough whitish wood. Bark, yellowish-brown with patches of grayish lichens, wrinkled, 1/50-1/7 inch thick, elliptical lenticels, furrows or abraded patches of cork (combined to form broad flat scales) light yellow and finely striate inner

	surface, dark green phelloderm, yellowish-green inner bark, short fracture and granular.
Leaves	Opposite, entire, smooth, glossy, thick, lanceolate, 1-3 inches long, almost evergreen.
Flowers	Large, red, glossy calyx, often in clusters of 2 to 3, nearly sessile, tubular, 1¼ inches long, 5 to 7 petals.
Fruit	Large pericarp, orange-size, thick reddish-yellow rind, short necked at top; acid pulp or membrane (edible, divides interior into 6-12 irregular cells), numerous seeds fastened to yellowish inner wall and filling the interior; seeds are angular, 1/2 inch long, edible, watery, pleasant flavor. Rind (dried) is curved, brittle, fragments, rough and yellowish-brown outside, paler and pitted inside (seed depressions).
Root	(Bark) Yellowish-brown, transversely curved pieces, irregular cork patches, conchoidal depressions; dark yellow internally, medullary rays extending nearly to outer surface. Powder: Yellowish-brown.
Taste	astringent, bitter, nauseous.
Odor	Slight.

Parts used:
Root bark (3 times stronger in alkaloids than stem bark), stem bark, flowers, fruit rind, seeds.

Therapeutic action:
Anthelmintic (taeniafuge, vermifuge), astringent, refrigerant, antibilious, anticancerous. Seeds: demulcent, cooling.

Medicinal uses:
Worms (tape, round, pin) diarrhea, leucorrhea, hemorrhage, intermittent fever, cancerous and other ulcers of mouth, throat, uterus, and rectum, sore throat, biliousness, spongy gums, loose teeth.

Preparations:
Decoction (bark); fluid extract, infusion (fruit rind, flowers), powder, tincture; the fresh or dried herb may be used.

Dosage:
Due to its potency, pomegranate should be given in small doses as indicated.

Decoction	(bark) 3 ounces every 4 hours.
Fluid Extract	(root bark) 1/4-2 teaspoons.
Infusion	(flowers, fruit rind) 6-8 fluid ounces.
Powder	(flowers, fruit rind) 1-2 grams.
Powder	(bark) 325-1,300 milligrams
Tincture	5-40 drops

ADMINISTRATION

Oral

Worms (tape, round, pin): Follow the procedure given on page 117; or, use the anthelmintic decoction (see "FORMULAS"). The powder may be used, but the decoction is preferred.

Diarrhea, hemorrhage, cancerous and other ulcers of the mouth, throat, uterus, and rectum, chronic dysentery: Use the fruit rind or flowers.

Skin

Sore throat: Use the fruit rind or flowers as a gargle.

Vaginal

Leucorrhea, douche: Use the fruit rind or flowers as an injection.

FORMULAS

Anthelmintic Decoction

4 ounces	Pomegranate root bark, cut (Punica Granatum)
3 pints	Distilled or D-cell water

Preparation: Simmer the herb in the water for 1 hour; strain, return the liquor to the cleansed vessel and reduce by simmering to 1 pint; strain, sweeten.

Dosage: 1/2 teacupful (3-4 ounces) every 4 hours.

Note: Results should be obtained within 24 hours; this can be taken in connection with the procedure given on page 117 or the patient can fast and clean the bowels with an appropriate cathartic the previous day, and afterwards an antibilious cathartic should be given.

Growth characteristics:
Perennial; found mostly in temperate and subtropical climates around the world, native of western Asia; grows widely in Mediterranean countries, southern United States, etc.; flowers June September.

AMERICAN WORMSEED or JERUSALEM OAK
(Chenopodium anthelminticum; C. ambrosioides; CHENOPODIACEAE)

Common names:
Jerusalem oak, American wormseed, wild wormseed, stinking weed, goose foot,

Jesuit's tea, Jerusalem tea; Anserine Vermifuge (Fr.); Amerikanischer Wurmsamen (Ger.); Herba Sancti Mariae, apasote, pazote (Span.).

Identifying characteristics:

Stem	Herbaceous, angular, coarse, stout, erect, furrowed or grooved, branched, 2-5 feet high.
Leaves	Alternate, yellowish-green, oblong-lanceolate, gland-dotted beneath (with small resinous particles), toothed (upper ones entire and tapering at both ends), slightly petioled.
Flowers	Small, very numerous, same color as leaves, in clusters of dense leafy, globular spikes (in the axis of slender, lateral, leafy branches), 5-cleft calyx, ovate and pointed lobes.
Fruit	Small, irregular (obtusely angled), depressed globular, size of pin head, perfectly enclosed in the calyx, greenish-gray or greenish-yellow or brown, glandular, 1/12 inch in diameter, membranous pericarp. Seed; small, smooth, glossy, solitary, lenticular, brownish-black, obtusely edged, albumen contains curved embryo.
Root	Branched.
Taste	Acrid, bitter, astringent, turpentine-like.
Odor	Strong, peculiar (camphoraceous) and resembling eucalyptus, aromatic.

Part used:
Seeds, oil, herb.

Therapeutic action:
Anthelmintic (vermifuge), antispasmodic, febrifuge, nervine, aromatic, expectorant, emmenagogue, tonic, diffusive, stimulant, diuretic, cardiac stimulant, diaphoretic. The leaves and seeds of Jerusalem oak were an old American Indian remedy for worms and painful menstruation. The powdered seeds are one of the best vermifuge remedies in nature. The seeds are rich in a volatile oil that is a useful expectorant for pulmonary complaints. It increases the power of the heart, and promotes secretions of the bronchi, kidneys, and skin.

Medicinal uses:
Round worms, hookworm (oil), tapeworm (especially good for children), intermittent fevers, hysteria, chorea, nervous affections, painful menstruation, pulmonary congestion, bronchitis, asthma, flatulent dyspepsia, chronic malaria.

Preparations:
Decoction, fluid extract, infusion, juice, oil, powder, tincture. Do not use the oil during pregnancy, because of its potent emmenagogic effect.

Decoction	Simmer 1 oz. of the fresh plant for 20 minutes in 1 pint of water.
Infusion	Make tea from the bruised leaves; covered to preserve volatile oil.

Juice	Express the juice from the fresh plant.
Oil	The seed is very high in the medicinally valuable volatile oil.
Powder	The seed should be bruised or powdered before using.

Dosage:

Decoction	1 tablespoonful to 2 fluid ounces
Fluid Extract	1/2-1 teaspoonful
Infusion	2 fluid ounces
Juice	1 tablespoonful
Oil	3-20 drops; children: 3-10 drops
Powder	1/4-2 teaspoonfuls (1-8 grams); for children: 1-2 grams
Tincture	1/2-1 fluid teaspoon

ADMINISTRATION

Usually the powdered seeds in honey, syrup, or jam is the favored method, but the other forms are also good.

Oral

Round worms: Give 1-2 grams of powdered seeds or 3-10 drops of oil to children; and generally give 1-2 teaspoonfuls of the powdered seed or 10-20 drops of oil to adults; the powdered seeds should be administered according to the procedure indicated on page 117. Also the fluid extract, fresh juice, decoction, or electuary (1-2 grams of powder for children) may be used.

Pulmonary congestion, asthma, painful menstruation: Use herb decoction.

FORMULAS

Round worms

1 ounce	American wormseed (Chenopodium anthelminticum)
1 ounce	Pink root (Spigelia marilandica)
1 ounce	Manna, exudation (Fraxinus Ornus)

Preparation: Pour 1 quart of boiling-hot water over the herbs, cover well, and steep for 1 hour; strain, sweeten, bottle and keep in a cool place.

Dosage: 4 ounces 4 times daily on an empty stomach.

Potter's emmenagogue

1 part	American wormseed (Chenopodium anthelminticum)
1 part	Black hellebore root (Helleborus niger)
1 part	Valerian root (Valeriana officinalis)

1 part   Mugwort herb (Artemisia vulgaris)

Preparation: Steep (covered) 1 teaspoonful of mixed herbs to each cupful of boiling hot water.

Dosage: 2-3 fluid ounces (warm).

Growth characteristics:
Perennial or annual (depending on the climate); found in almost all parts of the United States, native of Central and South America, West Indies, also found in Europe and North Africa, cultivated in Maryland for the oil; grows along roadsides and in waste places, about dwellings and in manured soils; flowers July-September.

Collection:
The fruits ripen successively in autumn and should be gathered in October.

Sister plants:
-Mexican Tea (Chenopodium ambrosioides; Herba Botryos Mexicanae; CHENOPODIACEAE); fruit or seed, herb: medicinally similar to Jerusalem oak and resembles it, except that it is more strongly aromatic, leaves more deeply toothed (lower ones almost pinnatifid) spikes more elongated, usually leafless; found in Europe and Asia.
-Feather Geranium or Jerusalem oak or Ambrosia (Chenopodium Botrys; CHENOPODIACEAE); herb: worms, catarrh, asthma; leaves on the small plant resemble oak leaves in shape and appearance (even turning red and yellow like oak leaves), are 1 inch long, the leaves diminish to almost nothing as the plant grows 2-3 feet high, and feathery branches develop; self-sows profusely; native to Europe and Asia.

KOUSSO or KUSSO
(Brayera anthelmintica; Hagenia abyssinica; ROSACEAE)

Common names:
Kousso, Kusso, Cusso, Kooso, Cossoo.

Identifying characteristics:

Stem	Beautiful ornamental tree, 20 to 40 feet high, round rusty branches, yellowish, flattened, furrowed, hairy, glandular, brownish cork, nodes, large pith.
Leaves	Alternate, crowded imparipinnate, 10 to 12 inches long; leaflets are oblong, acute, serrate, sessile, 3 to 6 pairs, 3 to 4 inches long.
Flowers	Monoecious (unisexual—both staminate and pistillate flowers on same plant), greenish-yellow, becoming purple (pistillate), small,

	brats, turbinate calyx, purple-veined bractlets, 1/2 inch across, 5 petals, 20 fertile stamens (staminate), 1 broad and hairy stigmas (pistillate); inflorescence is usually sold in the form of a reddish- brown cylindrical roll about 12 inches long and 2½ inches in diameter, consisting of the female or pistillate flowers. The staminate or male flowers are easily distinguished by their green color, fertile stamens and outer hairy sepals, whereas the pistil late flowers are a dark red color (the staminate are much less active). Powder: Brownish.
Taste	Bitter, acrid.
Odor	Balsamic.

Parts used:
Fresh or dried flowers (pistillate preferred); also herb, unripe fruit.

Therapeutic action:
Anthelmintic (taeniafuge), cathartic, astringent. Kousso is generally quick and effective, and is safe, but it is sometimes slightly nauseous, and occasionally may excite heat, followed by vomiting (rare) or diuresis. Since its purgative power is often insufficient to expel the head of the parasite, a brisk antibilious cathartic is often necessary if the bowels do not move within 4 hours.

Medicinal uses:
Tape worms (both types).

Preparations:
Fluid extract, infusion, powder.

Dosage:

Fluid Extract	2-4 fluid teaspoons
Infusion	See "FORMULAS."
Powder	1-2 teaspoons taken successively.

ADMINISTRATION

Kousso is more effective if you abstain from food and drink lemon juice freely before and after the dosage. If a bowel movement does not occur within 4 hours, take a brisk antibilious cathartic.

FORMULAS

Anthelmintic infusion of Kousso

3/4 ounce	Kousso flowers (Brayera anthelmintica)
1 pint	Distilled or D-cell water

Preparation: Pour the boiling-hot water over the herb, cover, and steep for 15 minutes (do not strain).

Dosage: Stir up the powder and drink the whole in 3 doses, 10 minutes apart.

Congenial combinations:
Kousso is combined effectively with male fern.

Growth characteristics:
Perennial; found in Abyssinia, North-Eastern Africa; grows 3,000-8,000 feet in the tablelands and mountains.

Drying and preservation:
The flowers are often powdered, but owing to its high price it is apt to be adulterated, so the flower in the whole or cut form is advisable.

PINK ROOT or CAROLINA PINK or WORMGRASS
(Spigelia marilandica; LOGANIACEAE)

Common names:
Pink root, Carolina pink, wormgrass, Indian pink, Maryland pink, American worm grass, Carolina wormroot, Maryland wormroot, American wormroot, starbloom.

Identifying characteristics:

Stem	Several, smooth, simple, rounded below, square above, 1 to 2 feet high, purplish.
Leaves	Few, opposite, sessile, ovate-lanceolate (acuminate at apex, tapering at base), smooth.
Flowers	Few, large, scarlet red externally, yellow within, long and club shaped corollas that terminate in spreading, star-like petals, borne in a brilliant red-pink spike on one side of stem above the leaves, surrounding the fruit.
Fruit	Double capsule, many-seeded.
Root	Rhizome, horizontal, dark brown, cup-shaped scars above (from stems of previous years), numerous root lets beneath, 2/5 to 2 inches long, 1/12 to 1/2 inch thick, knotty, tortuous, short and brittle fracture, whitish wood and dark brown pith internally, spiral markings in cells of wood; rootlets, thin, brittle, long, lighter colored than rhizome. Powder: grayish-brown.
Taste	Bitter, sweetish, pungent, somewhat nauseous.
Odor	Slightly aromatic.

Part used:
Root, herb.

Therapeutic action:
Anthelmintic (taeniafuge, vermifuge) for adults and children. It is safe and harmless as long as it is administered properly. It works for both tapeworms and round worms; usually a purgative agent such as senna is added, which speeds and aids its action.

Medicinal uses:
Tapeworms, round worms.

Preparations:
Fluid extract, infusion, powder, tincture. Pink root is usually combined with purgatives such as senna, and/or in formulas with other anthelmintic agents. The strength deteriorates rapidly with age.

Dosage:
Because of the potency of pink root, take care to administer as indicated.

Fluid Extract	1/4-1 fluid teaspoon
Infusion	6-8 ounces morning and night; children: 1 tablespoon morning and night
Powder	1-2 teaspoons; children (4 years and over), 650-1,300 milligrams
Tincture	1/2-1 fluid teaspoon

FORMULAS

Compound infusion of pink root

1 ounce	Pink root or herb (Spigelia marilandica)
1/2 ounce	Senna leaves (Cassia acutifolia; C. angustifolia)
1/2 ounce	Fennel seeds (Foeniculum vulgare)

Preparation: Pour 1 pint of boiling hot water over the herbs, cover, steep for 20 minutes, strain, sweeten.

Dosage: 1 teacupful morning and evening; children, 1 tablespoonful morning and evening.

Pink root anthelmintic powder
(children especially)

2 teaspoons	Pink root, powder (Spigelia marilandica)
2 teaspoons	American wormseed, powder (Chenopodium anthelminticum)
1.3 grams	Cascara sagrada, powder (Rhamnus purshiana)

Preparation: Mix well and divide into 12 equal doses (about 1 gram each).

Dosage: Children, 1 dose 3 to 4 times daily until the whole is taken (mix with honey, syrup, molasses, jelly). Repeat within a week or so to destroy young worms that have possibly hatched from eggs left in the intestines. If there is itching in the rectum, it can be relieved by a small enema (an injection) of warm water in which garlic or onions have been crushed and then strained. Always keep the outside of the rectum clean with soap and water. Itching in the sexual organs may indicate that the worms have migrated to these parts, and you can give the foregoing injection in these parts.

Note: Any good cathartic such as mandrake, senna, or cascara sagrada may be used, but we do not recommend castor oil internally. In using these more potent herbs, do not overdose the patient; when instructions are followed, they are safe and reliable.

Round and pin worms

1 ounce	Pink root, powder (Spigelia marilandica)
1 ounce	American wormseed, crushed seeds (Chenopodium anthelminticum)
1 ounce	Senna leaves (Cassia acutifolia; C. angustifolia)
1/2 ounce	Balmony (Chelone glabra)
1 teaspoonful	Anise (aniseed), crushed seeds (Pimpinella anisum)

Preparation: Steep the herbs in 1 quart of water for 2 hours; strain, sweeten, bottle and keep in a cool place.

Dosage: 3 ounces 3 to 4 times daily; children, 2 fluid ounces 4 times daily on an empty stomach.

Worm tea

1/2 ounce	Pink root (Spigelia marilandica)
1/2 ounce	Male fern, root (Dryopteris Filix-mas)
1/2 ounce	Santonica, crushed seeds (Artemisia santonica)
1/2 ounce	Senna leaves (Cassia acutifolia, C. angustifolia)
1/2 ounce	Fennel seeds, crushed (Foeniculum vulgare)
1/2 ounce	Manna, exudation (Fraxinus Ornus)

Preparation: Be sure to bruise the roots and crush the seeds if not using the powdered herbs. Pour 1 quart of boiling-hot distilled water over the herbs, cover, and steep for 20 minutes; strain, sweeten well, bottle and keep in a cool place.

Dosage: 1 teacupful (6 ounces) 2 to 4 times daily; children, 2 tablespoonfuls to 2 fluid ounces 3 to 4 times daily (according to age, etc.).

Growth characteristics:
Perennial root, annual stems; found in southern and southwestern United States; grows in rich, dry soils on the edges of woods, flowers May-July.

Collection:
Gather the entire herb in autumn (it is easier to distinguish the root with the herb attached than the root alone, which is sometimes adulterated).

Sister plants:
-Demerara Pink Root or Wormgrass (Spigelia anthelmia; LOGANIACEAE); root: therapeutic action is stronger than pink root; found in West Indies and northern South America, growing abundantly in the tropics, it is an annual with similar habits to pink root, grows up to 2 feet high, leaves are lanceolate below, broad and almost ovate above, in whorls of 4, flowers are light reddish and 1/2 inch long, rhizome is short and blackish externally and whitish internally with long, thin roots, the taste is bitter and acrid, and the odor is nauseous; it has long been used by native Indians as a worm remedy, but its potency indicates caution and that it be administered in smaller dosages than pink root.
-Carolina Pink or Georgia Pink (Phlox Carolina); root: similar but less valued as an anthelmintic to that of pink root; rhizome is rather coarse and straight, brownish-yellow with a straw-colored wood underneath, readily removable bark.
-Smooth Phlox (Phlox glaberrima); root: resembles pink root and is used in some localities as an anthelmintic, the Phlox varieties are confused for and form an adulteration of pink root.
-Mountain Phlox (Phlox ovata); root: it is used in some localities and sometimes offered for pink root.

TANSY or BITTER BUTTONS
(Tanacetum vulgare; COMPOSITAE)

Common names:
Tansy, bitter buttons, parsley fern, hindheal, buttons, bachelor's buttons, English cost, scented fern, ginger, ginger plant, Johnson's remedy, cheese; Tanaisie, Herbe amere, Barbotine (Fr.); Rainfarn, Wurmkraut, Reinfahren (Ger.); Tanasia, Tanacato commune, Aniceto, Daneta, Frangia, Tanacetro (Ital.); Tanaceto, Hierba Iombriguera (Span.).

Identifying characteristics:
Stem — Erect, leafy, tough angular (obscurely hexagonal), grooved, 1 to 3 feet tall, striated, often reddish.
Leaves — Alternate, dark green, deeply and pinnately cleft into narrow and toothed segments (feathery), about 6 to 8 inches long, about 4 inches wide, about 12 segments on either side and a terminal one, attached to a toothed midrib, smoothish, segments are obtuse, oblong, serrate,

	glandular.
Flowers	Small, heads found (button-like), golden yellow, flat, or tubular florets packed within a depressed involucre, borne in dense terminal, flat-topped corymbs, naked (flowers appear as if all the petals have been pulled off, leaving only the central florets), convex receptacle.
Fruit	Small and oblong achene (seeds), 5-6 ribs, crowned with pappus.
Root	Fibrous, creeping.
Taste	Bitter, pungent.
Odor	Strong, characteristic, aromatic, disagreeable.

Part used:
Herb, seed.

Therapeutic action:
Anthelmintic (vermifuge, the seed), tonic, emmenagogue, diaphoretic, stimulant, diuretic, nervine (relaxant), vulnerary, aromatic, stomachic, antispasmodic, carminative. Mixed with elder leaves it serves as an effective fly repellent, and it is valued for relieving pain and inflammation in local applications. The leaves may be used as a flavoring agent.

Medicinal uses:
Expels worms, menstrual problems (amenorrhea, leucorrhea, dysmenorrhea), intermittent fevers, colds, flu, hysteria, colic, nervous affections, ague, kidney problems, jaundice, dropsy, heart palpitation, flatulence, spasms, eruptive skin diseases, rheumatism, ulcers, tumors, sprains, bruises, inflammation, wounds, freckles, sunburn, sciatica, inflamed eyes, toothache, dyspepsia, poor digestion, nausea, weak veins, gout, dysentery.

Preparations:
Decoction, fluid extract, infusion, powder, solid extract, tincture. Tansy is an aromatic that possesses a valuable volatile essential oil that is very medicinal that should be preserved with care.

Dosage:

Decoction	1 tablespoonful to 6 ounces
Fluid Extract	1/2-2 fluid teaspoons
Infusion	2-8 fluid ounces 2 to 3 times daily
Powder	1-3 grams
Solid Extract	325-650 milligrams
Tincture	1/2-1 fluid teaspoon

ADMINISTRATION

Give in small and repeated doses: extra large doses may cause venous congestion and resultant discomfort to the abdominal organs.

Oral

Worms: Take 3-6 ounces of the infusion (especially of the crushed seeds) night and morning, following the cleansing procedure given on page 117 or fasting during the time.

Hysteria, nervous affections, kidney problems: Take 2 fluid ounces of the infusion repeated frequently (5-6 times daily).

Low fevers, ague, colds: Take small and frequent dosages of the warm infusion.

Heart trouble, palpitation: Make a decoction by simmering the herb 10 minutes, take 2 fluid ounces 4 to 5 times daily.

Spasms, flatulence, stomach disorders: Take the infusion, making sure to preserve the volatile essential oils which possess much of the medicinal potency.

Gout: Take the infusion of the green herb (as indicated), or an infusion of dried seeds and flowers (1 teaspoonful 2 to 3 times daily), or decocted syrup of the root, fasting during the treatment.

Skin

Eruptive diseases (chicken pox, smallpox, measles, etc.): Use the infusion or decoction as a wash, etc.

Sprains, bruises, inflammations, rheumatism, sciatica, etc.: Bruise and apply the green leaves, or use the infusion as a fomentation, wash, etc.

Flies, insect repellent: Use a preparation combined with elder leaves.

FORMULAS

Infusion of tansy

1 ounce	Tansy herb, cut (Tanacetum vulgare)
1 pint	Distilled or D-cell water

Preparation: Boil the water and pour it boiling-hot over the herb, cover and steep 10 to 15 minutes; strain, sweeten to taste, bottle and keep in a cool place.

Dosage: From 2 fluid ounces 5 to 6 times daily to 6 ounces 2 to 3 times daily. Small children, reduce dosage according to age.

Potter's vermifuge

1 part Tansy herb or seeds (Tanacetum vulgare)
1 part Wormwood herb (Artemisia absinthium)
1 part Santonica or levant wormseed (Artemisia santonica)
1 part Camomile flowers (Chamaemelum nobile)

Preparation: Steep 10-15 minutes (while tightly-covered) 1 teaspoonful of the mixed herbs to each cupful of boiling-hot water; strain.

Dosage: 2 ounces 3 times daily (see also "Dr. Shook's formula", page 119).

Growth characteristics:
Perennial; native of Europe, brought to America by early colonists and is found in many parts of the United States (especially along roadsides, in waste places, etc., in the East and Midwest); flowers July-September. Tansy can be grown in every herb garden in this country, as it thrives in almost any soil; it may be propagated and increased either spring or autumn by slips or dividing the creeping root (plant at least 1 foot apart), which will overspread the ground in a short time if allowed to remain undisturbed.

Collection:
Cut the herb close above the roots when it first comes into flower.

Drying and preservation:
Handle as with other aromatics, being careful to preserve the volatile oils.

Sister plants:
-Double Tansy (Tanacetum vulgare var. crispum; COMPOSITAE); herb: cultivated and possesses similar therapeutic properties and medicinal uses as tansy; leaves are twice pinnatifid and curled, native of Southern Europe.
-(Tanacetum Balsamita; Pyrethrum Tanacetum; COMPOSITAE); herb: similar therapeutic properties and medicinal uses as tansy; strong odor, bitter taste, native of Southern Europe, cultivated.

PUMPKIN SEEDS
(Cucurbita pepo; Semen Peponis; Semina Curcurbitae; CUCURBITACEAE)

Common names:
Pumpkin seeds, pumpkin, cold seeds; Cucurbitae Semina Praeparata, Pumpkin melon, English melons, millions (Br.); Semences de Potirons, Citrouille (Fr.); Kuerbissamen, Kurebisterne (Ger.); Semillas de calabaza comun (Span.).

Identifying characteristics:

Stem	Trailing, rough, hollow, hairy, 10-30 inches long, branched tendrils.
Leaves	Large, 10-20 inches long, 6-12 inches wide, green, obtusely cordate (heart-shaped), hispid (covered with stiff and bristly hairs), palmately 5-lobed, serrate, petioles 3-8 inches long.
Flowers	Large, yellow, 2-5 inches wide, bell-shaped, axillary, monoecious.
Fruit	Large, yellow, round, oblong, 10-20 inches in diameter, furrowed, smooth, fleshy internally with seeds. Seed: broadly elliptical, ovate, 3/5-5/6 inches long, 1/4-3/8 inch broad, 1/12-1/8 inch thick yellowish-white, smooth, shallow groove near margin, often transparent fragments of adhering pulp; short fracture, seed coat of white coriaceous (tough) outer layer and membranous (sometimes dark green) inner layer, whitish embryo, small conical hypocotyl, planoconvex cotyledons. Powder: Yellowish-white.
Taste	Bland, oily.
Odor	Slight when crushed.

Part used:
Ripe seeds (best when fresh).

Therapeutic action:
Anthelmintic (taeniafuge, vermifuge), diuretic, nutritive.

Pumpkin seed expels both tape and round worms. Some herbalists advocate the removal of the outer husk, and others contend that the whole should be taken. The active principle is in the acrid and resinous envelope immediately surrounding the embryo. Make an emulsion or simply take the crushed seeds for worms. The infusion of the crushed seeds is a diuretic.

Medicinal uses:
Worms (tapeworm, roundworm), renal problems (urinary complaints).

Preparations:
Infusion, crushed seeds. Best when fresh seeds are used. Infusion: Steep 1 ounce of crushed seeds for 15-20 minutes in 1 pint of boiling hot water.

Dosage:

Infusion	1 teacupful or more (up to 1 pint daily).
Crushed seeds	1-2 ounces or more

ADMINISTRATION

There is no harshness, so a larger dosage will not be harmful if necessary.

Oral

Worms: Take 1 pint of emulsion (2 ounces of seeds crushed in honey and water) in 3 doses at 2 hour intervals; or take 1-2 tablespoonfuls of the crushed seeds in honey, syrup, etc., in 3 doses at 2 hour intervals. The patient should fast during the treatment, then take an appropriate cathartic several hours after the last dosage (or follow procedure on page 117).

Urinary complaints: Take the infusion, 1 teacupful 3 to 4 times daily.

FORMULAS

The Four Greater Cold Seeds remedy
(catarrhal affections, bowel and urinary disorders, fever, etc.)

1 part Pumpkin seeds, crushed (Cucurbita pepo)
1 part Ground seeds, crushed (Cucurbita maxima)
1 part Watermelon seeds, crushed (Citrullus lanatus; C. vulgaris)
1 part Cucumber seeds, crushed (Cucumis sativus)

Preparation: Triturate with water and make into an emulsion.

Dosage: 1 teacupful 3 to 4 times daily.

Growth characteristics:
Annual; native of tropical Africa, and cultivated in the warmer and temperate climates around the world; needs ample water either by rainfall or irrigation.

Collection:
Separate the seeds from the fleshy fruit when ripe, wash to remove pulp, dry or crush and use. The outer seed coating (testa or husk) may be removed before using or the whole may be ground fine and taken.

Drying and preservation:
The seeds are more potent when used matured and fresh, but may be dried and stored in appropriate containers.

Sister plants:
-Watermelon seed (Citrullus lanatus; C. vulgaris; RUTACEAE) (older texts may use Cucurbita citrullus, Cucumis citrullus; CUCURBITACEAE); seeds: similar therapeutic value and medicinal uses as pumpkin seeds; fruit: fevers (Potter's gives a good cooling formula that consists of equal parts of watermelon seeds, common melon seeds, and cucumber seeds), urinary affections (especially strangury), dropsy, hepatic congestion, intestinal catarrh; very large and edible fruit; seed is flat, ovate, 1/2 inch long, blackish, marbled, or orange-brown, ungrooved, blunt on the edge. Cultivated in temperate and warmer regions around the world.

-Common Melon or Musk Melon or Casaba (Cucumis melo; CUCURBITACEAE): seeds, fruit: similar therapeutic properties as the watermelon and pumpkin, and cultivated in the same regions.

SANTONICA or LEVANT WORMSEED

(Artemisia santonica (Linn.); A. cina (Berg.); A. pauciflora; A. Lercheana; A. maritima var. pauciflora; A. maritima var. Stechmanniana; A. Chamaemelifolia; COMPOSITAE)

Common names:
Santonica, Levant wormseed, Alepo wormseed, Tartarian southern wood, Semen contra vermes; Semen-contra d'Alep, Barbotine (Fr.); Flores Cinae, Zitworbluetensamen, Wurmsamen (Ger.); Semenzina (Ital.).

Identifying characteristics:

Stem	Small and semi-shrubby plant; branching from crown, several (6-8) erect, flowering, 1 foot high, leafy at first, woolly or glabrous.
Leaves	Bipinnatisect, 1/2 inch long, woolly when young, afterward grayish.
Flowers	Heads (commonly called "seeds"), 1/12-1/6 inch long, 1/25 inch wide, grayish-green or yellowish-green (turning brownish with age), oblong-ovoid, slightly flattened, obtuse, smooth, glossy; each has 12-18 oblong-obtuse scales closely overlapping each other and bearing minute yellow glands on their surface; broad midribs enclose 3-5 rudimentary florets, without pappus; at first glance when dried, the unexpanded flower heads appear as brownish ridged seeds.
Root	Knotty, fibrous.
Taste	Bitter, aromatic.
Odor	Characteristic, strong, camphoraceous.

Parts used:
Unexpanded flower buds or heads.

Therapeutic action:
Anthelmintic (taeniafuge, vermifuge), stimulant, emmenagogue.

Medicinal uses:
Worms (tape, round, thread or seat or pin).

Preparations:
Decoction, fluid extract, infusion, powder.

Dosage:

Decoction	1 tablespoonful-2 ounces.
Fluid Extract	1/2-1 fluid teaspoon.

Infusion	2-4 ounces.
Powder	650 milligrams-2 grams.

ADMINISTRATION

At times it will change the urine to a yellowish (acid) or reddish (alkaline) tint; follow the procedure given on page 117.

FORMULAS

This herb may be substituted as an anthelmintic in formulas where American wormseed or Jerusalem oak is used.

Growth characteristics:
Perennial; a Russian variety of Sea Wormwood native to North Turkestan, Siberia, and Chinese Mongolia on the vast plains of Kirghiz (especially near Chimkent).

Collection:
Gathered before the flower bud expands in July-August, forwarded to the great fair of Nizhnee-Novgorod, then to market via Moscow, Leningrad, Western Europe.

Drying and preservation:
The flowers exposed to light and air soon become brown and inactive, and hence should be preserved in appropriate dark and air-tight containers.

Allied plants:
Mexican Tea, Jesuit's Tea, or American Wormseed (Chenopodium anthelminticum; C. ambrosioides; CHENOPODIACEAE); seeds, oil, also herb: both the American and European remedies are referred to simply as "wormseed," and even though they are therapeutically similar as anthelmintic agents and are often used as substitutes, they should be carefully distinguished.

HYSSOP
(Hyssopus officinalis; LABIATAE)

Hyssop is treated in Chapter 7, "Diaphoretic Herbs" page 254. An infusion of hyssop is extremely useful where worms are found, and often no other remedy is necessary.

For a listing of alternative anthelmintic herbs, which may be used when the foregoing are not available, please see Chapter 17, "Herb Alternatives," page 638.

CHAPTER 4

THE ASTRINGENT HERBS

Astringents, or constringents, promote greater density and firmness of tissue, as compared to cathartics or laxatives. These herbs constringe, contract, and condense the cellular structures of muscles, arteries, nerves, etc. They also lessen or powerfully arrest blood hemorrhages from the lungs, renal organs, bowels, etc. by coagulating the albumin; and they lessen or arrest excessive perspiration or night sweats from lymphatic glands and skin tissues. Astringents are generally mucus cleansers, and they are used externally to contract and strengthen a relaxed or weakened condition of muscular fiber. In case of sores in the mouth, or loose teeth, where the gums need to be firmed up, astringents do excellent work. Some astringents are stimulant; others are sedative. Astringents also vary in strength.

BAYBERRY or WAX MYRTLE
(Myrica cerifera; M. caroliniensis; MYRICACEAE)

Common names:
Bayberry, wax myrtle, myrica, wax berry, candle berry, tallow bush, bayberry vegetable tallow tree, myrtle, tallow shrub, candle berry myrtle, American vegetable wax; Arbre a la cire, Myricae Cortex Cirier (Br.); Arbre a suif (Fr.); Wachgagel Wachsmyrte (Ger.); Albero della cera, Pianta della cera, Mortella cerifera (Ital.); arrayan brabantico (Span.).

Identifying characteristics:

Stem	Dense evergreen shrub, branching 2-4 feet high; bark has grayish, peeling epidermis that covers a hard, reddish-brown layer beneath, quilled and 1/16 inch thick, the inner surface is slightly fibrous with a granular fracture.
Leaves	Lanceolate, shining dark green, sometimes resinous, dotted on both sides, entire, fragrant when rubbed.
Flowers	Aments or catkins (unisexual, without calyx or corolla, staminate are yellow and longer, pistillate are greenish and short).
Fruit	Drupes or small globular berries in groups (growing close to the branches similar to juniper), at first green then become crusted with a greenish-white wax, hard stone with two-lobed and two-seeded kernel, gunpowder-like grains on outside of stone and under the wax covering.

Rootbark	Scaly, grayish and brownish, 1/25-1/10 inch thick, occasional warts, lenticels (cortical pores), striated, a brownish inner surface,quills. Powder: reddish-brown.
Taste	Astringent, bitter, pungent (acrid).
Odor	Characteristic, slightly aromatic.

Parts used:
Bark (preferably the rootbark), wax (from the berries), leaves.

Therapeutic action:
Bark: astringent, tonic, alterative, cholagogue, diuretic, sialagogue, emetic (large doses), hemostatic, styptic, vulnerary, errhine, sternutatory, discutient. Wax: mildly astringent, somewhat narcotic. Leaves: astringent, aromatic.

Some herbalists consider bayberry and lobelia as the most useful herbs in botanic medicine. Bayberry forms the base for the famous Composition Powder, which comes as near to being a cure-all as anything we have. Bayberry is a powerful stimulant, astringent and tonic, influencing the alimentary tract, toning and promoting glandular activity, all the while thoroughly cleansing and restoring the mucous secretions to normal function.

Bayberry is an effective deobstruent, and it is a useful cleansing tonic for the liver. Its stimulant properties affect the whole circulatory system, especially the arterial and capillary circulation, with a toning action on the tissues. Its astringent action is very potent, yet it does not dry the mucous membranes as the inorganic chemical agents such as alum do.

Bayberry is an excellent tonic for the uterus (especially during pregnancy), and is a valuable agent for arresting hemorrhage of the uterus, bowels or lungs. When used with cayenne, it is very effective in reviving the heat in the body and in inducing diaphoresis.

Medicinal uses:
Sore throat, cold extremities, chills, narcotic poisoning, emesis, hemorrhage (uterus, bowel, lungs), menorrhagia, leucorrhea, goiter, diarrhea, dysentery, ulcers, spongy and bleeding gums, boils, carbuncles, gangrenous sores, adenoids, fevers, flu, colic cramps, jaundice, scrofula, catarrh of stomach, dyspepsia, weak digestion, sluggish liver, slow healing wounds, burns, polypus (nasal, laryngeal, uterine), sore throat, frog, thrush, trench mouth, inflamed tonsils, catarrhal deafness, alopecia (loss of hair), dandruff, tooth powder.

Preparation:
Decoction, fluid extract, infusion, powder, tincture. For wax, boil the berries in water; the wax will soon float on the surface and may be removed upon cooling and hardening. The wax is used as a base for astringent salves.

Dosage:

Decoction	2 fluid ounces 3 to 4 times daily.
Fluid extract	1/2-1 teaspoonful.
Infusion	1 cupful.
Powder	1/2-1 teaspoon.
Tincture	15-30 drops.

ADMINISTRATION

The warm infusion promotes perspiration and improves arterial and capillary circulation, with a toning of the tissues.

Anal

Diarrhea, dysentery: See "FORMULAS"; or simply use the tea in enema form.

Nasal

Nasal catarrh: See "FORMULAS."

Nasal or laryngeal polypus (adenoids): Snuff or blow powder up the nostrils 3 to 4 times daily. At first there is pain, then sneezing every 20 to 30 seconds, continuing for 5 to 10 minutes; there will be copious discharges of thick, viscid and often stringy mucus. The powder causes the adenoids to dry up—an adenoid being an inflamed condition of the mucous membrane.

Oral

Chills, stomach catarrh, indigestion, etc.: Use the decoction or infusion with a little cayenne.

Goiter: Use in doses of 10 grains 3 times daily; take orally and use as a fomentation on the throat.

Narcotic poisoning: Administer liberal doses of the strong infusion or decoction (which contracts the capillaries of the stomach), then follow this with a lobelia emetic.

Hemorrhage (uterus, bowels, lungs), leucorrhea: Use the infusion or decoction alone, or in combination with suitable stimulants (cayenne, ginger, etc.).

Poor circulation, relaxed tissues (loss of muscle tone): Use the warm infusion or decoction.

Colds, flu, fever, etc.: Use bayberry in combination with diaphoretics (yarrow, catnip, peppermint, sage, etc.); it is very effective.

Fevers, flu, hoarseness, sluggish circulation, colic, cramps, colds, etc.: Use the Composition Powder (See "FORMULAS").

Sore throat, inflamed tonsils, catarrhal deafness: Make a strong decoction solution (boil 2 ounces of the herb 15 minutes in 1 pint of water, strain and add sufficient glycerine to make up the pint, cool); spray the solution into the nose and throat every 1 to 2 hours during one day, then gradually extend the time between applications.

Frog, thrush, trench mouth: Spray mouth and throat with tea in atomizer. If too young or throat too sore to gargle, then drink 1 or 2 tablespoons each hour until relief.

Sore throat: Gargle thoroughly with the decoction until throat is clean, then drink a pint lukewarm to cleanse stomach.

Emetic for narcotic poisoning, etc.: Use 1 or more teaspoons of the powder in 1 teacupful of boiling hot water and drink hot (including the powder), and even better, mix some lobelia with it. This may cause some temporary pain and nausea.

Skin

Alopecia (loss of hair), dandruff: Use a strong decoction and rub in well at night; wash off in the morning, brush the hair thoroughly and apply again (add a few drops of lavender oil). This will quickly stop falling hair and remove dandruff.

Slow-healing burns or wounds, indolent ulcers: Dust on powder and bandage; change according to discharge.

Boils, carbuncles, gangrenous sores: Apply the powder in a poultice.

Ulcers, spongy and bleeding gums: Use the decoction as a wash.

Vaginal

Douche: Use a warm tea; it is cleansing to the membrane and toning to the tissues.

Vaginal or uterine polyps: Spray powder on growth, leave on for 6 to 8 hours, wash away and repeat.

FORMULAS

Decoction

1 ounce Bayberry root bark (Myrica cerifera)

1 pint Distilled or D-cell water

Preparation: Simmer the herb for 10 minutes; cool, but do not strain.

Dosage: 2 fluid ounces 3 to 4 times daily (stir and take powder and all).

Abscess, ague, chills, colds, poor circulation, blood poisoning

4 parts Bayberry root bark (Myrica cerifera)
1 part Pinus bark or hemlock spruce (Tsuga canadensis; Pinus canadensis)
1 part Ginger (Zingiber officinalis)
2 parts Cayenne (Capsicum frutescens; C. minimum)
2 parts Cloves (Syzygium aromaticum; Eugenia aromatica)

Preparation: Use 1 tablespoonful of the compound in 1 pint of boiling hot water; cover well and steep until cool, strain.

Dosage: 2 tablespoonfuls or more 3 times daily.

Dr. Thompson's canker remedy

1 part Bayberry root (Myrica cerifera)
1 part White pond lily (Nymphaea odorata)
1 part Pinus or hemlock spruce inner bark (Tsuga canadensis)

Substitutes: Sumac (bark, leaves, berries), red raspberry leaves, witch hazel leaves, marsh rosemary.

Preparation: Pound and mix well together; steep 1 ounce of the powder in 1 pint of boiling water; sweeten.

Dosage: 2 fluid ounces.

Administration: In a serious case, add 1 teaspoonful of cayenne and teaspoonful of nervine powder to each dosage; give 3 doses at intervals of 15 minutes; give the same compound by injection and repeat if necessary.

Dr. Thompson's Composition Powder

2 pounds Bayberry root bark (Myrica cerifera)
1 pound Pinus or hemlock spruce inner bark (Tsuga canadensis)
1 pound Ginger (Zingiber officinalis)
2 ounces Cayenne (Capsicum frutescens; C. minimum)
2 ounces Cloves (Syzygium aromaticum; Eugenia aromatica)

Preparation: Pound into a fine powder, sift through a fine sieve and mix well together; use 1 teaspoonful of the composition and 1/2 teaspoonful of honey in 3-4 ounces of boiling hot water and drink as soon as it is sufficiently cool (be sure the patient is well-covered in bed, or covered by a blanket).

Thompson commentary:

> This composition is calculated for the first stages, and in less violent attacks of disease. It is a medicine of much value, and may be safely used in all complaints of male or female, and for children. It is good for relaxation, dysentery, pain in the stomach and bowels and for removing all obstructions caused by cold, or loss of inward heat.
>
> By taking a dose on going to bed, and putting a hot stone to the feet, wrapped in wet cloths, it will cure a bad cold, and will generally throw off a disease in its first stages, if repeated two or three times. If the symptoms are violent, with much pain, add to each dose a teaspoonful of brandy, gum myrrh, and stimulant tincture (cayenne, ginger, gotu-kola) and half a teaspoonful of lobelia (vinegar base), and in nervous symptoms add half a teaspoonful of nerve powder [see "Nerve Combination" page 558]; at the same time give an injection of the same. If these should not answer the purpose, the patient must be carried through at a regular course of the medicine, as has been described.

Dr. Nowell's
Composition Powder preparation

4 ounces	Bayberry root bark powder, (Myrica cerifera)
2 ounces	Ginger, powder, (Zingiber officinalis)
1 ounce	Pinus or hemlock spruce inner bark powder (Tsuga canadensis)
1 teaspoon	Cloves powder (Syzygium aromaticum; Eugenia aromatica)
1 teaspoon	Cayenne, powder (Capsicum frutescens; C. minimum)

Preparation: Mix and pass through a fine sieve at least twice; use 1 teaspoonful in 1 cupful of boiling-hot water, sweeten; cover and allow to stand a few minutes.

Dosage: Drink the clear liquid, or Dr. Shook recommends stirring the mixture and drinking the powder too for its stimulating benefits. Some people drink this as a culinary tea to help prevent disease.

Composition Powder
(for seniors)

12 ounces	Bayberry root bark (Myrica cerifera)
12 ounces	Ginger (Zingiber officinalis)
6 ounces	White poplar; quaking aspen inner bark (Populus tremuloides)

4 ounces Pinus or hemlock spruce inner bark (Tsuga canadensis)
4 teaspoons Cayenne (Capsicum frutescens; C. minimum)

Preparation: Use the powder form or pound into a fine powder; mix and sieve as before; use 1 teaspoonful of the compound in a cupful of boiling-hot water.

Dosage: 1 cupful of the clear liquid.

Nowell commentary:

> This will help in cases where circulation is weak and obstructed, and is a good article where the aged need a stimulating drink and where the lumbar region is painful, as the combination will help the urinary tract.

Diaphoretic

8 parts Bayberry root bark, powder (Myrica cerifera)
4 parts Ginger, powder (Zingiber officinalis)
1/2 part Cloves, powder (Syzygium aromaticum; Eugenia aromatica)
1/2 part Cayenne, powder (Capsicum frutescens; C. minimum)

Preparation: Use 1 teaspoon of the compound powder in 1 pint of boiling water.

Dosage: 1 cupful warm at 15 minute intervals until the desired effect is obtained.

Diarrhea, dysentery, piles, hemorrhoids, colitis (cathartic injection)

1 part Bayberry root bark, powder (Myrica cerifera)
1 part African ginger (Zingiber officinalis) use more pungent African variety
1 part Pinus or hemlock spruce inner bark, powder (Tsuga canadensis)

Preparation: Pour 3 pints of boiling-hot water over 1 level tablespoonful of the compound; steep 10-15 minutes; add sufficient cold water to make 2 or 3 quarts; let settle and pour carefully into the syringe.

Administration: Have the patient lie on the right side so that the liquid may readily fill the colon; where the patient has a weak rectum and cannot hold the water, have him take the inclined position with the head lower than the hips; females with a retroverted condition of the uterus may take the knee-chest position, which will help turn the uterus over and allow the liquid to enter.

Hemorrhoids (suppository)

2 ounces Bayberry root bark, powder (Myrica cerifera)
1 ounce Pinus or hemlock spruce inner bark, powder (Tsuga canadensis)

1 ounce Golden seal, powder (Hydrastis Canadensis)
1 ounce Wheat flour or slippery elm powder

Preparation: Mix together and add sufficient glycerine to form into suppository of the size desired.

Administration: Insert 1 suppository at nighttime.

Mucus discharges
(ears, nose, vagina, urethra, or any other part)

1/2 ounce Bayberry root bark, powder (Myrica cerifera)
1 dram Bistort, tincture (Polygonum bistorta)

Preparation: Steep the bayberry in 8 ounces of boiling-hot water, strain; add the bistort and mix.

Dosage: 2 fluid ounces morning and night.

Sinus catarrh (profuse discharge)

1 part Bayberry root bark, powder (Myrica cerifera)
2 parts Golden seal, powder (Hydrastis Canadensis)

Preparation: Mix and sift through a fine sieve.

Administration: Use the powder as a snuff.

Sore mouth (gargle)

1 ounce Bayberry root bark (Myrica cerifera)
1/2 ounce Golden seal (Hydrastis Canadensis)
1/2 ounce Blue cohosh root (Caulophyllum thalictroides)
1/2 ounce Witch hazel bark (Hamamelis virginiana)

Preparation: Steep the herbs for 30 minutes in 1 pint (16 ounces) of boiling-hot water; strain, sweeten as desired.

Stomach tonic
(Dr. Coffin's Stomach Bitters)

4 ounces Bayberry bark (Myrica cerifera)
4 ounces Balmony (Chelone glabra)
2 ounces White poplar or quaking aspen inner bark (Populus tremuloides)
2 ounces Ginger (Zingiber officinalis)
1/4 ounce Cayenne (Capsicum frutescens; C. minimum)

1/4 ounce Cloves (Syzygium aromaticum; Eugenia aromatica)

Preparation: Mix all herbs in powder form; use 1 teaspoon of the compound in 1 cup of hot water; cover and steep a few minutes; sweeten to taste.

Dosage: 1 cupful warm 2 to 3 times daily.

Note: This is an excellent compound to correct the bile, create appetite, and correct flatulence and systemic debilitation from disease.

Growth characteristics:
Perennial; found in eastern North America from Canada to Florida, grows in dry woods and fields, also in thickets near swamps and marshes in the sand belt near the Atlantic Coast and on the shores of Lake Erie; flowers appear in May before the leaves are fully expanded.

Collection:
Gather in the latter part of the fall or early spring before it puts forth leaves, cleanse thoroughly and separate the bark from the wood with a hammer, mallet or club while fresh (when it is easily separated).

WHITE OAK, or TANNER'S OAK
(Quercus alba; FAGACEAE)

COMMON EUROPEAN OAK or ENGLISH OAK
(Quercus robur; Q. pubescens; Q. pedunculata; Q. sessiliflora; FAGACEAE)

BLACK OAK or SCARLET OAK
(Quercus velutina; Q. coccinea FAGACEAE)

RED OAK
(Quercus rubra; FAGACEAE)

The local Western Scrub Oak is part of the same family and its uses are the same.

Common names:
Oak, tanner's oak, tanner's bark, acorn tree, cups and ladles, Jove's nuts, mast, pipes, etc.; Bouvre, Rovere, Querciloa (Ital.); ruble (Span.).

Identifying characteristics:
Stems — White: Stately tree, 60-80 feet high, 3-8 feet thick, branched, pale brownish bark; stringy or roughly fibrous and uneven fracture, 1/12-2/5 inch thick, not readily powdered, does not tinge the saliva yellow when chewed.

	English: Tall tree, 80 to 100 feet high, bark and branches young tree are grayish, somewhat polished externally and brownish internally, fibrous fracture, rough inner surface projecting medullary rays. Black: Tall tree, 80-100 feet high, 3-4 feet thick, resembles white oak, only reddish-brown in color and it tinges the saliva a brownish-yellow color.
Leaves	White: Large, light green, smooth, glaucous (powdery coating) with prominent veins beneath, 4 to 6 lobed, petiolate, brownish when dry. English: Old leaves hairy (Q. pubescens), smooth leaves (Q. pedunculata, Q. sessiliflora). Black: Oblong and lobed, 6 to 8 inches long, mucronate (encasing in a sharp point).
Flowers	White: Monoecious (staminate and pistillate flowers on the same-plant), staminate catkins, small pistillate flowers. English: Pistillate flowers on pedicels or stalks (Q. pedunculata) sessile flowers (Q. sessiliflora).
Fruit	White: 1-seeded ovoid nut or acorn, base in cupule. English: On pedicels or stalks (Q. pedunculata), sessile (Q. sessiliflora). Black: Acorns, 1/2-3/4 inch long, 1/2 inch thick, shallow but thick cupule.
Taste	Strongly astringent.
Odor	Characteristic, slightly aromatic.

Parts used:
Mainly the inner bark; also the leaves, acorn, acorn cups.

Therapeutic action:
Strongly astringent, slowly antiseptic, slightly stimulant, tonic, hemostatic, antivenomous, febrifuge, anti-emetic, diuretic (lithotriptic), anthelmintic (vermifuge).

The white oak variety is preferred by herbalists, the English is therapeutically similar, and the red and black oak barks are generally used for external applications. There are some eighty species of oaks, ranging from shrubs (scrub) to trees, that may, with their acorns, be used similarly. Because of its powerful astringent properties, oak bark is used for both external and internal hemorrhages. It cleanses abraded surfaces of the skin and mucous membranes. It expels pinworms, increases the flow of urine, and removes gall and kidney stones. It has a cleansing and toning influence on the entire alimentary tract.

Medicinal uses:
Internal and external hemorrhage, leuko diarrhea, dysentery, prolapsus uterine, prolapsed anus, relaxed vagina, sore mouth, gums, ulcerated and inflamed throat, diphtheria, seminal emissions, ulcerated bladder, bloody urine, pin worms, inflammations, burning fevers, infections, uterine troubles, piles, varicose veins,

kidney and liver problems, goiter, hardened neck, tumors, swelling ulcers, hard tumors, sores, tetters, ringworm, scaly eruptions, catarrh, colon troubles, gonorrhea, gleet, stomach troubles, relaxed tissue, thrush, infant cholera, hemoptysis, phthisis, prolapsed uvula, gangrene, tooth powder, washes, poisoning.

Preparation:
Decoction, fluid extract, infusion, powder, tincture.

Dosage:

Decoction	2 tablespoons to 2 fluid ounces.
Fluid extract	1/2-1 teaspoonful.
Infusion	1 cupful.
Powder	325 mg.-1 gram.
Tincture	1/4-1/2 teaspoonful.

ADMINISTRATION

Anal

Colon trouble, prolapsed anus, diarrhea, dysentery, gonorrhea, gleet: Use the injection in small and frequent doses.

Oral

Diphtheria: Where one suspects a light attack, a gargle with oak bark, with a little cayenne or composition powder added to arrest further development.

Ulcerated and inflamed throat: Use the decoction as a gargle.

Pinworms: Drink 1 cupful of the infusion 3 times daily.

Bleeding at the mouth, spitting blood, vomiting: Drink a tea of the bark and powder of the cups.

Poisoning and venomous bites, ulcerated bladder, bloody urine: Use the powder of the acorns and/or the bark made into a tea.

Inflammations, infections, fevers: The distilled water from the leaf buds is excellent both externally and internally.

Leucorrhea: Use the infusion of the leaves.

Dysentery, diarrhea: Use small doses of the infusion.

Skin

Poisonous bites: Take the tea internally and apply a poultice or fomentation of the powdered acorns and inner bark externally.

Sore mouth and sore or spongy gums: Use the decoction as a wash.

Ulcers, sores, varicose veins, tumors, tatters, inflammation, ringworm, scaly eruptions, etc.: Use the decoction as a wash, and bathe 3 to 4 times daily (dilute for open sores); also a fomentation may be wrapped around the affected part and covered well with flannel.

Gangrene: Apply the powdered bark as a poultice.

Goiter: Apply a hot fomentation of a strong decoction of the inner bark of oak; bind over the swollen gland with woolen or flannel cloth and repeat as required.

Vaginal

Leucorrhea, prolapsus uteri, relaxed vagina, etc.: Use as a vaginal injection.

FORMULAS

Bleeding (lungs, stomach or bowels)

1 part White oak (Quercus alba), etc.
1 part Tormentil (Potentilla erecta)
1 part Shavegrass (Equisetum hyemale)
1 part Shepherd's purse (Capsella bursa-pastoris)

Preparation: Steep 1 ounce of the herbs in 1 pint of boiling-hot water.

Dosage: 2 or 3 tablespoonfuls each 1/2 hour as needed.

Cancerous sores (ointment)

1/2 ounce White oak (Quercus alba)
1/3 ounce Garden Sage (Salvia officinalis)
1/2 ounce Tormentil (Potentilla erecta)
1/3 ounce Shavegrass (Equisetum hyemale)
1 teaspoon Balm (Melissa officinalis)

Preparation: Simmer for 1/2 hour in 1 quart of water; strain, reduce to 1/2 pint by simmering; add 1/2 pound of honey, bring to a boil and skim off the scum; allow to cool.

Administration: Apply 2 times daily on sores.

Colitis

1 part White Oak inner bark (Quercus alba)
1 part Golden Seal (Hydrastis Canadensis)
1/4 part Myrrh gum resin (Commiphora myrrha, var. molmol)

Preparation: 1 teaspoonful of herbs to the cup of boiling water. Keep warm 15 or 20 minutes.

Dosage: Orally 2 tablespoonfuls 3 or 4 times a day; also by injection into anus.

Diphtheria (gargle)

1 part White oak inner bark (Quercus alba)
1 part Persimmon bark (Diospyros virginiana)
1 part Mullein leaves (Verbascum thapsus)

Preparation: Make a strong decoction; strain and add honey.

Administration: Use as a gargle.

Ulcerated tonsils

1 teaspoonful White oak inner bark (Quercus alba)
1 teaspoonful Persimmon bark (Diospyros virginiana)
1 teaspoonful Golden seal (Hydrastis Canadensis)

Preparation: Steep in 1/2 pint of boiling-hot water for 20 minutes.

Administration: Use the clear liquid as a gargle.

Diarrhea

1/2 ounce White oak leaves (Quercus alba)-or inner bark.
1/2 ounce Raspberry leaves (Rubus idaeus)
1/4 ounce Cinnamon, powder (Cinnamomum zeylanicum)

Preparation: Infuse in 1 pint of boiling-hot water; cover tightly until cool, strain.

Dosage: 2 fluid ounces 4 times daily. Infants: 1/2 teaspoonful. Children: 1 teaspoonful.

Growth characteristics:
Perennial; found in North America, Europe (a large proportion of the species grow

in the United States).

***Sister plants*:**
Oak Gall or Galla or Nutgall or Dyer's Oak (Quercus infectoria); excrescences on the young twigs (caused by the puncture and ova deposit of the wasp Cynips gallae-tinctoriae) contain 15-75% tannic acid and 5% gallic acid and are used for hemorrhages, diarrhea, dyspepsia, cholera, relaxed uvula, coryza, diphtheria, toothache, leucorrhea, chapped nipples, gleet, gonorrhea, ulcers, piles, chilblain, chronic bronchitis, whooping cough, phthisis (tuberculosis of the lungs), influenza, fissures, hemorrhoids, prolapsus of colon and uterus, vesical catarrh, spongy gums, tough skin around ingrowing toe-nails, nipples, etc.; use injection of infusion, gargle, etc.

RED RASPBERRY
(Rubus idaeus; R. strigosus; ROSACEAE)

Common names:
Red raspberry, American raspberry, wild red raspberry (R. idaeus is the cultivated variety; R. strigosus is the wild variety), hindberry; Hindbur (Ger.).

Identifying characteristics:

Herb	Erect and freely branched, 3 to 6 feet high, glaucous, spiny (covered with small, straight and slender prickles).
Leaves	Pinnate, stalked, 2 pairs of ovate leaflets and a larger terminal leaflets, rounded base, double serrate margins, abruptly pointed at apex, pale green above, grayish-white beneath with oppressed felted hairs, 2½-3½ inches long, 2-3 inches broad.
Flowers	Small, white pendulous (hanging) clusters of five with cup shaped corolla.
Fruit	Red berry, globular cluster of 20-30 small, rounded and succulent drupelets, numerous hairs, fleshy, red juice (sweet, pleasant, acidulous), small stony endocarps (pits).
Taste	Astringent.
Odor	None.

Parts used:
Leaves; also root bark, fruit.

Therapeutic action:
Leaves: astringent, tonic, stimulant, alterative, stomachic, anti-emetic, parturient, hemostatic, cathartic, antiseptic, anti-abortive, antigonorrheal, antileucorrheal, antimalarial. Fruit: Mildly laxative, esculent, antacid, parturient, refrigerant.

Red raspberry leaves are great for cleansing a canker condition of the mucous membranes in the alimentary tract, leaving the tissue toned. When taken regularly in pregnancy, the infusion will quiet inappropriate premature pains and produce a safe, speedy and easy delivery. Raspberry leaves stimulate, tone and regulate before and during childbearing, assisting contractions and checking hemorrhage during labor, relieving after-pains, then strengthening, cleansing, and enriching the milk of the mother in the post-delivery period.

Both the leaves and fruit are high in citrate of iron, which is the active alterative, blood-making, astringent and contractile agent for the reproductive area. The tea is a valuable and effective agent for female menstrual problems, decreasing the menstrual flow without stopping it abruptly. Raspberry leaves are soothing and toning to the stomach and bowels, with healing action to sore mouths, sore throats, nausea, aphtha, stomatitis, diabetes, diarrhea and dysentery. They are especially valuable in stomach and bowel complaints of children. Raspberry leaf tea is a specific for colds and flu.

Medicinal uses:
Constipation, nausea, diarrhea, dysentery, diabetes, pregnancy, uterine hemorrhage, parturition, uterine cramps, labor pains, cholera infantum, leucorrhea, prolapsus uteri, prolapsed anus, hemorrhoids, dyspepsia, vomiting, colds, fevers, intestinal flu, bowel complaint, thrush, relaxed sore throat, ophthalmia, sore mouth, sore throat, spongy gums, ulcers, wounds, gonorrhea.

Preparations:
Decoction, fluid extract, infusion, powder, tincture.

Dosage:

Fluid Extract	(leaves) 1-2 teaspoonfuls.
Infusion	1 teacupful at mealtimes, 3 times daily (hot or cold).
Powder	1-2 grams.
Tincture	1/2-1 teaspoon.

ADMINISTRATION

Anal

Diarrhea, dysentery, bowel complaints: See "FORMULAS."

Hemorrhoids, prolapsed anus: Inject 6 ounces and retain as long as possible.

Oral

Constipation: See "FORMULAS."

Parturition: Drink the warm infusion of the leaves along with a small amount of cayenne; or use the leaves in combination with lady slipper (Cypripedium calceolus var. pubescens) and add some cayenne where required; or add Composition Powder (see page 147-148) to the infusion.

Pregnancy: Drink the infusion regularly during and after the period of child-bearing. Many pregnant women drink this combination: Red raspberry leaves, alfalfa leaves, comfrey leaves (Symphytum officinale), and one of the mints. This can be taken fresh as a green drink or as a tea. It supplies minerals, tones up the uterus, and helps during parturition.

After-pains (childbirth), uterine hemorrhage, miscarriage preventive: Drink the raspberry leaf tea with a little Composition Powder (see page 147-148) in it.

Amenorrhea, dysmenorrhea: Drink the infusion of the leaves: 1 cupful at meal-time 3 times daily along with an intestinal tonic-laxative for 2-3 months or until the distressing symptoms have disappeared.

Children's stomach and bowel disorders: Give the infusion (strong); a little ginger (Zingiber officinalis), and pennyroyal (Metha pulegium) may be added.

Diabetes: See "FORMULAS."

Skin

Sore mouth and throat, thrush, spongy gums: Use the strong infusion as a wash and gargle.

Remove proud flesh, cleanse wounds: Apply the leaves with slippery elm bark powder (Ulmus rubra; U. fulva) as a poultice.

Ulcers, wounds: Use the infusion as a wash.

Vaginal

Leucorrhea, gonorrhea, inflamed mucous membrane, prolapsed or enlarged uterus: Use the strong infusion as a douche, or see "FORMULAS."

FORMULAS

Canker sores

2 grams	Red raspberry leaves (Rubus idaeus)
2 grams	Shavegrass (Equisetum hyemale)
2 grams	Agrimony (Agrimonia eupatoria)

Preparation: Pour 1 pint of boiling-hot water over the herbs and steep for 20 minutes tightly covered; strain.

Administration: Use as a mouthwash.

Dr. Coffin's Formula for Colic with Stoppage of the Bowels

1/2 pint	Raspberry leaf tea, strong infusion (Rubus idaeus)
1 teaspoonful	Lobelia, powder (Lobelia inflata)
1 teaspoonful	Cayenne, powder (Capsicum frutescens; C. minimum)
1/2 teaspoon	Myrrh, gum (Commiphora myrrha, var. molmol)
1/2 teaspoon	Valerian root, powder (Valeriana officinalis)

Preparation: Make the strong infusion of raspberry leaves, then add the other herb ingredients, mix thoroughly and let stand 1/2 hour (tightly covered); strain.

Administration: Inject 1/3 into the bowels at body temperature, repeat in 4 hours, and the remainder after another 4 hours. This will be followed by copious and frequent fecal discharges during the course of the next 8 hours. For the next few days, astringent and tonic herbs should be administered orally as the patient's stomach is able to retain them.

Constipation

1/2 ounce	Raspberry leaves (Rubus idaeus)
1/2 ounce	Mountain flax (Linum catharticum)
1/2 ounce	White poplar or quaking aspen inner bark (Populus tremuloides)
1/2 ounce	Dandelion root (Taraxacum officinale)

Preparation: Simmer gently in 1 quart of water and reduce to pint; strain.

Dosage: 2 tablespoonfuls 4 times daily.

Diabetes

1/2 ounces	Raspberry leaves (Rubus idaeus; R. strigosus)
3 teaspoons	Myrrh, tincture (Commiphora myrrha, var. molmol)
1 teaspoon	Cayenne, tincture (Capsicum frutescens; C. minimum)

Preparation: Infuse the raspberry leaves in 1/2 pint of boiling hot water, cover tightly until cool; strain and add the myrrh and cayenne, mix thoroughly; sweeten to taste with honey or sugar.

Dosage: 2 tablespoonfuls 3 times daily.

Erysipelas (St. Anthony's Fire)

1/2 ounce	Raspberry leaves (Rubus idaeus)

1/2 ounce	Yarrow (Achillea millefolium)
1/2 ounce	Elder flowers (Sambucus canadensis)
1/2 ounce	White poplar; quaking aspen inner bark (Populus tremuloides)
1/2 teaspoon	Cayenne, powder (Capsicum frutescens; C. minimum)
1/2 ounce	Licorice, powder (Glycyrrhiza glabra)

Preparation: Simmer the first 4 herbs in 1 quart of water and reduce to 1 pint; strain hot over the cayenne and licorice; mix together thoroughly; sweeten to taste.

Dosage: 2 fluid ounces every 1-2 hours, as the case requires.

Administration: When the patient is weak and fevered, give 1 cupful of Composition Powder tea (see page 147-148) every few hours. Frequently a gentle laxative is needed, and may be added to the formula. Bathe the affected parts in a decoction of elder flowers or chickweed (Stellaria media) using 2 ounces of the herb in 1 quart of water and simmer 10 minutes. For ulcerated blisters, use a slippery elm (Ulmus rubra) poultice and then apply chickweed ointment.

Eyewash

1/2 ounce	Raspberry leaves (Rubus idaeus)
1/2 ounce	Oak bark (Quercus alba, etc.)
1/2 ounce	Myrrh, tincture (Commiphora myrrha, var. molmol)

Preparation: Simmer the first 2 herbs for 5 minutes in 1 pint of water, strain, when cool add the myrrh and mix well.

Administration: Bathe the eye freely.

Excessive menstruation (menorrhagia)

2 parts	Raspberry leaves (Rubus idaeus)
1 part	Prickly ash (Zanthoxylum americanum)
1 part	Blue cohosh (Caulophyllum thalictroides)
1 part	Wild yam (Dioscorea villosa)
1/2 part	Cinnamon (Cinnamomum zeylanicum)

Preparation: Infuse 1 ounce of the compound for 20 minutes in 1 pint of water, cover tightly; strain and sweeten with honey to taste.

Dosage: 1/2-1 cupful 3 to 4 times a day.

Hysteria (general building tonic)

1/2 ounce	Raspberry leaves (Rubus idaeus)

1/2 ounce	White poplar; quaking aspen inner bark (Populus tremuloides)
1/2 ounce	Balmony (Chelone glabra)
1/2 ounce	Calumba root (Jateorhiza palmata)
1/4 teaspoon	Cayenne (Capsicum frutescens; C. minimum)

Preparation: Simmer the first 4 herbs in 1 quart of water and reduce to 1/4 pint; strain hot over the cayenne and cover until cool.

Dosage: 2-3 tablespoonfuls 3 to 4 times daily.

Indigestion

1/2 ounce	Raspberry leaves (Rubus idaeus)
1/2 ounce	European century (Erythraea centaurium)
1/2 ounce	Cleavers (Galium aparine)
1/2 ounce	Dandelion (Taraxacum officinale)
1 teaspoon	Ginger (Zingiber officinalis)

Preparation: Simmer the first 4 herbs in 1 quart of water and reduce to 1/4 pint; strain hot over the ginger, cover tightly until cool; sweeten to taste with honey, keep in a cool place.

Dosage: 3 tablespoonfuls (cool) 3 to 4 times daily.

Inflammation of the uterus

2 ounces	Raspberry leaves (Rubus idaeus)
1/2 ounce	Myrrh or gum myrrh, powder (Commiphora myrrha var. molmol)

Preparation: Simmer the raspberry leaves for 10 minutes in 1 pint of water, keeping the vessel tightly covered; strain, and when cool enough to use, add the myrrh and stir in well.

Administration: Inject 1/2 of the quantity into the womb every second day; this is both soothing and toning to the uterus.

Dr. Shook's healing douche (leucorrhea, gonorrhea, inflamed mucous membrane, prolapsed or enlarged uterus, etc.)

2 ounces	Raspberry leaves (Rubus idaeus)
15 drops	Sandalwood, oil (Santalum album)
8 ounces	Irish moss, mucilage (Chondrus crispus)
1 ounce	Glycerine

Preparation: Simmer the raspberry leaves for 15 minutes while tightly covered in 1½ pints of water; strain, add the remaining ingredients and shake together thoroughly.

Administration: Use as douche (make fresh each time).

Jaundice

1/2 ounce	Raspberry leaves (Rubus idaeus)
1/2 ounce	Barberry bark (Berberis vulgaris)
1/2 ounce	Agrimony (Agrimonia eupatoria)
1/2 ounce	Cleavers (Galium aparine)
1/4 ounce	Mountain flax (Linum catharticum)
1/4 teaspoon	Cayenne (Capsicum frutescens; C. minimum)

Preparation: Simmer the first 5 herbs in 1 quart of water for 15 minutes, strain hot over the cayenne and stir; sweeten to taste with honey or sugar; keep in a cool place.

Dosage: 2 fluid ounces 3 times daily.

Administration: Use diaphoretics and vapor baths to open the pores of the skin to facilitate waste elimination. Give the patient fresh orange juice freely and only a very light diet (no dried foods, meats, etc.). After the foregoing formula is used for some time, gradually increase the tonic ingredients (barberry, agrimony, European century, etc.) and leave out the mountain flax.

Leucorrhea (whites)

1 ounce	Raspberry leaves (Rubus idaeus)
1/2 ounce	Bethroot (Trillium erectum; T. pendulum)
1 ounce	Myrrh tincture (Commiphora myrrha, var. molmol)

Preparation: Simmer the first 2 herbs for 10 minutes in 1 pint of water, cover tightly; let stand until cool, strain, add the myrrh.

Administration: Use 1/3 pint warm as a vaginal douche 2 to 3 times daily.

Mumps

1 ounce	Raspberry leaves (Rubus idaeus)
1 ounce	Bayberry bark (Myrica cerifera)
1 teaspoonful	Ginger (Zingiber officinalis)

Preparation: Simmer the first 2 herbs while tightly covered for 10 minutes in 1 quart of water; strain hot over the ginger, cover and let stand until cool, sweeten to taste with honey, keep in a cool place.

Dosage: 2 fluid ounces 3 to 4 times daily.

Note: This condition is evidence of a faulty glandular system and toxicity in the body. This formula is splendid for cleansing the stomach and removing canker from the whole digestive tract, thereby leaving the body cleaner and enabling healing to take place.

Ophthalmia
(sore eye, inflammation of the eye)

1/2 ounce	Raspberry leaves (Rubus idaeus)
1/2 ounce	Agrimony (Agrimonia eupatoria)
1/2 ounce	Eyebright (Euphrasia officinalis)
1/2 ounce	Buckbean or bogbean (Menyanthes trifoliata)

Preparation: Simmer the herbs for 20 minutes in 1 quart of water while covered tightly; strain, sweeten to taste with honey, cool and keep in a cool place.

Dosage: 2 fluid ounces 4 times daily.

Note: If a laxative is needed to clear the bowels, add 1/4 ounce of senna (Cassia angustifolia, C. acutifolia) just a few minutes before straining the decoction.

Piles (English Ointment)

1/2 ounce	Raspberry leaves, powder (Rubus idaeus)
1/2 ounce	Yarrow flowers and stems, powder (Achillea millefolium)
3 ounces	Olive oil
1 ounce	Wheat germ oil
Sufficient	Beeswax

Preparation: Fold herbs into warm olive oil and stir for 15 minutes over heat. Add Wheat germ oil and enough beeswax (around 1/2 ounce) to eventually stiffen the ointment. Continue stirring over heat till the beeswax is melted, take off heat and, while still stirring, let cool till it begins to thicken. Pour off into clean container and let sit till it sets up, keep in a cool place.

Dosage: Use externally as needed.

Quinsy (inflammation of the throat)

1/2 ounce	Raspberry leaves (Rubus idaeus)
1/2 ounce	Agrimony (Agrimonia eupatoria)
1/2 ounce	Horehound (Marubium vulgare)
1/4 ounce	Barberry bark (Berberis vulgaris)
1/2 ounce	Senna leaves (Cassia angustifolia, C. acutifolia)

1 teaspoonful Cayenne (Capsicum frutescens; C. minimum)

Preparation: Simmer the first 5 herbs for 20 minutes in 1 quart water; strain hot over the cayenne and mix well, cover until cool; sweeten to taste with honey; keep in a cool place.

Dosage: 2 fluid ounces 4 times daily.

Administration: Give a vapor bath. Inhale the steam from a decoction of yarrow (2 ounces of the herb boiled 5 minutes in 1 quart of water) from a teapot spout or the small end of an inverted funnel. Foment the neck area with a cloth wrung out of tincture of cayenne infusion; keep warm and change every 1/2 hour if needed.

Parturition (labor)

1 ounce Raspberry leaves (Rubus idaeus)
1/4 teaspoon Composition Powder (see page 147-148)

Preparation: Infuse the herbs for 15 minutes in 1 pint of boiling hot water, cover tightly and let stand until cool; strain and sweeten to taste with honey.

Dosage: 1 teacupful every hour during labor.

Relaxed sore throat
canker in mouth or throat, spongy gums, etc.

1/2 ounce Raspberry leaves (Rubus idaeus, R. strigosus)
1/2 ounce Bayberry bark (Myrica cerifera)

Preparation: Infuse the herbs while tightly covered for 30 minutes in a pint of boiling-hot water; strain.

Administration: Use as a gargle and mouthwash as required.

Sore throat

1 ounce Raspberry leaves (Rubus idaeus)
1 ounce Cranesbill root (Geranium maculatum)
1 ounce Blackberry root (Rubus villosus)
1 ounce Culver's root or leptandra (Veronicastrum virginicum)

Preparation: Simmer the herbs in 3 quarts of water and reduce to 3 pints; strain, keep in a cool place.

Administration: Use as a gargle.

Dr. Coffin's Formula for Tuberculosis or Consumption

1/2 ounce	Raspberry leaves (Rubus idaeus)
1/2 ounce	Agrimony (Agrimonia eupatoria)
1/2 ounce	Barberry bark (Berberis vulgaris)
1/2 ounce	Cleavers (Galium aparine)
1/2 ounce	Ground ivy (Glechoma hederacea)
1/2 ounce	European century (Erythraea centaurium)
1/2 ounce	Horehound (Marubium vulgare)
1/2 teaspoon	Cayenne (Capsicum frutescens; C. minimum)
1/4 ounce	Licorice, powder or fluid extract (Glycyrrhiza glabra)

Preparation: Simmer the first 7 herbs while tightly covered in 1 quart of water; strain hot over the cayenne and licorice; cover until cool; sweeten to taste with honey; keep in a cool place.

Dosage: 2 fluid ounces 4 times daily (3 to 4 pints per week).

Administration: Also use 1/2-l teaspoonful of Acid Tincture of Lobelia (see page 400) in order to promote free expectoration, and sustain the lungs with sufficient oxygen with cayenne and chlorophyll; you can also use the stomach tonic (see bayberry "FORMULAS") and the antispasmodic powder (see skullcap "FORMULAS").

Congenial combinations:
Raspberry leaves make an excellent combination with slippery elm (Ulmus rubra; U. fulva) for cleansing wounds.

Growth characteristics:
Perennial; found wild and under cultivation in Canada and in almost all parts of northern and middle United States (where the fruit or berry is in great demand); grows in hedges and thickets and upon neglected fields; flowers in May and the fruit ripens June-August.

Sister plants:
-Blackberry or Bramble (Rubus villosus; ROSACEAE); bark, leaves, root bark berries; diarrhea, dysentery, hemorrhoids, leucorrhea, excessive saliva, atonic and relaxed condition of the stomach, intestines, larynx, and mucous tissues generaly.
-Black Raspberry (leaves, fruit); therapeutically similar to red raspberry.
-Thimble berry (Rubus occidentalis; ROSACEAE); leaves, fruit; therapeutically similar to red raspberry.

MULLEIN
(Verbascum thapsus; Verbasci filia; SCROPHULARIACEAE)

This valuable herb has effective astringent properties and is treated in detail on page 344.

WHITE POPLAR or QUAKING ASPEN
(Populus tremuloides; SALICACEAE)

This valuable herb is used in a number of formulas; more information may be found on page 491.

CRANESBILL / CROWFOOT / WILD GERANIUM / WILD ALUM ROOT
(Geranium maculatum; GERANIACEAE)

Common names:
Crow foot, wild geranium, wild alum root, spotted geranium, wild cranes bill, stork bill, dove('s) foot, American kino, American tormentilla, chocolate flower; Storchsnabel, Geranium (Ger.) geranipico de grulla (Span.).

Identifying characteristics:

Stem	Hairy, slender, round, simple or branching above, erect, grayish-green, 1-3 feet high, swollen at joints.
Leaves	Palmately lobed (5-7), opposite (stem), pale green with paler green spots, cleft and toothed at apex hairy petiolate, basal ones 3-6 inches wide and on stems 8-10 inches long.
Flowers	Purplish pink, pale magenta or lavender, large (1-1½ inches broad), solitary or pair, 5 entire petals, on elongated peduncles that spring from the forks of stems, calyx consists of 5 lapping and pointed sepals.
Fruit	Long, pendulous, sharp-pointed, imaginatively resembling a crane's bill; in maturity it ejects the seeds elastically, far from the parent plant.
Root	Horizontal, roundish, 1-4 inches long, 1/8-3/4 inch thick, knotty, somewhat bent, wrinkled, root scars, externally dark purplish-brown, internally light purplish-brown, short fracture, thin bark, large central pith. Powder: purplish-brown.
Taste	Strongly astringent.
Odor	None.

Parts used:
Root; also the herb (the root possesses the greatest potency and astringency).

Therapeutic action:
Astringent, tonic, styptic.

Cranesbill is an excellent and effective astringent with pleasant tonic properties. Its astringent action is powerful and non-irritating, well-suited for relieving relaxed and atonic conditions of the mucous tissues debilitated by copious discharges. The astringent action is weaker than oak bark (Quercus alba) and black catechu (Acadia catechu) but is stronger than witch hazel (Hamamelis virginiana). It is not nauseous, making it useful for infants and persons with sensitive stomachs. Cranesbill is moderately drying in action, and strengthens the stomach, kidneys, and the other internal organs.

Dr. Shook wrote this concerning cranesbill's use as a beauty aid for skin:

> We say, without fear of favor, that for removing wrinkles, astringing enlarged pores, checking the over activity of the sudoriferous and sebaceous glands in the skin, contracting enlarged and engorged capillaries in the skin that are brought about by excessive stimulation with hot packs, steaming, massage, and irritants which are employed in the usual procedure in so-called beauty parlors, there is no remedy equal to Geranium maculatum when properly combined and compounded into creams and lotions and perfumed with non-irritating and astringent oils, gums, resins, etc. (Shook, *op. cit.*, p. 118).

Medicinal uses:
Chronic diarrhea, chronic dysentery, menorrhagia, night sweats, catarrhal gastritis, inflammation, cholera infantum, hemorrhages, indolent ulcers, aphtha, ophthalmia, leucorrhea, gleet, hematuria, diabetes, excessive and chronic mucus discharges, mercurial salivation, relaxed uvula or vagina or rectum, chronic catarrh, internal wounds, hemorrhage of lungs (see "FORMULAS"), internal ulcerations.

Preparation:
Decoction, fluid extract, infusion, powder, tincture.

Dosage:

Decoction	1-2 teaspoonfuls in a little water.
Fluid Extract	30-60 drops.
Infusion	2-6 fluid ounces.
Powder	1-4 grams.
Tincture	30-60 drops.

ADMINISTRATION

Anal

Mucus discharges from the intestines, rectal problems: Combine equal parts of cranesbill and golden seal (Hydrastis Canadensis) and inject a small amount of a strong infusion into the rectum.

Diarrhea, dysentery, cholera infantum: Use the injection as required.

Piles: Inject 2-3 tablespoonfuls of the cranesbill decoction alone or the strong infusion in combination with golden seal (Hydrastis Canadensis) several times during the day and after each bowel movement.

Oral

Gastric ulcer, diabetes: Use cranesbill in combination with golden seal (Hydrastis Canadensis).

Diarrhea, dysentery, cholera infantum, bowel problems: Use the decoction or strong infusion in soymilk (tofu-milk).

Internal bleeding: Drink 2 ounces of the fluid extract (root) or decoction.

Bright's disease, incontinence of urine: Drink the decoction in combination with golden seal (Hydrastis Canadensis).

Skin

Sore, inflamed, or irritated throat: Use the decoction of the root as a gargle.

Relaxed or elongated uvula: Apply the fluid extract frequently or gargle with the decoction of the root.

Sore mouth, bleeding gums: Use the decoction or strong infusion as a mouth rinse.

Cuts, wounds: Use the decoction as a wash, or apply the bruised leaves directly on the affected part.

Nosebleed: Use the powder as a snuff; also see "FORMULAS."

Bleeding (wounds, cuts, tooth extraction): Sprinkle powder onto the affected area; rub powder into the tooth cavity. As a local styptic, apply the special strong decoction to the affected area on the lint or cotton without dilution.

Dry up mother's milk: Massage the decoction into the breast area.

Firm up and harden sore and tender nipples: Massage the decoction into the nipples only.

Female restorative powder (tonic for menstrual troubles, leucorrhea, etc.): See "FORMULAS."

Vaginal

Leucorrhea: Use cranesbill in combination with bistort (Polygonum bistorta) as a douche; or see "FORMULAS."

FORMULAS

Decoction of cranesbill

1 ounce	Cranesbill root, cut or powdered (Geranium maculatum)
1 ½ pints	Distilled or d-cell water

Preparation: Simmer for 20 minutes while tightly covered; strain, let stand until cool, bottle and keep in a cool place. For preserving this decoction with glycerine, reduce the strained liquid to 3/4 pint (12 ounces) by simmering, and add 4 ounces of glycerine, shake well together, keep in a cool place.

Dosage: 1-2 teaspoons in a little water (this is stronger than an infusion).

Uses: Severe hemorrhages, chronic catarrh, chronic mucus discharge from the mucous membranes, purulent leucorrhea, dysentery, purulent sore throat, indolent ulcers, severe bleeding piles, etc.

Special strong decoction
(Hemorrhage of the lungs, internal wounds, excessive menorrhagia)

4 ounces	Cranesbill root, cut (Geranium maculatum)
4 ounces	Comfrey root, cut (Symphytum officinale)
8 ounces	Glycerine

Preparation: Stir and soak the herbs for 6 hours in 2 quarts of distilled water; bring to a boil and simmer for 30 minutes; strain and press all liquid from the herbs, place the liquid into the cleansed vessel and reduce slowly by simmering to 1½ pints; when cool add 8 ounces of glycerine and shake well together; bottle and keep cool.

Dosage: 2 teaspoons to 1 tablespoonful in water.

Female restorative powder (tonic)

2 ounces	Cranesbill root, powder (Geranium maculatum)
4 ounces	White poplar; quaking aspen inner bark (Populus tremuloides)
2 ounces	Bistort root, powder (Polygonum bistorta)

2 ounces Bethroot, powder (Trillium erectum; T. pendulum)
1 ounce Golden seal root, powder (Hydrastis Canadensis)
1 ounce Balmony leaves, powder (Chelone glabra)
1/2 ounce Bayberry bark, powder (Myrica cerifera)
1 ounce Cloves, powder (Syzygium aromaticum; Eugenia aromatica)
2 ounces Ginger, powder (Zingiber officinalis)
1 teaspoon Cayenne, powder (Capsicum frutescens; C. minimum)

Preparation: Use fine powder, sieve and mix well together; use 1 teaspoonful in 1 cupful of hot water, sweeten with honey to taste, cover and steep for 10 minutes.

Dosage: 1 cupful 3 times daily.

Leucorrhea (injection)

1/2 ounce Cranesbill root, crushed or powdered (Geranium maculatum)
1/2 ounce Bethroot, crushed or powdered (Trillium erectum; T. pendulum)

Preparation: Infuse the herbs in 1 pint of boiling-hot water, cover tightly and let stand until cool enough to inject.

Administration: Inject a small quantity 3 times daily.

Nosebleed (epistaxis)

1 ounce Cranesbill root (Geranium maculatum)
1 ounce Bistort root (Polygonum bistorta)
1 ounce Raspberry leaves (Rubus idaeus) or substitute Avens herb or root (Geum urbanum)

Preparation: Simmer the herbs in 1 quart of water and slowly reduce to 1/4 pint; strain and sweeten to taste with honey.

Dosage: 1/2 cupful with 1/4 teaspoon of cayenne (Capsicum frutescens; C. minimum) every 2 hours. If the bleeding is severe, give the dose every 10 minutes until results are obtained.

Piles

1 ounce Cranesbill herb or root (Geranium maculatum)
1 ounce Ladies mantle herb (Alchemilla vulgaris)
1 ounce Shepherd's purse (Capsella bursa-pastoris)

Preparation: Simmer the herbs in 2 quarts of water and slowly reduce to 3 pints; strain and sweeten to taste with honey; bottle and keep in a cool place.

Dosage: 2 fluid ounces 3 times daily.

Pile ointment

1 ounce	Cranesbill root, crushed (Geranium maculatum)
1 ounce	Bistort root, crushed (Polygonum bistorta)
1 ounce	Pinus or hemlock spruce bark (Tsuga canadensis)
1 quart	Olive oil (Olea europaea)
6 ounces	Beeswax, yellow

Preparation: Place the herbs in the olive oil and heat in the oven for 1 hour at 135° F.; strain out the spent herbs and add the beeswax (melted) and mix thoroughly. When the mixture cools and solidifies sufficiently, keep in a cool place. If it is not solid enough, reheat and add more beeswax.

Administration: Apply to the affected areas.

Note: This is a good general purpose ointment.

Sore throat (gargle)

1/2 ounce	Cranesbill root (Geranium maculatum)
1/2 ounce	Bayberry bark (Myrica cerifera)
1/2 ounce	Golden seal root (Hydrastis Canadensis)
1/2 ounce	Marshmallow root (Althaea officinalis)
1/2 ounce	Wild indigo root (Baptisia tinctoria)
1/2 ounce	Rosemary herb (Rosmarinus officinalis)

Preparation: Simmer the herbs for 20 minutes tightly covered in 1/2 pints of water; strain and add 4 ounces of honey; bottle and keep in a cool place.

Administration: Use as a gargle as needed.

Ulcerations (stomach, intestines, bladder, genito-urinary organs, mucous membranes), gleet, gonorrhea, gastric and chronic catarrh, purulent ophthalmia

2 ounces	Cranesbill root, cut (Geranium maculatum)
4 ounces	Golden seal root (Hydrastis Canadensis)
4 ounces	Echinacea root, cut (Echinacea angustifolia)
8 ounces	Glycerine

Preparation: Soak the herbs for 6 hours in 3 quarts of distilled water; bring to a boil and simmer for 30 minutes; strain, return the liquid to the cleansed vessel and reduce by simmering to 1/2 pint; let stand until cool, add the glycerine (1½ pints) shake and mix well together, bottle and keep in a cool place.

Dosage: 1-2 teaspoonfuls in water 3 to 4 times daily.

Administration: Gonorrhea injection or douche: 1 tablespoonful in 1 large cup of warm water. Ophthalmia: 1 tablespoonful in 2 ounces of water, pour onto and saturate lint or cotton and bandage on the eyes (dilute with more water if too strong), keep on 2 hours followed by 1 hour rest, then make a fresh application.

Congenial combinations:
Tonics; Cranesbill combines well with golden seal (Hydrastis Canadensis).

Growth characteristics:
Perennial, native of North America, grows in almost all sections of the country, preferring rich open woods, low grounds, thickets and shady roadside, flowers April-July.

***Sister plants*:**
-Herb Robert or Red Robin or Dragon's Blood (Geranium robertianum; GERANIACEAE); herb: hemorrhage, gravel; grows in northeastern United States, flowers May-October with a 1/2 inch purplish rose, leaves and stems are strongly scented disagreeably.
-Meadow Cranesbill or English Cranesbill (Geranium dissectum; G. pratense GERANIACEAE) herb: hemorrhage, kidney problems, leucorrhea, diarrhea, etc.; possess similar therapeutic properties to Cranesbill (G. maculatum) small bright red flowers, stems swollen at joints and free-branched, dark green leaves almost palmately circular with 5-7 leaflets.

SUMAC(H) or SMOOTH SUMAC or SCARLET SUMAC
(Rhus glabra; ANACARDIACEAE)

Common names:
Sumac, sumach, smooth sumac, scarlet sumac, upland sumac, mountain sumac, dwarf sumac, sleek sumac, Pennsylvania sumac; Sumach, Sumac (Fr.); Sumach (Ger.); zumaque (Span.).

Identifying characteristics:

Stem	Woody shrub, 5-15 feet high, more or less bent, many straggling, large spreading branches, large pith, thin with smooth grayish bark with occasional reddish tint and small scattered warts.
Leaves	Alternate or imparipinnate, consisting of 6-31 leaflets lanceolate, acuminate, sharply serrate, shining and green above, whitish beneath (changes to a beautiful red in autumn).
Flowers	Greenish-red, in terminal panicles.
Fruit	Small dark red dupes or berries, in large clusters, flattened ovoid, velvety with short hairs (shiny crimson down), 1 very hard brown seed;

	in odorous, but has a pleasant sour astringent taste. Powder: brownish-red.
Root	Quilled, dull reddish-brown, scattered transversely-oval (bark) lenticels, whitish or brown fracture with transverse rows of minute blackish, linear oil cells.
Taste	Gummy, astringent.
Odor	None.

Parts used:
Bark (preferably root bark), berries; also leaves (of lesser potency than the bark and berries) and galls.

Therapeutic action:
Bark: Astringent, alterative, tonic, vulnerary, antiseptic. Berries: astringent, refrigerant, diuretic, emmenagogue, diaphoretic, cephalic.

Sumac is an effective astringent and a useful tonic for the bowels. It cleanses the alimentary tract and is especially useful in healing internal sores, ulcers and wounds on the mucous membranes.

Medicinal uses:
Relaxed bowel conditions, chronic diarrhea, intestinal hemorrhage, prolapsed uterus, prolapsed anus, leucorrhea, dysentery, gonorrhea. Berries: Sore throat, diphtheria, irritated bladder, pharyngitis, tonsillitis, spongy gums, ulcers, wounds, catarrhal conditions of the stomach and bowels, febrile diseases, incontinence of urine (enuresis), erysipelas, diabetes.

Preparation:
Decoction, fluid extract, infusion, powder, tincture.

***Dosage*:**

Decoction	2 tablespoonfuls to 2 fluid ounces.
Fluid Extract	1-2 teaspoons (bark and berries).
Infusion	2 fluid ounces 2 to 3 times daily.
Powder	1-2 grams.
Tincture	1/2-1 fluid teaspoon.

ADMINISTRATION

Anal

Prolapsus anus: Give injection of the infusion of the bark; also drink as tea.

Oral

Leucorrhea, scrofula, gonorrhea, syphilis, inward sores, wounds: See "FOR-

MULAS."

Diabetes, bowel complaints, catarrhal affections of the stomach, fevers: Drink the infusion of the sumac berries alone.

Fevers, irritated conditions of the bladder: Infuse the berries for 1/2 hour; strain and sweeten to taste; mix with fresh pineapple juice.

Relaxed bowel conditions, chronic diarrhea, intestinal hemorrhage: Drink the decoction of the bark, as it is more stimulating and tonic.

Skin

Erysipelas: Apply a poultice of raw sumac berries and golden seal (Hydrastis Canadensis).

Sore throat, diphtheria: Infuse the berries for 1/2 hour in a quantity of water, strain and sweeten to taste with honey; mix with fresh pineapple juice; use as a gargle.

Mouth affections (sores, canker), spongy gums: Use the infusion of berries as a mouth rinse.

Ulcers, wounds: Use the infusion of berries or decoction of bark as a wash.

Vaginal

Leucorrhea: Use an injection of the infusion of leaves; this has the same soothing influence and is equal to witch hazel (Hamamelis virginiana), but is more drying.

FORMULAS

Leucorrhea, scrofula, gonorrhea, syphilis, inward sores and wounds

1 part Sumac berries (Rhus glabra)
1 part Sumac bark (Rhus glabra)
1 part White pine bark (Pinus strobus)
1 part Slippery elm bark (Ulmus rubra; U. fulva)

Preparation: Soak 2 ounces of the herbs in 1 quart of distilled water for 30 minutes; simmer the herbs in the same water for 20 minutes; strain.

Dosage: 1-2 fluid ounces 3 to 4 times daily according to age.

Administration: Take internally as directed as well as externally as a fomentation or injection (douche or enema).

Incontinence or involuntary flowing of urine (enuresis)

1/4 ounce	Sumac berries (Rhus glabra)
1/4 ounce	Bethroot (Trillium erectum; T. pendulum)
1/4 ounce	Yarrow (Achillea millefolium)
1/4 ounce	Agrimony (Agrimonia eupatoria)
1/4 ounce	White pond lily (Nymphaea odorata)

Preparation: Simmer the herbs for 10 minutes in 1 pint of water; strain and sweeten to taste with honey; allow to stand until cool; bottle and keep in a cool place.

Dosage: 1 tablespoonful to 2 fluid ounces 3 to 4 times daily according to age.

Administration: In this condition, the nervous system should be toned with nervines, as the whole body is with tonics. Massage over the lumbar regions to stimulate the nerves to the bladder.

Quinsy

1 ounce	Sumac berries (Rhus glabra)
1 ounce	Agrimony (Agrimonia eupatoria)
1 ounce	Raspberry leaves (Rubus idaeus)
1 ounce	Garden sage (Salvia officinalis)
1 ounce	Cudweed (Gnaphalium obtusifolium)
1 ounce	Slippery elm bark (Ulmus rubra; U. fulva)
1/2 ounce	Myrrh gum (Commiphora myrrha var. molmol)
1 teaspoon	Cayenne (Capsicum frutescens; C. minimum)

Preparation: Place the first 6 herbs in 2 quarts of water and simmer down to 1 quart; strain while boiling hot over the myrrh and cayenne, stir and cover until cool; bottle and keep in a cool place.

Dosage: 3 tablespoonfuls 4 times daily.

Congenial combinations:
Sumac bark and berries combine well with tonics such as Golden Seal (Hydrastis Canadensis) and Agrimony (Agrimonia eupatoria).

Growth characteristics:
Perennial; found in Canada and the United States from the East to the West Coast; prefers thickets, woods and barren, rocky wasteland soils; it flowers June-July; the

fruit (berries) mature September-October. The bark and leaves contain 25-30% tannin and the galls 60-70% tannin, so these are cultivated commercially in Virginia and other states to make fluid extract for tanning, dyeing and other trade and chemical purposes.

Collection:
The berries should be gathered before the rain, as it washes away the valuable medicinal acid properties that are in the external downy efflorescence. The bark should be gathered in the fall. **Be careful to select the right species of Rhus, for many are highly poisonous**.

Sister plants:
Sweet Sumac(h), Fragrant Sumac, Sweet-Scented Sumac (Rhus aromatica, ANACARDIACEAE); root bark; incontinence or urine (enuresis), hematuria, leucorrhea, diabetes, diarrhea, dysentery, cystitis, night-sweats, menorrhagia.

GROUND IVY
(Glechoma hederacea; Nepeta glechoma; LABIATAE)

Common names:
Ground ivy, Gill-go-over-the-ground, Alehoof, haymaids, cat's foot, turn hoof, field-balm, runaway jack, running charlie.

Identifying characteristics:

Stem	Procumbent (prostrate, trailing), creeping, quadrangular, gray, hairy, unbranched, 6-24 inches long.
Leaves	Opposite at every joint, stalked (petiolate), somewhat kidney-shaped, deeply and obtusely crenate (rounded scallops), margins, purplish upper leaves, paler and gland-dome beneath, hairy on both sides.
Flowers	Bluish-purple, two-lipped, bloom 3-4 together in exile of upper leaves.
Roots	Issue at the corners of the jointed stems.
Taste	Bitter and acrid.
Odor	Strong, aromatic, unpleasant.

Parts used:
Whole herb.

Therapeutic action:
Astringent, diuretic, tonic, pectoral, stimulant.

Ground ivy is beneficial to the kidney and liver. Containing vitamin C, it is useful as an anti-scorbutic agent, and has also cured severe skin eruptions which medical treatment could not clear. It tones the stomach and is effective in pulmonary troubles generally. Sweetened with honey, ground ivy may be drunk liberally as a very cooling beverage.

Medicinal uses:
Deafness, sore eyes, kidney disorders, dyspepsia, scurvy, abscesses, gatherings, tumors, cough, pulmonary complaints, skin eruptions, sores, lead-colic, headache, nasal congestion.

Preparation:
Fluid extract, infusion, powder, tincture.

Dosage:

Fluid extract	1/2-1 fluid teaspoon.
Infusion	2 fluid ounces or more 3 to 4 times daily.
Powder	2-4 grams.
Tincture	1/4-1/2 fluid teaspoon (15-30 drops).

ADMINISTRATION

Oral

Cooling beverage: Use the infusion, 1 ounce of the herb to 1 pint of water, sweeten with honey and drink cool.

Lead-colic (from painting): Drink the infusion of the leaves.

Skin

Deafness, sore eyes: Drop expressed juice of ground ivy into the ears or eyes frequently.

Gathering of breasts, tumors, sores: See "FORMULAS."

Skin eruptions: Use the infusion as a wash.

FORMULAS

Gathering of breasts, tumors, sores
(poultice)

2 parts Ground ivy (Glechoma hederacea)
1 part Camomile flowers (Chamaemelum nobile; Anthemis nobilis)
1 part Yarrow, fresh (Achillea millefolium)

Growth characteristics:
Perennial; common to Europe and the United States; prefers woods and shady

places, waste grounds, dry ditches, under hedges, etc.

BISTORT or SNAKEWEED
(Polygonum bistorta; POLYGONACEAE)

Common names:
Bistort, snake weed, adderwort, odor wort, snake root, patient dock, dragonwort, sweet dock, red legs, Easter giant, columbrina.

Identifying characteristics:

Stems	Several long foot-stalks, 1-2 feet high.
Leaves	Bluish-green above with purplish tint underneath, somewhat long and broad, oval, resembling a dock leaf.
Flowers	Pale-hued, borne in a dense cylindrical spike from the top of the stem.
Root	Rhizome, S-shaped, bent upon itself (distorted), 2 inches long, 3/5 inch thick, externally blackish, reddish-brown within, depressed or channelled on the upper surface, transversely striated, convex, root-scars on the under surface, short fracture, thick bark, ring of small woody surface, short fracture, thick bark, ring of small woody wedges enclosing a pith of same thickness as the bark, numerous black thready rootlets from which the foot-stalk and leaves spring.
Taste	astringent.
Odor	None.

Parts used:
Rhizome or root.

Therapeutic action:
Astringent, styptic, diuretic, alterative, tonic, anthelmintic (vermifuge), anti-venomous.

Bistort is one of the most powerful astringents in botanic medicine. It cleanses canker and toxic matter from the mucous membrane of the alimentary canal, at the same time toning the entire tract. It influences the kidneys, firms up and tones internal and external tissue, and is a versatile styptic agent for hemorrhages.

Medicinal uses:
Diarrhea, dysentery, cholera, hemorrhage, mucus discharges, leucorrhea, sore and ulcerated mouth, spongy gums, smallpox, measles, pimples, jaundice, rupture, insect stings, snake bites, worms, cuts, wounds, amenorrhea, dysmenorrhea, incontinence (enuresis), bruises.

Preparation:
Decoction, fluid extract, infusion, powder tincture.

Dosage:

Decoction	1 teaspoon to 1 tablespoonful in a little water.
Fluid Extract	1/2-1 fluid teaspoon (30-60 drops).
Infusion	2 fluid ounces.
Powder	1-2 grams.
Tincture	1/2-1 fluid teaspoon (30-60 drops).

ADMINISTRATION

Anal

Diarrhea, dysentery, cholera: Dilute the decoction in a little water and use as an injection; also see "FORMULAS."

Oral

Enuresis (incontinence of urine): Combine bistort with other diuretic agents.

Internal canker, mucus discharges, jaundices, measles, smallpox, pimples, etc.: Bistort decoction, powder, etc. is very cleansing, astringing and toning. It can also be combined equal parts with red raspberry leaves (Rubus idaeus).

Hemorrhage: Use a strong decoction.

Sore and ulcerated mouth or gums, running sores, nasal problems: Use the decoction or infusion, etc. as a rinse or wash.

Insect stings, snake bites: Foment externally with a strong decoction; take stronger doses internally.

Cuts, wounds: Apply the powdered root directly to the injured part.

Vaginal

Menstruation (decreases or regulates flow): Use the diluted decoction as a douche.

Leucorrhea: Use the diluted decoction as an injection.

FORMULAS

Diarrhea

1 ounce	Bistort root, crushed (Polygonum bistorta)
1 ounce	Raspberry leaves (Rubus idaeus; R. strigosus)
1 teaspoonful	Composition powder (see page 147-148)

Preparation: Simmer the bistort root for 20 minutes in 1½ pints of water (covered tightly); pour the hot liquid over the raspberry leaves and composition powder (see page 147) and steep another 20 minutes well-covered; strain off the clear liquid, sweeten with honey to taste; when cool, bottle and keep in a cool place.

Dosage: 3 tablespoonfuls every 1/2 hour until the purging stops.

Diarrhea (infant syrup)

1 ounce	Bistort root, bruised (Polygonum bistorta)
1 ounce	Marshmallow root, bruised (Althaea officinalis)
1/4 ounce	Cloves (Syzygium aromaticum; Eugenia aromatica)
1/4 ounce	Angelica, powder (Angelica archangelica)
1/4 ounce	Ginger, powder (Zingiber officinalis)

Preparation: Simmer the first 3 herbs in 1½ pints of water and slowly reduce to 1 pint; add the last 2 herbs, simmer again for 10 minutes (cover well); remove from heat, let stand until cool, strain; preserve with vegetable glycerine (up to 8 ounces); bottle and keep in a cool place. If you do not have access to vegetable glycerine, make into a syrup by adding 12 ounces of brown sugar, bring to a boil, remove scum, let stand until cool; bottle.

Dosage: 1/2-1 teaspoonful, according to age.

Pile and general purpose ointment

1 ounce	Bistort root, crushed (Polygonum bistorta)
1 ounce	Cranesbill root, crushed (Geranium maculatum)
1 ounce	Pinus or hemlock spruce (Tsuga canadensis; Pinus canadensis)
6 ounces	Beeswax, yellow
4 ounces	Mutton suet
8 ounces	Lard, leaf
2 ounces	Olive oil (Olea europaea)

Preparation: Simmer the ingredients (except the oil) for 1 hour; strain and press; add the olive oil and keep mixing thoroughly until cool; keep in a cool place.

Administration: Apply as needed.

Tooth powder

1 part	Bistort root, powder (Polygonum bistorta)
1 part	Bayberry bark, powder (Myrica cerifera)
1 part	Orris root, powder (Iris florentina)

Preparation: Mix thoroughly.

Administration: Use as a tooth powder.

Growth characteristics:
Perennial; found in North America, northern Europe, Western Asia, grows in mountain meadows, flowers May-June.

Collection:
Gather in March when the leaves just begin to shoot.

Sister plants:
Smartweed or Waterpepper (Polygonum punctatum; P. hydropiper, P. hydropiperoides; POLYGONACEAE); herb: menstrual obstructions, amenorrhea, uterine problems, gravel (bladder), colds, coughs, skin irritation, kidney and bowel complaints, ulcers, appendicitis, cholera, sore mouth, erysipelas; it produces a sensation of heat in the stomach, increases the force of the heart, raises arterial tension, promotes surface warmth and the secretions of the bronchial, renal and uterine areas, and it is an efficient diuretic and emmenagogue; the plant is characterized by narrow, lanceolate leaves and slender spikes of small greenish-white or greenish-pink flowers.

WHITE POND LILY or WATER LILY
(Nymphaea odorata; Castalia odorata; NYMPHAEACEAE)

Identifying characteristics:

Stem	Not a true stem, see "Root."
Leaves	Floating, nearly round, 4-12 inches broad, slit at bottom, shiny green above, reddish and more or less hairy on under surface, petiole attached at center or lower surface; petioles and peduncles round and rubber-like, 4 main air-channels.
Flowers	Solitary, pure white or pinkish, 3-8 inches across, floating, very pleasantly fragrant; it is a relative to the lotus. The flower opens to the sun and closes again at night.
Root	Thick (about 2 inches in diameter), simple or with few branches, (stock) very long, circular leaf scars on upper side, remains of root lets on lower side, brown externally, grayish-white internally, spongy with scattered weed bundles.
Taste	Mucilaginous, astringent, bitter.
Odor	None.

Parts used:
Root (preferably fresh), also the leaves.

Therapeutic action:
Astringent, antiseptic, demulcent, tonic, anodyne, antiscrofulous, vulnerary,

deobstruent, discutient.

White pond lily is an excellent astringent agent for removing toxins from the system, while its content of mucilage has a very soothing effect to the mucous membrane lining and is toning to the tissues. It draws, cleanses, and relieves the pain and inflammation of ulcerated surfaces, both internally and externally, and has been successful in healing uterine cancer.

Medicinal uses:
Inflamed tumors, sores, sore and inflamed gums, thrush, bowel troubles (especially infants), leucorrhea, prolapsus uteri, relaxed vagina, ulceration of the cervix, inflammation, diarrhea, dysentery, bladder catarrh, prostate irritation, chafed surfaces, gonorrhea, uterine cancer, boils, abscesses, ulcers, tumors, infections, syphilis, scrofula, gleet, sore eyes, ophthalmia, putrid sore throat, bronchial troubles, dropsy, kidney troubles, painful swelling, canker, cuts, wounds, irritable chancres, excoriations of the prepuce and vulva.

Preparation:
Decoction, fluid extract, infusion, powder, tincture.

Dosage:

Decoction	1-2 tablespoonfuls or more.
Fluid Extract	1/2-1 fluid teaspoon (30-60 drops).
Infusion	2-4 tablespoonfuls 3 to 4 times daily between meals.
Powder	2 grams (approximately 1/2 teaspoonful or 30 grains).
Tincture	1/2-1 fluid teaspoon (30-60 drops).

ADMINISTRATION

Anal

Infant bowel troubles: Use the infusion as a warm injection.

Diarrhea, dysentery: Use the decoction without sweetening as a cool injection.

Oral

Cancer of the uterus: Drink the decoction and use the decoction as a vaginal injection.

Bladder catarrh, prostate irritation: Give the decoction alone, or combined with other suitable diuretic agents.

Skin

Poultice: Use the leaves and fresh roots, wash and clean thoroughly; crush or put through a mincer, heat in the oven on a plate or dish; place on some gauze or appropriate material and apply, change as often as necessary; a few drops of eucalyptol or eucalyptus oil will increase the drawing power.

Boils, tumors, scrofulous ulcers, ulcers of mouth and throat, inflamed skin and mucous membrane, infection, cancer: Apply a poultice of the fresh roots and leaves; also the strong decoction makes an excellent base for mixing other ingredients for application; the powder is often mixed equal parts with crushed flaxseed (linseed) or powdered slippery elm.

Bad legs and sores generally: The decoction makes an excellent lotion.

Putrid sore throat and canker: Use the decoction or infusion as a gargle.

Sore eyes, ophthalmia: Use the infusion as a wash.

Wounds, cuts: The bruised leaves applied directly are very healing.

Vaginal

Leucorrhea, prolapsus uteri, relaxed vagina, ulceration of the cervix, etc.: Use the decoction as an injection into the uterus.

Chafed surfaces, irritable chancres, excretions of the prepuce and vulva: Dust the powdered root onto the affected area.

FORMULAS

Inflammation of the uterus

1/2 ounce	White pond lily (Nymphaea odorata)
1/2 ounce	Comfrey root (Symphytum officinale)
1/2 ounce	Slippery elm bark (Ulmus rubra; U. fulva)
1/2 ounce	Uva ursi (Arctostaphylos uva-ursi)
1/2 ounce	Wild Yam root (Dioscorea villosa)
1 ounce	Licorice, juice or powder (Glycyrrhiza glabra)
1/4 teaspoon	Cayenne (Capsicum frutescens; C. minimum)

Preparation: Simmer all of the ingredients, except cayenne for 20 minutes in 1 quart of water; strain hot over the cayenne, cover and allow to cool; sweeten to taste, bottle and keep in a cool place.

Dosage: 2 fluid ounces 3 to 4 times daily.

Note: The patient should be careful not to lift heavy weights and to keep the feet warm and dry.

Leucorrhea (whites)

1 ounce	White pond lily (Nymphaea odorata)
1 ounce	Comfrey (Symphytum officinale)
1/2 ounce	Cranesbill (Geranium maculatum)
1/2 ounce	Female restorative combination (see page 169)

Preparation: Simmer the first 3 herbs for 20 minutes in 1 quart of water, add the Female restorative combination and simmer 5 minutes more, strain; add honey sweetening (to taste); allow to cool; bottle and keep in a cool place.

Dosage: 2 fluid ounces 3 times daily.

Congenial combinations:
White pond lily combines well with slippery elm and flax seed or linseed.

Growth characteristics:
Perennial; it is commonly found from Nova Scotia to Florida and Louisiana especially and elsewhere in the United States; grows in still water, pond marshes, lakes, slow and sluggish streams; flowers June September.

Collection:
The best time to gather it is in the fall of the year, when dry, and when the water in the fresh water ponds is low.

Sister plants:
English White Water Lily (Nymphaea alba: NYMPHAEACEAE); root, also leaves, used therapeutically similar to white pond lily (N. odorata).

TORMENTIL or SEPTFOIL
(Potentilla erecta; ROSACEAE)

Common names:
Tormentil, septfoil, cinquefoil (this common name more often refers to other species of the same genus), Thormantle, flesh and blood, bloodroot, biscuits, ewe daily, shepherd's knapert, shepherd's knot, English sarsaparillas, earth bank.

Identifying characteristics:

Stem	Freely-forked, 6-12 inches high.
Leaves	Lanceolate, serrate, lower leaves frequently stalked, upper ones derive directly from the stem and appear to encircle it.
Flowers	Bright yellow, distinctly separate petals, form an almost perfect Maltese cross when seen from above.
Root	Brown, hard and cylindrical, roundish elevations or swell pits, or

	depressed stem scars, tiny and thread-like (filiform) rootlets, short and light brownish-red fracture, small and distinct circles of wood bundles, large pith.
Taste	Bitterish, astringent.

Parts used:
Root (most frequently); also the herb.

Therapeutic action:
Astringent, tonic, hemostatic, styptic, antiseptic, antiputrefactive, nervine (sedative), discutient, resolvent, solvent of calcareous deposits.

Tormentil is a very powerful astringent, useful in toning relaxed bowels and in checking abnormal discharges. It heals relaxed and atonic mucous membranes. It relieves any griping pains of the stomach or intestines, and it will open obstructions of the lungs, spleen, etc.

Medicinal uses:
Diarrhea, relaxed bowels, sore or relaxed or ulcerated throat, sores, ulcers, leucorrhea, cuts, wounds, jaundice, piles, ague, smallpox, whooping cough, cholera, dysentery, prolapsus uteri, prolapsus ani, excessive menstrual flow, atonic intestines, hemorrhoids (protruding or internal), gleet, gonorrhea, prostate enlargement, hernia, tonsillitis, laryngitis, relaxed and elongated uvula, internal hemorrhages, nosebleed, inflamed eyes, purulent ophthalmia, varicose veins, bleeding cancerous tumors, wounds, toothache, warts, infectious gangrene.

Preparation:
Decoction, fluid extract, infusion, powder tincture.

Dosage:

Decoction	2 fluid ounces 3 times daily between meals.
Fluid extract	1 teaspoonful (1/8 of decoction)
Infusion	1 cupful.
Powder	1-4 grams.
Tincture	1/2-1 fluid teaspoon (30-60 drops).

ADMINISTRATION

Anal

Bleeding and internal hemorrhoids, bowel problems: Inject 3-4 ounces of the undiluted decoction and retain as long as possible.

Prolapsed anus: Apply the undiluted decoction onto a tampon, insert and allow to remain as long as possible.

Oral

Diarrhea: Drinking the infusion has been very successful for chronic cases.

Diarrhea, dysentery, cholera, leucorrhea, menorrhagia, hemorrhoids, hemorrhage: Give 2 fluid ounces every 1/2 hour until the excessive discharges are checked.

Skin

Cuts, wounds: Both the fluid extract and the powder applied to bleeding surfaces will serve as a powerful styptic.

Sore throat, relaxed uvula, spongy gums, etc.: Use the undiluted decoction as a gargle or mouthwash.

Sore and inflamed eyes: Saturate cotton with the infusion or decoction and bind on the closed eyes.

Warts, varicose veins, bleeding cancers, wounds, etc.: Apply the decoction as a fomentation, wrap with plastic bandage; when nearly dry, renew the application. Also drink the decoction internally.

Old sores, ulcers: Use the decoction as a wash.

Vaginal

Leucorrhea: Inject 3-4 ounces of the undiluted decoction into the vagina and retain as long as possible.

Prolapsed uterus: Saturate a tampon and insert, allow to remain as long as possible.

FORMULAS

Fluid extract of Tormentil

1 pound	Tormentil root, cut or granulated (Potentilla erecta)
1 gallon	Distilled or d-cell water
8 ounces	Glycerine

Preparation: Place the herb into the water and simmer for 1 hour; strain and set this liquid aside; pour 1 more gallon of water over the roots and simmer for 1 hour; strain and put the two quantities of liquid in a clean pot, reduce down to 1 pint; watch carefully toward the last (may take days); to be free from sediment, this should be filtered through a filter paper in a glass funnel (this may take a long time), add the glycerine; place in brown glass bottles and cork or cap securely. This should keep indefinitely, but if placed in clear glass and kept in light, it will rapidly lose its healing potency.

Dosage: Use 1/8 amount of the decoction dosage (1 ounce decoction dosage would be 1 teaspoonful fluid extract dosage or 1 pint decoction = 2 ounces).

Chronic hemorrhage

1 teaspoon	Tormentil root, powder (Potentilla erecta)
1 cup	Hops, infusion (Humulus lupulus)

Preparation: Stir the powder into the infusion.

Dosage: 1 teacupful cold 4 times daily.

Congenial combinations:
As is the case with other astringents (to soothe inflammed membrane), we sometimes combine tormentil with mucilaginous herbs, such as Irish moss, comfrey, marshmallow, etc.

Growth characteristics:
Perennial, native of Europe and naturalized in America; grows in dry pastures, moor land (extensive moist wastes, overladen with peat); flowers June-July.

Allied plants:
Cranesbill or Wild Geranium or Wild Alum Root (Geranium maculatum; GERANIACEAE); root, herb: similar therapeutic action. See page 166.

WITCH HAZEL
(Hamamelis virginiana; HAMAMELIDACEAE)

Common names:
Witch hazel, spotted alder, shaping hazel, winterbloom, snapping hazelnut, striped elder, pistachio, tobacco wood.

Identifying characteristics:

Stem	Woody shrub, several from same root, branching, 5-15 feet high, 3-6 inches in diameter, flexuous, knotty.
Bark	Smooth, grayish-brown with many lenticels, or reddish-brown with short ridges or scars, old bark somewhat scaly, corky layer easily removed; pale cinnamon, yellowish smooth, and finely striated inner surface, short (young) or tough and fibrous (old) fracture.
Leaves	Short, broadly obovate, 3¼-5 inches long, 2-2½ inches broad, alter-

	nate, acuminate, short petioles, pale or brownish-green, lighter underneath, serrate-dentate margins, feather-veined (prominent below), rather smooth above and hairy underneath. Powder: light green.
Flowers	Yellow, small calyx, 4 petals, appear in autumn when the leaves are falling, fringe and thread-like, clustered in the axis of branches.
Fruit	Nut-like capsule or pod, woody, maturing the next season and remaining with the flowers of the succeeding year.
Taste	Astringent, aromatic, bitter.
Odor	Slight and agreeable.

Parts used:
Bark and leaves; also the young twigs.

Therapeutic action:
Astringent, tonic, sedative, hemostatic, styptic, anti-phlogistic, anti-abortive.

Witch hazel is a valuable and soothing astringent, especially useful in hemorrhage of the lungs, stomach, nose, rectum, uterus, and kidneys. It is useful in threatened miscarriage, and it corrects problems with the venous structures and restores perfect circulation. It can be used locally or internally for hemorrhoids.

Medicinal uses:
Hemorrhage, diarrhea, gonorrhea, inflamed eyes, leucorrhea, relaxed vagina, prolapsus uteri, vaginal catarrh, varicose veins, hemorrhoids, nasal catarrh, nosebleed, piles, tumors, excessive menstruation (menorrhagia), bed sores, dysentery, throat troubles, leucorrhea, ulcers, venous congestions, local inflammations, threatened abortion, sprains, bruises, pruritus of eczema.

Preparation:
Decoction (bark), fluid extract, infusion (leaves, twigs), powder, tincture; the distilled fluid extract purchased at a drugstore is acceptable.

Dosage:

Decoction	2 fluid ounces.
Fluid Extract	1/2-1 fluid teaspoon (30-60 drops).
Infusion	1 teacupful or more as needed.
Powder	1-2 grams.
Tincture	1/2-1 fluid teaspoon (30-60 drops).

ADMINISTRATION

Anal

Hemorrhoids, diarrhea, dysentery: Give a rectal injection of the fluid extract (distilled aqueous extract) or decoction; take internally.

Piles: Give a rectal injection of the fluid extract or decoction; or combined with the leaves of pile wort or prince's feather or red cock's amaranth (Amaranthus hybridus var. erythrostachys), it is thought to be one of the most effective pile medicines known in the ointment or injection form. Dr. Thompson recommends using witch hazel combined with an appropriate stimulant.

Oral

Hemorrhage, threatened abortion, etc.: Drink the infusion freely.

Stomach bleeding: Drink the infusion of the dried leaves or chew them when green.

Skin

Sore and inflamed eyes: Use the liquid extract as an eye wash.

Varicose veins: Apply a lint bandage and keep it constantly wet with the fluid.

Nasal catarrh: Use the fluid extract or infusion in an atomizer, or mix it with Vaseline and apply with a camel brush up the nostrils.

Nosebleed: Snuff the tea up the nose.

Painful tumors, external inflammation, bed sores, gonorrhea: Apply as a poultice, fomentation, or wash.

Throat troubles: Use the fluid extract or tea as a gargle.

Vaginal

Leucorrhea, relaxed vagina, prolapsus uteri, vaginal catarrh: Use an injection of the distilled extract in warm water as a warm infusion.

FORMULAS

Nasal catarrh

1 ounce	Witch hazel, fine powder (Hamamelis virginiana)
1/2 ounce	White oak bark, fine powdered (Quercus alba)
1/2 ounce	Wild or choke cherry bark (Prunus serotina)

Preparation: Rub well together.

Administration: Use as a snuff.

Growth characteristics:
Perennial; indigenous to the Eastern United States and Canada; grows in damp woods, thickets, ponds, ditch banks in nearly all parts of the country; flowers September-November.

For a listing of alternative astringent herbs which may be used when the forego-ing are not available, please see Chapter 17.

CHAPTER 5

THE CATHARTIC HERBS

Cathartics hasten intestinal evacuations. There are various products on the market for this purpose, mostly inorganic substances that are irritating to the sensitive organs and often quite dehydrating. These are definitely harmful to the functional process and vibrancy in the body: mineral oils, saline purgatives (magnesium sulphate or Epsom salts, magnesium citrate, potassium sulphate, potassium tartrate, potassium bitartrate, sodium sulphate or Glauber's salt, sodium phosphate, sodium chloride, sodium tartrate, manganese sulphate, etc.), mercurous chloride or calomel, etc. Check labels on products to see their contents. These should never be used where natural and regenerative results are desired. Natural mineral waters from an organic source, such as Pluto water, may be used.

The botanical cathartics, however, speed up the physical evacuation processes, and are also powerful healers in cleansing, strengthening and toning the malfunctioning tissues and organs. These agents are classed into several categories according to their action:

Aperients or laxatives excite *moderate* peristalsis, and produce normal stool formation without griping or irritation. Many fruits are aperient, and the drinking of large quantities of water is also laxative. This category of evacuant agents is the one generally used for infants and very weak people. Aperients are mild and slow, and these generally should be administered at night before retiring to bed. Some of these agents, such as olive oil, have an affinity for the small intestines, while others, such as agar and cascara sagrada, act specifically upon the large intestines, and some, such as licorice, act upon the entire intestinal tract.

Cathartics or simple purgatives cause active peristalsis and stimulate the glandular secretions of the intestines, producing one or more semi-fluid bowel movements accompanied by some irritation and griping. These usually act within 8-12 hours and should be administered in the morning or between meals on an empty stomach. Some of these agents have an affinity for particular areas—such as the duodenum (mandrake root) or large intestines (aloes, senna, Turkey rhubarb).

Drastics or drastic purgatives act still more intensely, and produce violent peristalsis and watery stools with much griping pain. They irritate the mucous membrane, and weaken it by causing serum to exit from the intestinal vessels. In large doses these can cause inflammation, so use two foregoing categories of aperients and cathartics whenever possible. Whenever drastics are used, take only in combination with corrective and demulcent agents. This is a partial listing of drastics: castor oil, colocynth apple, crouton oil, gamboge, hedge hyssop, jalap, red bryony, white bryony.

Hydragogues or hydragogue purgatives are very active drastics and will remove large quantities of serum and water from the vessels, causing large watery discharges. This is a partial listing of hydragogues: dwarf elder root, gamboge, great celandine, red-berried elder bark, saltwort, stinking glad wine root.

Cholagogues or cholagogue purgatives stimulate a flow and discharge of bile, while, at the same time, producing a free purgation of green-colored or "bilious" and liquid stools. These act mainly on the duodenum and contract the bile ducts, which pour bile into the small intestine, but they do not necessarily increase the secretion of bile as hepatic agents, although some herbs are found in both categories.

Follow the instructions for each herb below, but you will also find the following summary guidelines given by Dr. Shook to be very helpful:

> Where the tonic effect is most indicated, use the bitters. Where the liver and gallbladder are involved, use the hepatics. Where a quick cleansing effect is desired, use rhubarb. For children, generally, there is no better remedy than licorice. For atonic and partially atrophied colon, either mandrake or Culver's root. For long continued treatment of constipation, use cascara sagrada. A study of each will guide you correctly.

CASCARA SAGRADA or SACRED BARK or CHITTEM BARK
(Rhamnus purshiana; RHAMNACEAE)

Common names:
Cascara sagrada, sacred bark, chittem bark, California buckthorn, Persian bark, bearberry, bear wood, chittimwood, holy bark, Christ's thorn; Rhamni Purshiani Cortex (Br.); Cascara Sagrada (Fr.); Amerikanisch Faulbaumrinde (Ger.).

Identifying characteristics:

Stem: Small tree, 15-20 feet high, pubescent (downy or hairy) twigs. Usually flattened, transversely curved pieces, occasionally quilled, 1/25-1/5 inch thick, dark brown or reddish-brown, longitudinally ridged (wrinkled), usually covered with light grayish or whitish lichen patches, sometimes numerous transverse lenticels (linear marks), occasionally moss; inner surface is longitudinally striate (very fine lines), somewhat smooth, transversely wrinkled, according to age it is yellowish, dark reddish-brown, or dark brown, short fracture with projections of vast-bundles in inner bark. Powder: Light brown-olive brown.

Leaves: Elliptical, finely serrate (saw-toothed), 2-6 inches long, 1-2 inches wide, obtuse or blunt apex (or with a short, sharp point), rounded or slightly heart-shaped base, somewhat pubescent or hair beneath, prominent veins, dark green, short petioles.

Flowers: Large umbels or clusters, small and greenish.

Fruit: Drupe or berry, black, ovoid, 3-seeded, 1/3 inch long, insipid or without taste.

Taste: Persistently bitter, slightly acrid, disagreeable and nauseous to many

	people.
Odor	Distinct, leather-like.

Parts used:
Dried bark, collected at least one year before using (due to the action of oxygen, the bark becomes more medicinally virtuous with aging.) The fresh bark definitely nauseates and gripes and should be avoided. The active bitter principles become more mild and more effective by aging through oxidation from 1 to 6 years. The longer it is aged, the milder it becomes in cathartic and tonic action.

***Therapeutic action*:**
Tonic, cathartic laxative to drastic purgative (according to dosage), alterative, hepatic, stomachic, febrifuge, nervine, antibilious, antidiabetic, peristaltic.

Cascara sagrada heals the entire alimentary canal, increasing the secretions of the stomach, liver, pancreas, and lower bowels. Dr. Shook calls it one of the very best and safest laxatives ever discovered; it is most beneficial to the gall ducts. This great herb is another valuable medicine we inherited from our Indian brothers. Cascara sagrada is not generally used as a one-time laxative. It produces large, soft and painless evacuations and, after extended usage, the bowels will function naturally and regularly from its tonic effects. The bitter principle is also a stimulant-tonic to all nerves it comes in contact with.

Medicinal uses:
Chronic constipation (children and adults), chronic gout, cardiac asthma, catarrh, dyspepsia, indigestion, mucus colitis, worms, high blood pressure, digestive complaints, liver problems (especially enlarged liver), piles, hemorrhoids, torpor of the colon, gallstones.

Preparations:
Decoction, fluid extract, powder, tincture. Only the aged bark should be used (the fracture becomes darker with aging).

Dosage:

Decoction	1 teaspoonful 3 to 4 times daily, 1 hour before meals.
Fluid extract	1/2-1 teaspoonful at night upon retiring to bed.
Powder	1-4 grams.
Tincture	5-20 drops.

ADMINISTRATION

Cascara sagrada is generally combined with other healing agents but may be given alone. It acts upon the large intestines, and when given at night, it produces a normal stool the next morning without griping. It operates in 6 to 10 hours and acts best when given on an empty stomach.

Oral

Chronic constipation: Take the dosage as indicated; this must be continued for several months as an intestinal tonic to produce permanent benefit.

Liver complaints, enlarged liver, dyspepsia etc.: Take the decoction as indicated.

Laxative: 20-25 drops of the fluid extract 3 times daily (gentle action) or 1/2-3/4 fluid teaspoon, then smaller dosages 3 times daily for prompt action on the lower bowels (also see "Lower bowel formula" on page 578).

FORMULAS

Decoction of cascara sagrada

4 ounces Cascara sagrada, cut (Rhamnus purshiana)
2 quarts Distilled or D-cell water, simmering

Preparation: Soak the herb for 12 hours in the water, then bring to a boil and simmer for 1 hour; strain and set this quantity of liquor aside; add fresh water to the herb and simmer for another hour; strain and mix the two quantities of liquid together; return the liquor to the clean pot and reduce by boiling down to 1 pint; allow to cool, bottle and keep in a cool place. Twenty-five percent glycerine may be added if desired.

Dosage: 1 teaspoonful 3 to 4 times daily, 1 hour before meals. Children: less, according to age.

Note: Regulate the dose to accommodate the bowels.

Fluid extract of cascara sagrada

1 pound Cascara sagrada bark, cut (Rhamnus purshiana)
1½ gallons Distilled or D-cell water
1/2 pint Glycerine

Preparation: Place the herb in 1 gallon of water and boil vigorously until the water just covers the bark, strain and set the liquid aside; cover the herb with another 1/2 gallon of water and boil again until the water just covers the bark strain and mix the two quantities of liquid together; return the liquid to the cleansed vessel and slowly reduce to 1/2 pint; this last part should be done in a double boiler to avoid burning and excessive heat; remove frown heat, stir in the glycerine well, allow to cool and bottle.

Dosage: 1/2-1 teaspoonful at night upon retiring; it is best to take this without sweetening if possible, as much of its medicinal virtue depends upon its bitterness; take for 3 to 6 months. Children: 5-15 drops in honey water.

CASE HISTORY

A new life through proper diet and herbs.
A man and his wife came to visit Dr. Christopher on their way through the area. When Dr. Christopher saw him the previous year on a business deal, the man was so bad that rigor mortis had almost set in. In fact, the medical doctors had refused to give him any more medication. He had a heart condition that had gone into dropsy, and his blood pressure was so high that he was just tottering around. There was so much mucus in his body that the tissue was completely loaded to suffocation. Knowing of Dr. Christopher's profession, he asked what could be done. Dr. Christopher started him off with a very simple procedure: he put him on nutritional herbs (fruits and vegetables—our Regenerative Diet) and on medicinal herbs.

A year later, the man had finished 8,000 miles of touring! He had the finest skin color you ever saw, and was so full of pep and energy. Tears dropped from his eyes when he saw Dr. Christopher again, because he was so happy to be alive. Dr. Christopher commented that these are the times that make it worth all of the trouble suffered to assure others of the legal right to use and obtain healing with medicinal herbs. This man was a living example of Dr. Christopher's chief message that health begins in the bowel. For when the colon is clean, when we are free from toxins in the eliminative system, then the whole body can be fed properly, and we begin to live!

Growth characteristics:
Perennial; grows from northern Idaho west to the Pacific, especially plentiful in northern California, Oregon, Washington, British Columbia. It is difficult to distinguish this from other similar species.

Collection:
The bark should be gathered in the spring from trunks and large branches, but it must be seasoned properly before using.

Drying and preservation:
Dry carefully for at least 1 year (3 is recommend). Continual maturing is advisable (up to 6 years).

Sister plants:
-Buckthorn or Purging Buckthorn or European Blackthorn or Black Alder or Alder Buckthorn (Rhamnus Frangula; RHAMNACEAE); dried bark (1-2 years old): chronic constipation (small doses 3 to 4 times daily), dropsy, costiveness, constipation, parasitic skin affections in pregnancy, gout, itch, etc. Ointment of fresh bark: appendicitis, rheumatism, worms, warts; its action is less powerful and certain than cascaras sagrada, and is milder than Turkey Rhubarb; slender

straggling bush of Europe and northern Asia (10-15 feet high) and senna.
-Common Buckthorn or Highwaythorn or Waythorn or Buckthorn Berries (Rhamnus cathartica; Baccae Spinae-crevinae; RHAMNACEAE); berries (fresh or dried): used chiefly in veterinary practice; small tree 10-15 feet high, short and thorny branches, greenish flowers, pea-sized ovoid fruit with 3-4 brown seed-like nutlets; native of Europe and northern Asia, naturalized to America.

Allied plants:
Quebracho (Aspidosperma quebracho; APOCYNACEAE); bark; bronchitis, asthma, pulmonary asthma, pulmonary complaints; dyspepsia, native of Chile; cascara sagrada contains two percent quebrachol, which is the valuable therapeutic agent in this herb (see above).

BARBERRY
(Berberis vulgaris; B. Canadensis; BERBERIDACEAE)

We will treat barberry as an effective and speedy tonic agent to the alimentary canal and liver on page 473.

BUTTERNUT or WHITE WALNUT
(Juglans cinerea; JUGLANDACEAE)

Common names:
Butternut, white walnut, oil nut, oil nut bark, lemon walnut, Kisky Thomas nut.

Identifying characteristics:

Stem	Spreading tree, 30-50 feet high, trunk about 4 feet thick, smooth, light Greg bark, durable wood; bark (inner 1/8-1/4 inch thick, short fracture with brown fibers alternating with the white medullary rays and white cellular tissue.
Leaves	Imparipinnate, 12-20 inches long, 7-8 pairs of leaflets, leaflets are oblong-lanceolate, finely serrate.
Flowers	Staminate and pistil late.
Fruit	Dark-colored hard nut (drupe), 2 inches long, green turning brown, hairy, viscid; contains a thick and oily kernel that is pleasantly flavored and edible.
Root	(Inner bark) 1/8-2/5 inch thick, quills and curved strips, deep brown, outer surface smooth and warty, smooth inner surface, striate, short and weak fracture. Powder: dark brown.
Taste	Bitter, astringent, and slightly acrid.
Odor	Slightly aromatic.

Parts used:
Inner bark of root and trunk (the root bark is somewhat stronger than the trunk).

Therapeutic action:
Mild and stimulating hepatic, mild cathartic, tonic, anthelmintic (vermifuge), astringent, cholagogue, alterative.

Butternut bark is a valuable laxative remedy for the aged, middle-aged and delicate children where no drastic action is tolerated; its cathartic action resembles Turkey rhubarb. It gently purges and does not bind after operation. It is tonic to the entire intestinal tract and is especially beneficial to the lower bowels.

Medicinal uses:
Chronic constipation, dysentery, chronic diarrhea, worms, malaria, sluggish liver, fevers, colds, flu.

Preparations:
Decoction, fluid extract, powder, solid extract, syrup, tincture. Only alcohol will extract the astringent properties of the bark.

Dosage:

Decoction	1 tablespoonful 3 to 4 times daily.
Fluid extract	1-2 fluid teaspoons.
Powder	4 grams.
Solid Extract	325-650 milligrams
Syrup	1 tablespoonful 1 to 2 times daily.
Tincture	10-20 drops.

ADMINISTRATION

Oral

Chronic constipation: Use the aqueous extract which is free of astringency.

Diarrhea, dysentery: The astringent properties of the alcohol extract is best for these problems; use 1-2 teaspoons.

Laxative tonic: See "FORMULAS."

Hemorrhoids: Give daily doses as called for by the case.

FORMULAS

Fluid extract of butternut bark

2 ounces Butternut bark, powder (Juglans cinerea)

1 pint	Alcoholic menstruum (50% alcohol, 40% water, 10% glycerine)

Preparation: Macerate for 10 days in combined liquids, filter and bottle in dark bottles.

Dosage: 1-2 teaspoonfuls.

Syrup of butternut bark # 1

1 pound	Butternut inner bark, crushed (Juglans cinerea)
1/2 dram	Ginger, fluid extract (Zingiber officinalis)
2 ounces	Rectified spirit of wine or alcohol
4 ounces	Honey or yellow D sugar

Preparation: Simmer the herb gently for 20 minutes in 2 quarts of water; strain off the liquid and set aside; add 1 quart of water to the herbs and gently boil another 20 minutes; strain off the liquid and add to the first batch; add 1 pint of water to the herbs and boil vigorously for 10 minutes; strain, pour all the liquids into a clean pot and reduce by slow simmering (evaporation) to 12 fluid ounces (3/4 quart); add the honey, and allow to cool; when cool, stir in the ginger and rectified spirit of wine or grain alcohol (if using sugar: add the sugar, bring to a simmer and remove scum; strain and allow to cool).

Dosage: 1 tablespoonful 1 to 2 times daily.

Syrup of butternut bark #2

1/2 ounce	Butternut bark, fluid extract (Juglans cinerea)
4 ounces	Honey or yellow D sugar
10 ounces	Water, boiling hot

Preparation: Mix the ingredients thoroughly and bottle; keep in a cool place.

Dosage: 1 tablespoonful 2 times daily.

Mild laxative tonics

1 part	Butternut bark, powder (Juglans cinerea)
1 part	Oregon grape root, powder (Berberis aquifolium)
1 part	Licorice root, powder (Glycyrrhiza glabra)
1 part	Senna leaves (Cassia acutifolia; C. angustifolia)

Preparation: Steep 1-2 heaping teaspoonfuls of the mixture for each cupful of boiling hot water; strain.

Dosage: 1 teacupful at bedtime or as desired.

Laxative

6 ounces	Butternut, syrup (Juglans cinerea)
1 ounce	Wahoo, fluid extract (Euonymus atropurpureus)
1/2 ounce	Cascara sagrada, fluid extract (Rhamnus purshiana)
2 teaspoons	Licorice, fluid extract (Glycyrrhiza glabra)
1 teaspoon	Ginger, essence (Zingiber officinalis)

Preparation: Mix the ingredients thoroughly and bottle.

Dosage: 1 teaspoonful morning and night.

Growth characteristics:
Perennial; grown in the United States and Canada as an indigenous forest tree (especially the mountains of Georgia).

Collection:
When the inner bark is uncovered, it is pure white; but upon exposure to air and light, it turns yellow and finally a deep brown.

Sister plants:
-Black Walnut (Juglans nigra; JUGLANDACEAE); leaves, inner bark, fruit (nut), green husk of unripe nut: contains organic iodine that is much more antiseptic and healing than the usual poisonous iodine used for infections, cuts, etc.; germicide, powerfully sudorific and febrifuge (strong infusion). It is heavily laden with potassium iodine, which is a recognized universal remedy for scrofula, syphilis, diphtheria, and other forms of bad blood.

Inner bark: besides being cathartic, is a fibrin solvent (potassium sulphate), muscle and nerve food (magnesium sulphate), and food for hair, nails, skin, nerve sheath, and periosteum (silica). Black walnut is used for bleeding surfaces or moist skin diseases (apply powdered leaves), nosebleed and catarrh (spray the nasal passages or insert a saturated tampon of cotton), leucorrhea, diarrhea, hemorrhoids, etc. (use injections every 3-4 hours), internal ulcerations, inflammations, bleeding piles, worms of all types, dysentery, relaxed and ballooned intestines, syphilis, scrofula, eye diseases, prolapsed uterus, varicose veins, ulcers, tumors, cancer, abscesses, boils, carbuncles, acne, eczema, itch, shingles, sore throat, tonsillitis, relaxed uvula, falling hair, dandruff, ringworm, hoarseness (very valuable as a gargle).

The infusion of leaves and bark should be steeped for 15 minutes and taken in 2 fluid ounce doses; the strong infusion of leaves and husks should be macerated in warm or hot water for 1 hour; the husks make a valuable alcohol tincture.

-English Walnut (Juglans regia; JUGLANDACEAE); leaves, green husk or rind of unripe fruit, inner bark: similar therapeutic characteristics and medicinal uses as black walnut. Use a decoction of the leaves for leucorrhea and meningitis. Use a decoction of the leaves, rind, or bark to check mammary secretion, ulcers, diarrhea, sore mouth, tonsillitis, uterine hemorrhage, and carbuncles.

MOUNTAIN FLAX or PURGING FLAX
(Linum catharticum; LINACEAE)

Common names:
Mountain flax, purging flax, dwarf flax, fairy flax, mill mountain.

Identifying characteristics:

Stem	Several, simple, 2-3 inches high, slender, straight, sometimes branched toward the upper part, glaucous, resembles chickweed at first glance. Leaves Small, opposite (lower), alternate (upper), entire, lower are obovate, higher are lanceolate.
Flowers	Small, white, 1/3-1/4 inch diameter, five-parted with serrate sepals, pointed petals arranged in a forked and loose panicles.
Root	Small, thready.
Taste	Bitter and acrid.
Odor	None.

Parts used:
Herb.

Therapeutic action:
Cathartic (laxative to simple purgative), demulcent, tonic, hepatic, anticatarrhal.

Mountain flax is similar to senna, preferred by some because it does not gripe to the same extent (it rarely gripes, but to make sure, add a little carminative or stimulant such as peppermint leaves). It is excellent for torpor of the liver, and is effective against colds.

Medicinal uses:
Torpid liver, jaundice, obstinate constipation, digestive problems, gravel, dropsy, muscular rheumatism, catarrhal affections.

Preparations:
Decoction, fluid extract, infusion, powder, tincture.

Dosage:

Decoction	1 tablespoonful 3 to 4 times daily.
Fluid extract	1/2-1 fluid teaspoon.
Infusion	2 fluid ounces 3 to 4 times daily.
Powder	1-3 grams.

Tincture 10-30 drops.

ADMINISTRATION

Oral

Gravel, dropsy: Give in combination with appropriate diuretics.

Digestive problems: Give in combination with tonics and stomachics (such as gentian, calumba, etc.), see "FORMULAS."

Obstinate constipation: Use with a mild corrective agent (such as ginger or peppermint leaves), or in combination with other appropriate healing agents.

FORMULAS

Digestive and intestinal cleansing tonic

1 ounce	Mountain Flax (Linum catharticum)
1 ounce	Buckbean or bogbean herb (Menyanthes trifoliata)
1 ounce	Meadowsweet herb (Filipendula ulmaria)
1/2 ounce	Ginger root, crushed (Zingiber officinalis)

Preparation: Simmer while tightly covered for 15 minutes in 1 quart of water; strain, cover, allow to cool, bottle and keep in a cool place.

Dosage: 3 tablespoonfuls 3 times daily.

Growth characteristics:
Annual, grows in waste and peat land, meadows, pastures, etc.; flowers June-September.

Collection:
Gather in July when in flower.

Sister plants:
Flaxseed or Linseed (Linum usitatissimum; LINACEAE); dried ripe seed: cough, bronchitis, inflamed mucous membranes (respiratory, digestive, and urinary organs), renal and vesical irritation, catarrh, dysentery, gravel, strangury; a decoction best brings out the oil for enemas, coughs, asthma, pleurisy, etc.; use the oil for scalds, burns, piles, laxative (corrective for purgatives), erysipelas, irritated surfaces, etc.; poultice with slippery elm bark (Ulmus rubra; U. fulva) and lobelia seed (Lobelia inflata) for ulcers, boils, enlarged glands, swellings, pneumonia, tumors, carbuncles, old sores. When carelessly preserved (especially in the ground form), it is subject to insect attack; it should not be used after one year for best results. The seeds yield 30-40% linseed oil and about 6% mucilage.

TURKEY RHUBARB or CHINA RHUBARB
(Rheum palmatum; R. officinale, POLYGONACEAE)

Common names:
Turkey rhubarb, China rhubarb, East India rhubarb; Rhei Rizoma (Br.); Rhubarbe de Chine (Fr.); Rhizoma Rhei, Rhabarber (Ger.); Reibarbo (Span.).

Identifying characteristics:

Stem	Aerial, persists through the winter, after a few years reaches 1 foot high and 4-6 inches thick; many branches 10-15 inches long, blunt summit, dark brown coat from withered scales (ocrea) and leaf bases, internally fleshy (semi-pulpy), yellowish juice.
Leaves	Very large, 2-4 feet long and broad, petioles 10-12 inches long and 1-1 inches thick (solid), palmately-veined, 5-7 lobed, subspherical, reticulate (netted veins), pubescent (hairy, downy), pale green, very large stipples.
Flowers	Flowering stems or branches, several, 5-10 feet high, green, smooth-ish, thick, hollow, striate; clusters of 7-10 catkin-like compound panicles, greenish-white, 1/4 inch long.
Fruit	Small clusters, crimson-red, triangular (winged at each angle), 1/2 inch long, 1/4 inch broad, solitary seed.
Root	Sub-cylindrical (barrel-shaped), conical, irregular, 2-7 inches long, rhizome 1-4 inches thick, hard, smooth, moderately heavy, yellowish brown (with lighter striations and occasional small patches of brown cork, more or less covered with yellowish- brown powder), uneven fracture, stellate vascular bundles, granular yellowish mottled (blotched) surface. Powder: Yellowish- brown.
Taste	Bitter, astringent, gritty when chewed, tinges the saliva yellow.
Odor	Aromatic, agreeable.

Parts used:
Dried rhizome or root, deprived of most of its bark (periderm tissue).

Therapeutic action:
Cathartic (aperient to brisk purgative, according to dosage), hepatic, cholagogue, astringent, tonic, stomachic, antibilious, sialogogue, vulnerary, anthelmintic, peristaltic.

Turkey rhubarb, given in small doses, is a valuable stomach tonic, increasing saliva and the flow of gastric juice, improving the appetite, promoting the action of the liver and flow of bile without astringing the intestines, and facilitating absorption throughout the system. As a cathartic, it increases the circulation of the glands by the intestinal canal and increases peristalsis by stimulating the muscular layer of the bowel; in larger doses (2-3 grams), it produces copious yellow, pultaceous (mushy, soft) stools in 6-8 hours, with considerable hepatic stimulation and some griping (although the larger doses may occasionally produce quite severe griping, the herb will never inflame the digestive mucous membrane).

Turkey rhubarb is highly esteemed as a laxative tonic for children and infants because of the milk-like quality of its action; it acts chiefly on the duodenum, and generally does not clog or produce an after-constipation as so many of the active cathartics do. The tonic and astringent action following evacuation makes Turkey rhubarb a valuable healing remedy for diarrhea due to irritating matter in the bowel; it removes the irritating substance, the after-astringent properties check the diarrhea, and then it tones the tissue and corrects the accompanying atonic indigestion.

It is also a particularly suitable mild laxative agent for hemorrhoids with constipation; you can check the astringent after-action by taking 2-4 teaspoons nightly of olive oil. It will act as a cathartic by simply applying locally to ulcers, moist or abraded skin, or in poultices to the abdomen. The urine of a patient taking Turkey rhubarb will often become quite red, which is the alkaline urine acting upon the yellow matter of the root. It is a most valuable and reliable organic friend for stimulating, cleansing, and toning the vital alimentary and intestinal areas.

Medicinal uses:
Diarrhea, dysentery, weakened digestion (atonic dyspepsia), hemorrhoids, cholera infantum, threadworms, jaundice, scrofula (with distended bowels), abdominal pains, salivation.

Infantile troubles: Turkey rhubarb has enjoyed a good reputation for infantile digestive and intestinal troubles.

Scrofula: Turkey rhubarb is very beneficial to children with distended bowels.

Atonic Dyspepsia: Turkey rhubarb very materially assists digestion, creating healthy action of the digestive organs when they are in a condition of torpor and debility.

Salivation: Turkey rhubarb will often cure this problem.

Hemorrhoids: Turkey rhubarb is particularly suitable for this condition.

Diarrhea, Constipation: Turkey rhubarb is useful in both conditions.

Preparations:
Fluid extract, infusion, powder, solid extract, syrup, tincture. For instructions on infusion, powder (compound), and syrup, see "FORMULAS."

Dosage:
Fluid extract 10-30 drops.

Infusion	2 fluid ounces 3 times daily, after meals.
	Children: 1 teaspoon to 1 tablespoonful according to age.
Powder	100-200 milligrams.
Solid extract	100-200 milligrams.
Tincture	1/2-1 teaspoonful (fluid dram).

ADMINISTRATION

Large doses are a simple and safe evacuant; small and frequent doses are a tonic hepatic. It is often compounded with aromatic or stimulant agents to eliminate possible griping, especially in the larger doses.

Oral

Mild cathartic, abdominal pains: Use some form of Turkey rhubarb compounded with ginger, or aromatics (cinnamon, cloves, nutmeg, licorice, anise, cardamon, etc.).

Acute diarrhea: Give the syrup of Turkey rhubarb according to the dosage specified (see "FORMULAS").

Liver and jaundice problems: See "FORMULAS."

Nausea, vomiting: See "FORMULAS."

FORMULAS

Infusion of Turkey Rhubarb

1 ounce	Turkey rhubarb root, cut (Rheum palmatum)
1¼ pints	Distilled or D-cell water

Preparation: Pour boiling hot water over the herb and steep in a hot place for 20 minutes; strain, allow to cool, bottle, and keep in a cool place. This may be preserved by adding 25% (1/4 part) glycerine if desired.

Dosage: 2 fluid ounces 3 times daily, after meals. Children: 1 teaspoonful to 1 tablespoonful, according to age.

Compound of Turkey Rhubarb and Ginger

2 ounces	Turkey rhubarb root, powder (Rheum palmatum)
1/2 ounce	Ginger root, powder (Zingiber officinalis)

Preparation: Mix the powders thoroughly together until uniform.

Dosage: Stir 1/4-1/2 teaspoonful of the compounded powder into 2 fluid ounces of water; stir and drink, powder and all. Children: Do not give to infants under 5 because it is too powerfully stimulant.

Syrup of Turkey rhubarb

4 ounces	Turkey rhubarb root, cut (Rheum palmatum)
2 quarts	Distilled water
3 pounds	Yellow D sugar (or 1-2 pounds of honey)
4 ounces	Glycerine

Preparation: Simmer the herb in the distilled water for 80 minutes; strain, return the liquid to the clean pot and reduce by simmering to 1 pint; add the sugar or honey while stirring and simmer slowly for 5 minutes (skim if necessary as the scum rises to the surface); remove from heat and when clear add the glycerine; allow to cool, bottle, and keep in a cool place.

Dosage: 1 tablespoonful 3 to 4 times daily. Children: less, according to age.

Dr. Shook's liver and jaundice compound

50 grains	Turkey rhubarb root, solid extract (Rheum palmatum)
60 grains	Aloe leaf, solid extract (Aloe vera)
40 grains	Fringetree, solid extract (Chionanthus virginica)
20 grains	Culver's root, solid extract (Veronicastrum virginicum)
10 grains	Wahoo bark, solid extract (Euonymus atropurpureus)
10 grains	Poke root, solid extract (Phytolacca americana)
2 grains	Nux vomica seeds, solid extract (Strychnos nux vomica)

Note: 1 grain is equal to 65 milligrams

Preparation: Mix thoroughly (use finely-powdered material), pass through a small-meshed sieve; fill into 40 capsules (dividing equally); this would be about 5 grains per capsule.

Dosage: 1-2 capsules 1 to 2 times daily, according to the laxative action desired.

Uses: According to Dr. Shook, this formula is especially useful in biliousness, sluggish or torpid liver, constipation of long standing, catarrh of the stomach, bowels and gall bladder. It is beneficial in dizziness, sick headache, nausea and gassy conditions of the stomach and bowels.

Inactive bowel (injection)

1/2 teaspoon	Turkey rhubarb, powder (Rheum palmatum)

1/2 teaspoon Myrrh or gum myrrh, powder (Commiphora myrrha)
1/2 teaspoon Ginger, powder (Zingiber officinalis)

Preparation: Infuse the herb into 1/2 pint of hot water, allow to cool to body temperature.

Administration: Inject into the bowels. This will generally bring about a bowel movement and will often cause the patient to sweat as well, which is also helpful.

Nausea, vomiting (especially during pregnancy)

1 teaspoon Turkey rhubarb (Rheum palmatum)
1 ounce Spearmint herb (Mentha spicata)
1 teaspoon Cinnamon bark (Cinnamomum zeylanicum; C. Loureirii)
1 teaspoon Cloves (Syzygium aromaticum; Eugenia aromatica)

Preparation: Simmer the first 2 herbs slowly for 10 minutes in 1 pint of water with the lid tightly on; pour hot over the cinnamon and cloves, cover tightly and allow to cool; strain, sweeten to taste, bottle and keep in a cool place.

Dosage: 2 tablespoonfuls every 1/2 hour.

Rheumatism

1 ounce Turkey rhubarb, fine powder (Rheum palmatum)
1 ounce Guaiacum gum, fine powder (Guaiacum officinale)
1 ounce Cayenne, fine powder (Capsicum frutescens; C. minimum)

Preparation: Mix well.

Dosage: 1 level teaspoonful in sorghum or molasses at night; or 3-6 #00 capsules every night. This helps the bowels but will also assist the circulation and the blood stream.

Growth characteristics:
Perennial; native of western and central China, Tibet; Flourishes best at 8,000-10,000 feet elevation in the Himalaya and other mountains, on the shady side of damp ravines, with northern exposure; most of the supply came from Hankow on the Upper Yang-tse, with the Shensi rhubarb being the most expensive and undoubtedly the best (East India variety). The Turkish variety (no longer on the market) consists of the best rhizome formerly, was shipped from Chinese Tartary via Siberia to Turkish ports (hence the name). The Shensi variety has a characteristic orange color and agreeable odor; the Canton variety has a smoky odor, is bitter, and ocher yellow; and the Shanghai variety has a smoky odor and is light yellow. These plants resemble our garden rhubarb.

Collection:
The rhizome is dug when the plant is 8-10 years old in the autumn (Tartary rhubarb is collected in the springtime).

Drying and preservation:
The roots and core layer are removed from the rhizome; it is cut into segments (to aid in drying), perforated, strung on cords and suspended in the shade or under cover (house roofs, eaves, etc.) to be cured by the circulating air. This process takes about one year and results in an 80% loss in weight. Those varieties having a smoky odor indicates various types of high-temperature drying which is medicinally undesirable (usually have broad ridges, blackish grooves, heavy disagreeable odor). Experienced persons can detect both the variety and quality of Turkey rhubarb by the odor. Since it is subject to insect attack, the herb should be kept in tightly closed containers; beware, however, that some persons use cotton saturated with chloroform or carbon tetrachloride as insecticides.

***Sister plants*:**
-European Rhubarb (Rheum rhabarbarum; R. rhaponticum; R. undulatum, etc.: POLYGONACEAE); rhizome: medicinally similar, but weaker, than the Turkey rhubarb; cultivated in Europe, Asia Minor, and Siberia, cut to resemble the Turkey or China rhubarb, but lacks the outside white meshes, with the medullary rays interrupted, narrow and nearly straight, paler color, weaker odor, and the taste is less gritty and more mucilaginous (it is rarely imported). This herb is generally cultivated as a pie-plant.
-English Rhubarb (Rheum australe; R. emodi; POLYGONACEAE); rhizome (root): similar but milder in action to Turkey or China rhubarb; it is especially useful in infantile stomach troubles and looseness of the bowels, acts as a laxative in fairly large doses; the bark is generally not removed; R. australe has dark (blackish) veins and R. rhabarbarum shows red veins, with pinkish fracture.

SENNA, ALEXANDRIAN or NUBIAN
(Cassia acutifolia; C. Senna; C. Lenitive; C. officinalis; C. aethiopica; C. Orientalis; LEGUMINOSAE (subfamily CAESALPINIOIDEAE)

SENNA, EAST INDIAN or TINNEVELLY
(Cassia angustifolia; C. elongate; C. medica; LEGUMINOSAE (subfamily CAESALPINIOIDEAE)

Common names:
(1) Alexandrian senna, Nubian senna, Tripoli senna, senna Alexandrina, mountain senna; Sennae Folia (Br.); Sene—d'Alexandrie (Fr.); Alexandrinische Senna (Ger.); Senna Jebel (Arab.).
(2) East Indian senna, Tinnevelly senna, Arabian senna, Bombay senna, Mecca senna, Mocha senna, senna Indica; Sene de I'Inde—de Tinnevelly, Feuilles de

Sene (Fr.); Folia Sennae, Sennesblaetter, Indische Senna (Ger.).

Identifying characteristics:

Stems	Alexandrian: Small shrub, 2-3 feet high, erect, woody, whitish, branching.
Leaves	East Indian: Small shrub, similar to Alexandria. Alexandria: alternate, paripinnate (4-5 pairs), gland less footstalks, 2 small pointed stipules at base.
Leaflets	(Cassia acutifolia) lanceolate ovate, (terminating in a point), entire, brittle, pale grayish-green, short oppressed hairs (more numerous on lower surface), 4/5-1 inches long, 1/5-1/4 inch broad, broadest below the midrib. East Indian: Similar to Alexandrian. Leaflets (Cassia angustifolia) yellowish-green, paler beneath, smooth above, slightly hairy; more abruptly pointed, broader near the middle and proportionately longer than the Alexandrian leaves, 5-8 pairs. Powder: Light green.
Flowers	Alexandrian: Large, yellow, maxillary race me, clustered at apex. East Indian: Similar to Alexandria.
Fruit	Alexandrian: Few, legume or pod, 2 inches long, 3/4 inch broad, thin, broadly elliptical, reniform (kidney-shaped), dark green, membranous out, smooth, indehiscent, 6-7 celled, each with a heart-shaped, ash-colored seed. East Indian: similar to the Alexandrian, except that it is a trifle longer and narrower, darker, and has the base of the style prominent on the upper edge.
Taste	Mucilaginous, bitter, tendency to nauseate. Tea made from Nubian pods is tasteless.
Odor	Characteristic, somewhat tea-like, tendency to nauseate.

Parts used:

Leaves, pods. (The Arabs preferred the pods of Nubian senna, as they contain 25% more cathartic principle than the leaflets, and have no resin or volatile oil (hence are free of griping); they are non-nauseous to the most delicate stomach.

Therapeutic action:

Cathartic (pods: laxative, leaflets: simple purgative), slightly stimulating, anti-bilious, anti-periodic, tonic.

Senna is a somewhat prompt cathartic that acts on nearly the entire intestinal tract, and especially the lower bowel, that is, the colon and large intestine, so it is very suitable in cases of habitual constipation. It acts locally on the intestinal wall, increasing peristaltic movements and intestinal secretions (except biliary); and from 2-6 hours following administration, it produces copious yellow stools, but not water evacuations, which causes griping and flatulence (leaves only), but does not bind or constipate afterwards. The odor is nauseous to many persons, but the griping and nausea are modified by adding some corrective, such as cloves, ginger, cinnamon, coriander, fennel, manna, etc. It then becomes well adapted for children, elderly persons and delicate persons. The coloring matter in senna is readily absorbed, and within 2-30 minutes after administration, it appears as a reddish tint on the urine.

The Alexandrian leaves and pods are generally preferred by herbalists over the East Indian variety, as they are milder yet equally certain in action. The cathartic action of senna is intensified when combined with tonic herbs, but senna should not be used where there is an inflamed condition of the alimentary canal or intestines, hemorrhoids, piles, intestinal hemorrhage, etc. When senna is given in small doses, it will not tire the system.

Medicinal uses:
Habitual costiveness, chronic constipation, dyspepsia, disordered stomach, biliousness, jaundice, eruptive diseases, diphtheria, fevers, fissure ani.

Preparations:
Decoction, fluid extract, infusion, powder, syrup, tincture. The longer the leaves are macerated in water, or if the herb mass is tightly pressed, the more acrid and resinous principle will be extracted, producing more of a griping action.

Dosage:
Small doses will not tire the system; extra large doses will cause vomiting and purging but there are no after-effects.

Decoction	Teaspoonful doses, generally in combination with other agents such as licorice root (Glycyrrhiza glabra).
Fluid extract	10-30 drops.
Infusion	2 fluid ounces, as desired.
Powder	500 mg.-4 grams.
Syrup	1/2-4 teaspoonfuls (fluid drams).
Tincture	1/2-4 fluid teaspoon.

ADMINISTRATION

Always give some aromatic or stimulant, such as ginger, peppermint, cloves, coriander seed, etc. in combination with senna to prevent griping and to modify the nauseous characteristics; it is also more palatable given cold. The use of bitters or tonics will intensify the action of senna.

Oral

Children's laxative: See "FORMULAS."

Diphtheria, tonsillitis: In these problems and other acute cases where the bowels are constipated, use Dr. Lyle's recipe (see "FORMULAS"), or simply use senna and ginger; use the children's laxative formula for very young children.

FORMULAS

Infusion of senna (leaves)

2 ounces Senna leaves, cut (Cassia acutifolia; C. angustifolia)
1 teaspoon Ginger root, sliced, cut or powder (Zingiber officinalis)

Preparation: Pour 1 pint of boiling-hot water over the herbs, cover tightly and allow to steep 1 hour, strain through muslin or cheesecloth (but do not press, unless stronger action is desired); bottle and keep in a cool place.

Dosage: 2 fluid ounces, as desired.

Infusion of senna (pods)

6-12 pods (adults) Senna (Cassia acutifolia)
3-6 pods (children) Senna (Cassia acutifolia)
1/4 teaspoon Ginger root, powder (Zingiber officinalis)

Preparation: Place the pods in a glass of lukewarm or cold water and allow to soak about 12 hours; strain. Ginger is not necessary but will assist the action.

Dosage: 2-8 fluid ounces taken at night. This will act mildly but thoroughly on the whole intestine.

Syrup of senna

8 fluid ounces Senna tea (Cassia acutifolia; C. Angustifolia)
2 teaspoons Coriander oil (Oleum Corandri; Coriandrum sativum)
1/2-3/4 ounces Simple syrup or honey

Preparation: Mix thoroughly.

Dosage: 1-4 teaspoonfuls.

Compound of senna
(stronger than simple infusion)

1 part Senna leaves, powder (Cassia acutifolia, C. angustifolia)
1 part Mandrake root or May apple, powder (Podophyllum peltatum)
1 part Cloves, powder (Syzygium aromaticum; Eugenia aromatica)

Preparation: Mix the powders thoroughly.

Dosage: 1-2 teaspoons in honey, syrup, capsules, or infused in water.

Dr. Lyle's antibilious and purging compound

2 ounces	Senna leaves, powder (Cassia acutifolia; C. angustifolia)
4 ounces	Jalap root, powder (Ipomoea purga; I. Jalapa; Exogonium Jalapa)
1/4 ounce	Ginger root, powder (Zingiber officinalis)

Preparation: Mix thoroughly.

Dosage: 1/2-1 teaspoon in a cupful of water, with or without sweetening (can be given in honey, capsule, etc.). The smaller doses given every 3 hours will influence the liver more than the bowels and therefore, can be taken as desired. The larger dose will produce speedy action in the bowels (2-3 hours), and relieve the liver and gall ducts; be sure to keep the patient quiet.

Dr. Nowell's antibilious and purging compound

1 teaspoon	Senna leaves, rubbed or broken, about 25 leaves (Cassia acutifolia; C. angustifolia)
1/4 teaspoon	Ginger root, powder (Zingiber officinalis)
1 teaspoon	Honey or molasses (if these are not available use sugar)
1 slice	Lemon

Preparation: Place the ingredients into a cup and pour over 1/3 cupful of boiling hot water, cover and allow to stand a while.

Dosage: Drink the whole amount while warm (leave the powder). This makes a very pleasant drink and can be given to children.

Children's laxative and tonsillitis (Young children)

1 part	Senna leaves (Cassia acutifolia, C. angustifolia)
1 part	Red raspberry leaves (Rubus idaeus)
1 part	Pennyroyal herb (Hedeoma pulegioides)

Preparation: Infuse 1 teaspoonful of the mixed herb in 1 cupful of boiling hot water; cover and allow to stand until lukewarm; sweeten.

Dosage: Give a strong and as frequently as required.

Black Draught
compound infusion of senna

1 ounce	Senna (Cassia acutifolia; C. angustifolia)
1 ounce	Gentian root (Gentiana lutea)
1/4 ounce	Aromatic herb (Cardamon seeds, Coriander seeds, Fennel seeds, Seville orange rind, etc.)
1 quart	Boiling, distilled water

Preparation: Pour boiling hot water over the herbs and let steep for 20 minutes while covered tightly.

Dosage: 2 fluid ounces, as desired.

Growth characteristics:
Perennial; native of southern Arabia and the interior of Africa; Alexandrian derives its name from its port outlet, Alexandria, Egypt, and comes chiefly from Nubia (Sennaar, Kordofan) and from Timbuktu and forwarded to the Nile to Cairo and then to the Mediterranean port; East Indian original from Arabian seeds, and it grows luxuriantly under cultivation in southern India (with Tinnevelly furnishing the finest and purest leaflets), and is exported from Tuticorin, Madras, and a lesser quality from Bombay.

Collection:
The senna plants yield two annual crops of leaflets, with the largest and best at the end of the rainy season in September, and the smaller in April during the dry season. The natives cut down the entire plant (Alexandria variety), place it on rocks for drying by direct exposure to the hot sun, strip off the leaflets, pack them in palm-leaf bags and transport them by camel to the market ports; there the leaflets are garbled (sifted of foreign matter, adulterations), and placed into large bales for exportation.

Drying and preservation:
The leaflets are dried quickly by direct exposure to the hot sun (but brown leaflets and adulterated material indicate inferior processing).

***Sister plants*:**
Wild Senna or Port Royal or Jamaica Senna (Cassia obovata; CAESALPINIOIDEAE); leaflets: this variety has similar therapeutic characteristics and uses as the official varieties of Cassia, but is considered less valuable; it grows wild on the sandy soil in Egypt, Nubia, Abyssinia, Tripoli, Senegal, Arabia, India, and is cultivated in Jamaica; this was the first senna introduced into Europe, by the Moors as early as the 9th century, and it was wildly cultivated in the 16th century; the leaflets are obovate, obtuse, in 5-7 pairs.

American Senna or Wild Senna or Locust Plant (Cassia marylandica LEGUMI-

NOSAE (subfamily CAESALPINIOIDEAE); leaflets; worms (combine with other anthelmintics), biliousness, bad breath; valued almost as highly as the official variety, and is an effective, mild, and less expensive substitute; grows from New England to South Carolina west to Nebraska and the Gulf States flourishing in rich sandy or moist soils, swamps, along river banks and roadsides; it is a handsome and bushy plant, growing 3-8 feet tall, has alternate green, and pinnately-compounded leaves (usually 8 pairs of oblong leaflets resembling those of locust), and yellow flowers with brown centers in loose maxillary clusters on the upper part of the plant, bearing a narrow, flat and curving pod that is 3-4 inches long.

American senna can be cultivated as a beautiful garden plant in your medicinal garden; it is propagated by seed or seedling. Old seed is difficult to grow, but it self-sows freely and gives innumerable seedlings that may be separated by root division in the spring, and should be placed in light moist, sandy soil in a sunny spot. American senna flowers July-September, and the leaflets are generally gathered during the flowering season.

Purging Cassia (Cassia fistula; LEGUMINOSAE (subfamily CAESALPINIOIDEAE); unripe fruit bark; constipation, costiveness, promote bile flow—usually combined with aromatics and carminatives; grows in East Indies, Egypt, naturalized in West Indies and South America; handsome tree that grows 30-50 feet high, gray bark, paripinnate leaves (6-7 pairs of ovate leaflets, 2-6 inches long), easily recognized by the hanging racemes of brilliant yellow flowers, fruit is a chestnut-brown, cylindrical pod, 10-20 inches long with 25-100 transverse compartments, each with a brown seed embedded in blackish-brown pulp (prune-like odor and nauseating sweetish taste).

LICORICE

(Glycyrrhiza glabra; G. glandulifera; LEGUMINOSAE)

Licorice root is treated on page 387 as a very valuable expectorant and demulcent agent. Licorice root is also one of our most valuable cathartic herbs. It is laxative or mildly purgative (according to the dosage taken) to the entire intestinal tract, and in moderate dosage it will produce frequent liquid stools without griping within 3-12 hours (3-6 hours when given on an empty stomach). It modifies the action of drastic cathartics, and it is especially useful for dry or inflamed mucous tissues. It is healing to the glandular system. There are few herbs in nature that can equal its action for hemorrhoids. This is a great healer for both children and adults.

MANDRAKE or MAY APPLE
(Podophyllum peltatum; BERBERIDACEAE)

Common names:
Mandrake, may apple, American mandrake, wild mandrake, raccoon berry, yellow berry, hog apple, Indian apple, devil's apple, ground lemon; Rhizome de Podophyllum (Fr.); Fussblattwurzel (Ger.).

Identifying characteristics:

Stem	Pale green, simple, round, smooth, erect, 1/2-1 feet high, branches at about 1 foot into two petioles that are 3-6 inches long and each support a single leaf.
Leaves	Two (one on each petiole near the summit), large, palmately (5-7) and deeply lobed or cordate lobes, peltate (stem attached lower surface instead of the base or margin), coarsely-toothed apex, smooth yellowish-green on top and paler underneath, petiole resembles the webbed foot of a duck.
Flower	Solitary and borne in the fork of the petioles, large (2 inches broad), white, nodding, somewhat fragrant.
Fruit	White, yellowish berry, (lemon color) ovoid, fleshy, soft 1-2 inches long, flavor resembles the strawberry and is edible (and hence, some of its names).
Rhizome	Roots, long, horizontal, running (creeping) root stock, dark reddish brown, knotty joints (annulate nodes, 1½-2 inch intervals), subcylindrical (compressed on upper and lower surfaces 1¼-3 inches long, 1/12-1/3 inch thick, depressed stem-scar above with numerous root-scars or brittle roots (1-3 inches long) beneath at the joints or nodes, short and mealy fracture, whitish pith, light brown cork, wood with yellowish vascular bundles. Powder: Yellowish-brown.
Taste	Rhizome: disagreeably bitter, acrid.
Odor	Unpleasantly strong and nauseating (fresh), slight (dry).

Parts used:
Root and resin (the resin is the active principle).

Therapeutic action:
Cathartic (hydragogue), cholagogue, hepatic, antibilious, alterative, tonic, emetic, diaphoretic, resolvent, anthelmintic (germicide), deobstruent, astringent, sialogogue, anti-rheumatic, anti-syphilitic, antiscrofulous.

As a cathartic, mandrake is the slowest but surest acting, and it will continue acting for hours and sometimes days after one stops taking it. It acts mainly on the duodenum and increases intestinal secretion and flow of bile in very small doses. In larger doses, it causes copious watery stools, griping and nausea within 10-20 hours, resembling jalap in intestinal irritation, but slower acting. It is not usually taken alone but is combined with other less active laxatives such as licorice and cascara sagrada. **Mandrake should never be given in overdose and should not be combined with quick or brisk cathartics.**

Medicinal uses:
Bilious troubles (vomiting), dropsy, congestion of the liver, constipation, torpid liver, lead poisoning, diarrhea, catarrhal or malarial jaundice, intermittent and remittent fevers, dyspepsia, headache, rheumatism, syphilis, scrofula, typhoid fever, prolapsed rectum (prolapses ani), uterine diseases, pin worms, cancer.

Preparations:
Decoction, fluid extract, infusion, powder, syrup, tincture.

Dosage:
Be exact in giving the dosage as indicated; as the larger than prescribed doses will produce copious watery stools, griping, and nausea, and possibly convulsions and coma, especially in children. The first dose should be small, to determine how much is required to achieve activation of the bowels with safety and without purgation; then the dose should be increased or decreased to suit the case.

Decoction	(compound) 2 teaspoons to 1 tablespoonful cold (according to case) 2 times daily (morning and evening).
Fluid Extract	5-30 drops.
Infusion	1-2 tablespoonfuls COLD, 3 to 4 times daily.
Powder	325 mg.-2 grams.
Syrup	(compound) 2 teaspoons to 1 tablespoonful 2 to 3 times daily. Children: 1/2-1 teaspoonful in water.
Tincture	5-30 drops.

ADMINISTRATION

Mandrake should be given in the quantities and manner as explained under "Dosage." It is powerful, and it should never be given in too large or too frequent doses. Give cold at all times. *Do not give during pregnancy.*

Oral

Liver disorders: Use the compound decoction (see "FORMULAS") or take about 500 milligrams of powdered mandrake and 325 milligrams of powdered cloves (Syzygium aromaticum; Eugenia aromatica) in honey.

Constipation, laxative, worms, dyspepsia, dropsy, rheumatism, scrofula, syphilis, uterine disorders, etc.: Use the compound decoction or other suitable formulas.

Jaundice: Use the compound syrup.

FORMULAS

Compound decoction of mandrake root

1 teaspoonful	Mandrake root or May apple, cut (Podophyllum peltatum)
1 teaspoonful	Ginger root, cut or powdered (Zingiber officinalis)
4 ounces	Glycerine

Preparation: Place the herbs in 1½ pints of distilled or D-cell water and boil slowly or simmer for 10 minutes; strain and stir in the glycerine; allow to cool, place in brown bottles, and keep in a cool place.

Dosage: 2 teaspoons to 1 tablespoonful cold (according to case) 2 times daily (morning and evening). Children: reduce above dosages, giving only enough to gently activate the bowels and produce loose (not watery) stools 2 to 3 times daily.

Infusion of American mandrake

1/2 oz	Mandrake root or May apple, cut (Podophyllum peltatum)
1 pint	Distilled or d-cell water

Preparation: Bring the water to a boil and pour it over the root; allow it to steep while cooling (20 to 25 minutes); strain, sweeten to taste, bottle and keep in a cool place.

Dosage: 1-2 tablespoonfuls cold 3 to 4 times daily.

Compound syrup of mandrake

1 ounce	Mandrake root or May apple, cut (Podophyllum peltatum)
1 ounce	Licorice root, cut (Glycyrrhiza glabra)
1 ounce	Ginger root, cut (Zingiber officinalis)
1½ pounds	Yellow D sugar

Preparation: Place the herbs in 3 pints of cold water and soak for 2 hours; bring the water to a boil and simmer slowly for 20 minutes; strain, return the liquid to the clean pot and reduce by simmering to 1 pint; add the sugar, bring to the boil, allow to cool, bottle, and keep in a cool place.

Dosage: 2 teaspoons to 1 tablespoonful 2 to 3 times daily.

Administration: Regulate the dose to suit the bowels, trying to affect a soft, molded stool and avoiding any tendency to diarrhea. The formula is slow working, but if persisted in for a time, it will act with certainty in clearing jaundice conditions and restoring the liver to normal function.

Dr. Nowell's compound liver capsule

1 ounce	Mandrake root or May apple, powder (Podophyllum peltatum)
1/2 ounce	Culver's root, powder (Veronicastrum virginicum)
1 ounce	Dandelion root, powder (Taraxacum officinale)
1 ounce	Gentian root, powder (Gentiana lutea)
1/2 ounce	Golden seal root, powder (Hydrastis Canadensis)
1/4 ounce	Cayenne powder (Capsicum frutescens; C. minimum)

Preparation: Mix the powders well and place in #0 capsules.

Dosage: 2-3 capsules 2-3 times daily, as required.

Constipation capsule #1

1/2 ounce	Mandrake root or May apple, powder (Podophyllum peltatum)
1/2 ounce	Turkey rhubarb, powder (Rheum palmatum)
1/4 ounce	Myrrh or gum myrrh, powder (Commiphora myrrha)
1/4 ounce	Cayenne powder (Capsicum frutescens; C. minimum)

Preparation: Mix the powder thoroughly, fill into #0 capsules.

Dosage: 1 with meals, 2 upon retiring at night (vary to suit bowel movements).

Constipation capsule #2

1 ounce	Mandrake root or May apple, powder (Podophyllum peltatum)
1 ounce	Socotrine aloes, powder (Aloe Perryi)
1/2 ounce	Turkey rhubarb, powder (Rheum palmatum)
1/2 ounce	Golden seal root, powder (Hydrastis Canadensis)

Preparation: Mix thoroughly and put into #00 capsule.

Dosage: 2 capsules 3 times a day, more or less as needed.

Inflammation of the liver

All herbs are to be used in powder form:

1 teaspoonful	Mandrake root or May apple (Podophyllum peltatum)
2 teaspoonfuls	Culver's root (Veronicastrum virginicum)
1 teaspoonful	Blood root (Sanguinaria canadensis)
2 teaspoonfuls	Dandelion root (Taraxacum officinale)

Preparation: Mix the powder thoroughly and place into #0 capsules.

Dosage: 1 capsule nightly upon retiring to bed.

Syphilis

2 ounces	Mandrake root or May apple (Podophyllum peltatum)
2 ounces	Poke root (Phytolacca americana)
2 ounces	Yellow dock (Rumex crispus)
2 ounces	Sassafras (Sassafras albidum)
2 ounces	Blue flag (Iris versicolor)
2 ounces	Elder flowers (Sambucus canadensis)
3 ounces	Caraway seed (Carum carvi)
2 pounds	Yellow D sugar (or 3/4 pound of honey)

Preparation: Place the herbs in an appropriate vessel; add 1 pint of alcohol, and sufficient water to cover the herbs; place the vessel in a warm place and macerate for 3-4 days; pour off 1 pint of the liquid, then add 1 pint of water to the remainder and reduce by simmering to 1 pint; strain, stir in 2 pounds of yellow D sugar, allow to cool; mix the two quantities of liquid together, bottle, and keep in a cool place.

Dosage: 1 tablespoonful 3 to 4 times daily, before meals and at bedtime.

Congenial combinations:
Combine mandrake with corrective agents such as ginger, cascaras sagrada, licorice, flax seed, certain tonics, etc.

Mandrake combines well in stomach, liver, and bowel problems with tonic laxatives, such as balmony, Oregon grape root, barberry, calumba, gentian, golden seal, etc.

Growth characteristics:
Perennial; found throughout most of the United States; grows in rounded or irregular patches or clusters of 100 or more plants (10-20 feet broad), preferring low, shady places, rich and moist woods, in the open on heavy soils, etc.; flowers May-June; fruit matures August-October.

Collection:
The root should be dug soon after the fruit has ripened.

Sister plants:
-Indian Podophyllum (Podophyllum hexandrum; P. emodi; BERBERIDACEAE); rhizome; similar but stronger therapeutic action than mandrake; grows in the Himalaya Mountains of India Kashmir); cylindrical stem scars crowded on upper surface, numerous roots beneath; collected in autumn.
-White Bryony or English Mandrake (Bryonia dioica; B. alba; CUCURBITACEAE); use this herb with great caution, it is very potent.
-Blue Flag or Flag Lily or Water Flag (Iris versicolor; IRIDACEAE).

WAHOO
(Euonymus atropurpureus; CELASTRACEAE)

Common names:
Wahoo, wa-a-hoo, spindle tree, burning bush, Indian arrowroot, pig wood, Indian arrow, bitter bush, arrow wood, strawberry tree, euonymus, fusoria, skewer wood, prick wood, gutter; Fusain, Bonnet-de-pretre (Fr.); Spindelbaume (Ger.).

Identifying characteristics:

Stem	Small ornamental shrub or bush, smooth branches, white wood, 5-15 feet high, greenish layer under epidermis, usually lichens or outer surface. Powder (stem-bark): Greenish.
Leaves	Lanceolate-ovate, finely serrate, acute, 2-5 inches long.
Flowers	Dark purple comes.
Fruit	Crimson capsule, smooth, 4-lobed.
Root	Usually transversely curved pieces, sometimes quilled, 1/25-1/6 (bark) inch thick, 4/5-3 inches long, light weight, ash gray with blackish ridges or patches, wrinkled, soft scaly cork, transverse lenticels (fissures); inner surface is smooth, grayish-white, striated porous fracture is friable (fragile, crumbly), short with silky fiber. Powder: Light brown.
Taste	Sweetish, bitter, acrid, unpleasant.
Odor	Slight, distinct.

Parts used:
Rootbark (stronger and preferred), bark, fruit (berries).

Therapeutic action:
Cathartic (aperient), tonic, alterative, cholagogue, hepatic stimulant, expectorant, antiperiodic, astringent, antibilious.

Wahoo is an excellent and persisting laxative agent, with an action similar to Turkey rhubarb, but milder. It must be administered in small doses; however, as the larger dosages will be purgative and irritating to the intestines. Its expectorant action makes it a useful agent for lung affections and it is particularly effective in correcting liver disorders during and following fever. Wahoo has a beneficial action on the pancreas and spleen, and is slightly diuretic. It stimulates the appetite and increases the flow of gastric juice.

Medicinal uses:
Habitual constipation, bilious cough, rheumatism, dropsy, torpid liver, pulmonary affections, dyspepsia, fevers, jaundice, biliousness, skin troubles.

Preparations:
Decoction, fluid extract, infusion, powder, tincture.

Dosage:
Wahoo should be given in small doses, as larger doses are purgative and irritating; always administer cold.

Decoction	1-2 fluid ounces, 2 to 3 times daily.
Fluid extract	1/2-1 teaspoonful.
Infusion	1 cupful 2 to 3 times daily.
Powder	1/2-1 teaspoon.
Tincture	10-40 drops.

ADMINISTRATION

Oral

Rheumatism, dropsy: Combine wahoo with appropriate alterative herbs.

Habitual constipation: Combine wahoo with butternut bark (Juglans cinerea), or use alone.

Torpid liver, gall bladder, pancreas; jaundice, biliousness, skin disorders: Use the hepatic formula (see "FORMULAS") or combine wahoo with other appropriate agents.

FORMULAS

Decoction of wahoo

1 ounce	Wahoo root-bark, cut (Euonymus atropurpureus)
1 pint	Distilled or D-cell water
4 ounces	Glycerine (when longer preservation is desired)

Preparation: Soak the herb for 2 hours in the water; bring to a boil and simmer 20 minutes, strain, allow to cool, add the glycerine (if longer preservation is desired); bottle and keep in a cool place.

Dosage: 1-2 fluid ounces cold, 2 to 3 times daily.

Hepatic

1 part	Wahoo, fluid extract (Euonymus atropurpureus)
4 parts	Ginger, syrup (Zingiber officinalis)

Preparation: Mix thoroughly.

Dosage: 1 teaspoonful 2 to 3 times daily.

Growth characteristics:
Perennial; found mainly east of the Mississippi River in the United States, southern Europe, Great Britain, Japan; grows in woods, thickets, river bottoms; flowers in June.

Sister plants:
Strawberry Bush or Wahoo (Euonymus Americana; ANACARDIACEAE); root bark, medicinally equal to E. atropurpureus in therapeutic action and uses; low or trailing bush with crimson capsules; also grows in woods, thickets, river bottoms in many sections of the United States, flowers in June.

BALM OF GILEAD or BALSAM POPLAR or TACAMAHAC
(Populous balsamifera; P. gileadensis; P. candicans; P. nigra; SALICACEAE)

Common names:
Balm of Gilead, balsam poplar, tacamahac, tacamahac poplar.

Identifying characteristics:

Stem	Large tree, 50-70 feet high, about 13 inches in diameter; branches are smooth, round, and deep brown.
Leaves	Ovate, gradually tapering, pointed apex, deep green above, smooth on both sides. Buds are conical (narrowly ovate), pointed, closely imbricated (overlapping) scales, brown, glossy, up to 4/5 inch long and 1/12-1/5 inch thick, glutinous (sticky) with fragrant resin, abundant oleoresin and salicin crystals internally.
Taste	Balsamic and slightly bitter, somewhat unpleasant.
Odor	Aromatic (incense-like), pleasant.

Parts used:
Bark, buds.

Therapeutic action:
Bark: cathartic (laxative to simple purgative), tonic, stimulant, diuretic, antiscorbutic, stomachic, resolvent, discutient, alterative, expectorant.
Buds: stimulant, tonic, diuretic, expectorant, nephritic, demulcent, emollient, vulnerary, counter-irritant, antirheumatic, antiscorbutic, cathartic (laxative to simple purgative), peristaltic, nutritive.

Medicinal uses:
Bronchitis, nephritis, catarrh, rheumatism, bad blood (scurvy), coughs, pulmonary and chest complaints, stomach troubles, skin diseases, kidney and bladder diseases, chronic constipation, dry and debilitated intestines, sore throat, cholesterol, inflammation of the mucous membranes in the alimentary canal, gout, colds, cuts, wounds, burns, eczema, sprains, bruises, dandruff, etc.

Preparations:
Decoction, fluid extract, infusion, oleo-resin, powder, solid extract, tincture. The fragrant resinous matter that covers the buds (of this and other balsams) is easily separated in boiling water; it is soluble in alcohol, olive and other oils, but not in water.

Dosage:

Decoction	1-2 tablespoonfuls.
Fluid extract	1-2 teaspoonfuls nightly, adjust to bowel movement.
Infusion	1 teacupful 1 to 2 times daily.
Oleo-Resin	1 tablespoonful (in lemon juice, honey, etc.) 3 to 4 times daily between meals.
Powder	1-2½ grams.
Solid extract	325-650 milligrams.
Tincture	2-4 fluid teaspoons.

ADMINISTRATION

Add ginger whenever there are any griping pains.

Anal

Babies' chafed skin: Apply the ointment gently over the sore surface; then apply the finely-powdered slippery elm bark over this.

Hemorrhoids: Apply the ointment to the affected parts.

Oral

Dry cough, sore throat: Beat up 1/2 teaspoonful of ointment with 1 teaspoonful of honey and take internally (it will give almost instant relief).

Tonic, digestive, resolvent, discutient; scurvy, constipation, urinary problems, nephritis, bronchitis, etc.: Use the decoction or fluid extract of the bark.

Scurvy: Use either the bark or the buds.

Cholesterol, inflammation, ulceration, gall stones, biliary calculi, constipation, wounds, etc.: Use the oleo-resin in the buds (see "FORMULAS").

Coughs, colds, pulmonary problems: Use the oleo-resin of the buds in combination with expectorants.

Skin

Inflammation (swollen glands or joints), dry and scaling skin, chapped hands, bruises, athlete's foot, dandruff, burns, dry eczema, infected wounds, itching affections, impetigo, psoriasis, pityriasis, sore throat, sore or tender feet, sprains, ulcers, varicose ulcers, etc.: Use the ointment (see "FORMULAS"); for skin diseases, burns, wounds, etc. apply on lint and bandage.

Sore throat: Gargle with an infusion of the buds.

FORMULAS

Fluid extract of balm of Gilead bark

1 pound	Balm of Gilead bark, cut (Populous balsamifera; P. gileadensis)
1 gallon	Distilled or D-cell water
1 pint	Glycerine

Preparation: Boil the herb slowly in an open pot for 30 minutes, using half the water; strain, set the liquid aside and return the herb to the clean pot; use the remaining water and simmer until about 3 inches of the water has evaporated; strain, return both quantities of liquid to the clean pot; slowly reduce to 1 pint, remove from heat, add the glycerine, and allow to cool; bottle, and keep in a cool place. This will keep indefinitely without decreasing in potency.

Dosage: 1-2 teaspoonfuls nightly upon retiring (regulate dosage accordingly to obtain a soft, molded stool 2 to 3 times daily); the average dosage is 1 teaspoonful, but as cases differ it is best to start with small doses.

Oleo-resin of balm of Gilead buds

1 ounce	Balm of Gilead Buds (Populous balsamifera; Populus gileadensis)
1 pint	Olive oil, pure (Oleo (olea) europaea; Oleum olive)

Preparation: Heat the oil almost to the boiling point; steep the buds in the hot oil for 1 hour (keep the oil hot, but not boiling); strain through appropriate cloth or a fine stainless steel mesh strainer, allow to cool, bottle and keep in cool place.

Dosage: 1 tablespoonful (in lemon juice, mixed into honey; etc.) 3 to 4 times daily between meals. Children: 1-2 teaspoonfuls, according to age.

Separating oleo-resin from balsam poplar buds

2 ounces	Balsam poplar buds (Populous balsamifera)
1 quart	Distilled or D-cell water

Preparation: Boil the herb slowly for 30 minutes without stirring; have a pan of cold water ready, and as the resinous matter rises to the top of the boiling water, skim it off carefully and place it into the cold water (avoid skimming the buds); when the resinous material no longer rises, the buds and boiling water can be discarded (it may separate perfectly after simmering just 5 minutes or it may take up to 30 minutes); then remove the resin; use an appropriate alcohol or oil solvent to make the oleo-resin soluble.

Balm of Gilead ointment

Quantity of	Oleo-resin from 2 ounces of the buds of balm of Gilead (oleo-resin balsamifera, Populous balsamifera)
3½ ounces	Castor oil (Oleum Ricinous, Ricinus communis)
1/2 ounce	Eucalyptol (Eucalyptus Globulus)
1 pound	Anhydrous lanolin (wool fat)

Preparation: Heat the castor oil, eucalyptol and lanolin until uniformly mixed; add the balm of Gilead oleo-resin and stir until dissolved and bubbles removed; pour into preheated jars, place caps over jars to keep out any dust in the air (but do not close until quite cold), allow to cool without disturbing; chill in a refrigerator for 1-2 hours, keep in a cool place.

Administration: Cleanse the parts by washing well with biodegradable soap, rinsing well, and drying. Massage in the ointment well 5-10 minutes, wiping off any excess thereafter (to avoid smearing grease on bed or clothing).

Congenial combinations:
Any of the following herbs (in equal parts) may be added to Balm of Gilead (Populous balsamifera): anise root or sweet cicely (Osmorhiza longistylis), chickweed (Stellaria media), colts foot (Tussilago farfara), horehounds (Marrubium vulgare), hyssop (Hyssopus officinalis), licorice (Glycyrrhiza glabra), lobelia (Lobelia inflata), and/or red sage (Salvia colorata).

Growth characteristics:
Perennial; found in United States and Canada.

Collection:
The leaf-buds must be gathered before opening.

Drying and preservation:
The oleo-resin of the leaf-buds should be separated as soon as possible and made into an appropriate solution or preparation.

Sister plants:
Poplars, Balms: The oleo-resinous substance in the leaf-buds of these plants are similar in therapeutic action and medicinal uses.

BALMONY
(Chelone glabra; SCROPHULARIACEAE)

This has already been treated as a tonic, see page 505. It also works on the liver and intestinal areas.

CULVER'S ROOT or BLACK ROOT or TALL SPEEDWELL
(Veronicastrum virginicum; Leptandra Virginca; Eustachya purpurea; E. alma; SCROPHULARIACEAE)

Common names:
Culver's root, black root, speedwell, Culver's physic, tall speed well, physic root, tall veronica, leptandra, St. veronica's herb; Veronique (Fr.); whorlywort, Leptandrawurel, Anrenspreis (Ger.); Veronica (Span.).

Identifying characteristics:

Stems	Simple, straight, erect, 2-6 feet high, smooth or downy, angular, herbaceous, usually unbranched.
Leaves	Whorled, clusters of 3-9, lanceolate or oblong, acuminate tapering to a point), 3-4 inches long, sharply serrate.
Flowers	Small, white (rarely bluish), tubular, numerous, nearly sessile, crowded in dense spike-like racemes 3-9 inches long (usually several spikes at the top of stem or from upper axis), 4-lobed calyx (petals), 2 protruding stamens.
Fruit	Capsule, small, compressed, many-seeded.
Rhizome	Horizontal rhizome, irregular, nearly cylindrical, grayish-brown, and woody, somewhat branched, 1¾-4 inches long, 1/6-1/2 inch thick, annulate root rings 1/8-1/4 inch apart (from circular scars of bud-scales), numerous stem scars above, coarse (wiry, brittle) rootlets on sides and beneath, short horny (tough, woody) fracture, thin wood, thin and resinous bark, large pith, more or less hollow. Powder: Yellowish-brown.
Taste	Bitterish, acrid.
Odor	Characteristic.

Parts used:
Dried rhizome and roots, never fresh.

Therapeutic action:
Cathartic (laxative to simple purgative, according to dose), relaxant hepatic, tonic, alterative, emetic, diaphoretic, anthelmintic, vermifuge, antiseptic, astringent, antiscrofulous, anti-syphilitic, depurant, deobstruent.

The active principles in Culver's root are similar to mandrake, but Culver's root acts more on the duodenum, where mandrake acts more powerfully on the liver; they are often combined in the same preparation. Culver's root is a gentle relaxant/tonic to the liver, best given in small and repeated doses. Its certain action is evident by the rapid change in the biliary color in the eyes and skin, even though the bowels are apparently not affected. It does act specifically, however, on the intestinal secretions as noted, generally producing a positive and non-griping action in 10-15 hours. Add a carminative or corrective agent to avoid potential nausea or griping problems. It is an excellent tonic for the stomach, and it is valuable for purifying the blood and removing toxins and congestion in a mild, natural manner.

Medicinal uses:
Liver disorders, typhoid, dysentery, jaundice, eruptive skin troubles, chronic constipation due to insufficient biliary and intestinal secretions, duodenal atony (intestinal indigestion), scrofula, syphilis, impure blood, stomach disorders, fevers (typhus, typhoid, rheumatic), diarrhea, cholera infantum, worms.

Preparations:
Decoction, fluid extract, infusion, powder, tincture. Do not use the fresh root due to its violent and irritating action.

Dosage:

Decoction	1 tablespoonful to 2 fluid ounces before meals.
Decoction	(compound) 2 teaspoons to 1 tablespoon (according to bowel condition). Children: 1/2-1 teaspoonful, as required.
Fluid extract	1/2-1 fluid dram (teaspoonful)
Infusion	(compound) 1 tablespoon nightly in 2 fluid ounces of water. Children: This is usually not given to children.
Infusion	3-4 tablespoonfuls every 3 hours, until it operates.
Powder	1-3 grams.
Tincture	1/2-1 fluid teaspoon.

ADMINISTRATION

Best results are generally obtained with small and frequent doses.

Oral

Jaundice, torpid liver: Culver's root may profitably be used alone, 3-5 drops of fluid extract (add cayenne where the pulse is weak); or you can combine it with positive hepatic stimulants such as mandrake or bitter root, see "FORMULAS."

Scrofula, syphilis: Give non-purgative doses.

Intermittent fevers: Give the decoction.

Worms: Use alone or combine with golden seal (Hydrastis Canadensis).

FORMULAS

Decoction of Culver's root

1 ounce Culver's root, cut (Veronicastrum virginicum)
1 pint Distilled or D-cell water

Preparation: Pour the boiling hot water over the herb and simmer for 10 minutes; allow to cool; strain, bottle and keep in a cool place.

Dosage: 1 tablespoonful to 2 fluid ounces before meals.

Compound decoction of Licorice and Culver's root

1 ounce Culver's root, cut (Veronicastrum virginicum)
4 ounces Licorice root, cut (Glycyrrhiza glabra)
4 ounces Vegetable glycerine

Preparation: Boil the herbs slowly for 20 minutes in 3 pints of water; strain and return the liquor to the cleansed vessel and reduce slowly to 3/4 pint; remove from heat and add the glycerine; allow to cool, bottle, and keep in a cool place.

Dosage: 1 tablespoonful to 2 fluid ounces 3 to 4 times daily (if desired, this may be taken without difficulty in much larger doses). Children: 1 teaspoon to 1 tablespoonful, according to age, etc.

Liver secretory and excretory problems

1 ounce Culver's root, cut (Veronicastrum virginicum)
1 ounce Mandrake or May apple, cut (Podophyllum peltatum)
1/2 ounce Ginger root, powder (Zingiber officinalis)

Preparation: Simmer the first 2 herbs for 20 minutes in 1 quart of water; strain hot over the ginger, cover and allow to cool; strain; sweeten to taste, bottle and keep in a cool place.

Dosage: 1-3 tablespoonfuls 3 to 4 times daily, as required.

Hepatic tonic

4 teaspoons Culver's root, fluid extract (Veronicastrum virginicum)
1/2 teaspoon Golden seal, fluid extract (Hydrastis Canadensis)

15 drops	Gentian, fluid extract (Gentiana lutea)
Sufficient	Ginger, syrup (Zingiber officinalis)

Preparation: Mix thc first 3 ingredients together and add sufficient syrup of ginger to make 4 ounces; bottle and keep in a cool place.

Dosage: 1/2-1 teaspoonful 3 to 4 times daily.

Growth characteristics:
Perennial; found in eastern, southern and central United States; grows in low grounds, rich and moist woods, thickets, meadows; flowers June-September.

Collection:
Gather in the fall of the second year.

Sister plants:
Common Speedwell (Veronica officinalis; SCROPHULARIACEAE); herb; urinary problems, calculi, rheumatism, tuberculosis, gout, hemorrhage, skin diseases, scurvy, cough, catarrh; procumbent and creeping woody stem, sends up branches at joints 3-10 inches high, 4-parted flowers in maxillary racemes, pale blue corolla with dark blue stripes; found in northern and north central United States, grows under trees and in shady spots where grass will not grow, spreads rapidly and makes a good ground cover; can be propagated by seed or root division in almost any soil or location, excellent for rock gardens and flower borders.

BITTER ROOT or SPREADING DOGBANE or WANDERING MILKWEED (Apocynum androsaemifolium; APOCYNACEAE)

Common names:
Bitter root, spreading dog bane, milkweed, dog bane, flytrap, honey-bloom, milk ipecac, wandering milkweed, bitter dog bane, western wallflower, catch-fly.

Identifying characteristics:

Stem	Smooth, elegant, shrub by, 2-6 feet high, forked branches, leafy, spreading; exudes milky juice when any part of the plant is wounded.
Leaves	Opposite, broadly ovate, narrow at base, 2-3 inches long, 1 inch wide, dark green above paler and somewhat hairy beneath, entire.
Flowers	Delicate pink corolla, veined with a deeper shade, fragrant bell-shaped, about 1/3 inch broad, 5-cleft calyx, borne in loose terminal comes; somewhat similar to the flower of lily-of-the-valley; serves as a trap to flies and certain insects.
Fruit	Twin pods, about 4 inches long.
Root	Rhizome, 1/8-1/4 inch thick, pale brown, transversely wrinkled and cracked bark, readily separated from white woody center; groups of

	stone cells in outer bark. Powder: Light brown.
Taste	Bitter and astringent.

Parts used:
Root.

Therapeutic action:
Cathartic, emetic (large doses), tonic, diuretic (lithotriptic), stimulant, detergent, diaphoretic (sudorific), expectorant, cardiac stimulant, hepatic stimulant, depurant.

Bitter root has a slow, persistent and extensive influence on intestinal digestion and elimination, stimulating the secretory functions of the liver (liver tubuli), gall ducts, gall cyst, and also the muscular and mucous coats of the kidneys and bowels. It is excellent for torpid conditions of the bowels, and it will produce a soft stool within 6-8 hours, but is not recommended for irritated or sensitive conditions.

Medicinal uses:
Jaundice, dyspepsia, cardiac dropsy, kidney problems, liver problems, typhoid and other fevers, relaxed bowels, poor digestion, dropsy, worms, syphilis , rheumatism, neuralgia, diabetes, chronic Bright's disease, gall stones, diseases of the joints and mucous membranes, constipation.

Preparations:
Fluid extract, infusion, powder, tincture. The root tends to deteriorate with age.

Dosage:
Large doses are emetic and tend to gripe.

Fluid extract	10-30 drops every 3 to 4 hours.
Infusion	2-3 tablespoonfuls 6 times daily.
Powder	260 mg.-2 grams.
Tincture	10-20 drops.

ADMINISTRATION

Give in smaller and frequent doses as an alterative or tonic; use peppermint, ginger, aniseed, or other carminatives to offset possible griping.

Oral

General tonic, debility, dyspepsia: Take 5 grains (325 milligrams) of powder 3 times daily; it has also been used successfully in combination with yellow parilla (Menispermum canadense).

Jaundice: Give 3-5 drops of fluid extract every 2 to 3 hours combined with tincture of cayenne or some syrup of ginger, in water, etc.

Cardiac dropsy: Give 325 mg.-1 gram of powder 3 times daily.

FORMULAS

Liver tonic

All herbs to be used in powder form:

1½ ounces	Bitter root (Apocynum androsaemifolium)
1/2 ounce	Culver's root (Veronicastrum virginicum)
2 ounces	White poplar or quaking aspen bark (Populus tremuloides)
1/4 ounce	Ginger root (Zingiber officinalis)
2 ounces	Golden seal root (Hydrastis Canadensis)
1/4 ounce	Cayenne fruit (Capsicum frutescens; C. minimum)

Preparation: Mix the powders well and place in #00 capsules.

Dosage: 1-2 capsules after each meal.

Growth characteristics:
Perennial; found from Canada to Florida to the mid-West; grows best in dry, sandy soils, in fields, thickets, beside roads, lanes, and walls; flowers June-July. It usually grows associated with dog bane or Canadian hemp (Apocynum cannabinum), so it should be distinguished with care (see "Sister Plants").

Drying and preservation:
The root tends to deteriorate with age, so the supply should be renewed each season unless preserved in an appropriate form (fluid extract, tincture, etc.).

Sister plants:
Dogbane or Canadian Hemp or Black Indian Hemp (Apocynum cannabinum; A. pubescens; APOCYNACEAE; LAURACEAE); root; cardiac dropsy, intermittent and remittent fevers, amenorrhea, leucorrhea, emetic (500 mg.-2 grams), renal dropsy, dyspepsia; it has similar therapeutic properties and medicinal uses as bitter root, but its action is slightly different; the root bark is often sold for bitter root, but has a yellowish wood, is longitudinally wrinkled, and has no groups of stone cells in the outer bark; bitter root has a more spreading stem, broader leaves, thinner and tougher rhizome with a central pith, thinner bark with groups of stone cells, and the flower is pinkish (rather than dog bane's greenish-white cymes); do not substitute for bitter root.

For a listing of cathartic herbs which may be used when the foregoing are not available, please see Chapter 17.

CHAPTER 6

THE DIAPHORETIC HERBS

The diaphoretics are one of the most important of all herb groups.
They induce perspiration in the following ways:

They enter the circulation, and are then thrown off by the sweat glands; they stimulate the local nerve-fibers to these glands to increase action. Herbs providing this action are Virginia snake root, senega, sassafras, sarsaparilla, jaborandi, etc.

They influence the peripheral sensory nerves, which relax and dilate the superficial capillaries and vessels. They primarily influence the surface circulation and then the whole circulation, and perspiration is a result of the increased blood flow. Herbs and therapies providing this action are cayenne, mustard, lobelia, ipecac, etc.; also vapor baths, Turkish baths; wet packs, cold sheet treatment, etc.

They stimulate the sweat glands indirectly by stimulating the cells in the central nervous system (the spinal cord and medulla), from which the nerve fibers controlling the action of the sweat glands originate. Herbs characterizing this action are lobelia, jaborandi, etc.

Dr. Nowell states:

> In a condition where the system is hot and the skin dry, with a pulse that is full and frequent, a relaxing diaphoretic should be used; but if the heart impulse were weak, and the skin cold, we should use a stimulating diaphoretic working from the center to maintain the heart.

Setaceous or oil glands work in conjunction with the sudoriferous glands. These give pliancy and softness to the skin. When these glands are not functioning properly the skin becomes hard and chafed. Here we need to do more than produce perspiration; the setaceous glands must also be stimulated. Conditions requiring this action include scarlatina and eczema. The seeds of burdock (Arctium lappa) and of sunflower (Helianthus annuus) are excellent for this. They should be given in hot infusion.

Diaphoresis, or sweating, is one of the most certain means of restoring health in a great number of cases; for when the millions of pores in the skin are closed, the bloodstream soon becomes impure, poisoning the whole system. In the past, when people could not afford a physician, it was common knowledge that they could induce perspiration to help cure their sick.

The old herbal practitioners were wonderfully successful because they sought to equalize the circulation. They made the vapor bath famous, along with herbal diaphoretics; there is nothing more effective than the vapor bath to treat fevers, inflammation, colds, congestions, etc.

You should think of diaphoresis in any case where general circulation is involved such as inflammation of the lungs, pleurisy, peritonitis, inflammation in the stomach, spleen, bowels, kidneys, bladder, uterus or brain. It makes little difference where the trouble may be, diaphoresis is practically essential when you need to equalize the circulation. Maintain a frequent outward flow of blood, and you will have your patient on the highway to recovery.

Of course, diaphoretics must be given warm. If given cold, they will, as a general rule, influence the kidneys. Have the bowels as clean as possible. If the bowels are not clean, use an injection of warm water to clean them. Your diaphoretics will then act quicker. Cold drinks should not be given between doses. Never overdo diaphoresis to the point of exhausting the patient, causing oppressed breathing and tremulous pulse.

Hot water alone is a diaphoretic. Combined with the potential power of herbal diaphoretics, it is one of the most valuable of healing tools. Whenever you treat illness, think first of a hot herbal bath and internal diaphoretics.

Cathartics should not be given just before or during the administration of diaphoretics.

Diaphoretics induce increased perspiration by influencing the sweat or sudoriferous glands. These herbs relax the sweat glands and increase perspiration. Their influence is mainly on the surface, opening the pores and thereby freely emitting body poisons and keeping the blood pure. The nervous system is also influenced, and ultimately the whole circulation is affected as a result of an increased blood flow. Accompany internal diaphoretics by stimulating baths and friction with a coarse towel or massage. The diaphoretics are one of the most important of all herb groups, because they clean the foul, mucus conditions from the entire body.

Sudorifics stimulate the sudoriferous or sweat glands, producing profuse and visible sweating that stand as beads upon the surface of the skin when taken hot; and they act beneficially as tonics when taken cold.

YARROW or MILFOIL
(Achillea millefolium; A. lanulosa; COMPOSITAE)

Common names:
Yarrow, milfoil, thousand leaf, nosebleed, millefolium, ladies' mantle, noble yarrows, thousand seed, old man's pepper; plumajillo (Span.).

Identifying characteristics:

Stem	Simple, angular, rough, hairy (the whole plant is hairy with white, silky, oppressed hairs), erect, 1-2½ feet high, grayish-green, branching toward the top.
Leaves	Finely-dissected dentate segments ("thousand leaf", feeder like appearance), narrowly oblong (lanceolate), alternate bipinnate, clasping stem at base, 3-4 inches long, 1 inch broad, glandular underneath, spread along the ground.
Flowers	Grayish-white or rose-colored, 4-6 ray florets (hard, close or dense, flat-topped and terminal compound clusters or corymbs).
Root	Horizontal (creeping root stock).
Odor	Pungently aromatic, faint, pleasant.
Taste	Bitter, astringent and rough, insipid.

Part used:
Herb (everything above ground).

Therapeutic action:
Diaphoretic, diuretic, stimulant, astringent, tonic, alterative, emmenagogue, vulnerary.

Yarrow, when administered hot and copiously, will raise the heat of the body, equalize the circulation, and produce perspiration. It opens the pores freely by relaxing the skin, and it purifies the blood of toxins. Yarrow regulates the liver and the secretions of the entire alimentary canal; it tones the mucous membrane of the stomach and bowels, and is healing to the glandular system. Yarrow will never weaken a patient, because of its tonic action.

Medicinal uses:
Fevers, eruptive diseases (measles, chicken pox, smallpox, etc.), hemorrhage of the lungs and bowels, dyspepsia, jaundice, piles, mucoid bladder discharges, incontinence of urine, chronic dysentery, typhoid fever, diarrhea (including infants), colds, obstructed perspiration, catarrh (especially of the respiratory tract), uterine problems (amenorrhea, menorrhagia, leucorrhea) suppressed urine, scanty urine, wounds, ulcers, colic, diabetes, Bright's disease, stomach gas, piles, relaxed throat, sore nipples, rheumatism, flatulence, fistulas, influenza (flu), congestive headache, ague, loss of hair.

Preparations:
Decoction, fluid extract, infusion, oil, powder, tincture.

Dosage:

Decoction	1/2 cupful.
Fluid Extract	1/2-1 teaspoonful.
Infusion	2-3 fluid ounces 3 to 4 times daily.
Oil	5-20 drops.
Powder	1/4-1/2 teaspoonful.
Tincture	1 tablespoonful, 3 to 4 times daily.

ADMINISTRATION

Anal

Diarrhea (infants): Inject 1 cupful or more of the infusion (according to age).

Hemorrhoids (piles), hemorrhage of the bowels: Use a clean enema, then inject the cool tea into the bowels (where there is pain, the tea should be about 112° F.); then inject 2 tablespoonfuls several times a day, and after each stool.

Oral

Colds: Take freely as a hot infusion at the beginning of a cold, alone or preferably in combination with other herbal remedies such as elder flowers and peppermint. It will break up a cold overnight or within 24 hours; wrap the feet in flannel that has been wrung out in apple cider vinegar, keeping it warm with a hot water bottle.

Fevers: For all types of fever, give 2-3 fluid ounces of yarrow decoction (see "FORMULAS") every 2 to 3 hours as hot as the patient can conveniently take it. Be sure to keep the bowels clean, using senna tea (Cassia acutifolia) if necessary.

Enuresis, bronchitis (and other respiratory affections): Drink the decoction cool.

False membranes in the small intestines: Yarrow is a very reliable agent to remove them; give 2-4 ounces of the decoction 3 to 4 times daily, 1 hour before meals.

Hemorrhage, spitting of blood: Drink the warm infusion; it will equalize the circulation and relieve the pressure from the ruptured vessel, allowing it to heal.

Skin

Old wounds, ulcers, fistulas: Use an ointment of yarrow; soaking and washing with the tea is also very beneficial.

Vaginal

Leucorrhea, inflammation of bladder: Yarrow makes an excellent douche for this problem; use cool.

FORMULAS

Infusion of Yarrow

1 teaspoon	Yarrow (Achillea millefolium)
1 cup	Boiling-hot water (preferably D-cell or distilled)

Preparation: Steep for 15 minutes in a warm place, cover with a saucer.

Dosage: 3-4 cups daily, 1 hour before meals and before retiring to bed.

Note: The quantity would be 1 tablespoonful for each pint.

Decoction of yarrow

1 ounce	Yarrow, dried (Achillea millefolium) or
4 ounces	Yarrow, green (Achillea millefolium)
1 quart	Distilled or d-cell water

Preparation: Place the herb in cold water, bring to a boil and simmer down to 1 pint of liquid; strain, cool, bottle and keep in a cool place.

Dosage: Give cool in 1/2 cup doses.

Hemorrhoids, fistula, false membranes in the small intestines

2 ounces Yarrow, dried (Achillea millefolium)
1 ounce Ginger, bruised or powder (Zingiber officinalis)

Preparation: Place in 4 quarts of water and bring to a boil, simmer down to 2 quarts of liquid; strain, and while hot add 2 lbs. of blackstrap molasses or 3 pounds sorghum; cool.

Dosage: 1/2 cup 4 times daily, before meals (cool).

Fever

1 ounce Yarrow (Achillea millefolium)
1 ounce Angelica (Angelica atropurpurea)

Preparation: Bring the herbs to a boil or pour 1 quart of boiling hot water over the herbs, simmer to 1 pint; strain, cool, bottle and keep in a cool place.

Dosage: 2 fluid ounces (warm) every 2 hours.

Hemorrhoids (piles)

2 parts Yarrow (Achillea millefolium)
1 part Mullein (Verbascum thapsus)

Preparation: Mix in boiling water, cover and steep till cool.

Dosage: 1 cup 2 to 3 times daily.

Enuresis (bed-wetting, incontinence of urine)

1/4 ounce Yarrow (Achillea millefolium)
1/4 ounce Bethroot (Trillium erectum, T. pendulum)
1/4 ounce Sumac berries (Rhus glabra)
1/4 ounce Agrimony or Sticklewort (Agrimonia eupatoria)
1/4 ounce White pond lily (Nymphaea odorata)

Preparation: Bring to a boil in 1 pint of water, simmer slowly for 10 minutes, strain, cool.

Dosage: 1 tablespoonful to 2 fluid ounces 3 to 4 times daily.

Note: Massage over the lumbar region to stimulate the nerves to the bladder.

Congenial combinations:
Yarrow combines well with ginger (Zingiber officinalis). It is a sure cure for fevers when combined with elder flowers (Sambucus canadensis or S. nigra) and peppermint (Mentha piperita). All of these are both stimulant and diaphoretic.

CASE HISTORY

Overnight recovery for flu:
The old-time herbalist never took the temperature of his patient when there was fever. Often he did not know what a clinical thermometer was. He placed a handful of yarrow in a jug, poured a pint of boiling water over it, and after allowing it to stand a few minutes, gave the strained tea to the patient as warm as it could be drunk. The result was free perspiration. Congestion was removed; the circulation was equalized. The treatment was easy, the results were sure, and the remedy was safe, simple and natural. Yarrow is just the same today as it was a thousand years ago. Dr. Christopher would gather it by the armful every year to use in his practice.

While away at a summer camp, Dr. Christopher's daughter caught a severe cold. Dr. Christopher went to the island for the weekend and found her in bed with a high temperature, headache, and the general symptoms of influenza or la grippe, the body aching and the child most restless. He had noted some yarrow growing a little distance from the cottage and went and gathered a handful. He did not weigh it. He had no scales. It was not necessary. It was not a harmful drug. He placed a bunch of the clean whole plant in a jug and poured over it about one and a half pints of boiling water, covered it for about five minutes, then poured off a cupful of the warm tea. He gave this to his daughter who, by the way, insisted that she would vomit if he made her drink the whole of it. Dr. Christopher told her that if the stomach rejected it, the result would be a cleaner stomach for the next dose. She drank the cupful.

He went into the kitchen and poured off a second cupful of the warm tea and gave this to her. She got it all down, and in a few minutes was perspiring freely. In half an hour she informed her father that she felt better and in the morning she was completely recovered. Dr. Christopher said, "You ask me what would I have done if there had been no yarrow there. I would have looked for sage, peppermint, hyssop or any other of the half a dozen other herbs which will do the work."

Growth characteristics:
Perennial; found throughout North America, in Europe and Asia; it grows by

road-sides, in wastelands, pastures, meadows, dry fields; flowers most of the summer and fall. The herb grows quite easily, and may be propagated by the creeping root stock or by root division. Every home medicinal garden should contain yarrow; it is also grown as a decorative wildflower, used both fresh and dried.

Collection:
Gather yarrows at the flowering stage.

Sister plants:
Sneezewort (Achillea Ptarmica); leaf; catarrh, epilepsy, uterine problems.

CAMOMILE or ROMAN CHAMOMILE
(Chamaemelum nobile; Anthemis nobilis; COMPOSITAE)

Common names:
Camomile, chamomile, Roman chamomile, double camomile, garden camomile, low camomile, ground apple, whig plant; Anthemis noble, Chamomile romaine (Fr.); Romisch Kamomile (Ger.); Camomilla odorosa (Ital.); Manzanilla (Span.).

Identifying characteristics:

Stem	6-12 inches high, hairy, round, furrowed, hollow.
Leaves	Pale green, bipinnate, sessile, with short, hairy, lacy and thread-like leaflets.
Flowers	Daisy-like, terminal, whitish or yellowish, ligulate florets surrounding a conical and solid receptacle (which is covered with lanceolate membranous scales).
Root	Strong and fibrous.
Odor	Agreeable.
Taste	Aromatic, very bitter.

Part used:
Flowers, herb.

Therapeutic action:
Diaphoretic (hot), stomachic, tonic (cold), antispasmodic, stimulant, carminative, nervine (sedative), emmenagogue, anthelmintic, anodyne, bitter aromatic, emetic (warm large dose), cathartic (large dose).

The camomile flowers are excellent for diaphoresis, bringing a good flow of blood to the skin surface. For those who find yarrow bitter, it is an excellent substitute. It acts quickly on the circulation, stomach, nerves, and uterus. It is an excellent stomachic, improving the appetite and aiding the digestion by increasing the vascularity (fluid conveyance) of the gastric mucous membrane. Camomile is very soothing to the nerves, and as a uterine agent it relieves congestion and stimulates the menstrual flow, when taken cold. As a poultice, it reduces swelling without drawing the poison to a head. Used as a hair rinse, it will keep the golden tints of the hair. Camomile is well-known for its soothing effects as well, helping to equalize the circulation and promote relaxation. In Europe, it is commonly used as a soporific (sleep-inducing herb).

Medicinal uses:
Colds, fevers (remittent, bilious, puerperal), painful and congested menstruation, bilious headache, indigestion, colic, spasmodic cough, bronchitis, pulmonary catarrh, acute dyspepsia, hysteria, nervousness, torpid liver, delirium tremens, rheumatism, ulcers, produces appetite, stomach weakness, kidney, spleen and bladder problems, expel worms, ague, dropsy, jaundice, sore and weak eyes (wash), open sores and wounds (wash), pains and swellings (poultice), gangrene (preventative), bruises, sprains, corns, earache, toothache, neuralgia.

Preparations:
Fluid extract, infusion, solid extract. Do not boil the flowers, as the volatile oils possessing much of the therapeutic value will escape. Also, be sure to cover well in preparation.

Dosage:

Fluid Extract	1/2-1 teaspoonful.
Infusion	1 tablespoonful to 2 fluid ounces.
Powdered flowers	1/2-1 teaspoonful 3 times daily (tonic).
Oil	1-3 drops.
Solid Extract	100-500 milligrams.

ADMINISTRATION

As a diaphoretic, use hot; as a tonic, use cold.

Oral

Colds, bilious fever: Give a warm infusion with a little ginger (Zingiber officinalis) added.

Digestive trouble: Steep 5-6 flowers for a few minutes in 1/2 cup of hot water and drink as soon as it is comfortable.

Skin

Pain, swellings, neuralgia: Apply as a poultice alone or combination with poppy heads (Papaver somniferum); see “FORMULAS.”

Toothache, earache, neuralgia: Apply in the form of lotion.

Bruises, sprains, callous swellings, corns: Apply as an ointment, in combination with bittersweet (Solanum dulcamara).

Sore and weak eyes, open sores and wounds: Use the tea as a wash.

FORMULAS

Bruises, swellings, neuralgia, toothache

1 ounce	Camomile flowers (Chamaemelum nobile; Anthemis nobilis)
3 heads	Poppy flowers (Papaver somniferum)

Preparation: Break up the poppy heads and mix together; pour on sufficient boiling hot water to make a poultice.

Administration: Apply as hot as possible.

Cystitis (fomentation)

2 ounces	Camomile (Chamaemelum nobile; Anthemis nobilis)
2 ounces	Ragwort or Squaw weed (Senecio jacobaea)
2 ounces	Wormwood (Artemisia absinthium)

Preparation: Simmer the herbs slowly in 5 pints of water for 15 minutes.

Administration: Foment as hot as possible. Give the composition tea (see page 147-148) as a diaphoretic agent freely until the patient sweats.

Colic

9 parts	Camomile (Chamaemelum nobile; Anthemis nobilis)
3 parts	Caraway (Carum carvi)
2 parts	Valerian (Valeriana officinalis)
2 parts	Peppermint (Mentha piperita)

Preparation: Use one teaspoonful of the combined mixed herbs to a cup of boiling water.

Administration: Foment abdominal area (warm as possible) and drink in 2 fluid ounce doses (as needed).

Relaxing nervine
(headache, neck, shoulder and muscular tension, irritability, nervousness or raw nerves, sleeplessness, female organs)

3-4 teaspoons	Camomile flowers (Chamaemelum nobile; Anthemis nobilis)

1 teaspoon	White poplar or quaking aspen (Populus tremuloides)
1/2 teaspoon	False unicorn, blazing star or helonias (Chamaelirium luteum)
1/2 teaspoon	Ladies slipper (Cypripedium calceolus var. pubescens)
4-8 drops	Lobelia, tincture (Lobelia inflata)
4-8 drops	Ginger, tincture (Zingiber officinalis)

Preparation: Bring 1 quart of water to a boil, stir in or pour over first four herbs; cover closely and steep 15 minutes; strain through cheesecloth and sweeten with honey; add the lobelia and ginger to each dosage in proportion before drinking.

Dosage: 1/2-1 cupful warm as required.

Congenial combinations:
Camomile combines well with ginger (Zingiber officinalis) as a diffusive agent.

Growth characteristics:
Perennial; grows low and spreads gracefully over the earth; thrives in dry, light, sandy soil in full sunlight. For plant propagation, use the seed, which germinates easily, root division, or layering of runners, and space the plants 6 inches apart. Camomile grows freely in moist conditions, contributes to the health of the soil, and keeps away obnoxious pests—for which characteristic it has been called "the plant's physician." Every home medicinal garden should grow camomile, especially homes with small children.

Collection:
Gather at the flowering stage.

Sister plants:
-English chamomile; tubular central florets; similar use.
-Scotch Chamomile; only an outer row of florets, similar use.
-German Chamomile (Matricaria chamomilla); flowers, herb: general debilitating fevers, colic, stomach cramps, flatulence, delirium tremens, local pains, toothache, earache, abscesses, sprains, rheumatism, etc.; therapeutically interchangeable with camomile (Chamaemelum nobile), but the German variety is considered more potent and superior to the American variety; similar in appearance, except the German variety has smooth, striated stems, leaflets that are small, smooth and linear, and the flower receptacle is hollow.

PLEURISY ROOT
(Asclepias tuberosa; ASCLEPIADACEAE)

Common names:
Pleurisy root, butterfly-weed, white root, wind root, orange root, orange milkweed, swallow-wort, tuber root, colic root, Canada root, asclepias.

Identifying characteristics:

Stem	Numerous (growing in bunches from the root), erect, 1-2 feet high, round, hairy, leafy, green or reddish, very little milky juice.
Leaves	Alternate, lanceolate, hairy, dark green above and pale beneath, seated on the stem.
Flowers	Numerous and erect (many-flowered in terminal clusters) beautiful bright orange-red, each singular flower resembles the common milkweed flower.
Fruit	Two long, narrow, green, erect, hoary pods, 2-5 inches long (at least one contains ovate seeds that are silky plumed terminally).
Root	Knotty crown, slightly annulate (faintly ringed), numerous interstock setting grooves. Fusiform (spindle-shaped), large 4-8 inches long, 1/5-2 inches thick, longitudinally wrinkled, orange-brown (turns grayish when kept too long), internally whitish, fleshy, thin bark, tough and uneven fracture, yellowish wood with bundles and medullary rays. The powder is yellowish-brown.
Odor	Slight (almost none).
Taste	When fresh, somewhat disagreeably acrid; when dried, bitterish or slightly bitter.

Part used:
Root.

Therapeutic action:
Powerful and relaxing diaphoretic (sudorific), diuretic, stimulant, expectorant, tonic, antispasmodic, mildly carminative, anodyne, cardiac depressant, nervine (slightly sedative), slightly astringent, mildly cathartic (large doses), emetic (large doses).

The North American Indians considered pleurisy root to be one of the "Great White Father's best gifts to the children of nature" because of its specific action for the lungs. And for all chest complaints, including pleural bronchitis, it assists expectoration, subduing inflammation rapidly, reabsorbing moisture from the tissues and serous cavities, and exerting a general and mild tonic effect on the whole system. It is one of the very best herbs for pulmonary catarrh and difficult or suppressed expectoration, through its beneficial influence on the mucous membranes and serous tissues. Pleurisy root influences the skin and circulation by relaxing the capillaries, relieving the heart and arteries of undue tension, and stimulating a slow and steady perspiration of the sudoriferous glands, so that excessive heat due to congestion in the skin is gradually eased.

Medicinal uses:
Chest and lung troubles, pleurisy, bronchitis, chronic cough, catarrh, asthma, eruptive diseases (specific), fevers (all types), dysmenorrhea, amenorrhea, spasmodic pain, dyspnea, pain, pneumonia, inflammatory rheumatism, dyspepsia, tuberculosis, diarrhea, colds, influenza, acute dysentery, kidney troubles, colic,

scrofula, ulcers, wounds, phthisis (tuberculosis of the lungs), gastralgia.

Preparations:
Decoction, fluid extract, infusion, powder, tincture.

Dosage:

Decoction	1/2-2 fluid ounces.
Fluid Extract	1/2-1 teaspoonful (30-60 drops).
Infusion	1-2 teacupfuls daily taken hot (6 fluid ounces = 1 teacupful).
Powder	1-4 grams 3 to 4 times daily.
Tincture	1/2-1 teaspoonful (fluid teaspoon).

ADMINISTRATION

Pleurisy root is quite harmless in correct doses, but is not recommended for children because of its powerful action. Do not use when the skin is cold and the pulse is weak, but use a more stimulating diaphoretic.

Oral

Pleurisy, bronchitis, pneumonia, inflammatory rheumatism: Give hot infusion while the patient is closely-covered in bed; repeat the dosage every 30 minutes until free perspiration is produced; apply hot cloths externally, wrung out in the infusion.

Fevers: In fevers where the skin is hot and pulse is rigid, pleurisy root is especially relaxing and sedative in its cleansing action.

FORMULAS

Fever

2 ounces	Pleurisy root, powdered (Asclepias tuberosa).
1/2 ounce	Ginger, powdered (Zingiber officinalis)

Preparation: Mix the herbs thoroughly; stir 1 teaspoonful into 1 cup of hot water, cover and allow to stand (steep) 10 to 15 minutes.

Administration: Drink warm, leaving the sediment.

Influenza

2 ounces	Pleurisy root, powdered (Asclepias tuberosa)
2 ounces	Goldenrod, powdered, (Solidago odora)
1/2 ounce	Ginger, powdered, (Zingiber officinalis)
1 teaspoon	Cayenne, powdered (Capsicum frutescens; C. minimum)

Preparation: Mix the herb powders thoroughly; use 1 teaspoonful of the powder per each cupful of hot water.

Administration: Give freely in warm infusion; as the patient improves decrease the amount of pleurisy root and add more cayenne.

Diaphoretic

2 ounces	Pleurisy root, powder (Asclepias tuberosa)
1/2 ounce	Thyme, powder (Thymus vulgaris)
1/2 ounce	Ginger, powder (Zingiber officinalis)
1/2 ounce	Sweet marjoram, powder (Origanum majorana)

Preparation: Mix the powders thoroughly and use 1 teaspoonful to each pint of water; steep in boiling hot water 10 to 15 minutes, cover closely.

Dosage: 1-2 fluid ounces every 45 minutes (hot).

Pleurisy

1 ounce	Pleurisy root (Asclepias tuberosa)
1/2 ounce	Hyssop (Hyssopus officinalis)
1/2 ounce	Comfrey root (Symphytum officinale)
1 ounce	Vervain (Verbena officinalis)
1 teaspoonful	Cayenne (Capsicum frutescens; C. minimum)

Preparation: Simmer the first 4 herbs slowly in 3 pints of water down to 1½ pints; strain over the cayenne.

Dosage: 3 tablespoonfuls every 2 to 3 hours, hot.

Administration: Foment the painful parts with hot cayenne tea; give vapor bath if the patient is not too weak; wrap the feet in cloths wrung out in apple cider vinegar and keep warm with a hot water bottle; nourish with slippery elm gruel (Ulmus rubra; U. fulva); keep the bowels clean with catnip injection (Nepeta cataria) when necessary.

Menstrual problems
(dysmenorrhea, amenorrhea)

1 ounce	Pleurisy root (Asclepias tuberosa)
1/2 ounce	Blue cohosh (Caulophyllum thalictroides)
1/2 ounce	Wild Yam (Dioscorea villosa)
1/4 ounce	Ginger (Zingiber officinalis)

Preparation: When powders are used, stir 1 teaspoonful of the mix in 1 cupful of hot water, cover with a lid and steep 10 minutes. When herbs are used, steep 1 ounce of the mixture in 1 pint of boiling hot water, cover and let stand 10 to 15 minutes; keep warm.

Dosage: When powders are used, drink the cupful warm, leaving sediments; when the herbs are used, give 2 fluid ounces every 4 hours.

Congenial combinations:
When the heart is palpitating or on the weak side, cayenne should be used in combination with pleurisy root; pleurisy root alone will quiet a heavy pulse and moisten dry skin, but a diffusive agent such as ginger will hasten the outward flow of blood in the capillaries.

Growth characteristics:
Perennial; indigenous to North America (particularly of the Southern States), some in South America; prefer dry, sandy and gravelly soil; flowers June-September.

BONESET
(Eupatorium perfoliatum; COMPOSITAE)

Common names:
Boneset, thoroughwort, Indian sage, crosswort, Joe pye weed, rheumatism root, vegetable antimony, sweating plant, teasel, ague weed, feverwort, fit plant.

Identifying characteristics:

Stem	Stout, tall (1-5 feet), round, rough, hairy, leafy, branching at the top.
Leaves	Opposite (but united at the base or clasping), lanceolate 3-8 inches long, 3/5-2 inches broad, crenate-serrate, green or gray-green, veined or reticulated above, resin-dotted on the under side. Powder: dark green.
Flowers	Composite dull-white, fluffy heads of 10-15 tubular flowers in flat-topped terminal comes spreading out from a scaly involucre (compound umber).
Root	Horizontal and crooked.
Odor	Faintly aromatic or fragrant.
Taste	Astringent and persistently bitter.

Parts used:
Dried leaves and flowering tops.

Therapeutic action:
Diaphoretic (sudorific), tonic, febrifuge, expectorant, nervine, stimulant, diuretic, antispasmodic, aperient, emetic (large doses warm), anti-periodic, stomachic, bit-

ter.

Boneset is another of our great Indian remedies, cleansing to the stomach, liver, bowels, uterus, and skin; and though it manifests great power, it is harmless. Boneset is a sudorific tonic in its action on the skin, and it stimulates the secretion of bile by the liver, as well as the gallbladder. It is similar to camomile in action.

Medicinal uses:
Fevers (all types), influenza, catarrh, skin diseases, dyspepsia, constipation, night sweats, indigestion, bilious conditions, jaundice, muscular rheumatism, bronchitis, sore throat, chills, emesis, general debility.

Preparations:
Fluid extract, infusion, powder, solid extract, tincture.

Solid Extract: Boil the herb in water for 15 minutes to make a strong decoction; then evaporate the decoction to a solid extract and make into pills. Boiling down the herb to make a solid extract removes the relaxing properties of Boneset, leaving a medicinal material which is a stimulant, antispasmodic, and tonic remedy of great importance. However, this procedure requires constant watching and skill in preparing.

Dosage:

Fluid Extract	1/2-1 teaspoonful.
Infusion	2 fluid ounces 3 to 4 times daily.
	Children: 1 teaspoonful to 1 tablespoonful, according to age.
Powder	500 mg.-1 gram.
Solid Extract	325-650 milligrams.
Tincture	10-40 drops (2/3 teaspoonful).

ADMINISTRATION

Give the infusion cold as a tonic, diuretic; give the infusion warm as a diaphoretic emetic (large doses).

Oral

Emesis: Give a large dose of the strong infusion as hot as can be comfortably swallowed, which will also induce an evacuation of the bowels.

Bilious colic: Give 2 fluid ounces (warm) every 1/2 hour until vomiting results; then, after 1/2 hour give a small dose as a tonic (cold), and every 2-3 hours thereafter.

Influenza, colds, fevers, etc.: Give the patient 1/2-1 teacupful hot, every hour until freely perspiring and the fever begins to subside; then give in smaller dose as a tonic (cold) every 2 to 3 hours and keep closely-covered in bed 24 to 48 hours until all signs of the fever are gone.

Muscular rheumatism: Give in small, tonic doses; this is one of the best known remedies for this problem.

Bilious remitting fevers, yellow fever, night sweats, indigestion, etc.: Give 1 solid extract pill every 2 to 3 hours.

FORMULAS

Infusion of Boneset

1 ounce Boneset (Eupatorium perfoliatum)
1¼ pints Distilled or d-cell water

Preparation: Boil the water and, while boiling, pour over the herb, cover and place in a warm place for 20 minutes to steep; strain, cool, bottle and keep in a cool place.

Dosage: 2 fluid ounces 3 to 4 times daily.

Epilepsy #1

1 part Boneset (Eupatorium perfoliatum)
1 part Blue vervain (Verbena hastata)

Preparation: 1 teaspoonful to cup of combined herbs in boiling hot water.

Dosage: 1 cup 3 times a day, children less according to age.

Epilepsy #2

1 part Boneset (Eupatorium perfoliatum)
1 part Blue vervain (Verbena hastata)
1 part Water pepper (Polygonum hydropiperoides)
1 part Camomile (Chamaemelum nobile; Anthemis nobilis)

Preparation: Combine and mix herbs, use 1 teaspoonful to cup of boiling water.

Dosage: 1 cup 3 times a day or 1/2 cup 6 times a day, children according to age.

Influenza

1½ ounces Boneset (Eupatorium perfoliatum)

1½ ounces	False Boneset (Eupatorium cannabinum)
1 ounce	Vervain (Verbena officinalis)
1 ounce	Culver's root or leptandra (Veronicastrum virginicum)
1 ounce	Agrimony or sticklewort (Agrimonia eupatoria)

Preparation: Place 1 ounce of the above herbs in 1 pint of water, simmer for 10 minutes; strain.

Dosage: 4 tablespoonfuls (hot) every 2 to 3 hours.

Enteric or intestinal fever

1 ounce	Boneset (Eupatorium perfoliatum)
1 ounce	Twin leaf (Jeffersonia diphylla)
1 ounce	Prickly ash (Zanthoxylum americanum, Z. fraxineum)
1 ounce	False unicorn, blazing star or helonias (Chamaelirium luteum)

Preparation: Simmer the herbs in 3 pints of water for 20 minutes; strain.

Dosage: Give warm 2-4 tablespoonfuls every 1 to 2 hours.

Liver complaints, bowel constipation

1 part	Boneset, powder (Eupatorium perfoliatum)
1 part	Butternut, powder (Juglans cinerea)

Preparation: Use in capsule form or in an infusion (cool).

Dosage: 1 teaspoonful (1 dram) doses.

Jaundice, constipation

1 ounce	Boneset, fluid extract (Eupatorium perfoliatum)
1 ounce	Butternut, fluid extract (Juglans cinerea)
4 ounces	Ginger, syrup (Zingiber officinalis)

Administration: Give 1 teaspoonful 3 to 4 times daily.

Growth characteristics:
Perennial; native of North America, grows throughout the United States from Canada to Florida and west to Texas and Nebraska. Boneset is found in low meadows, on banks of streams, borders of swamps, but it will grow well in almost any soil or location; it flowers August-September; propagate by sowing the seed when ripe early in the autumn, or by root division in the spring; thrives best in light, moist, rich and well-drained soil, grow in sunlight, and space about 12 inches; protect during the winter with a straw mulch.

Sister plants:
-Gravel Root (Eupatorium purpureum; COMPOSITAE); properties similar to Boneset; see page 246.
-False Boneset (Eupatorium cannabinum); properties similar to Boneset.
-Rough Boneset or Wild Horehound (Eupatorium verbenaefolium; E. teucrifolium); properties similar to Boneset.

BLESSED THISTLE or HOLY THISTLE
(Cnicus benedictus; Carduus sanctus; C. benedictus; Carbenia benedicta; Centura benedicta; COMPOSITAE)

See page 497.

THYME
(Thymus vulgaris; LABIATAE)

Common names:
Thyme, common thyme, garden thyme, whooping cough herb; Herba Thymi, Thymain, Thymolum, Tomillo (Span.); Thymiansaeure (Ger.).

Identifying characteristics:

Stem	Small undershrub, numerous stems; procumbent or trailing at base, 6-12 inches high, quadrangular stem and branches, pubescent (downy or covered with soft, fine hairs), purplish shoots, pale brown bark, almost evergreen.
Leaves	Opposite, small, 1/3 inch long, 1/16 inch broad, elliptic (lanceolate or arrow-shaped), grayish-green, short-stalked reflexed at margin, strongly aromatic, numerous. Powder: light green.
Flowers	Small, lavender, arranged on leafy and whorled spikes, bilabiate.
Odor	Aromatic.
Taste	Strong, pungent and spicy.

Part used:
Herb.

Therapeutic action:
Diaphoretic (hot), tonic, antiseptic, antispasmodic, carminative, emmenagogue, nervine sedative, vulnerary, anthelmintic (germicide).

The oil is a stimulant, tonic, emmenagogue, antispasmodic, and germicide. Warning: In excessive doses, it is emetic, depressive and exhaustive.

Thymol: stimulant, antiseptic, deodorant, disinfectant, anthelmintic (germicide), parasiticide, antipyretic, local anesthetic. It is anesthetic to the skin and mucous membranes; has paralyzing effect on the ends of sense nerves.

Thyme is an old-time household remedy with a very healing and antiseptic action, especially for respiratory, stomach, uterine and bowel problems. It also has a soothing sedative action on the nerves. It is powerful, yet harmless and non-poisonous, and will eliminate all infection, destroy worms, and take away all foul odors. It will restore health to children who are debilitated and exhausted by whooping cough. It forms the basis for the world-famous Listerine antiseptic compound. There are over 60 varieties of thyme, but Thymus vulgaris is the best for both medicinal and culinary purposes.

Medicinal uses:
Menstrual obstructions (dysmenorrhea, amenorrhea), headaches, nightmares, colic, flatulence, asthma, lung problems, whooping cough, febrile condition (fevers), stomach weakness, dyspepsia, stomach cramps, diarrhea, bronchitis, cough, wounds, toothache, bad odor (deodorant), rheumatism, gout, scabies, indolent ulcers, throat irritations (gargle), spasms, hysteria.

Oil: Chlorosis, diarrhea, bronchitis, gleet, gonorrhea, leucorrhea, neuralgia, rheumatism, vesical catarrh, externally for baths, earache, gangrene, itch or scabies (lotion), muscular rheumatism, sores, ulcers (especially the odor), toothache (apply on cotton).

Thymol: Fetid (foul-smelling) bronchitis, cancer, diarrhea, dysentery, diphtheria, diabetes, gonorrhea, leucorrhea, conjunctivitis, ozaena, otorrhea, rhinitis, stomatis, skin diseases (psoriasis, eczema, etc.), typhoid fever, uterine lochia.

Preparations:
Elixir, fluid extract, infusion, oil, powder, tincture. Infusion: Do not boil and keep closely covered, due to the highly medicinal volatile oil.

Dosage:

Elixir	1-2 teaspoonfuls.
Fluid extract	10-60 drops (1 teaspoonful).
Infusion	2 fluid ounces 3 to 4 times daily.
Oil	1-5 drops (always use in small doses when used internally).
Tincture	1/2-1 teaspoonful.

ADMINISTRATION

Thyme is generally given in combination with other remedies. The infusion is preferred for children.

Oral

Menstrual problems (dysmenorrhea, amenorrhea), fevers, whooping cough, asthma, bronchitis, etc.: Give a warm infusion; for small children, give small and frequent doses.

Stomach weakness, dyspepsia, flatulence, spasms, diarrhea; Give a cold infusion.

Whooping cough: Mix 1 part of the infusion with 1 part honey (1 teaspoonful to 1 tablespoonful); give when the cough is troublesome.

FORMULAS

Whooping cough

2 grams	Thyme (Thymus vulgaris)
5 grams	Mistletoe (Viscum album)

Preparation: Infuse in 1 pint of water; strain.

Dosage: 1 tablespoonful each hour or as needed. Children: adjust according to age.

Compound antiseptic oil
(a good substitute for Listerine)

1/2 teaspoon	Oil of thyme or Olium thymi (Thymus vulgaris)
1 teaspoon	Thyme (Thymus vulgaris)
1/2 teaspoon	Eugenol (Caryophyllus aromaticus; Eugenia aromatica)
1/2 teaspoon	Menthol (Mentha piperita)
1/2 teaspoon	Eucalyptol (Eucalyptus Globulus)
15½ ounces	Olive oil (Olea europaea)

Preparation: Gently heat the olive oil until quite warm (not too hot), stir in the other ingredients until dissolved and clear, cover and allow to cool; bottle and cap.

Dosage: May be taken internally or used externally with amazing results. Internally: 1 teaspoonful in 1 cupful of water, sweetened with 1 tablespoonful of honey 3 to 4 times daily; good for infectious bronchitis, diarrhea, cancer, diabetes, dysentery, ulcerations, gonorrhea, leucorrhea, vesical catarrh, diphtheria, stomatitis, typhoid fever, uterine lochia, worms, syphilis.

Externally *(Dosage)*: For skin diseases, ulcers, cancers, gangrene, putrid sores, etc. apply on lint or cotton and cover, changing the application as often as necessary; for ulcerated or sore throat, swab the throat, apply outwardly and cover with flannel; for rheumatism, sciatica, lumbago, stiff joints or muscles, rub in well and cover to retain heat; for fetid or foul-smelling feet, wash the feet well, then rub in the oils well (5 minutes for each foot); nasal spray, make an emulsion with equal parts of lime water.

Children *(Dosage)*: An emulsion oil; the oils are always better suited to the delicate stomachs of children and certain adults, sweetened with honey to make it more palatable.

Congenial combinations:
Thyme combines well with flax seed or linseed (Linum usitatissimum), or acacia or gum Arabic (Acacia Senegal).

Growth characteristics:
Perennial; native of southern Europe, from Portugal to Greece; naturalized in the United States and cultivated in gardens for culinary purposes, grows wild in the mountains; flowers all through June. Propagate by seed indoors and transplant the seedlings (only the Thymus vulgaris variety is easy to germinate), layering, cuttings, or root division, spacing 10 inches apart; grows best in light, sandy, limy and well-drained soil, in raised beds and in full sunlight (it needs plenty of sunshine), or it will thrive indoors in a sunny window (grown in a 5-inch pot or box); keep well-clipped to prevent getting too woody and renew or replace periodically with a new plant. Thyme is very hardy, but it should be protected in winter by a leafy covering or mulch; often if the top is frozen, it will put out new green shoots. It is very easy to grow, and belongs in every home medicinal garden.

Collection:
Clip the tops at the full state of bloom (June).

Drying and preservation:
Be careful, as much of the medicinal value in thyme is due to its volatile oil.

Sister plants:
-Mother of Thyme or Wild Thyme (Thymus serpyllum; LABIATAE) herb; convulsive coughs, whooping cough, catarrh, sore throat; it resembles Thymus vulgaris, but the leaves are 1/8 inch broad tapering below, green, ciliate at the base and not recurved at the margins, prominent veins on the under surface, weaker odor.
-Lemon thyme (Thymus citriodorus; LABIATAE) broader leaves and not recurring at margins.
-Caraway (Thymus Herba-barona; LABIATAE) leaf; culinary.
-(Thymus azoricus; T. caespititius; LABIATAE); leaf; culinary.
-(Thymus zygis; LABIATAE); leaf; culinary.

HYSSOP
(Hyssopus officinalis; LABIATAE)

Common names:
Hyssop (there seems to be no other).

Identifying characteristics:

Stem	Sub-shrub, 1 to 2 feet high, woody at the base, rod-like branches, almost evergreen.
Leaves	Opposite, nearly sessile, smooth, dark green and punctual (dotted) on each side, linearly lanceolate, about 1 inch long and 1/8 inch broad, hairy on the margin.
Flowers	Purplish-blue (seldom white or pink), in maxillary tufts or spikes arranged on one side (4 stamens).
Odor	Aromatic, spicy and misty.
Taste	Pungent, spicy and somewhat bitter.

Part used:
Herb.

Therapeutic action:
Diaphoretic (sudorific), diuretic (lithotriptic, nephritic, etc.) stimulant, expectorant, aromatic, tonic, anthelmintic (vermifuge), aperient, carminative, pectoral, febrifuge, vulnerary.

Hyssop promotes a gentle diaphoresis of the skin, relieving pain and healing the kidneys, bladder and spleen. Its virtues are largely due to a volatile oil which is stimulative, carminative and sudorific. It will influence the bowels with a gentle movement, and its stimulating properties are a pleasant tonic and relief to the mucous lining of a weak stomach and to dryness in the bowels. Hyssop is an excellent expectorant and has been used for generations in pulmonary complaints. Its stimulant properties increase blood circulation and equalize the blood pressure.

Medicinal uses:
Colds, coughs, fevers, bronchitis, hoarseness, sore or ulcerated throat, lung troubles, eruptive diseases (scarlet fever, smallpox, chicken pox, etc.), kidney and liver affections, tuberculosis or consumption, asthma, chronic catarrh, black eye, bruises, quinsy, high blood pressure, scrofula, gravel, stomach complaints (gastric debility, dyspepsia, flatulence, etc.), dropsy, dyspnea, epilepsy, expel worms, eye trouble, inflammation, germicide for body lice.

Preparations:
Fluid extract, infusion, powder, tincture.

Dosage:
Fluid extract 1/2-2 teaspoonfuls.

Infusion	2 fluid ounces taken frequently (as often as every hour).
Powder	1/4-1/2 teaspoon taken frequently (as often as every hour).
Tincture	1/2-1 fluid teaspoon.

ADMINISTRATION

Hyssop is usually given in warm infusion, taken frequently; generally it is used in combination with other remedies.

Oral

Sore or ulcerated throat: Use a warm gargle.

Fevers, bronchitis, etc.: Give 2 fluid ounces warm every hour; it acts as a mild diaphoretic, relieves the kidney and bladder, gently influences the bowels, pleasantly soothes the lining of the stomach; sponge daily with vinegar and warm water.

Asthma: Brew the green tops in soup, or give the warm infusion.

Eruptive diseases: Give 2 fluid ounces of the infusion every hour; or combine with marigold flowers; sponge down with vinegar and warm water.

Kidney and liver affections, etc.: Give the infusion cold.

Worms: Give the tea 3 times daily before meals.

Skin

Cuts, inflammations, black eye, wounds: Bruise the green herb or leaves and apply to the affected area as a poultice.

Rheumatism, bruises, contusions: Apply a fomentation of the infusion from the leaves externally, and keep warm with moist heat.

FORMULAS

Fever, inflammation of throat
(opens pores, equalizes circulation)

1/2 ounce	Hyssop (Hyssopus officinalis)
1/2 ounce	Vervain (Verbena officinalis)
1/2 ounce	Raspberry leaves (Rubus idaeus)
1/2 ounce	Centaury (Erythraea centaurium)
1 teaspoonful	Cayenne (Capsicum frutescens; C. minimum)

Preparation: Simmer the first 4 herbs in 1 quart of Distilled or d-cell water for 20 minutes; strain hot over the cayenne.

Dosage: 1 teaspoonful (warm) every hour.

Administration: Give hot (preferably) or cold; also wrap the feet with a cloth wrung out in apple cider vinegar and keep warm with a hot water bottle.

Whooping cough

1/2 ounce Hyssop (Hyssopus officinalis)
1/2 ounce Raspberry leaves (Rubus idaeus)
1/2 ounce Turkey rhubarb (Rheum palmatum)
1/4 ounce Bayberry bark (Myrica cerifera)
1/2 ounce Thyme (Thymus vulgaris)

Preparation: Simmer the first 4 herbs slowly in 1½ pints of water for 15 minutes; pour over the thyme and steep 1/2 hour, covered; strain.

Dosage: 2 teaspoons for children under 6 years old (can be increased for older children); be sure to keep the feet warm and dry.

Congenial combinations:
Hyssop combines well with horehound (Marrubium vulgare), which is a stimulating tonic and diaphoretic.

Growth characteristics:
Perennial; common to Europe and the United States, raised principally in gardens, grows best in well-drained; limy and warm soil, and in partial shade (but it can be grown in direct sunlight); blooms from July to frost, and it makes a lovely hedge; propagate by seed (easy germination), cuttings, or root division in the spring.

GARDEN SAGE or SAGE
(Salvia officinalis; LABIATAE)

Common names:
Garden sage, sage, meadow sage.

Identifying characteristics:
Stem — Semi-shrubby, 2 feet high, pubescent (hairy), quadrangular, gray, branched.
Leaves — Grayish-green, soft and furry, petiolate (stalked), 1¼-3 inches long and 3/4 -1 inch broad, oblong-lanceolate (rounded at ends), both surfaces strongly reticulated (netted with veins) which are pebbly to the

	touch, crenelate or scalloped at the margins.
Flowers	Cymes, blue with white and purple (on woolly stalks), lipped, the whorls are on terminal spikes.
Odor	Aromatic.
Taste	Pungent, aromatic, bitter, astringent.

Part used:
Leaves.

Therapeutic action:
Diaphoretic (sudorific), aromatic, stimulant, tonic, emmenagogue, astringent, vulnerary, antiseptic, digestive, nervine (sedative), brain stimulant, expectorant, antispasmodic, anthelmintic (vermifuge), condiment, anaphrodisiac.

Garden sage is an excellent diaphoretic when used hot, opening the pores quite freely, but be sure the patient remains well-covered, because cold and congestion may result from exposure during or after diaphoresis. It is very soothing and quieting to any excitement of the nerves and brain. It is a good astringent and is very stimulating as a gargle. It promotes a strong blood circulation within the system. Sage is a substitute for quinine, and is more effective. There are over 500 species of this plant, of which a large number have either medicinal or culinary value.

Medicinal uses:
Febrile conditions (fevers), indigestion, flatulence, ulcers of the mouth and throat, excessive mucus discharge, excessive salivation, nasal catarrh, suppresses or dries up mammary secretions, excessive sexual desire, sexual debility, indurated sores, dyspepsia, quinsy, spermatorrhea, kidney and liver troubles, nerve troubles, hysteria, pneumonia, relaxed throat, laryngitis, tonsillitis, nasal sores, gum strengthener, teeth cleanser, hair tonic (grows hair, removes dandruff), expels worms, stops hemorrhage of wounds, cleanses sores and ulcers.

Preparations:
The medicinal virtues can be extracted by infusion. There is considerable volatile oil in the leaves, so never boil. Fluid extract, infusion, powder, tincture.

Dosage:

Fluid extract	1/2-1 teaspoonful.
Infusion	2 fluid ounces 3 to 4 times daily.
Powder	1-2 grams.
Tincture	1/4-1 teaspoonful (20-60 drops).

ADMINISTRATION

Oral

Nightsweats: Drink 1 cupful of cold sage tea 2 times daily.

Relaxed uvula, ulcerated throat, quinsy, laryngitis, tonsillitis: Use equal parts of the sage infusion and apple cider vinegar as a gargle; also see "FORMULAS."

Nervous troubles, delirious fevers: Give the infusion warm.

Pneumonia: Clear the bowels, give 3-5 cupfuls of hot infusion 1/2 hour apart. Keep well covered in bed.

Skin

Bleeding wounds, indurated sores, ulcers: Use the infusion as a wash or fomentation; or bruise the fresh leaves and use as a poultice.

FORMULAS

Infusion of garden sage

1 ounce	Sage leaves, cut (Salvia officinalis)
1¾ pints	Distilled or d-cell water
4 ounces	Pure glycerine

Preparation: Boil the water and pour it over the herb, cover and steep 20 minutes in a warm place; strain, add glycerine, bottle and keep in a cool place.
Dosage: 2 fluid ounces 3 to 4 times daily.

Throat gargle mouth wash

1 ounce	Sage leaves, cut or powder (Salvia officinalis)
2 ounces	Honey (wild honey when possible)

Preparation: Steep in 1 pint of hot, but not boiling, water and cover until cool; strain. If a more stimulating gargle is desired, use 1 cupful of water and 1 cupful of apple cider vinegar in the preparation, instead of 1 pint of water.

Stomach tonic

1 gram	Garden sage (Salvia officinalis)
3 grams	Wormwood (Artemisia absinthium)
1 gram	Juniper berries (Juniperus communis)
2 grams	Peppermint (Mentha piperita)

Congenial combinations:
Garden Sage combines well with sumac berries (Rhus glabra).

Growth characteristics:
Perennial, native of southern Europe but cultivated universally in gardens. It

grows best in warm, limy, sandy or stony soil, but it will thrive even in poor soil if it gets plenty of sunshine. Sage flowers in June and July. Propagate sage by seed (it will self-sow freely), cuttings, or root division in well-drained and limy or sandy soil in the full sunshine; it requires cultivation and soil enrichment, and the plant should be renewed or replaced periodically.

Collection:
Gather during the flowering season and dry carefully to preserve volatile oil.

Sister plants:
All of the following, like garden sage, produce perspiration in the warm infusion, and check excessive sweating in the cold infusion:
-Chia-seed (Salvia columbariae; LABIATAE); seed: aromatic, bitter, Mexico.
-Meadow sage (Salvia pratensis; LABIATAE); leaf: diaphoretic, expectorant; Southern Europe.
-Red sage or Purple-topped sage (Salvia colorata); herb; lung trouble, asthma, coughs, colds, bronchitis, fevers (all types), sore throat, tonsillitis, diphtheria, female troubles, flatulence, biliousness, liver cleanser, nervousness, nervous headache, eruptive diseases (measles, scarlet fever, smallpox, chicken pox, etc.); therapeutic substitute for garden sage (similar in appearance, with reddish leaves and stems).

CATNIP or CATNEP
(Nepeta cataria; LABIATAE)

Common names:
Catnip, catmint, nip, catsup, cat's-wort, field balm.

Identifying characteristics:

Stem	Erect, square, 2-5 feet high, downy (covered with very fine whitish, hairs), gray, branching.
Leaves	Opposite, heart-shaped (cordate-ovate, oblong with pointed apex), petioled or stalked, 1-2½ inches long, finely scalloped margins (incise-serrate), green upper surface, grayish-green undersurface with whitish hairs. Powder; grayish-green.
Flowers	Small whitish or mauve blossoms, dotted with crimson (purple), in dense spikes, bilabiate or two-lipped (lower lip has 3 lobes, finely crenate, crenulate, or scalloped, upper lip is straight and notched).
Odor	Faintly aromatic and mint-like, but characteristic.
Taste	Bitter, pungent, aromatic, mint-like.

Part used:
Herb, leaves.

Therapeutic action:
Aromatic, relaxant, diffusive, stimulant, diaphoretic, emmenagogue, antispasmodic, nervine, sedative, carminative, anodyne, refrigerant, antacid.

Medicinal uses:
Convulsions, restlessness, hysteria, chlorosis, colic, amenorrhea, toothache, nervous headache, flatulence, deranged stomach, spasms, prevent griping, insanity, fevers, fits, expel worms, suppressed urination, colds.

Preparations:
Fluid extract, infusion, powder, tincture. Never boil catnip, as much of the therapeutic value is in the volatile oil.

Dosage:

Fluid extract	1/4-1 teaspoonful as needed.
Infusion	2 fluid ounces to a cup as needed.
Powder	1/4-1/2 teaspoonful as needed.
Tincture	1/2-1 teaspoonful as needed.

ADMINISTRATION

Anal

Convulsions, nervousness, colic, fevers, expel worms, bowel problems, (infants and children): Give a warm injection of the infusion (see "FORMULAS").

Hysteria, nervous headache, invagination of the bowels: A warm high enema of catnip infusion will bring relief.

Oral

Pain, flatulence, acidity, spasms: Give 2 tablespoonfuls frequently; children: 2-3 teaspoonfuls.

Fevers, hysteria, nervousness, etc.: Use the warm infusion.

Suppressed urination: Take the infusion cold.

FORMULAS

Soothing and quieting baby remedy

3 parts	Catnip (Nepeta cataria)
2 parts	Balm (Melissa officinalis)
2 parts	Marshmallow (Althaea officinalis)

Preparation: 1 teaspoonful of herbs to a cup of boiled, distilled water, steep 10 to 15 minutes; strain.

Dosage: 1 teaspoonful or more as needed.

Colic (injection)

1 ounce	Catnip herb (Nepeta cataria)
1 ounce	Pleurisy root (Asclepias tuberosa)

Preparation: Steep about 10 to 15 minutes in 1 pint of water that had been brought to the boil; strain.

Administration: Use about 2 ounces lukewarm in an injection.

Fever compound

1 ounce	Catnip, powder (Nepeta cataria)
1 ounce	Pleurisy root, powder (Asclepias tuberosa)
1 ounce	Lobelia, powder (Lobelia inflata)
1/2 ounce	Composition powder (see page 147-148).

Preparation: Mix thoroughly; place 1 teaspoonful in 1 cupful of boiling hot water; cover and steep a few minutes, sweeten.

Dosage: 1/4 cupful every 1½-2 hours.

Note: In case of depressed or low vitality, add Virginia snake root (Aristolochia serpentaria) or Canada snake root (Asarum canadense).

Congenial combinations:
As a diffusive stimulant, ginger (Zingiber officinalis) will intensify the therapeutic action of catnip.

Growth characteristics:
Perennial; native of Asia, Europe, and naturalized to the United States; it is a hearty herb and found abundantly wild; flowers June-September. Propagate by seed in the fall or spring (easy germination, viable 4-5 years), or by root division in the spring, spacing 15 inches; grows best in rich, dry, sandy soil (without lime), in full sunlight; needs little care and attention.

Collection:
By gathering the plants (cutting back) in July, a second crop may be had in the fall.

SPEARMINT
(Mentha spicata; M. viridis; LABIATAE)

Common names:
Spearmint, mint, mackerel mint, lady's mint, brown mint, lamb mint, pea mint, common garden mint, sage of Bethlehem; Herba Menthae Romanae, Herba Menthae Acuta (Br.); Menthe romaine, Menthe verte, Baume vert (Fr.); Gruene Minze, Roemische Minze (Ger.); Herba buena, Yerba buena (Span.).

Identifying characteristics:

Stem	2-4 feet high, 1/25-1/8 inch thick, acutely quadrangular, smooth (nearly glabrous), often tinged with purple, characteristic opposite branches.
Leaves	Nearly sessile, ovate-lanceolate, bright green, 2/5-3/5 inches long, sharply and unequally serrate, smooth upper surface and strongly ribbed (glandular), hairy on the under surface, wrinkled. Powder: green (closely resembles peppermint).
Flowers	Small, nearly white or bluish-purple tint, in maxillary whorls, approximated (interrupted or crowded) so as to form a tapering and leafless spike.
Root	Has elongated suckers, by which it multiplies extensively.
Odor	Slightly pungent and characteristic.
Taste	Aromatic and characteristic taste, not followed by a cooling sensation in the mouth.
Note	Peppermint is distinguished from spearmint by the following characteristics: Peppermint leaves are broader, shorter, and a much darker shade of green. Chewing the leaves of peppermint, a pronounced cooling sensation is experienced when inhaling breath.

Part used:
Herb, oil.

Therapeutic action:
Diaphoretic, diuretic (lithotriptic), stimulant, carminative, antispasmodic, aromatic, nervine (sedative), condiment, nephritic, anti-emetic.

The therapeutic properties of spearmint are similar to peppermint (Mentha piperita), but as it is much milder, it is to be preferred in disorders of infancy, culinary purposes, confectionery, perfumery, etc. It has a gentle diaphoretic action of mild perspiration, and as a diuretic it is very beneficial to the kidney, bladder (especially for suppression of urine). Spearmint is a very soothing and quieting agent for the nerves and stomach, and it is added to many compounds because of its carminative properties and pleasant taste.

Medicinal uses:
(Same as peppermint, but much milder.) Colic, flatulence, dyspepsia, spasms,

dropsy, nausea, vomiting, gravel in bladder, urinary problems (suppression, painful or scalding), hemorrhoids, inflammation of kidneys and bladder, soothes and quiets the nerves, stomach disorders, etc.

Preparations:
Fluid extract, infusion, oil, powder, tincture. Never boil as the important volatile oils will dissipate and be lost.

Dosage:

Fluid extract	1/4-1 teaspoonful.
Infusion	2 fluid ounces.
Oil	1-3 drops.
Powder	1-4 grams.
Tincture	1/2-1 fluid teaspoon.

ADMINISTRATION

Anal

Hemorrhoids: Inject small amounts of the infusion into the rectum.

Oral

Vomiting and nausea of pregnancy: Use alone, or for an excellent combination, see "FORMULAS."

Colic, flatulence, hysteria: Give an infusion, and add ginger to intensify and accelerate the action (see "FORMULAS").

FORMULAS

Nose Ointment
(asthma, nasal catarrh and irritated mucous membrane)

1 part	Oil of Spearmint (Mentha spicata)
1 part	Oil of Peppermint (Mentha piperita)
Sufficient	Vaseline

Preparation: Mix the oils in Vaseline to proper potency (sufficiently astringent in its action).

Administration: Apply into the nostrils with a pencil brush.

Colic, flatulence, hysteria

3 parts	Spearmint (Mentha spicata)

1 part Ginger (Zingiber officinalis)

Preparation: Mix and infuse 1 teaspoonful to each cupful of hot water.

Dosage: Drink the clear tea and leave the sediment.

Vomiting and nausea of pregnancy

1/2 ounce Spearmint (Mentha spicata)
2 teaspoons Cloves (Syzygium aromaticum; Eugenia aromatica)
2 teaspoons Cinnamon (Cinnamomum zeylanicum)
2 teaspoons Turkey rhubarb (Rheum palmatum)

Preparation: Infuse in 1 pint of boiling hot water, cover 20 minutes; strain.

Dosage: 3-4 tablespoonfuls every 30 minutes.

Congenial combinations:
Combine ginger (Zingiber officinalis) with spearmint to intensify and accelerate its action.

Growth characteristics:
Perennial; flowers August-September; easy to grow, must be restrained because of a rapidly spreading and running root stock; best start from a root, needs ample moisture, and grows best in filter sunlight for part of the day; thrives indoors at temperatures less than 65° F. It is thought to be a cultivated form of Horsemint (Mentha longifolia; M. sylvestris).

Collection:
Gather just as the flowers appear (for oil, just after the flowers have expanded).

***Sister plants*:**
-Peppermint (Mentha piperita; LABIATAE); see page 459.
-Hyssop (Hyssopus officinalis); see page 254.
-(Mentha cardiaca; M. gentilis; LABIATAE); sometimes sold as spearmint, but leaves are smaller, and the whorls of flowers are distant and leafy.
-Curled Mint (Mentha crispa; M. aquatica; LABIATAE) cultivated form of spearmint.

For alternative diaphoretic herbs which may be used when the foregoing are not available, see Chapter 17.

CHAPTER 7

THE DIURETIC HERBS

Urine is excreted by the kidneys. The fluid part of the urine is formed by some of the blood passing into the tubules of the kidneys and the glomeruli (where the capillary blood vessels and the tubules meet) which are situated at the cortex. As this fluid passes along the tubules, it becomes filled with dissolved waste substances that are removed from the blood by the direct action of the cells lining the tubules. The action of the kidneys is further described by Deschauer as follows:

> The duty of the kidneys are best described by calling them the filters of the blood. Your blood flows constantly through your kidneys to be purified or filtered. You might be surprised to learn that more than 500 grains of waste matter, acids and poisons have to be moved from the blood through the kidneys every 24 hours. You can easily see, therefore, that on this filtering and eliminating depends your health to a very great extent. Let the kidneys fail to function properly and nature will call

> your attention to it right away. You will feel depressed and tired, restless at night, and pains in the back will show up. There might be scanty urine or a desire to urinate frequently. Your head will ache and many other aches and pains will be making their appearance. You really cannot be surprised that you do not feel well.
>
> Just figure your kidneys would do only half the work and eliminate only 250 grains of waste, what will become of the other 250 grains? They will be carried back into your blood and poison your system. Watch, therefore, your kidneys and deal with even minor irregularity promptly.

To avoid trouble, be careful with your diet. Meat consumption as a protein source causes more stress on the kidneys than do the equivalent vegetable sources. The average American's daily consumption of meat far exceeds the requirements for protein. This causes an excess of uric acid and protein that must be disposed of on top of the daily metabolic waste. This overload causes cellular damage in the kidneys and throws them out of commission.

Our kidneys cannot talk, they just have to stay mum until a hundred and one bodily disorders start us looking around for some mysterious cause of serious trouble. Then, as a rule, it is too late to apologize to the kidneys.

Diuretic herbs are used to:

Remove waste and poisonous materials from the blood; remove waste fluids from the tissues and cavities of the body, and maintain the action of the kidneys and stimulate the normal excretory functions. This is especially valuable when the kidneys are impaired (due to acute fevers, congestion, Bright's disease, etc.). diuretic herbs lessen irritation of the genito-urinary tract, where the urine is excessively concentrated or acid; they dilute the urine; relieve the distress or uric acid concretions by a solvent or flushing action, and eliminate uretic solids. diuretic herbs alter morbid conditions of the renal excretions; they are antiseptic.

Some diuretics increase the flow of urine by stimulating the cells in the kidney to excrete more urine, while others improve the blood circulation in the kidneys so that the fresh blood brings more fluids and wastes to be eliminated, which forms into urine.

Renal secretion is increased by raising the local pressure by dilating the afferent vessels, or increasing the renal blood-supply and circulation through raising the general arterial pressure by increasing the action of the heart. This is performed by such herbs as black cohosh, Canadian hemp, lily of the valley, squill, broom tops.

Other herbs work by stimulating the secreting cells or nerves of the kidney tissue. These include such herbs as buchu, uva ursi, juniper berries, corn silk, guaiac, fennel, cubeb, copaiba, pareira, matico, sandalwood, pipsissewa, etc.

When diuretics act upon renal solids (dissolving biliary concretions, calculi, stones or gravel) in the excretory passages, they are called lithotriptic. They are called antilithics when they prevent the fomentation of urinary and biliary concretions in the urinary passages. The herbalist must know which diuretics influence the excretion of solid materials (sediment, gravel, etc), as these should be administered in combination with demulcent agents such as marshmallow, couchgrass, etc. which will soothe any irritation and forestall any stress that may arise during the elimination process.

Take diuretics during the day, on an empty stomach, avoiding all physical exertion for the fastest diuretic action. But do not drive the kidneys in your haste to heal them, as often renal troubles originate elsewhere.

Bile: When bile shows in the urine, treat the liver.

Bed-wetting: In nearly all cases, this is a nervous condition; the nerves are frayed and the kidneys are delicate.

Constipation: The kidney irritation and backlogging of toxins may be due to constipation in the bowels, so see that these are in good order.

Dropsy: This is a sign that the kidneys are partially paralyzed and are not eliminating the urine sufficiently, so the diuretic agent should be used in combination with a diffusive stimulant such as Jamaica ginger or Virginia snake root or even cayenne.

Female problems: For female urinary problems, the cause may be in the genital area, which is very interrelated, so treat that area also.

PARSLEY
(Petroselinum crispum; P. sativum; Carum petroselinum; Apium petroselinum; UMBELLIFERAE)

Common names:
Parsley, garden parsley, rock parsley, common parsley, march.

Identifying characteristics:

Stem	Smooth, erect, furrowed, jointed and branching stem, 2 feet high.
Leaves	Bright green, biternate, on long petioles; the leaflets are wedge shaped.
Flowers	White or greenish, rounded petals that are barely emarginate.
Root	Conical or spindle-shaped, fleshy, yellowish, about 5 inches long and

	1/2 inch broad.
Fruit	Ovoid and crescent-shaped, 1/12-1/8 inch long, brownish on aging, 2 mericarps, aromatic when seeds are bruised.

Parts used:
Whole herb; root, leaves, seeds.

Therapeutic action:
Culinary, aperient, diuretic (lithotriptic), tonic, antispasmodic, aromatic, expectorant, antiperiodic (juice), carminative (seeds), emmenagogue (seeds), febrifuge (seeds), vulnerary.

This herb is used freely in food and for garnishing dishes (where it is likely more nutritive than the concoctions to which it lends color), that it is a very reliable and an old diuretic remedy is very much ignored today. If used properly, parsley will work on the gall bladder and remove gall stones. Parsley is a specific for the adrenal glands, is powerfully therapeutic for the optic nerves, the brain nerves, and the whole sympathetic nervous system. The fluid extract or juice is an excellent tonic for the blood vessels, particularly the capillaries and arterioles. It is rich in vital minerals and contains more iron than any other green leafy vegetable. It is especially high in vitamins A and B, and it contains three times the potency of C than do citrus juices.

It is a remarkable remedy for expelling watery poisons, excess mucus, flatulence, for reducing swollen and enlarged glands, etc.

Medicinal uses:
Dropsy, gall bladder problems, gall stones, gravel, aches in the lumbar region, menstrual obstructions, jaundice, urinesis, kidneys (congestion, irritation, inflammation), amenorrhea, dysmenorrhea, nephritis, cystitis, intermittent fevers (fresh juice, seeds), hepatitis, obstruction of liver and spleen, female problems, insect bites and stings, swollen glands, swollen breasts, cancer preventative, difficult urination, strangury (painful urination), syphilis, gonorrhea, dry up nursing mother's milk, catarrh of bladder, anemia, tuberculosis, rheumatism, arthritis, acidosis, obesity, high blood pressure, catarrh, dyspepsia, halitosis.

Preparations:
Decoction, infusion, fluid extract, oil.

Decoction: Use the roots only. Infusion: Used for preparing the seeds and leaves. When the parsley is dried, use 1 teaspoonful to each cupful of water; and if it is green, use a larger amount; a handful of the green to a pint of water. Always cover the steeping herb.

Dosage:
Parsley must be taken in larger quantities as a decoction and infusion.

Decoction	1/2 cupful 3 to 4 times daily (root).
Infusion	1 cupful 3 to 4 times daily (herb).
Fluid extract	1 teaspoonful (root & seeds)
Oil	3-5 drops per day.
Apiol	3-10 drops.

ADMINISTRATION

Oral

Gall stones: Take 1 pint of the infusion daily.

Kidney, bladder, dropsy: Make at least 2 quarts of the parsley root strong decoction and drink copiously.

Dangerous suppression of urine: 3-6 oz. of the decoct(hot) every hour.

Parsley green drink and tea: Parsley is terrific when blended with other greens as a green drink. The herb in tea form acts rapidly, whereas the capsules are slower. In some cases, we can not take enough parsley (or any other herb) to do us any good by just eating it in the raw form. Instead of using parsley straight, just make a tea with it. If you are using parsley as a juice, use it moderately; it is very highly concentrated and potent and will work very quickly on the system. It will throw out the poisons too fast if used excessively and can cause serious upsets.

Skin

Dropsy: Mix equal parts of parsley root tea and glycerine, saturate cloths and apply to swollen areas; keep patient warmly-covered in bed with tepid air circulation; this brings water through the skin and helps relieve the burden on the kidneys. At the same time, give the parsley root tea without the glycerine as a drink, 1/2 cupful each hour.

Concussions, swollen breasts, enlarged glands: Apply a poultice of bruised leaves.

Dry up nursing mother's milk: Apply a poultice of bruised leaves to the breasts.

FORMULAS

Gall stones

1 ounce	Parsley, dried (or 3 ounces fresh) (Petroselinum crispum)
1/2 ounce	Wild Yam, fluid extract (Dioscorea villosa)
1/2 ounce	Fringetree, fluid extract (Chionanthus viriginicus)

Preparation: Infuse the parsley in 1 pint of boiling hot water, cover and let stand until cool; strain and add the wild yam and fringetree; mix thoroughly.

Dosage: 2 tablespoonfuls 3 to 4 times daily.

Note: This will assist greatly in liquefying the bile and ease colic pains.

Backache

1 part	Parsley root (Petroselinum crispum)
1 part	Carrot tops-garden variety (Daucus carota, var. sativus)
1 part	Celery tops (Apium graveolens)
1 part	Skunk cabbage root (Symplocarpus foetidus)
1 part	Juniper berries (Juniperus communis)
2 parts	Senna (Cassia acutifolia, C. Marilandica)
1/2 part	Wahoo bark (Euonymus atropurpureus)

Preparation: Mix thoroughly; then use 1 teaspoonful of mixture to the cup of water and simmer 10 to 20 minutes.

Dosage: 2 fluid ounces 3 or 4 times daily.

Bladder stones

1 part	Parsley leaves (Petroselinum crispum)
1 part	Cleavers (Galium aparine)
1 part	Juniper berries (Juniperus communis)
1 part	Flaxseed (Linum usitatissimum)
1/2 part	Ginger (Zingiber officinalis)

Preparation: Infuse in boiling water, cover and let stand until cool, and strain.

Dosage: 1 or 2 tablespoonfuls 3 times a day.

Kidneys

1 part	Parsley (Petroselinum crispum)
1 part	Juniper berries (Juniperus communis)
1 part	Buchu (Agathosma betulina; A. crenulata; Diosma ericoides)
1 part	Flax seed (Linum usitatissimum)

Preparation: Infuse one teaspoonful of well mixed herbs to each pint of boiling water, cover and let stand until cool, and strain.

Dosage: 2 fluid ounces every one or two hours until relief; then reduce as required.

Void urine

1 part Parsley (Petroselinum crispum)
1 part Juniper berries (Juniperus communis)

Preparation: 1 teaspoonful to the cup of mixed herbs infused in boiling hot water, cover and let stand until cool, and strain.

Dosage: 2 fluid ounces or more each hour until relief.

Female troubles

1 part Parsley leaves (Petroselinum crispum)
1 part Buchu (Agathosma betulina; A. crenulata; Diosma ericoides)
1 part Black Haw bark (Viburnum prunifolium)
1 part Cramp bark (Viburnum trilobum; V. Opulus)

Preparation: Using 1 teaspoonful to the cup of mixed herbs, simmer slowly 5 to 10 minutes.

Dosage: 1/2 cupful or more morning and night. More just prior to menstrual period.

Babies soothing syrup (stomach and bowel pains, aches, cramps, colic, spasms, convulsions, flatulence, common ailments)

2 ounces Parsley seed, crushed or powdered (Petroselinum crispum)
2 ounces Caraway seed, crushed or powdered (Carum carvi)
2 ounces Rhubarb, cut and dried (Rheum rhabarbarum)
1 ounce Cinnamon bark, powdered (Cinnamomum zeylanicum)
1½ pounds Yellow D or Brown sugar
2 ounces Essence of peppermint (Mentha piperita)
1 quart Distilled or d-cell water

Preparation: Soak the herbs 12 hours in the water; bring to a boil, cover and simmer slowly for 1 hour; strain and return to clean pot; add the sugar and peppermint; cover and let stand until cold; bottle, cap tightly keeping in a cool and dark place.

Dosage: 1 teaspoonful of syrup to the cup of distilled or D-cell water, or in a cup of mint tea.

CASE HISTORY

Knowledge by divine assistance.
A Dr. Christopher case history in his own words: I had a personal acquaintance,

a Mrs. Hanger, who came here from England in her twenties. She was very sickly so her husband told her to go to the doctor (they were poor and childless at the time). She did, and returned home very discouraged and unhappy. The doctor had told her, "You have a kidney infection which is a very progressive type and there is nothing we can do to heal it; you will have possibly six months to live."

While at home meditating, she heard a knock at the front door. There stood a bearded man in a gray suit. He asked, "Sister Hanger, may I have a glass of water?" She told him, "certainly," although she didn't know him. She gave him the glass of water, and he said, "Sit down, I want to talk to you a minute, Sister Hanger." She wondered how he knew her name. He continued, "I would like to help you if you would like me to.

"You have just come from the doctor's and he told you that you have a bad kidney condition. Well, you are from England, and you have brought your herbs with you. You have a little herb garden out in the back in which you have a nice stand of parsley. Now, if you will take a handful of parsley each day and put it into a pint of water, cover and steep it, and drink it in regular doses during the day, it will heal your condition. The doctor told you that you have only six months to live, but I will tell you what you will see; you will see another depression." He went on and told her all the things she would see, "There will be a Third World War, but you won't see this one; it will be after you go." When he had finished the short interview, something momentarily distracted her attention and in that instant he disappeared.

Well, I spoke at her funeral; and it wasn't six months after she was supposed to die; she was eighty-six years old, and she had raised a number of wonderful children.

Good for kidney infections.
Dr. Christopher had several students testify in herbology classes as to the value of parsley, among which was the following:

> I talked to a man who went into the hospital for infection. He was there six weeks and it was costing $45.00 a day for the drugs they gave him. Then someone told his wife to take him some parsley. The doctor said, "Well, it won't hurt him, but it won't help him." He was released from the hospital after he had taken it for one day; it had started to drain the infection he had.

Growth characteristics:
Annual herb, biennial root, it is a native of Europe, but is cultivated universally in the civilized world (both outdoors and indoors). Propagates by seed best in autumn or spring, but has slow and uncertain germination. It grows best in medium-rich, deeply dug soil, in partial shade; does not transplant satisfactorily; soak seed for 24 hours before planting, sow on surface and tamp with a flat board; thin

unwanted seedlings and keep leaves clipped for thick growth; cut off flower stalks that appear the second year in order to preserve plants. It self-sows quite well if some of the plants are left to go to seed, so that you can have a constant supply.

JUNIPER BERRY
(Juniperus communis; PINACEAE)

Common names:
Juniper berry, juniper bark, juniper bush, ginepro, enebro; Fructus (Baccae); Juniperi (Br.); Genievre, Baies de Genievre (Fr.); Wachholderbeeren (Ger.).

Identifying characteristics:

Trunk	Evergreen shrub, main limbs 6-15 feet long (some often prostrate), many close branches.
Leaves	Narrow, whorls of three, 1/2 inch long, deep green, sharp pointed, channeled.
Fruit/Berry	Nearly globular, 3/10-2/5 inch diameter, purplish-black (ripens second year after bloom), blue-gray bloom 3-furrowed or triangular line at apex (from the cohesion or junction of the 3 fleshy bracts forming the fruit), internally it is loosely fleshy with many schizogenous cavities; contains 3 ovate seeds. Powder: dark brown.
Odor	Aromatic.
Taste	Sweet and pleasant, then bitter.

Part used:
Usually the berries; also the oil (from the berries and wood), leaves, bark.

Therapeutic action:
Diuretic, diaphoretic, aromatic, stimulant, carminative, anodyne, emmenagogue, stomachic, antiseptic.

Juniper increases the appetite, aids digestion, and as its major use, increases the flow of urine. It is a stimulating diuretic, so it is especially beneficial in eliminating passive congestion of the kidneys resulting from heart problems, and for removing waste products from the bloodstream. Juniper is a great healer to the kidneys, urinary passages, bladder. It is a counter-poison and a strengthener of the brain, memory, and optic nerve. It was a major herb for some American Indian tribes, notably the Seminoles, who used it for many illnesses.

Medicinal uses:
Renal dropsy, vesical catarrh, sciatica, retention of urine, swollen joints, rheumatic pains, lumbago, chest problems, leucorrhea, gravel, bladder discharges, retention of uric acid, kidney problems (acute or chronic), ague, poisoning, leprosy (Hansen's disease), gonorrhea, gleet, scurvy, immunization.

For renal dropsy, avoid taking too large doses, as the stimulating effect may irritate the urinary passages; usually administered in combination with demulcent agents.

Preparations:
Decoction, elixir, fluid extract, infusion, oil, solid extract, tincture.

Dosage:

Infusion	2 ounces 3 times daily; children: 1 teaspoon 3 times daily.
Fluid extract	1/2-1 teaspoon.
Oil Berries	1-3 drops.
Wood	1-5 drops.
Powder	1 teaspoon to the cup of liquid.
Solid extract	325 mg.-1 gram.
Tincture	5-20 drops.

ADMINISTRATION

For kidney complaints, etc, juniper is rarely given alone but is usually given in conjunction with other herbs. It is most often taken in infusion form. Do not use juniper in an acutely inflamed condition unless it is combined with gravel root.

Oral

Backache or lumbago, kidney problems: Use the infusion in the form of tea, or the oil on a little sugar (for lumbago, see below).

Immunization: Juniper is a good disease preventative, and may be used as a spray or fumigation. When exposed to contagious diseases, chew the berries or use as a gargle in a strong infusion form.

Suppression of menstrual flow (from cold and exposure): Give the infusion in 2 fluid ounce doses every 3 to 4 hours.

Acute rheumatism, sciatica, lumbago: Combine with gravel root.

Leucorrhea: Combine juniper with other herbs as douche (see "FORMULAS").

FORMULAS

Infusion of juniper berries

1 ounce	Juniper berries, cut or crushed (Juniperus communis) when necessary, the leaves may be substituted for the berries
1 pint	Distilled or d-cell water.

Preparation: Boil the water and, while boiling, pour it over the berries; steep 10 minutes; cool, strain, bottle, and keep in a cool place.

Dosage: 2 ounces 3 times a day. Children: 1 tablespoonful 3 times a day.

Bright's disease (chronic nephritis)

1 part Juniper berries (Juniperus communis)
1 part Blue cohosh (Caulophyllum thalictroides)
1 part Couchgrass (Agropyron repens)
1 part Buchu (Agathosma betulina; A. crenulata; Diosma ericoides)

Preparation: Mix well; then use 1 teaspoonful of combined herbs to a cup of boiling water. Steep until cool.

Dosage: 2-3 tablespoonfuls 4 times a day.

Diaphoretic

2 parts Juniper berries, powder (Juniperus communis)
1 part Parsley seed, powder (Petroselinum crispum)
1 part Rest harrow, powder (Ononis spinosa)

Preparation: Mix thoroughly; use 1 teaspoonful and steep in 1 pint of boiling hot water. When cool enough to drink, use.

Dosage: 2 fluid ounces each hour, then reduce as needed.

Retention of urine

1 part Juniper berries (Juniperus communis)
1 part Shavegrass (Equisetum arvense)
1 part Dwarf elder root (Sambucus Ebulus)
1 part Oat straw (Avena sativa)
1 part Black currant leaves (Ribes nigrum)

Preparation: Pour 1 teacupful of boiling water over 1 teaspoonful of combined herbs. Steep till cool.

Dosage: 2-3 tablespoonfuls each 1/2 hour to hour, until relief. Place castor oil or Parsley fomentation hot, over kidney bladder area.

Dropsy

4 ounces Juniper berries, crushed (Juniperus communis)
8 ounces Parsley seed, crushed (Petroselinum crispum)

3 pints Distilled or d-cell water

Preparation: Pour the boiling water over the herbs; cover and steep 30 minutes in a hot place; strain and, while hot, add 25% of the volume in glycerine.

Dosage: 2 teaspoons to 2 fluid ounces; give warm every 3 hours until the fluid flows freely; after the danger is passed, reduce the dosage immediately to 2 teaspoons.

Diuretic (infusion)

1/2 ounce Juniper berries, crushed (Juniperus communis)
1/2 ounce Buchu (Agathosma betulina; A. crenulata; Diosma ericoides)
1/2 ounce White poplar or quaking aspen bark (Populus tremuloides)
1/2 ounce Marshmallow root (Althaea officinalis)
2 pints Distilled or d-cell water

Preparation: Simmer in distilled water for 15 minutes at low heat; strain.

Dosage: 3-4 tablespoonfuls 3 to 4 times daily.

Note: In preparing the herbs be sure that the water does not boil as Buchu leaves lose their potency when boiled.

Nephritis

1/2 ounce Juniper berries (Juniperus communis)
1/2 ounce Tansy (Tanacetum vulgare)
1/2 ounce Cleavers (Galium aparine)
1/2 ounce White poplar bark (Populus tremuloides)
1/2 ounce Uva ursi (Arctostaphylos uva-ursi)
1 teaspoonful Cayenne (Capsicum frutescens; C. minimum)

Preparation: Simmer slowly in 2 pints of water down to 1 pint; strain hot over cayenne.

Dosage: 2 tablespoonfuls 4 times daily.

Note: Watch the bowels.

Dysuria (retention of urine)

1 ounce Juniper berries (Juniperus communis)
1 ounce Cleavers (Galium aparine)
1 ounce Marshmallow (Althaea officinalis)
1 ounce Tansy (Tanacetum vulgare)

1 ounce	Buchu (Agathosma betulina; A. crenulata; Diosma ericoides)
1/4 teaspoon	Cayenne (Capsicum frutescens; C. minimum)

Preparation: Simmer the first 4 herbs for 20 minutes in 1 quart of water; pour hot over the buchu and cayenne, cover and steep for 10 minutes; strain.

Dosage: 2 fluid ounces every 2 hours.

Administration: Wrap the feet with cloth soaked in apple cider vinegar and warm with a hot water bottle. Give the patient slippery elm gruel.

Note: If this formula does not give relief, the obstruction is possibly caused by a stone, so add 1 ounce gravel root (Eupatorium purpureum) to the formula.

Diuretic (fluid extract)

1 ounce	Juniper berries (Juniperus communis)
1 ounce	Gravel root, fluid extract (Eupatorium purpureum)
2 ounces	Jamaica ginger (Zingiber officinalis)

Preparation: Mix herbs thoroughly.

Dosage: 1 teaspoonful 4 times a day.

Congenial combinations:
Juniper combines well with marshmallow root. Juniper is usually combined with other diuretics (such as gravel root, uva ursi, cleavers, buchu, broom, parsley, peach leaves).

CASE HISTORY

Healing by obedience to divine prescription.
In N. B. Lundwall's book, *Assorted Gems of Priceless Value,* there is an attested account by Elizabeth J. Barney concerning her mother, who was about to die of an apparent kidney ailment during a pioneer journey at the beginning of this century. The wagon caravan stopped because of her and made camp for the night, intending to bury the rapidly-declining woman in the morning. A stranger suddenly was seen approaching the camp, and he told the husband (the father of the lady attesting to the account) to go and gather juniper berries and leaves growing in the vicinity and to "mix them together, steep them and give them to your wife and you can be on your way within an hour." Then the stranger said he had to go, and at that moment something drew the people's attention away, and during that instant he disappeared. The prescription was obeyed, and the woman revived miraculously, helped prepare the breakfast, and continued on the journey completely healed. So you will find that these herbs will not only repair the body as with a "divine touch," but they restore our faith in the Supreme Maker.

Growth characteristics:
Perennial; grows in North America, Europe, Asia, North Africa. This is a very common shrub that grows in dry woods, on hills and mountain slopes from Canada south to New Jersey and west to Nebraska, and in the Rocky Mountains south to New Mexico and Arizona.

Collection:
Do not use the first year berries which are green and acid; use only the second year berries, which are dark and almost deep purple.

Drying and preservation:
Juniper may be preserved for longer periods of time by drying or in the tincture form.

GRAVEL ROOT or QUEEN OF THE MEADOW or JOE-PYE
(Eupatorium purpureum; E. maculatum; E. ternifolium; COMPOSITAE)

Common names:
Gravel root, queen of the meadow, Joe-Pye, trumpet weed, purple thoroughwort, kidney root, tall boneset, gravel weed, jopi weed, hemp weed.

Identifying characteristics:

Stem	Tall and graceful, 3-6 feet high, 1 inch broad, green or purplish, purple band about 1 inch broad at each leaf joint, leafy, and usually branching toward the top.
Leaves	Whorls of 3-6 (usually 4), oblong (ovate to lanceolate) 8-10 inches long and 4-5 inches broad, thin and rough, petiolate, coarsely serrate, downy underneath.
Flowers	Pale (dull magenta, lavender pink, or whitish in color), slightly fragrant, very numerous tubular florets in large terminal, loose and compound clusters (soft, fringe blooms).
Rhizome (root)	Very hard and tough, 1/2-1 inch in diameter, wood is nearly whitish, bark is thin and grayish-brown, often hollow in the center with wide medullary rays, short lateral branches are crowded with tough, woody roots about 1/12 inch wide and several inches long.
Odor	Slightly fragrant, resembling old hay.
Taste	Slightly bitter and aromatic, faintly astringent and acrid, but not unpleasant.

Part used:
Rhizome (root); also the leaves and flowers.

Therapeutic action:
Diuretic (lithotriptic), nervine, stimulant, astringent, tonic, relaxant.

Gravel root is used principally for the urinary-genital areas, influencing the kidneys, liver, bladder, prostate gland and uterus. It relaxes moderately, stimulates, and tones the pelvic viscera and mucous membranes, helping to cast off any sediments that have settled on surfaces. It is good used alone or in combination with other herbs. It earned its name for its powerful solvent effect on stony deposits in the kidneys; here it can do the work alone, but its effects are improved with other herbal agents in combination. Gravel root can be used for any kidney and urinary problem, and it is also great as a tonic and stimulant. As a nervine, it influences the entire sympathetic nervous system.

Medicinal uses:
All chronic renal disorders (kidneys, bladder, urethral channels, etc.), hematuria, gout, rheumatism, dropsy, acute and chronic gonorrhea, backache, weak pelvic organs, chronic cystitis, strangury, Bright's disease, gravel, bladder stones, diarrhea, neuralgia, lame back, nerve relaxant, female troubles, diabetes, prostate troubles, bloody urine, febrile conditions.

Preparations:
Decoction (root), fluid extract, infusion (leaves, flowers), powder, tincture.

Dosage:

Decoction	1 tablespoon to 2 fluid ounces 3 to 4 times daily. Children: 1 teaspoonful to 2 fluid ounces (according to age, vitality, etc.).
Fluid extract	1/2-1 teaspoon.
Infusion	2 fluid ounces.
Powder	1/4-3/4 teaspoons.
Tincture	1/2-1 teaspoon.

FORMULAS

Seldom will you find a formula made for gravel or stone deposits that does not include the valuable gravel root herb.

Decoction for gravel root

1 ounce	Gravel root, cut (Eupatorium purpureum)
1 pint	Distilled or d-cell water
2 ounces	Pure glycerine

Preparation: Soak the root for 2 hours in the water, then bring to a boil and simmer for 20 minutes; strain and cool, bottle and store in a cool place. If the preparation is to be preserved over a period of time, add the glycerine after straining and while still hot.

Dosage: 1 tablespoonful to 2 fluid ounces 3 to 4 times daily. Children: 1 teaspoonful to 1 tablespoonful (according to age, etc.).

Pelvic troubles

1½ ounces Gravel root (Eupatorium purpureum)
1 ounce Squaw vine (Mitchella repens)
1 ounce Golden seal (Hydrastis Canadensis)

Preparation: Simmer in 2½ pints of water for 20 minutes, strain.

Dosage: 3 tablespoonfuls 3 times daily.

Note: The fluid extract may be used for the preparation in the same proportions, mix thoroughly; give 1/2-1 teaspoonful 3 times daily.

Strong decoction of gravel root for cystitis and kidney troubles (solvent of phlegm, fibrin, etc.)

4 ounces Gravel root, cut (eupatorium purpureum)
3 pints Distilled or d-cell water
4 ounces Glycerine

Preparation: Simmer for 30 minutes in a saucepan, strain, and add the glycerine, return to the heat and reduce to 1 pint by simmering; cool, bottle, and keep in a cool place.

Dosage: 2 teaspoons to 1 tablespoonful 3 times daily between meals (larger doses are also safe); children: 1 teaspoonful or less 3 times daily.

Gravel, Stones or Calculi

1 ounce Gravel root (Eupatorium purpureum)
1/2 ounce Wild carrot (Daucus carota)
1/2 ounce Meadowsweet (Filipendula ulmaria)
1/2 ounce Marshmallow (Althaea officinalis)
1/2 ounce Uva ursi (Arctostaphylos uva-ursi)
6 ounces Honey (use up to 8 oz. if needed)

Preparation: Simmer 20 minutes in 1 quart of distilled water, strain over honey.

Dosage: 2-3 fluid ounces 3 times daily.

Administration: Drink also weak composition tea (see page 147-148) with soymilk (tofu-milk); take care to avoid drinking hard water.

Prostate urinary troubles

1 part Gravel root, powder (Eupatorium purpureum)

1 part Marshmallow root, powder (Althaea officinalis)
1 part Parsley, powder (Petroselinum crispum)
1 part Juniper berries, powder (Juniperus communis)
1 part Lobelia, powder (Lobelia inflata)
1 part Cayenne, powder (Capsicum frutescens; C. minimum)
3 parts Golden seal, powder (Hydrastis Canadensis)

Preparation: Mix thoroughly, and use 1 teaspoonful for each cup of water or put the powder mixture in #00 capsules.

Dosage: In emergency, drink 1/2 cup frequently during the day; or take two #00 capsules in the morning and again at night.

Note: The above was one of Dr. Christopher's favorite formulas and was used successfully many times over the years.

Women's genital area

Use the same herbs and formula for "Prostate urinary trouble," above and add the following herbs:
1 part Squaw vine, powder (Mitchella repens)
1 part Raspberry leaves, powder (Rubus idaeus)
1 part Blessed thistle, powder (Cnicus benedictus)

Congenial combinations:
Gravel root combines well with the herbal agents for female problems, such as squaw vine. Gravel root combines well with golden seal.

CASE HISTORY

Enuresis-the problem of bed-wetting.
A Dr. Christopher case history in his own words: The kidney is very sensitive and sometimes malfunctions from fear or panic. Children quite often have bed-wetting problems when their nervous systems are damaged, and I have seen acute kidney problems from other causes. Tommy is a bed-wetter, and his parents bring him to me to see what is the problem. I, in checking the iris of the eye, not only find the invariable severe nerve rings, but in the kidney area we also find scar tissue where the kidney has been bruised. Why? Because he couldn't keep from wetting his bed and he got paddled for it. And instead of on the buttocks, it was just a little higher on the kidney area. We have seen kidneys torn loose from the body and floating because of these severe beatings, which have been called "spankings." Many parents do not realize it, because such is a lack of education, but the greatest part of enuresis trouble is from the nerves. And a lot of it is psychosomatic, so we have given quite a few severe lectures to the parents before we have started working on the child.

Cleanser of the urinary tract.
A Dr. Christopher case history in his own words: About a year ago, we had the case of a man who was to be sent back to the Mayo Clinic for a prostate operation. It was serious enough that the doctors there wanted to handle it. We had to put the catheter in to get the liquid to flow at all, and the man was in great pain. And even with this mechanical assistance, the pumping was very slow. This man agreed to do anything we suggested, so we changed his diet. That was the roughest "medicine" we could have given him, as he was a big eater of the orthodox foods. But we changed his diet and put him on the gravel root herb (the "Prostate urinary troubles" formula on page 280-281).

Not more than six weeks had gone by before he happily told me, "I now have the fountain of youth. This is the happiest that any man could ever be. It has been many, many years since I've had this freedom and no pain." He was so enthusiastic about this miracle taking place within him that he said, "I would think that I can go on straight raw food now that I've got started, and it will go faster." But we counseled, "No, please don't, because the mucus will break loose so fast that we need to slow it down, so at least 1/3 of your foods should be baked or steamed." Well, he went ahead with the raw diet anyway. The mucus came fast and furious, and one string of mucus from the urinary tract was so long and painful that he thought he was going to have triplets with all that he went through.

Growth characteristics:
Perennial root; the herb is indigenous to North America, and is common from New Brunswick to Florida and westward to Manitoba and Texas. It grows in moist soils, meadows, woods and low grounds. The flowers blossom in August and September.

UVA URSI or BEARBERRY
(Arctostaphylos uva-ursi; ERICACEAE)

Common names:
Uva ursi, bearberry, upland cranberry, universe vine, mountain cranberry, mountain box, wild cranberry, bear's grape, kinnikinnick, mealberry, sagackhomi; arbutus uva-ursi, fox berry, barren myrtle, Uvae Ursi Folia (Br.); Bousserole, Raisin d'Ours (Fr.); Baerentrauben blaetter (Ger.); Coralillo (Mex.).

Identifying characteristics:
Stem — Low evergreen shrub, creeping stem, young branches rising obliquely upward several inches, woody, smooth bark.

Leaves — Leathery, alternate, obovate-lanceolate, 1/2-1/15 inch long and 1/5-1/2 inch broad, rounded at apex, shiny and dark green on upper surface and finely reticulated with sunken veinlets, coriaceous (tough and leather like), and yellowish-green undersurface, on short petioles.

	Powder: olive green.
Flowers	Pinkish-white, 3-15 together on racemes, reddish calyx.
Fruit	Bright red drupaceous berry, fleshy, 1/4 inch broad, 5 seeded, resemble currants in appearance and clusters, ripen in the winter.
Root	Long and fibrous.
Odor	Dried leaves are odorless until pulverized, whereupon it is like dried grass, or aromatic and faintly tea-like.
Taste	Astringent and somewhat bitter.

Part used:
Leaves.

Therapeutic action:
Diuretic (antilithic, lithotriptic), astringent, soothing tonic, mucilage, nephritic, antiseptic, disinfectant. In larger doses, emetic, purgative, parturient.

Uva ursi has a specific healing action upon the genito-urinary organs, especially in cases of gravel or ulceration of the kidneys or bladder. It is of great value in kidney and bladder problems, where it soothes, strengthens and tones the mucous membranes of the urinary passages. It is a solvent to uretic calculi deposits. Uva ursi stimulates kidney activity, and it has a slight antiseptic effect on the mucous membranes. The leaves are powerfully astringent (due to a 6-8% tannic acid composition) and, according to old herbal works (wherein it was known by the name of "arbutus"), were used as such as early as the thirteenth century.

Medicinal uses:
Catarrh of the bladder, leucorrhea, gonorrhea, gleet, backache, kidney and bladder congestion or ulceration, enuresis, prostate weakness, urethritis, cystitis, gravel, chronic nephritis, incontinence of urine, dysuria, strangury, uterine hemorrhage, syphilis, rheumatism, anemia, chronic diarrhea, menorrhagia, urinary calculi, bronchitis, cardiac dropsy, diabetes, Bright's disease, dysentery, piles, hemorrhoids, pussy and bloody discharges, uterine ulceration, female problems.

Preparations:
Fluid extract, infusion, powder, tincture.

Dosage:

Concentrate	1/2-1 teaspoonful.
Fluid extract	1/2-1 teaspoonful.
Infusion	2 fluid ounces 3 to 4 times daily.
Powder	500 mg.-2½ grams.
Tincture	10-30 drops.

ADMINISTRATION

Uva ursi is usually taken orally in tea form.

Anal

Piles, hemorrhoids: Use the tea or diluted tincture as a wash.

Oral

Uva ursi is often used alone, but it is also good in combination with other healing agents.

Enuresis, or bed-wetting: With a child, when you first start off with uva ursi, don't expect the cure to be instantaneous from one night to the next morning. The problem has been a long time coming on, and this herb will assist with the regulation of the problem. Whenever a child lies sleeping on his back, pressure irritates the kidneys, and that is when the bed-wetting generally takes place. So we always prescribe that a ball of cotton (or cloth rolled into a ball), large enough to make an uncomfortable protrusion, be taped or fastened to the bed clothes or pajamas right in the small of the back. Then, when the child is asleep and unconsciously rolls from the side onto the back, he will roll back to the side position again. This will keep the child off his back and thereby lessen the irritation and help speed the healing process.

Vagina

Uterine ulceration, infection: Use the infusion or diluted tincture as a douche.

FORMULAS

Infusion of uva ursi leaves

1 ounce	Uva ursi leaves, cut (Arctostaphylos uva-ursi)
1 pint	Distilled or d-cell water.

Preparation: Boil the water and, while boiling, pour over the leaves, cover and steep 10 minutes; strain, cool, bottle, and keep in a cool place.

Dosage: 2 fluid ounces 3 to 4 times a day before meals.

Kidney and bladder

8 teaspoons	Uva ursi, cut or powder (Arctostaphylos uva-ursi)
2 teaspoons	Mountain mahogany or Sweet birch, cut or powder (Betula lenta)
8 teaspoons	Couchgrass, cut or powder (Agropyron repens)
4 teaspoons	Buchu leaves, cut or powder (Agathosma betulina)
2 teaspoons	Juniper berries, cut or powder (Juniperus communis)
3 teaspoons	Prince's pine, cut or powder (Chimaphila umbellata)
3 teaspoons	Shavegrass, cut or powder (Equisetum hyemale)

2 teaspoons Celery seeds, crushed or powder (Apium graveolens)

Note: The above mixture will make 20 doses.

Preparation: Add 1 dose to 3 cups of boiling water, and simmer 2 to 3 minutes, then steep 10 minutes and strain; or steep 1/2 hour in hot water and sweeten with honey; or divide 1 dose into 3 parts and take in water, honey, jelly or jam. Warning: Be sure not to boil Buchu leaves, as this removes the volatile oil and renders them useless.

Dosage: Take 1/3 of 1 dose before or after meals.

Gravel, obstructure and suppression of urine, bed-wetting, catarrh of bladder, inflammations

1/2 ounce Uva ursi (Arctostaphylos uva-ursi)
1/2 ounce White poplar or quaking aspen bark (Populus tremuloides)
1/2 ounce Marshmallow root (Althaea officinalis)

Preparation: Infuse in pint of boiling water for 20 minutes, strain.

Dosage: 3 tablespoonfuls 3 times daily.

Cystic catarrh, prolapsed uterus, flaccid vagina or uterus

1 ounce Uva ursi (Arctostaphylos uva-ursi)
1 ounce Squaw vine (Mitchella repens)
1½ ounces Dandelion root (Taraxacum officinale)

Preparation: Simmer in 1 quart of distilled or d-cell water for 20 minutes, strain.

Dosage: 3-4 tablespoonfuls 3 times daily.

Enuresis or bed-wetting (teas)

1 ounce Uva ursi (Arctostaphylos uva-ursi)
1/2 ounce White poplar or quaking aspen bark (Populus tremuloides)
1/2 ounce Sumach berries (Rhus glabra)
1/2 ounce Yarrow (Achillea millefolium)

Preparation: Simmer in 1 quart of distilled or d-cell water for 20 minutes, strain.

Dosage: 3 tablespoonfuls 3 times daily.

Enuresis or bed-wetting (capsules)

1 part	Uva ursi, powder (Arctostaphylos uva-ursi)
1 part	White pond lily, powder (Nymphaea odorata)
1 part	Yarrow, powder (Achillea millefolium)
1 part	Sumach berries, powder (Rhus glabra)
1 part	White poplar or quaking aspen bark, powder (Populus tremuloides)
1 part	Ginger, powder (Zingiber officinalis)
3 parts	Golden Seal, powder (Hydrastis Canadensis)

Preparation: Mix thoroughly and place in #00 capsules; or, use 1 teaspoonful of the mixture in 1 cupful of warm water.

Dosage: Give the child 1 #00 capsule 3 times a day; or, 1/2 cupful of tea 3 times daily.

Lumbago

1 ounce	Uva ursi (Arctostaphylos uva-ursi)
1 ounce	Goldenrod (Solidago odora)
1/2 ounce	Prince's pine (Chimaphila umbellata)
1/2 ounce	Licorice root or juice (Glycyrrhiza glabra)
1 ounce	Buchu (Agathosma betulina; A. crenulata; Diosma ericoides)
1 teaspoonful	Cayenne (Capsicum frutescens; C. minimum)

Preparation: Simmer slowly the first 4 herbs in 3 pints of water, then pour hot over the Buchu and cayenne and steep covered until cool, strain.

Dosage: In the day drink 2 fluid ounces 3 times daily and one hour prior to going to bed, drink 6-8 ounces of warmed tea.

Note: If there is constipation, add 1/4 ounce cascara bark.

Nephritis (inflammation of the kidneys)

1/2 ounce	Uva ursi (Arctostaphylos uva-ursi)
1/2 ounce	Cleavers (Galium aparine)
1/2 ounce	Juniper berries (Juniperus communis)
1/2 ounce	Marshmallow (Althaea officinalis)
1/2 ounce	Buchu (Agathosma betulina; A. crenulata; Diosma ericoides)
1 teaspoonful	Cayenne (Capsicum frutescens; C. minimum)

Preparation: Simmer the first 4 herbs for 20 minutes in 1 quart of water, then strain hot over the Buchu and cayenne.

Dosage: 2 fluid ounces every 1 to 2 hours.

Note: With the exception of marshmallow (the demulcent), wild carrot or tansy may be substituted for any of the above ingredients.

Administration: Also give the patient a tea made of slippery elm or linseed.

Nephritis

1 ounce	Uva ursi (Arctostaphylos uva-ursi)
1 ounce	Tansy (Tanacetum vulgare)
1 ounce	Wild carrot (Daucus carota)
1 ounce	Pellitory-of-the-wall (Parietaria officinalis)
1 ounce	Marshmallow root (Althaea officinalis)
1 teaspoonful	Cayenne (Capsicum frutescens; C. minimum)

Preparation: Simmer slowly in 2 quarts of water down to 1 quart, strain hot over the cayenne.

Dosage: 3 tablespoonfuls every 2 hours.

CASE HISTORY

Do cleanse, but gradually.
A Dr. Christopher case history in his own words: We had a case in Salt Lake where a man, who for the first time in years was beginning to enjoy the health that comes from cleansing, decided that the more aggresive he cleansed the better his health would be. He went too far, and his system sought to void a long string of mucus from the urinary track. He was so full of mucus that his system could not take it out normally, and it completely stopped the eliminative channel. He had to use a catheter to get it started again, but now he flows very freely. Do not drive the cleansing organs through over-dosage. You must cleanse these delicate areas in the body gradually; when you drive them excessively, damage can be caused.

Growth characteristics:
Perennial evergreen, found in Northern Europe, Asia, North America; grows in sterile, sandy and gravelly soil and in pine woods, south of New Jersey and west to California. The flowers appear June-September, but the berries do not ripen until winter.

Sister plants:
-Manzanita or California Manzanita (Arctostaphylos glauca); used like uva ursi.
-(Arctostaphylos polifolia and A. mucrocifera); in Mexico, used like uva ursi.

WILD CARROT
(Daucus carota; UMBELLIFERAE)

Common names:
Wild carrot, queen Anne's lace, bird's nest root, bee's nest plant.

Identifying characteristics:

Stem	Branching, tough and bristly (stiff hairs), 1-3 feet high.
Leaves	Obovate, bipinnate with acute segments (fringe foliage cut into fine divisions), hairy.
Flowers	Circular umbel (concave like a bird's nest), of small unequal, white (sometimes pinkish-gray), lacy, and numerous flowers in a compound, with one central floret that is often dark crimson.
Root	Tapering and conical, fleshy, yellowish-white, sweetish (edible), and aromatic.
Fruit	Oval, flat, 1/6 inch long, grayish-brown, margined with prickles and tipped with 1-3 bristles.
Odor	Aromatic.
Taste	Pungent, resembles the garden carrot.

Part used:
Whole herb.

Therapeutic action:
Stimulant, diuretic, stomachic, deobstruent, anthelmintic (vermifuge).

Wild carrot is highly valuable for gravel, stricture, or any obstruction in the urinary passages or bladder. It will often cure when all other means have failed.

Medicinal uses:
Dropsy, retention of urine, gravel, bladder problems, flatulence, nephritic complaints, ulcer, amenorrhea, eczema, itching, liver disorders, cancer, painful urination (strangury), dysmenorrhea, abscesses, carbuncles, scrofula, bad wounds, colic.

Preparations:
Decoction, fluid extract, infusion, powder, tincture.

Dosage:

Decoction	2-4 tablespoonfuls 3 to 4 times daily.
Fluid extract	1/2-1 teaspoonful.
Infusion	2 fluid ounces.
Powder	1-2 grams.
Tincture	1/2-1 teaspoon.

ADMINISTRATION

The most usual form is the infusion or tea.

Oral

Dropsy: See "FORMULAS."

Skin

Ulcers, abscesses, carbuncles, sores, bad wounds: Use grated as a poultice.

FORMULAS

Dropsy

1¼ ounce	Wild carrot (Daucus carota)
1½ ounce	Haircap moss (Polytrichum juniperum)
1 ounce	Watermelon seeds, crushed (Citrullus lanatus; C. vulgaris)

Preparation: Simmer in 3 pints of Distilled for 20 minutes, strain.

Dosage: 2 tablespoonfuls every 2 hours. With this, use vapor or steam bath 2 to 3 times a week.

Cystitis (inflammation of the bladder)

1/2 ounce	Wild carrot (Daucus carota)
1/2 ounce	Uva ursi (Arctostaphylos uva-ursi)
1/2 ounce	Juniper berries (Juniperus communis)
1/2 ounce	Tansy (Tanacetum vulgare)
1/2 ounce	Licorice root or juice (Glycyrrhiza glabra)
1/2 ounce	Buchu (Agathosma betulina; A. crenulata; Diosma ericoides)
1 teaspoonful	Cayenne (Capsicum frutescens; C. minimum)

Preparation: Simmer slowly the first 5 herbs for 20 minutes in 1 quart of water; strain hot over the cayenne and buchu.

Dosage: 2 fluid ounces 4 to 6 times daily.

Administration: Where necessary, cleanse the bowels with catnip injection (1 ounce steeped in 1 quart of boiling hot water); then after a few minutes add 1/2 teaspoonful composition powder (see page 147-148) and inject when lukewarm. Also this bowel action may be accomplished with 1/4 ounce of barberry bark or cascara bark added to the above formula.

Inflammation of the kidneys

1/2 ounce	Wild carrot (Daucus carota)
1/2 ounce	Pellitory-of-the-wall (Parietaria officinalis)
1/2 ounce	Uva ursi (Arctostaphylos uva-ursi)
1/2 ounce	Dandelion root (Taraxacum officinale)
1/2 ounce	Marshmallow root (Althaea officinalis)
1/2 ounce	White poplar bark (Populus tremuloides)
1 teaspoonful	Cayenne (Capsicum frutescens; C. minimum)

Preparation: Simmer the first 6 herbs slowly in 1 quart of water down to 1 pint; strain over the cayenne.

Dosage: 3 tablespoonfuls every hour until patient is eased, then every 2 hours.

Administration: At the same time, apply hot packs of flannel wrung out in hot water across the kidneys and the lumbar region.

Growth characteristics:
Biennial; found in the eastern half of the United States and Canada, and in Europe and Asia; it grows in wastelands, field borders, and roadside and flowers June-September. Wild carrot is considered to be a pest to the farmer, joy to the flower lover, and refreshment to nature's hosts (flies, beetles, bees, and wasps—especially the paper-nest builders).

Wild carrot and garden carrot not the same species: The name "wild carrot" probably originated from the popular belief that the garden carrot, which the Dutch introduced into England during Queen Elizabeth's reign, was derived from this wild species. The characteristic taste and smell, being similar, may have lent support to this myth. But botanists have failed to develop an edible vegetable from this wild root; and when the cultivation of the garden carrot lapses a few generations, it reverts to another ancestral type that is a species quite distinct.

GARDEN CARROT

(Daucus carota, var. sativus; domestic types: Oxheart, Chantenay, Nantes, etc.; UMBELLIFERAE)

Therapeutic action:
Nutritive, tonic, alterative, diuretic (lithotriptic). The garden carrot is reputed to do anything medicinally that the wild carrot will do, but the wild carrot is a little stronger in its potency. The garden carrot is more readily accessible and flavorful.

John B. Lust, in his book, *The New Ray Juice Therapy* quotes the learned

Ragnar-Berg on carrots:

> They have some protein, are rich in carbohydrates, potassium, sodium and calcium, there is a high alkali excess, a trace of iodine and a good proportion of all vitamins. They constitute a powerful cleansing food. A large amount of carrot carbohydrate is one of the most effective means of changing the intestinal flora from a putrefactive to a non-putrefactive type.

Medicinal uses:
Tonsillitis, colitis, appendicitis, anemia, gravel, acidosis, blood poisoning, faulty circulation, ulcers, rheumatism, indigestion, increase milk secretion, poor teeth (high in calcium), acne, adenoids, cancer, etc.

Preparations:
Juiced or whole (raw or cooked). The juice is preferred, as the healing factors are sufficiently concentrated to supply the system with what is needed.

Dosage:
Juice 1-6 pints a day.

ADMINISTRATION

The juice is taken orally, or is used as a wash or in a poultice form externally.

CASE HISTORY

Snowbound and healthy.
Dr. Christopher commented: The garden carrot is one of the great foods of all time. A little town in Idaho had its main crop in carrots, and they did so well there that every farm was in carrots. This was still in the "horse and buggy days" and the area was quite isolated, so when fall came, the people would harvest the carrots and take them down to a larger town and trade for supplies for the winter. But one particular winter they got snow-bound before they could take the carrots down, so over that winter they had raw carrots, fried carrots, grated carrots, juiced carrots, carrot salads. That is about all they lived on. And you know, that was the first year in the history of that town that there was no sickness, not even a case of sniffles! Well, the next year, being pretty smart people, they didn't take the chance of getting snow-bound again, so they hurried down early to get their usual dietary staples of refined, devitalized foods and, of course, they had their regular sickness. That year they kept their local doctor in business.

Loretta Foote
Dr. Christopher reminisced about Dr. Loretta Foote: she was one of the sweetest women we ever knew; and all she did was try to help people. She was an herbalist, and when we had our offices on First South in Salt Lake City, she was on our

staff as the obstetrician. She delivered thousands of babies, most of them in the home; in fact, our five were delivered in our home by natural childbirth, assisted by Dr. Loretta Foote.

Dr. Foote had a friend, a very prominent lady of Salt Lake City, who was told by her doctors that she was dying of cancer. When Dr. Foote found out, she put her friend on a carrot juice diet. This was before the days of mechanical juicers. Dr. Foote grated carrots for her with the old "knuckle-skinner" (grater) and squeezed out the juice by hand with cloths, until she would get a quart or so every day (and sometimes 2 to 3 times per day), so you can imagine how much dedicated effort this took. Dr. Foote fed this to her friend, and she was completely cured, to the astonishment of the doctors.

This woman later wrote a booklet on how she was healed of cancer, and we have one of the very, very few copies left in existence. Then she sponsored Dr. Foote in a health store, the first health store in America, and they went broke! So this appreciative lady said, "They don't want us here; let's go to the coast." Many of you have been to the coast and have seen the many, many juice bars and health food stores—well, these two great ladies started the first health store and juice bar on the coast, the first ones that were successful in the United States. And these started to gain in popularity. Later Dr. Foote returned to Salt Lake City and started another health food store, and this time it was a success. Here is a wonderful pioneer lady who did wonders with the juice of our common garden carrot!

The carrot poultice is good for man or beast.
A Dr. Christopher case history in his own words: Traveling from our office in Evanston, Wyoming, a number of years ago, I had to go over to Woodruff on a house call, to a family that was very, sick. They improved so rapidly and were so pleased with our program that it was with some reluctance and embarrassment that the man said to me "Would it insult you if we asked you something about an animal?" I said, "No, we're good for man or beast." He said that he had a favorite horse outside that got tangled up in the barbed wire. "The vet was here yesterday and used the last ointments, salves and things that he knew about, and then he said there was only one thing more to do; since the gangrene is setting in, we will need to shoot the horse."

Well, this lovely animal was part of the family. They had quite a few children, and they still loved the horse, so he said "What can we do?" So we went out and looked at the horse's leg. I said "All right, you have been taking carrot juice and you have some pulp there and a ton or so of carrots that you have brought in from your field, just grind up carrots and make a great big poultice and cover that horse's leg. That will do him good, and then give the horse all the carrots it can eat." Within seven days time that horse's leg was completely healed. The flesh was fully restored.

CLEAVERS or CLIVERS
(Galium aparine; RUBIACEAE)

Common names:
Cleavers, clivers, goosegrass, hayriffe, erriffe, burweed, goosebill, cleaverwort, bed straw, catch weed.

Identifying characteristics:

Stem	Succulent, weak, procumbent, quadrangular, 2-6 feet high, hairy at the joints.
Leaves	Lanceolate, 1/2 inch long and 1/4 inch wide, in rings of six, backward bristly hairs at the margin.
Flowers	Small, white, scattered.
Fruit	Nearly globular burr, 1/8 inch diameter, covered with hooked bristles.
Odor	Unpleasant in the green state, none when dried.
Taste	Slightly saline, acrid, astringent and bitter.

Part used:
Whole herb above ground.

Therapeutic action:
Diuretic (lithotriptic), antiscorbutic, tonic, aperient, alterative, refrigerant.

Cleavers is a soothing, relaxing and diffusive diuretic which influences the kidneys and bladder. It acts mildly upon the bowels. As cleavers is powerful, it should not be given where there is a tendency for diabetes, where there may be kidney weakness.

Medicinal uses:
Gravel, scalding urine, bladder irritation, dropsy, scrofula, cancer, ulcers, scurvy, suppressions of urine, obstruction of urinary organs, gonorrhea, sore nipples, wounds.

Preparation:
Fluid Extract, infusion, powder, tincture.

Dosage:

Fluid extract	1/2-1 teaspoonful.
Infusion	2-4 fluid ounces (cold) 3 to 4 times daily.
Powder	1 teaspoonful to the cup in boiling water.
Tincture	1/2-1 teaspoonful.

ADMINISTRATION

Where possible, the infusion form is recommended.

Oral

Acute gonorrhea: Bruise the fresh herb thoroughly in a mortar, then express the juice with strong pressure and take 1/2-1 fluid ounce every 4 to 6 hours.

Skin

Breast tumors: Use the expressed juice mixed with linseed meal, and apply to the breast; take 1 teaspoonful of the juice while fasting in the morning.

Cancer: Apply a poultice of the bruised green herb, and take 2 ounces of the expressed juice 3 times daily.

Sore nipples and green wounds: Apply the expressed juice and take internally 1 tablespoonful of the juice 3 times a day.

FORMULAS

Dropsy (adult)

1/2 ounce	Cleavers (Galium aparine)
1/2 ounce	Raspberry leaves (Rubus idaeus)
1/2 ounce	Agrimony (Agrimonia eupatoria)
1/2 ounce	Juniper berries (Juniperus communis)
1/2 ounce	Wild carrot (Daucus carota)
1/2 ounce	Barberry (Berberis vulgaris)
1/2 teaspoon	Cayenne (Capsicum frutescens; C. minimum)

Preparation: Simmer the first 6 herbs in 3 pints of water down to 1½ pints. Strain over the cayenne.

Dosage: 2 tablespoonfuls 4 times daily.

Note: Use centaury and calumba as tonics to build up the digestion and to strengthen the system.

Administration: Give patient a vapor bath every second day, giving 1/2 cup of composition tea (see page 147-148) while in the bath, which will open the pores to throw off toxins and relieve the kidney load. After the bath, rub down thoroughly with a towel that has been soaked in cold apple cider vinegar, wrap the feet in a cloth soaked in apple cider vinegar, and keep them warm with a hot water bottle. Take your regular dosage of cayenne 3 to 4 times daily (best before meals).

Dropsy (child)

1/2 ounce	Cleavers (Galium aparine)

1/2 ounce	Juniper berries (Juniperus communis)
1/2 ounce	Centaury (Erythraea centaurium)
1/2 ounce	Raspberry leaves (Rubus idaeus)
1/4 ounce	Senna (Cassia acutifolia)
1/2 teaspoon	Ginger, powder (Zingiber officinalis)

Preparation: Steep in 1 quart of boiling hot water; let stand until cool, strain.

Dosage: 1 tablespoonful 4 times daily.

Note: This may also be flavored with a little aniseed water or essence of aniseed. With dropsy, watch the kidneys, and strengthen the digestive system. Sponging the body with cold water and apple cider vinegar is an excellent skin tonic.

Congenial combinations:
Cleavers is better when combined with marshmallow.

Growth characteristics:
Annual; common to Europe and the United States. It grows in cultivated grounds, in moist thickets, and along river banks. It flowers from June to September.

Sister plants:
Small Cleaver (Galium tinctorium); nervine, antispasmodic, expectorant, and diaphoretic.

BUCHU

(Agathosma betulina; A. crenulata; Diosma ericoides; D. betulina, Barosma betulina, B. crenulata, B. serratifolia; RUTACEAE)

Common names:
Buchu, bookoo, buku, bucku, bucco; Buchu Folia; Folia Bucco, Diosmae, or Barsomae (Br.); Beuilles de Bucco, Booko, Buchu (Fr.); Buccoblaetter, Buchublatte (Ger.).

Identifying characteristics:

Stem	Woody shrub, 1-4 feet high, many branches, young twigs, covered with immersed oil glands.
Bark	Stiff, angular, smooth, purple.
Leaves	Round Buchu (Agathosma betulina); opposite, flat, about 1 inch long, rhomboid-ovate outline, with a blunt recurved apex (this is the preferred variety). Oval Buchu (A. crenulata); crenelated margin and blunt, but the apex is not recurved. Long Buchu (Diosma ericoides); serrate margin and truncate apex (this variety has only about 1/2 the amount of volatile oil as the foregoing two varieties.

Flowers	Solitary and pink.
Fruit	Ovate, capsule, 3/8 inch long and 1/2 inch broad, 5-seeded.
Odor	Aromatic, resembles peppermint.
Taste	Camphoraceous.

Part used:
Leaves.

Therapeutic action:
Diuretic, diaphoretic, stimulant, aromatic, antiseptic, tonic, astringent, carminative, vulnerary. In large doses, its action is emetic and cathartic.

Buchu is a mild aromatic and a tonic diuretic that is slightly diffusive and stimulating, which heals all chronic complaints of the genitourinary tract. It increases the quantity of urine (which becomes darker and strongly aromatic) and urinic solids. At the same time it acts as a tonic, astringent and disinfectant to the mucous membranes and diminishes their secretion into the urinary channel. Buchu increases the pulse rate, stimulates the appetite by influencing the mucous membrane of the stomach, soothes the pelvic nerves, and produces slight moisture on the skin. It is effective in chronic irritability of the bladder when there is a frequent desire to urinate.

Medicinal uses:
Backache, gravel, dropsy, aching of penis, myelitis, cystitis, urethritis, lithiasis, chronic bronchitis, prostate complaints, atonic dyspepsia, chronic rheumatism, skin affections, gleet, gonorrhea, inflamed prostate, retention or incontinence of urine, feeble digestion, flatulence, inflammation or catarrh of bladder, congestion of prostate, renal discharges, spermatorrhea, leucorrhea, diabetes (first stage), irritation of urethral mucous membrane, painful urination.

Preparations:
Fluid extract, infusion, powder, solid extract, tincture.

Be careful not to boil buchu, as the volatile oil which contains much of the therapeutic value will effervesce and escape, rendering it inert medicinally.

Dosage:

Fluid extract	1/2-1 teaspoonful.
Infusion	1 cupful 3 to 4 times daily.
Powder	500 mg.-1 gram 3 times daily.
Solid extract	325 mg.-1 gram.
Tincture	1/2 teaspoonful.

ADMINISTRATION

Give a strong cold infusion to increase the flow of urine, as in the case of stoppage of urine, and a warm infusion to soothe the nerves and as a gentle diaphoretic. There will be a sense of heat in the stomach, which gradually diffuses over the body. The warm infusion will soothe an inflamed and enlarged prostate gland and irritation of the urethral membrane.

FORMULAS

Inflammation of prostate (gonorrhoea, leucorrhoea)

1 ounce Buchu (Agathosma betulina; A. crenulata; Diosma ericoides)
1/4 ounce Juniper berries, crushed (Juniperus communis)
1/4 ounce Cubeb (Piper Cubeba)
1/4 ounce Uva ursi (Arctostaphylos uva-ursi)

Preparation: Infuse in 1½ pints of distilled or d-cell water pouring the boiling water over the herbs, cover until cold, strain.

Dosage: 3-4 tablespoonfuls 3 times daily.

Kidneys

2 parts Buchu (Agathosma betulina; A. crenulata; Diosma ericoides)
2 parts Uva-ursi (Arctostaphylos uva-ursi)
1 part Juniper berries (Juniperus communis)

Preparation: Infuse 1 teaspoonful in 1 cup boiling water; cover until cool, strain.

Dosage: 2 fluid ounces 3 or more times a day as required.

Dropsy

1 part Buchu leaves (Agathosma betulina; A. crenulata; Diosma ericoides)
1 part Hydrangea (Hydrangea arborescens)
1 part Broom tops (Cytisus scoparius)
1 part Couchgrass (Agropyron repens)
1 part Uva ursi (Arctostaphylos uva-ursi)
2 parts Saw Palmetto berries (Serenoa repens)

Preparation: Mix herbs well, then take one teaspoonful of combined herbs to cup of boiling hot water; steep until cool.

Dosage: 2 fluid ounces 3 or more times a day as required.

Gravel, kidney and bladder problems

1 ounce	Buchu, powder (Agathosma betulina; A. crenulata)
1/2 ounce	Uva ursi, powder (Arctostaphylos uva-ursi)
1 ounce	Parsley root, powder (Petroselinum crispum)
1 ounce	Gravel root, powder (Eupatorium purpureum)
1/2 ounce	Ginger, powder (Zingiber officinalis)

Preparation: Mix thoroughly. Infuse 2 ounces of powder in 1 quart of boiling hot water; cover and let stand until cool; strain.

Dosage: 3 tablespoonfuls 4 to 5 times daily.

Congenial combinations:
For pelvic nerves, aching back and loins: Use Buchu in combination with squaw vine (Mitchella repens) or unicorn root (Aletris farinosa).

Growth characteristics:
Perennial; imported from South Africa, where it grows in stony, hilly valleys of the mountains of the south west region in Cape Colony. It does not grow prolifically, but it can be cultivated in gardens.

Sister plants:
(Barosma eckloniana); has similar properties to Buchu.

Allied plants:
-Prickly ash (Zanthoxylum americanum; Z. Clava-Herculis); see page 469.
-Rue (Ruta graveolens); see page 321.

BURDOCK SEEDS
(Arctium lappa; Lappa minor; COMPOSITAE)

Common names:
Lappa, clothbur, thorny burr, fox's clote, beggars buttons, hardock, harebur, hurburr, turkey burr seed, bardana.

Identifying characteristics:
Burdock root is treated in Chapter 2 (see page 70), so we will only give information on the burdock seed, the burr or achene, here.

Fruit	Achene, globoidal, 1/2-1 inch broad, imbricated scale, with hooked extremities that adhere to almost anything they touch. The seed is obovate-oblong, angular, slightly curved, 1/4 inch long, brownish gray, wrinkled.

Part used:
Burr or seed.

Therapeutic action:
Diuretic, alterative, tonic, nervine, diaphoretic.

Medicinal uses:
Dropsy, inflamed kidneys and bladder, scalding urine, mucus discharges from the bladder, skin problems, eczema, boils, carbuncles, psoriasis, abrasions, burns, wounds, ulceration.

Preparations:
Crush the seeds for best results.

Dosage:

Infusion	Take in small doses, 2 fluid ounces 4 to 6 times daily.
Powder	2 teaspoonfuls 3 times daily.
Tincture	1/4-1/2 teaspoonful 3 times a day.
Decoction	2 teaspoons to 1 tablespoonful in some water 3 to 4 times daily between meals.

ADMINISTRATION

Skin

Ulcers, wounds, etc.: Dust the finely-powdered seed on the surface.

FORMULAS

Strong decoction for difficult skin diseases (eczema, pityriasis, psoriasis, etc.)

2 ounces	Burdock seeds, crushed or powdered (Arctium lappa)
2 quarts	Distilled or d-cell water
8 ounces	Glycerine

Preparation: Simmer seeds in water for 30 minutes; strain (this is an infusion), return to heat and simmer down to 1 pint (this is a decoction); cool, add the glycerine, mix thoroughly, bottle and keep in a cool place.

Dosage: 2 teaspoons to 1 tablespoonful in some water 3 to 4 times daily between meals. Very young children: 5-10 drops in water; older: 1 teaspoonful.

Note: For swollen glands or joints, take the infusion and use it to saturate lint, linen or cotton and apply warm to the area.

Eczema, scarlatina, etc.

1 part Burdock seeds, crushed (Arctium lappa)
1 part Sunflower seeds, crushed (Helianthus annuus)

Preparation: Steep herbs 10-15 minutes, strain.

Dosage: Give hot infusion 1 cupful 3 times daily.

Virtuous salve

3 parts Burdock seed, strong decoction (Arctium lappa) more or less
1 part Irish moss (Chondrus crispus)
1 part Anhydrous lanolin

Preparation: Add sufficient burdock seed decoction for uniform consistency, and mix in thoroughly.

Administration: Apply on lint and cover.

Skin problem

1/2 ounce Burdock seeds or root (Arctium lappa)
1/2 ounce Cleavers (Galium aparine)
1 ounce Fumitory (Fumaria officinalis)
1 ounce Wood sanicle (Sanicula europaea)

Preparation: Simmer slowly in 3 pints of Distilled or d-cell water down to 1½ pints, strain.

Dosage: 2 fluid ounces 3 times daily.

Growth characteristics:
Biennial found in the northern regions of the United States; the burr and seed appear and mature on the second year plant on the extended stem that reaches up to 5 feet high. It is found along the roadsides and in waste places, usually wherever stinging nettle is found.

Collection:
Gather after the seed has matured in the Fall of the second year's growth.

For alternate diuretic herbs to be used when the foregoing are not available, please see chapter 17.

CHAPTER 8

THE EMMENAGOGUE HERBS

The female generative organs may be divided into two groups, internal and external. The former, or internal organs, are the parts found within the pelvis: ovaries, Fallopian tubes or oviducts, uterus; and the latter, or external organs, are grouped under the name "vulva:" mons veneris, Labium majus, Labium minus, clitoris, vestibule, hymen, and urinary meatus. Most female troubles occur in the internal system, so we emphasize that here.

The UTERUS or womb is the organ of gestation or pregnancy—a hollow, pear-shaped, muscular organ, about 3 inches long, 2 inches wide, and 1 inch thick, situated in the pelvis between the bladder and the rectum. It receives and holds the fertilized ovum, carries the fetus during development and increases in size to 1 foot in length and 9-10 inches across, and then is the chief expelling agent during parturition or childbirth. Afterwards, the uterus rapidly reduces to a small size, but not as small as before pregnancy.

The uterus is a fixed organ, suspended within the pelvic cavity by means of ligaments—so when the bladder is full, the uterus is pushed backward, and when the rectum is enlarged, it is pushed forward. A change of posture affects the position of the uterus, and in pregnancy it normally becomes raised somewhat into the abdominal cavity; however, the upper rounded portion of the uterus, or fundus, is inclined slightly forward and the external orifice downward and slightly backward.

The uterus is divided into three portions: the fundus, the body, and the cervix or neck. The fundus is the upper and broad portion, the body is the middle and gradually narrowing portion, and the cervix or neck is the constricted or contracted part that extends to the vagina. The orifice or opening communicating the uterus with the mucous membrane is continuous with that of the vagina, while the outer surface of the fundus and body is covered with peritoneum.

For menstrual obstruction resulting in the absence, delay, retardation, or suppression of menstruation or amenorrhea, use herbs such as cramp bark, blue cohosh, black cohosh, etc. and formulas such as that found under cramp bark, pleurisy root, etc.

For retention of the menses at puberty, or chlorosis, also known as green sickness, resulting in the failure to menstruate, with accompanying symptoms of sallow skin, loss of appetite, lumbar pains, stomach acidity, constipation, nervous upset, and general constitutional derangement, improve the digestion, build up the whole system, and remove the obstruction; the formulas found under pennyroyal, blessed thistle, catnip, etc. are good for these conditions.

For profuse menstruation or menorrhagia, too frequent or too excessive menstrual flow, or a flow continuing longer than normal, with accompanying symptoms of lumbar pains, bearing down in the abdomen, possible nervous irritation, frequent constipation, etc. use the female corrective formulas found under red raspberry, true unicorn, etc.

Painful menstruation or dysmenorrhea, a condition of weakness in the generative organs from colds and general body weakness, with accompanying severe pains at the time of menstruation in the abdomen, loins and back, calls for equalization of the circulation with warm composition tea (see page 147-148), pennyroyal, etc. or the corrective formulas given under squaw vine, cramp bark, pleurisy root, etc.

For inflammation of the womb, or uteritis, which is due variously to colds, adhesions, blows, etc. with the patient suffering from pains in the womb and across the back and an irritated nervous system, the pains may be alleviated with repeated hot fomentations across the affected area, making a decoction of 2 ounces camomile flowers and 6 poppy heads, simmered for 10 minutes in 3 quarts of water, and using internal teas of the formulas found under red raspberry, white pond lily, etc.

Whites or leucorrhea, which is often accompanied by inflammation of the uterus, itching of the outer genital organs, a whitish to creamy discharge, pains in the small of the back and loins, headache, constipation, irritated nervous system, etc. is both disagreeable and weakening to the system. For this use the vaginal injections of herbs such as witch hazel, and the formulas given under red raspberry, white pond lily, etc.

There are some 150 herbs classed as promoting menstrual normalcy. But merely knowing that there is menstrual difficulty is not enough; we can only cure it by eliminating the cause. Where there has been a recent cold which has resulted in congestion, a relaxing diaphoretic may be all you need, and often only a few doses of composition powder (see page 147-148) are needed to remove a cold and the resultant congestion. General weakness may be the source of chronic suppression. In this case, the female organs may be built up by tonics and stimulating diaphoretics until health is restored. However, **never administer drastic cathartics or strong purgatives where there is menstrual difficulty**; this may greatly complicate and worsen the condition, but the natural remedies that we provide in the Lower Bowel tonic (see page 578) will always be beneficial and easy to take.

Emmenagogues are female correctives which provoke, stimulate, and promote the menstrual flow and discharge. Properly used, emmenagogues will readjust the entire reproductive areas, so that the menstrual flow and discharge will be the normal minimum, instead of excessive or lacking.

SQUAW VINE or PARTRIDGE BERRY
(Mitchella repens; RUBIACEAE)

Common names:
Squaw vine, partridge berry, checker berry, winter clover, deer berry, partridge vine, hive vine, one berry, twin-berry, Mitchella vine, squaw berry.

Identifying characteristics:
Stem Evergreen herb, slender, trailing or creeping, 1 to 2 feet long, smooth,

	deep furrow on one side, light green, rooting at joints, numerous erect branches. Powder: grayish-green.
Leaves	Evergreen, dark, shiny lower surface, opposite, smooth, coriaceous (tough, leather-like), small 3/8 inch long, 1/2 inch broad, entirely ovate (slightly cordate), clover-like, flat, sometimes white veined, short petiole.
Flowers	Waxy, cream-white (pink in bud, often tinged with red), pink-tipped, velvety, in pairs at ends of branches, 1/2 inch long, united ovaries, very fragrant (lilac-scented), 4-lobed calyx, funnel-shaped corolla, bearded within, 4 stamens inserted on corolla throat, 1 style.
Fruit	Berry-like drupe, scarlet-red, double, 4-seeded, small, edible, nearly tasteless, dry.
Root	Perennial rhizome, brownish, thread-like; fibrous roots; fine roots arise from joints in creeping stem.
Taste	Astringent, slightly bitter.
Odor	Faint.

Part used:
Herb or vine.

Therapeutic action:
Parturient, emmenagogue, diuretic, astringent, tonic, alterative.

This great herb is another legacy from our American Indians, who held it in high esteem as a uterine tonic during pregnancy and as an aid during parturition. It makes childbirth safe and wonderfully easy. It is highly beneficial for all uterine complaints and is most effective as a female regulator. In labor, it is reputed by some herbalists to be better than red raspberry leaves (these two herbs make a good combination). Squaw vine has very valuable diuretic, tonic and alterative properties, resembling those in prince's pine or pipsissewa (Chimaphila umbellata) and black haw (Viburnum prunifolium), for which it is often substituted, or used in combination.

Medicinal uses:
Childbirth, uterine troubles (menorrhagia, amenorrhea, dysmenorrhea, leucorrhea, etc.), dropsy, diarrhea, suppression of urine, sore eyes, urinary complaints, dysentery, gonorrhea, sore nipples, gravel, rheumatism, etc. Squaw vine when taken weeks before childbirth (better still, when taken all during pregnancy) will make the birth process much easier and safer.

Preparations:
Decoction, fluid extract, infusion, powder, tincture.

Dosage:

Decoction	2 fluid ounces 2 to 3 times daily.
Fluid extract	1/2-1 teaspoonful (fluid teaspoon).

Infusion	1 teacupful 2 to 3 times daily.
Powder	1-3 grams.
Tincture	5-60 drops.

ADMINISTRATION

Anal

Diarrhea, dysentery: Use the infusion or decoction as an injection.

Childbirth: Use the infusion of the herb alone, or in combination with red raspberry leaves.

Uterine problems, dropsy, rheumatism, diarrhea, urinary complaints: Use the infusion of the herb alone, in combination with cramp bark, prince's pine, black Haw, or as indicated in an appropriate formula (see "FORMULAS").

Skin

Sore eyes (especially infants): Combine squaw vine in infusion with equal parts of red raspberry leaves and witch hazel leaves and use as a wash; wild strawberry leaves may be substituted for witch hazel leaves.

Sore nipples: See "FORMULAS."

Vaginal

Leucorrhea: For mild cases, the infusion or decoction will serve as well as an injection.

FORMULAS

Dysmenorrhea (painful menstruation)

1/2 ounce	Squaw vine (Mitchella repens)
1/2 ounce	Red raspberry leaves (Rubus idaeus)
1/2 ounce	Uva ursi leaves (Arctostaphylos uva-ursi)
1/2 ounce	Golden seal root (Hydrastis Canadensis)
1/2 ounce	White poplar or quaking aspen inner bark (Populus tremuloides)

Preparation: Simmer the herbs in 1 quart of water down to 1½ pints; strain, sweeten, allow to cool, bottle and keep in a cool place.

Dosage: 2 fluid ounces 3 to 4 times daily.

Administration: Where there is general weakness, build up the constitution.

Equalize the circulation with composition tea or other appropriate stimulant; give 1 teacupful warm, and if pain continues, repeat every hour until patient perspires freely. This may be accomplished with warm pennyroyal tea; where there is cold and congestion, give a vapor bath followed with the composition tea. Relieve the bowels with the Lower Bowel tonic or with a gentle laxative agent. The Female Corrective Powder (see page 315 or 588) may be substituted for this formula.

Dysmenorrhea (painful menstruation)

2 parts Squaw vine (Mitchella repens)
2 parts Red raspberry leaves (Rubus idaeus)
2 parts Rue herb (Ruta graveolens)
2 parts White pond lily root (Nymphaea odorata)
1 part Black cohosh root (Cimicifuga racemosa)
1 part Uva ursi leaves (Arctostaphylos uva-ursi)
1 part Ginger root (Zingiber officinalis)
1 part Camomile flowers (Chamaemelum nobile; Anthemis nobilis)
1 part Spearmint herb (Mentha spicata)

Preparation: 1 teaspoonful of combined herbs infused with boiling water; cover tightly and cool.

Dosage: 2 fluid ounces every 2 hours or as needed.

Female Disorders

4 parts Squaw vine (Mitchella repens)
1 part Blue cohosh root (Caulophyllum thalictroides)
1 part Cramp bark (Viburnum trilobum; V. Opulus)
1 part False unicorn root or helonias (Chamaelirium luteum)

Preparation: Simmer slowly 5 minutes 1 teaspoonful to the cup.

Dosage: 1 cup 3 times a day.

Leucorrhea

2 parts Squaw vine (Mitchella repens)
2 parts Cramp bark (Viburnum trilobum; V. Opulus)
2 parts Black haw root bark (Viburnum prunifolium)
2 parts Prickly ash bark (Zanthoxylum americanum)
1 part False unicorn root, blazing star, helonias (Chamaelirium luteum)
1 part Blue cohosh root (Caulophyllum thalictroides)

Preparation: 1 teaspoonful of combined herbs to the cup; simmer slowly 5-10 minutes.

Dosage: 1/2 cup three times a day.

Menopause (change of life)

2 parts Squaw vine (Mitchella repens)
2 parts White poplar or quaking aspen inner bark (Populus tremuloides)
2 parts American Pennyroyal (Hedeoma pulegioides)
2 parts Mexican damiana leaves (Turnera aphrodisiaca)
3 parts Bethroot or wake robin root (Trillium erectum; T. pendulum)

Preparation: Pour boiling water over herbs: 1 teaspoonful of herbs to the cup.

Dosage: 1 cup three times a day.

Sore nipples

2 ounces Squaw vine, preferably fresh (Mitchella repens)
1/2 pint Olive oil
Sufficient Beeswax

Preparation: Make a strong decoction of the herb in 1 pint of water; strain, add the olive oil and beeswax and slowly reduce quantity until it is the consistency of a soft salve; allow to cool.

Administration: Anoint the nipple each time the baby is removed from the breast.

Congenial combinations:
ALTERATIVES: Squaw vine has valuable alterative properties.
ASTRINGENTS: Squaw vine will be most beneficial when combined with other astringents.
DIURETICS: Squaw vine will be very useful in combination with these agents, especially where there are accompanying uterine problems.
TONICS: Squaw vine has excellent tonic virtues, with an especial affinity for the reproductive area.

HEALTH NOTE: *Do not remove tonsils.*
Many medical practitioners believe that they can improve on the creation of God by removing what they deem as "useless" or "harmful" organs. Tonsils should NEVER be removed, rather, the body should be cleansed of the toxins which are creating the problem. The tonsils are very vital to the body, as is any other organ. They are the last refinery that guards the reproductive system from toxic wastes in the body. Removing the tonsils will lessen fertility, and the likelihood of trouble in the prostate glands and ovaries, etc. is greatly increased.

Growth characteristics:
Perennial; found in most of North America to the Rocky Mountains; grows in

swampy places and dry woods (usually in the latter); flowers April-June, and sometimes in autumn; leaves remain green throughout the winter. Blachan observes that squaw vine is usually found "spread at the foot of forest trees," but when "transplanted to the home garden in closely packed, generous clumps, with plenty of leaf mold, or, better still, chopped sphagnum, about them, they soon spread into thick mats in the rocky, the hardy fernery, or about the roots of rhododendrons, the taller shrubs that permit some sunlight to reach them. No woodland creeper rewards our care with greater luxuriance of growth."

Collection:
Squaw vine is best used fresh, but it may be dried.

Sister plants:
Black haw or Stagbush or Sweet viburnum or American Sloe (Viburnum prunifolium; RUBIACEAE); see page 433.

Allied plants:
Prince's pine or Pipsissewa (Chimaphila umbellata; PYROLACEAE)

TANSY or BITTER BUTTONS
(Tanacetum vulgare; COMPOSITAE)

Tansy has a number of compatible properties that makes it a valuable agent for various female complaints. It is one of the best remedies for menstrual problems. Refer to page 134.

EUROPEAN PENNYROYAL or PUDDING GRASS
(Mentha pulegium; LABIATAE)

Common names:
European pennyroyal, pudding grass, pennyroyal, run-by-the-ground, lurk-in-the-ditch, piliole-rial.

Identifying characteristics:
There are two varieties—*decumbens* and *erecta*.

Stem — Decumbens: weak, prostrate, bluntly quadrangular, 3-12 inches long, readily take root at lower joints or nodes.
Erecta: stiffly erect or sub-erect, bluntly quadrangular, 8-12 inches high, much branched.

Leaves — Opposite, oval (egg-shaped), 1-1½ inches long, 1/2 inch broad, faintly serrate, grayish-green, shortly stalked, deep green, nearly smooth, more or less hairy on both sides, stand out stiffly at right angles to

	stem.
Flowers	Pale or lilac blue to reddish-purple, whorled maxillary clusters of 10-12, rising as tiers one above the other at each node, tubular calyx, bi-labiate, 4-lobed corolla.
Fruit	Seed, light brown, oval, very small.
Root	Horizontal, creeping underground (in masses as with other mints), fibrous.
Taste	Characteristic, mint-like.
Odor	Pungent, mint-like.

Part used:
Herb, oil.

Therapeutic action:
Emmenagogue, tonic, diaphoretic, stimulant, carminative, anthelmintic, depurant, detergent, vulnerary, antivenomous, antispasmodic, sedative, condiment.

Pennyroyal is a very reliable and effective emmenagogue, especially for retarded or obstructed menstruation due to a sudden chill or cold. Dr. Nowell claimed that pennyroyal, taken warm with a vapor bath, is almost a specific cure. Pennyroyal has an agreeable and warming influence on the stomach, excellent for feverish conditions, bronchial congestion, eruptive diseases (measles, smallpox, etc.). It is soothing and relaxing to conditions with spasms, nervousness, and crossness. It is antivenomous and has been reputed to purify water. For some, pennyroyal can cause irritation in the genitourinary tract and may possibly cause reflex uterine movements. This is why **pennyroyal should not be used during pregnancy**. Prepared in apple cider vinegar, it is excellent to treat wounds and to cleanse the skin, even in such vile conditions as leprosy. The oil of pennyroyal is a first-rate protection against insect bites from mosquitoes, gnats, and other pests.

Medicinal uses:
Amenorrhea, menorrhagia, nausea, colds, pneumonia, flu, fever, flatulence, spasms, colic pains, nervousness, hysteria, disordered stomach, measles, pulmonary congestion, dizziness, ulcers, bruises, black-eye, whooping cough, leprosy, insect and snake bites, tuberculosis, headache, griping, etc.

Preparations:
Fluid extract, infusion, oil, powder, tincture. Due to its rich volatile oil (on which much of its medicinal effectiveness depends), pennyroyal should never be boiled, and care should be taken to cover the infusion.

Dosage:
Do not take during pregnancy; taken best in smaller and repeated doses.

Fluid extract	1/4-1 fluid teaspoon.
Infusion	2 fluid ounces to 1 teacupful 3 to 4 times daily.
Oil	1-3 drops.

Powder	1-4 grams.
Tincture	1/4-1 fluid teaspoon.

ADMINISTRATION

Oral

Menstrual problems, spasms, hysteria, flatulence, colic, chills, nausea, nervousness, feverish colds, disordered stomach, measles, etc.: Give the infusion in teacupful (6 fluid ounce) doses, repeated frequently (every 1 to 2 hours); when the herb is unavailable, 1-3 drops of the oil in warm water is excellent.

Infant sniffles: Give 1 teaspoonful or less of the infusion 3 times daily, nursing mother drink 2 fluid ounces 3 times daily.

Venomous bites, stings, etc.: Drink the infusion made from an alcohol tincture, and apply the tincture on the wound. A poultice of the freshly bruised herb is also highly recommended.

Bruises, foul ulcers, black eye, facial burns, skin problems, leprosy, etc.: Make an apple cider vinegar tincture with the freshly bruised herb; apply as a fomentation externally and drink internally.

Colds, pneumonia, flu: See "FORMULAS."

Whooping cough: Drink 1 teaspoonful to 1 tablespoonful of the fresh, sweetened juice.

Skin

Bruises, foul ulcers, facial burns, etc.: See above.

Fainting, dizziness: Apply the tincture preparation with apple cider vinegar to the nostrils.

Mosquitoes, gnats, fleas, etc.: Freely apply the oil, diluted with olive oil; it makes a first-rate insect repellent.

FORMULAS

Croup

1 ounce	Pennyroyal herb (Mentha pulegium; Hedeoma pulegioides)
2 teaspoons	Lobelia, Acid tincture (Lobelia inflata) (see page 400)

Preparation: Infuse the pennyroyal in 3/4 pint of boiling hot water for 10 minutes; be sure to cover tightly. You may use it sooner when necessary. Cool sufficiently so that the liquid will not burn the patient; add the acid tincture of lobelia (see page 400), sweeten.

Dosage: 2 fluid ounces every 1/2 hour until relief is obtained, then less often and regulated to the needs of the patient.

Administration: Croup is inflammation of the larynx and windpipe accompanied by spasmodic cough and great difficulty in breathing; a loose membrane forms in the windpipe or trachea which can choke the patient, and the attacks are often sudden, with a harsh cough, rapid pulse, impeded breathing, and the face may be flushed with fever. It is caused by wet feet, damp clothes, sudden changes in temperature, etc. where the vitality of the system is greatly lowered and results in inflammatory congestion and obstruction. Raise the body heat, relax the spasms, and stimulate the blood through the parts as rapidly as possible. Use a hot mustard and cayenne foot bath (in a vessel deep enough to get the water up part of the legs), and hot flannel fomentation of cayenne (1 teaspoonful in 2 quarts of water).

Amenorrhea (suppressed menstruation)

1 part Pennyroyal herb (Mentha pulegium; Hedeoma pulegioides)
1 part Motherwort herb (Leonurus cardiaca)
1 part Blue cohosh root (Caulophyllum thalictroides)
1 part Life root or golden ragwort root (Senecio aureus)
1 part Thyme herb (Thymus vulgaris)

Preparation: Infuse 1 cup of boiling water over 1 teaspoonful of herbs.

Dosage: 1/2 cup each 2 hours.

Colds, pneumonia, flu

1 part Pennyroyal herb (Mentha pulegium, Hedeoma pulegioides)
1 part Elder flowers (Sambucus canadensis, S. nigra)

Preparation: 1 teaspoonful to the cup of boiling water; infuse and cover tightly till cool enough to drink.

Dosage: One pint to the dose; keep patient well covered in bed. Repeat until sweating profusely.

CASE HISTORY

Powerful body revitalization.
Dr. Christopher emphasized the importance of strengthening the reproductive sys-

tem while healing the entire body. He had a case where a young lady was very afraid of marriage. She would have menstrual periods every two weeks or so and be in bed 6 to 7 days each time. She was weak, anemic, and could hardly sit up in bed. Dr. Christopher used the Lower Bowel tonic (see page 578) to clean out her bowels, put her on the Cleansing Program, the Regenerative Diet and emmenagogue herbs, and within just six weeks she was feeling wonderful and looking beautiful. She gained weight, took on the glow of health, and was the happiest person in the world. Not long after this, she married and later entered motherhood normally with a healthy baby. These herbs have great power in bringing order and strength to the generative system for new life in both the mother (or father) and the prospective child (embryo).

Growth characteristics:
Perennial; indigenous to Great Britain and Europe, naturalized to a large part of the civilized world and frequently found in herbal gardens in times past; grows best in strong and moist soils on the borders of ponds and streams (the *decumbent* variety does well in moist clay soil and in partial shade); in warmer climates it makes a useful ground cover and where it is subject to winter kill it may be taken indoors *(decumbent variety)* as a trailing house plant; it is easily grown by seed, but the common propagation is by root division in the fall or spring, and more rarely by cuttings; in planting space 5-6 inches apart; flowers July-August. The *erect* variety of European pennyroyal has pale or lilac blue flowers and the *decumbent* variety has more purplish ones; annual; grows best in dry, sandy, and open places in full sunlight and is very fragrant.

Sister plants:
-American Pennyroyal or Squaw Mint (Hedeoma pulegioides; LABIATAE); herb; **do not use during pregnancy;** similar therapeutic properties to European pennyroyal (both are referred to as simply "pennyroyal"), flatulence, colic, indigestion, diarrhea, bronchitis rheumatism, amenorrhea, corrective for overuse of purgatives, fevers, colds, consumption, leprosy, toothache, jaundice, dropsy, cramps, convulsions, headache, ulcers, mouth sores, snake and insect bites, itch, griping, nausea, bruises, black eye, wounds, nervousness, hysteria, skin diseases.
-(Hedeoma piperita; LABIATAE); herb; grows in Mexico and is used much the same as peppermint.
-(Hedeoma thymoides; LABIATAE); herb; grows in Texas, has a more agreeable odor.
-Horsemint (Monarda punctata; LABIATAE); herb (leaves, tops): flatulence, colic, nausea, rheumatism, neuralgia, diarrhea, nervousness, fevers, renal problems, menstrual difficulties, etc.; annual; stem, downy, 2-3 feet high, branched; leaves, opposite, lanceolate, serrate, punctuate (dotted with minute spots), about 2 inches long, nearly smooth, stalked; flowers: yellow and spotted red with pinkish bracts (which are sessile), maxillary tufts, downy and tubular, 5-toothed calyx, bi-labiate corolla; pungent and bitterish taste, aromatic odor similar to thyme.

BLESSED THISTLE or HOLY THISTLE
(Cnicus benedictus; Carduus sanctus; C. benedictus; Carbenia benedicta; Centaurea benedicta; COMPOSITAE)

In ages past, it has had a high reputation as a "hal'al," a heal-all. It should be taken in repeated doses of 2 fluid ounces so as to avoid the emetic action of large doses. Taken cold, it is a tonic; taken warm, it is diaphoretic and emmenagogue. It is wonderful for increasing milk production in nursing mothers. It may be eaten fresh like watercress, juice or herb; and there are a number of other thistles that have been used as substitutes. This is a valuable herb in this category. See page 497.

FALSE UNICORN or HELONIAS
(Chamaelirium luteum (Gray); Helonias dioica (Pursh.); H. lutea (Ait.); C. Carolinianum (Willd.); Veratrum luteum (Linn.); LILIACEAE)

False unicorn root is one of our very best stimulative tonics to the reproductive organs, a valuable corrective for all types of female disorders (as well as male) in the genitourinary area. This herb is turned to time and again to prevent miscarriage. It is helpful with impotence, kidney and liver problems, etc. See page 512.

CRAMP BARK or HIGH CRANBERRY
(Viburnum trilobum; V. Opulus var. americanum; CAPRIFOLIACEAE)

Cramp bark is possibly the best female regulator-relaxant agent that we have for the uterus and ovaries, and is especially useful for painful and difficult menstruation and for nervous affections that threaten abortion during pregnancy. See page 430.

TRUE UNICORN ROOT or STAR GRASS or COLIC ROOT
(Aletris farinosa; LILIACEAE)

Common names:
True unicorn root, star grass, colic root, blazing star, starwort, ague root, crow corn, unicorn root, aloe root, ague grass, black root, bitter grass, bettie grass, devil's bit; Aletris Farineau (Fr.); Mehlige Aletria (Ger.).

Identifying characteristics:
Stem — None (only flower stem).
Leaves — Radical, star-shaped, sessile (lying flat on the ground), lanceolate,

	acute, 3-4 inches long, 1 inch broad, ribbed, smooth and flat, pale colored, thin, coriaceous (tough and leather-like), slightly sheathing at base.
Flowers	Bell-shaped, oblong, white, indumentum on outer surface (a dense woolly pubescence giving a dusted mealy appearance—*farinose);* each plant sends up a simple (with remote scales), erect flower stem 1-3 feet high, that is topped with a spiked raceme bearing the short-stalked flowers.
Fruit	Triangular (ovate, tapering), and coriaceous capsule, enclosed in a persistent envelope, contains numerous ovate, ribbed, albuminous, fleshy, and oily seeds.
Rhizome	Grayish-brown, flattish on upper surface and densely covered with the tufted remains of leaf-bases and circular stem-scars, convex, 4/5-1 inches long, 1/5-2/5 inch thick, indistinctly jointed, short and mealy fracture (white, light brown or yellow, and slightly fibrous), twisted fibro-vascular bundles; rootlets; numerous, tough, wiry, flexuous, glossy black, about 3 inches long, on sides and beneath, brownish when first dried. Powder: Yellowish-brown.
Taste	Peculiar, sweetish, bitter (intensely bitter at first, but losing a great part of the nauseous bitterness with age).
Odor	Very faint, acetous.

Parts used:
Dried rhizome and rootlets (the fresh article is emetocathartic and somewhat narcotic, which properties are largely lost with drying).

Therapeutic action:
Tonic, stimulant, emmenagogue, stomachic, diuretic, carminative, sialogogue, antirheumatic, emetocathartic (large doses).

True unicorn root is a very valuable tonic for the female regenerative organs. It is also a good general tonic, especially effective for cases of habitual miscarriage due to chronic weakness. It may be safely used during the entire period of pregnancy. Due to its powerful uterine stimulative properties, it has proved valuable in cases of sterility and impotence, sometimes achieving healing results within a few weeks; but the more difficult cases must be given for a few months. As it increases the possibility of conception, it should be avoided where frequent pregnancy is undesirable. True unicorn root is soothing to the gastric area, especially useful where the stomach is upset in pregnancy. It resembles false unicorn.

Medicinal uses:
Dysmenorrhea, menorrhagia, chronic uterine weakness, general debility, sterility, impotence, nausea, chronic rheumatism, dropsy, colic, flatulence, habitual miscarriage, hysteria, dyspepsia, stomach derangements.

Preparations:
Decoction, fluid extract, powder, tincture. Use the dried root only.

Dosage:
Give in small doses, as large ones will produce nausea.

Decoction	1/2-2 fluid ounces 3 to 4 times daily.
Fluid extract	1/2 fluid teaspoon (30 drops).
Powder	650 milligrams.
Tincture	5-15 drops.

ADMINISTRATION

Give in small and repeated doses.

Oral

Sterility, impotence: Give the decoction over an extended period of time, a few weeks to several months.

Chronic uterine weakness, debility: See "FORMULAS."

Dysmenorrhea, menorrhagia, etc.: Give the dosages as indicated 3 to 4 times daily.

FORMULAS

Dr. Nowell's female corrective powder

1 ounce	True unicorn root (Aletris farinosa)
2 ounces	White poplar, quaking aspen inner bark (Populus tremuloides)
1 ounce	Golden seal root (Hydrastis Canadensis)
1/2 ounce	Black cohosh root (Cimicifuga racemosa)
1/2 ounce	Cinnamon bark (Cinnamomum zeylanicum; C. Loureirii)
1/2 ounce	Jamaica ginger root (Zingiber officinalis)
1/2 teaspoon	Cayenne (Capsicum frutescens; C. minimum)
8 ounces	Sugar (powdered loaf or yellow D)

Preparation: Mix the herbs well together; use 1 teaspoonful to each 2-6 fluid ounces of boiling hot water, cover and steep 10 to 15 minutes; or place in #00 capsules.

Dosage: 2 fluid ounces 4 times daily; or 1 #00 capsule 4 times daily.

Note: This is a good tonic compound, especially for debility and irregular menstrual periods, and it is also useful for loss of appetite, weakness, and irregularities in the menstrual flow.

Female tonic

1 part True unicorn root (Aletris farinosa)
1 part Squaw vine herb (Mitchella repens)

Preparation: 1 teaspoonful of combined herbs to the cup of boiling water; infuse, strain after 20 minutes.

Dosage: 1/2 cup 3 to 6 times in a day.

Female tonic

1/4 ounce True unicorn root (Aletris farinosa)
1/4 ounce Cramp or black haw bark (Viburnum trilobum; V. prunifolium)
1 ounce Squaw vine herb (Mitchella repens)
1/4 ounce Wild yam root (Dioscorea villosa)

Preparation: Simmer the herbs for 20 minutes in 1 quart of water; strain, sweeten to taste; allow to cool, bottle and keep in a cool place.

Dosage: 2-3 tablespoonfuls 3 times daily.

Leucorrhea (whites)

1 ounce True unicorn root (Aletris farinosa) or preferably False unicorn root, blazing star, or helonias (Chamaelirium luteum)
1 ounce White poplar or quaking aspen inner bark (Populus tremuloides)
1 ounce Bethroot, birthroot or wake robin (Trillium erectum; T. pendulum)
3/4 ounce Squaw vine herb (Mitchella repens)
3/4 ounce Cramp bark (Viburnum trilobum; V. opulus)
1/2 ounce Sacred bark (Rhamnus purshiana)
1/2 ounce Pimento or allspice berries (Pimento officinalis)
1/4 ounce Blue cohosh root (Caulophyllum thalictroides)

Preparation: Simmer the herbs for 10 minutes in 1 quart of water; sweeten to taste, add 2 tablespoonfuls glycerine, allow to cool, bottle, and keep in a cool place.

Dosage: 1 tablespoon before each meal and at bedtime.

Menopause (change of life)

1 part True unicorn root (Aletris farinosa)
1 part Lady slipper or nerve root (Cypripedium calceolus var. pubescent)
1 part Black cohosh root (Cimicifuga racemosa)

Preparation: Simmer 1 teaspoonful to the cup of water 5-10 minutes slowly. Steep 15 minutes and strain.

Dosage: 1/2-1 cup three times a day.

Growth characteristics:
Perennial; indigenous to the United States from Florida northward; grows in low grounds at the edges of wet sandy woods (especially near the seashore); flowers May-August.

Allied plants:
False Unicorn root, blazing star, or Helonias (Chamaelirium luteum; LILIACEAE) see page 512. These two herbs have certain similar tonic and emmenagogue characteristics, but there are other differences and generally we consider false unicorn root to be the superior emmenagogue.

BLUE COHOSH or PAPOOSE ROOT or SQUAW ROOT
(Caulophyllum thalictroides (Michx.); Leontice thalictroides (Linn.); BERBERIDACEAE)

Common names:
Blue cohosh, papoose root, squaw root, blueberry root, women's best friend, blue ginseng, yellow ginseng.

Identifying characteristics:

Stem	Round, smooth, glaucous (waxy with frosty appearance), 1-3 feet high, purple when young.
Leaves	Large, biternately or triternately (at summit) compounded, smooth, glaucous; leaflets-oval, 2-3 inches long, 3-5 lobed, pale beneath, petiolate.
Flowers	Small, greenish-yellow, on a panicle.
Fruit	Dry and nauseous berries; 1-2 seeds the size of a large pea.
Rhizome	Horizontal, brownish-or yellowish-gray, 3-10 inches long, 1/5-3/5 inch thick, crowded with numerous cup-shaped stem-scars above, curved, tortuous (twisting), knotty with short branches, then, tough, internally whitish to yellow, narrow woody rays, central pith running longitudinally, tough, and woody fracture; rootlets: pale brown or yellowish-gray, tough, tangled or matted below and often concealing the rhizome, about 1/25 inch thick and up to 8 inches long. Powder: light brown.
Taste	Sweetish, then bitter, acrid and pungent.
Odor	Slightly fragrant, sternutatory.

Parts used:
Rhizome and roots.

Therapeutic action:
Stimulant (diffusive, relaxant), nervine (sedative), antispasmodic, parturient, emmenagogue, tonic, diaphoretic (sudorific), diuretic, anthelmintic, demulcent, anti-rheumatic.

Dr. Shook wrote:

> This is a very old Indian remedy. They believed it to be the best parturient in nature, and it was the habit of their women to drink the tea several weeks before labor . . . this exceedingly valuable Herb is well called 'woman's best friend' for the reason that it is much more reliable and far less dangerous in expediting delivery in those cases where labor is slow, very painful, and does not bring about natural delivery. As you well know, these distressing cases are many, and great exhaustion sometimes results from delay, through debility, fatigue, or lack of uterine nervous energy. Blue cohosh in infusion or decoction taken warm will accomplish a particularly easy parturition, if given for some hours just previous to the time.

It is an excellent nervine and antispasmodic, which makes it very useful for various pulmonary, neural, and muscular affections. Blue cohosh contains the following vital mineral elements: potassium, magnesium, sodium, phosphorus, salts of potash, calcium, iron and silicon. Many more persons, male and female, will experience healing wonders, as they use it as a single remedy or in synergistic combination with other appropriate herbs.

Medicinal uses:
Female complaints (leucorrhea, amenorrhea, spasmodic dysmenorrhea, cramps, vaginitis or vaginal inflammation, uterine subinvolution, deficient labor-pains, spasmodic after-pains, spasmodic pains in the uterus or other sympathetic organs at any time), fits, colic, spasms, hysteria, rheumatism, ague, epilepsy, worms, colds, nervous exhaustion, neuralgia, dropsy, palpitation of the heart, high blood pressure, diabetes, hiccough, whooping cough, spasmodic asthma, puerperal convulsions, nervous affections.

***Preparations*:**
Decoction, fluid extract, infusion, powder, solid extract, tincture.

Dosage:

Decoction	2-4 teaspoons (according to case) 3 to 4 times daily.
Fluid extract	10-30 drops (1/6-1/2 teaspoonful).
Infusion	2 fluid ounces 3 to 4 times daily between meals.
Powder	325 mg-2 grams.

Solid extract 325-650 milligrams.
Tincture 1/2-1 fluid teaspoon.

ADMINISTRATION

Oral

Amenorrhea (due to severe shock): Give 2 fluid ounces of the decoction in hot water, while the patient is resting completely relaxed.

Renal problems, fever (diaphoretic), worms, rheumatism, dropsy, hysteria and nervous exhaustion (due to shock or accident): Use the warm decoction.

Worms: Use the warm infusion or decoction after fasting.

Recent colds (children): Give 2 teaspoons to 1 tablespoon of the infusion in 1/2 teacupful of sweetened hot water, while closely covered in bed; if the first dose does not produce free perspiration within an hour, repeat hourly until it is produced.

Spasms: Give larger or repeated doses until relief is obtained.

Parturition: Give the infusion or decoction warm several hours previous to the time of delivery, and during delivery as needed. Midwives commonly give it to bring on contractions. If it is time to give birth, blue cohosh greatly enhances labor. If it is not yet time, it does not act. The extract or tincture is most useful in childbirth, when a woman may not feel like taking cups of tea.

Constipation, congested liver, low fever: Give the warm infusion or decoction in combination with boneset (Eupatorium perfoliatum).

Bronchial catarrh: See "FORMULAS."

FORMULAS

Decoction of blue cohosh

2 ounces Blue cohosh, cut (Caulophyllum thalictroides)
1 quart Distilled or D-cell water
3 ounces Glycerine

Preparation: Place the ingredients in an appropriate vessel and simmer for 20 minutes, strain, press the herb, sweeten to taste, allow to cool, bottle, and keep in a cool place.

Dosage: 2 teaspoons to 1 tablespoon or more, according to age, 3 to 4 times daily.

Infusion of blue cohosh

1 ounce Blue cohosh root, cut (Caulophyllum thalictroides)
1 pint Distilled or D-cell water

Preparation: Boil the water and pour over the cut root; cover and steep for 15-20 minutes; strain.

Tincture

3 ounces Blue cohosh root, powdered (Caulophyllum thalictroides)
1 pint Grain alcohol

Preparation: Macerate for 2 weeks and be sure to shake well daily; filter and place in brown bottles.

Dosage: 1/2-1 fluid teaspoon.

Bronchial catarrh

1 ounce Blue cohosh root, cut (Caulophyllum thalictroides)
1 ounce Comfrey root, cut (Symphytum officinale)
1/2 ounce Pleurisy root, cut (Asclepias tuberosa)
2 teaspoons Lobelia herb (Lobelia inflata)
1/4 ounce Ginger root (Zingiber officinalis)

Preparation: Infuse the herbs in 1 quart of boiling hot water, cover tightly and keep warm for 20 minutes; strain, sweeten to taste; allow to cool, bottle and keep in a cool place.

Dosage: 1-2 tablespoonfuls 3 to 4 times daily.

Menopause (change of life)

1 part Blue cohosh root (Caulophyllum thalictroides)
1 part Lady slipper or nerve root (Cypripedium calceolus var. pubescens)
1 part Hyssop herb (Hyssopus officinalis)
1 part Chestnut leaves (Castanea sativa; C. dentata; Fagus castanea)

Preparation: Simmer 1 teaspoon to the cup of water 5 minutes.

Dosage: 1/2 cup 3 to 6 times daily.

Growth characteristics:
Handsome perennial found in Canada and in almost all parts of the United States; grows near running streams and in low, moist and rich or swampy grounds; flow-

ers May-June; seed ripens in August (a decoction of which resembles coffee in flavor).

RUE or GARDEN RUE
(Ruta graveolens; RUTACEAE)

Common names:
Rue, garden rue, herb-of-grace, German rue, herbygrass, herb of repentance, countryman's treacle; Fue des Jardins (Fr.), Gartenraute (Ger.); Ruta (Ital.); Ruda (Span.). Note: Do not confuse this with goat's rue (Galega officinalis), for the common names can be deceiving, but this is an entirely different plant of another family.

Identifying characteristics:

Stem	Unusual and beautiful plant; woody, cylindrical, branched, 2-3 feet high, bluish shoots in spring, turning purplish or brown in winter.
Leaves	Blue-green, evergreen, lacy, alternate, bi- or tripinnate; leaflets: 1/2-1 inch long, 1/4 inch wide, crenate (round scallops), thick, pellucid-punctuate (dotted with numerous immersed, translucent, small and round oil-glands), oblanceolate, wedge-shaped below.
Flowers	Bright yellow or greenish-yellow, situated on terminal panicles, many, 1/2 inch across, 5 wavy petals (in curved at tips, situated on a disk), gland-dotted ovary.
Fruit	Capsule—4-5 lobed, numerous black seeds (all parts active).
Taste	Extremely bitter, acrid, and nauseous.
Odor	None—but when pinched or bruised, it emits a powerful and disagreeable aromatic scent.

***Parts used*:**
Herb, leaves, oil.

Therapeutic action:
Stimulant, emmenagogue, antispasmodic, antiseptic, anthelmintic (germicide), nervine (stimulant), carminative, disinfectant, anti-rheumatic, tonic, emetic, aromatic, anti-venomous, rubefacient, counter-irritant, diuretic. It is also a wonderful aid for functional inactivity of both the uterus and ovaries.

Rue is excellent in hysterical and spasmodic affections. It is beneficial as a carminative, and when taken in small doses (always give rue in small doses) it is a good stomachic, stimulant, and tonic.

A British herbalist, Mrs. Level, wrote in her book, *Elixirs of Life:*

> It is said to bestow second sight, and it certainly preserves ordinary

> sight, by strengthening the ocular muscles. It acts upon the periosteum and cartilages, and removes deposits that through age are liable to form in the tendons and joints—particularly the joints of the wrist. It cures the lameness due to sprains, aching tendons, particularly flexor tendons, and pain in the bones of the feet and ankles.

Rue should never be given during pregnancy, and when given after meals it is likely to produce emesis.

Medicinal uses:
Female complaints (amenorrhea, dysmenorrhea, uterine atony, menorrhagia), hysteria, colic, flatulence, convulsions, stomach canker, spasms, whooping cough, spasmodic croup, typhoid fever, malaria fever, nervous headache, dizziness (vertigo), hysterical spasms, palpitation of the heart, sciatica, delayed menstruation, ague, fits, rheumatism, painful joints, earache, ophthalmia, eye inflammation, coughs, epilepsy, stomach trouble, griping, nervousness, worms, insanity, gout, poison, chronic bronchitis, sprains, glandular enlargements, scaly eruptions.

Preparations:
Fluid extract, infusion, oil, powder, tincture.

Rue has a very active medicinal and volatile oil, so never boil rue (except under certain specified conditions for fomentation). Water will have much more effect extracting these medicinal virtues than alcohol.

Dosage:

Fluid extract	1/2 teaspoon.
Infusion	6 fluid ounces during the day (2 fluid ounces taken between meals but not within 1/2 hour before or following a meal); or up to 2 fluid ounces every 1 to 2 hours in extreme cases.
Oil	15 drops.
Powder	1-2 grams.
Tincture	5-20 drops.

ADMINISTRATION

Note of caution: Rue is a potent healer, but in large doses it has powerful ecbolic and abortifacient action that can be most detrimental to the health and life of the user (producing inflammation and nerve derangement), so care must be taken to use the appropriate and indicated dosage. If there is any doubt as to whether or not the delay in menstruation might be conception, avoid rue and use another safe emmenagogue. Never use rue during pregnancy.

Oral

Menstrual problems, uterine atony, etc.: Use the infusion of rue (up to 2 fluid ounces every 1 to 2 hours) in combination with any of the indicated correctives which intensify the stimulative and antispasmodic action, while greatly modifying the ecbolic tendency.

Stomach disorders, systemic debility, circulatory congestion, etc.: Take small doses of the infusion at least 1 hour before meals.

Typhoid and malarial fevers: Give in small and repeated dosages.

Nervous nightmares: Take a small quantity of freshly extracted juice.

Nervous headache, dizziness (vertigo), hysterical spasms, palpitation: Chew 1 to 2 freshly-picked leaves.

Skin

Headache: Apply the freshly-bruised leaves to the temples.

Chronic bronchitis, glandular enlargements, scaly eruptions: Apply fomentation or compresses of a strong decoction to the chest or affected area.

Sciatica, gout, rheumatism, painful joints, bruises, sprains: Apply the freshly bruised leaves, or a fomentation of the strong decoction, or the compound oil to the affected area (see "FORMULAS").

Poisonous bites, stings, plants: Apply the juice of rue to the affected part, and chew several fresh leaves or drink the infusion internally.

Earache: Warm and place several drops of compound oil into the ear.

Ophthalmia, eye inflammation: Apply the compound oil to the eye on cotton.

FORMULAS

Infusion of rue

1 ounce Rue, cut (Ruta graveolens)
1/4 pints Distilled or D-cell water

Preparation: Boil the water and pour it immediately over the herb, cover tightly and allow it to stand in a hot place for 10-15 minutes; strain, allow to cool (preferably covered), sweeten to taste, bottle and keep in a cool place.

Dosage: 6 fluid ounces during the day (2 fl. oz. taken between meals—but not within 1/2 hour before or following); or up to 2 fluid ounces every 1 to 2 hours in extreme cases.

Note: If this is very nauseous to the individual, it can be made acceptable and palatable by adding an equal quantity of infusion of marjoram (Origanum vulgare) to the above preparation.

Compound oil of rue and olive

1 part	Oil of rue (Oleum Ruta; Ruta graveolens)
10 parts	Olive oil (Oleum olivae; Olea europæa)

Preparation: Shake well together.

Dosage: 1-5 drops (internally); it also makes an excellent external application.

Stimulative antispasmodic compound

1 ounce Rue herb, cut (Ruta graveolens)
1 ounce Any one of the following:
- Wintergreen herb (Gaultheria procumbens)
- Cinnamon bark (Cinnamomum zeylanicum; C. Loureirii)
- Fennel seed (Foeniculum vulgare)
- Caraway seed (Carum carvi)
- Anise seed (Pimpinella anisum)
- Marjoram herb (Origanum vulgare)

Preparation: Same as infusion of rue (Including the same quantity of water).

Dosage: See foregoing preparation.

Congenial combinations:
Rue combines well with carminatives, which modify its ecbolic tendency and augment its stimulant and antispasmodic characteristics.

Growth characteristics:
Perennial; native of Europe, cultivated in gardens in the United States; grows best partially sheltered and dry; situated in poor, rather heavy and well-drained soil (preferably lime, chalk or clay), but it grows almost anywhere, though it is not as hardy and more subject to winter kill in rich soil. Rue is easily propagated by (1) seeds—broadcast seeds into bed, weed and care until about 2 inches high, transplant to new beds and allow eighteen inches spacing; (2) cuttings—take from young shoots in the spring, insert in a shady border until well rooted, transplant; (3) rooted slips—take in the springtime and transplant. Rue blooms June-September.

Collection:
Gather rue before the medicinal potency in the leaves and young shoots goes into

the flower (June-September).

Drying and preservation:
Take sufficient precautions to preserve the medicinally valuable volatile oil carried in the oil glands dotting the herb.

HISTORICAL USE

Rue branches have been hung in rooms as a fly repellent due to the powerful and disagreeable scent of the bruised leaves; formerly the country people of England made the rue leaves into a conserve with treacle (molasses), then fed the leaves to cattle to cure croup and other diseases. There is an old and interesting tradition that rue grows best that has been "stolen" from another garden.

MOTHERWORT or ROMAN MOTHERWORT
(Leonurus cardiaca; LABIATAE)

Common names:
Motherwort, Roman motherwort, lion's tail, throwwort, lion's ear.

Identifying characteristics:

Stem — Square (angles prominent below), erect, branching, purplish, 2-5 feet high, stout, leafy.

Leaves — Opposite, dark green, rough, downy; and, according to Grieve:

> very closely set, the radical ones on slender, long petioles, ovate, lobed and toothed, those on the stem, 2 to 3 inches long, petioled, wedge-shaped; the lower roundish, palmately five-lobed, the lobes trifid at the apex, the upper three-fid, coarsely serrate, retic ulately veined, the veinlets prominent beneath, with slender, curved hairs. The uppermost leaves and bracts are very narrow and entire, or only with a tooth on each side.

Flowers — Dull purple-pink, pale purple, or white, small clustered in thick whorls in axis of upper leaves, 6-15 flowers in a whorl, sessile, short tubular and bell-shaped calyx for 5 rigid awl-like teeth, bi-labiate corolla with upper lip slightly arched and having numerous long and woolly hairs without; the lower lip is 3-lobed, spreading and spotted; the tube has an oblique ring of hairs inside, 4 twin like stamens, with the front ones longer and reaching under the upper lip (anthers are sprinkled with hard, shining dots), style is 2-cleft at summit, rigid and bristly calyx (an important distinguishing characteristic).

Fruit — Oblong achenium.

Taste — Very bitter.

Odor — Slightly pungent (acrid, pricking).

Part used:
Herb.

Therapeutic action:
Emmenagogue, diaphoretic, tonic, nervine, antispasmodic, cardiac tonic, cathartic (aperient), hepatic, diuretic.

From *Potter's Cyclopaedia:*

> Is especially valuable in female weakness and hysteria, acting as a tonic to the generative organs and allaying nervous irritability. It promotes the flow of the menses, and generally braces up the uterine membranes. It will be found useful as a simple tonic in heart diseases or weakness and in recovery from fevers when other tonics are inadmissible. It is a useful and calming tonic that strengthens the heart, allays nervous irritability, and induces quiet and passivity of the whole nervous system. And not only is its tonic action beneficial to the heart and uterine membrane, but to the gastrointestinal tract as well.

Medicinal uses:
Nervous irritability, amenorrhea, dysmenorrhea, uterine atony, vaginitis, heart troubles (weak and nervous heart, palpitation, endocarditis, pericarditis, intermittent pulse, etc.), spasms, fits, epilepsy, chorea (St. Vitus' dance), low fevers, influenza, colds, chills, indigestion, nerve exhaustion, hysteria, delirium tremens, fainting, neuralgia, spinal disease, pulmonary congestion, liver affections, suppressed urine, cramps, convulsions, painful joints, etc.

Motherwort vies for the honor of being the best heart tonic known. It calms and supports the heart and nerves, and may be used in large doses. Motherwort is beneficial as a healing tonic in recovery from debilitating fever where other tonics are inadmissible; it is a good diaphoretic.

Preparations:
Decoction, fluid extract, infusion, powder, solid extract, syrup, tincture.

Dosage:
Larger doses may be given if desired.

Decoction	1-2 tablespoonfuls 3 to 4 times daily.
Fluid extract	1/2-1 fluid teaspoon.
Infusion	2 fluid ounces 3 to 4 times daily.
Powder	1/2-1 teaspoonful.
Solid	325 mg.-1 gram.
Syrup	1 tablespoonful 3 to 4 times daily.
Tincture	1/2-1 fluid teaspoon.

ADMINISTRATION

Oral

Gastro-intestinal indigestion: Give the tonic (see "FORMULAS") as indicated.

Delayed menstruation: Give the syrup (see "FORMULAS"), in hot water (especially near the time), and when a normal flow has been reinstated give the dosage cold (as a tonic). The infusion too is always good.

Heart troubles: Give the syrup dosage cold every 3 hours until relief has been obtained, then 3 to 4 times daily as indicated. For chronic conditions, this should be taken as a tonic for several weeks or months (it is perfectly harmless and may be taken freely).

Epileptic fits, nerve exhaustion: Follow the instruction for heart troubles.

Influenza, severe colds, low fevers: Give 2 tablespoonfuls of the syrup in 1/2 pint of very hot water (as hot as can be taken), watch for beads of perspiration to appear on the forehead within 1 hour; if they do not, repeat the dose until the patient is perspiring freely (this is a specific and effective cure).

Skin

Chest cold, cramps and pains: Foment over the affected area, and take as a warm tea internally.

Vaginal

Vaginitis: Use the infusion or decoction as a vaginal douche.

FORMULAS

Syrup of motherwort (delayed menstruation, uterine tonic, acute and chronic heart troubles, epileptic fits, nerve exhaustion, chorea or St. Vitus' dance, spasms, nervous twitching, etc.)

4 ounces	Motherwort herb, cut (Leonurus cardiaca)
1 quart	Distilled or D-cell water
2 pounds	Yellow D or raw sugar (or 1 pound of honey)

Preparation: Place the herb into the cold water and allow it to soak for 6 hours; bring the water to a boil and let it simmer for 20 minutes; strain and return the liquid to a clean vessel, stir in the sugar and simmer for 5 minutes (removing any scum that may arise); set aside and allow to cool; bottle and keep in a cool place. Note: Honey (approximately 1 pound) may be used instead of sugar without the need for simmering.

Dosage: 1 tablespoonful 3 to 4 times daily.

Compound infusion (heart tonic, etc.)

2 ounces Motherwort herb, cut (Leonurus cardiaca)
1 ounce Hawthorn berries, cut (Crataegus laevigata) or substitute any of the following:
Asparagus root or seed (Asparagus officinalis)
Bugleweed herb (Lycopus americanus)
Lily-of-the-valley herb (Convallaria majalis)
Cactus Grandiflorus or Night Blooming Cereus, fresh succulent stem (Selenicereus grandiflorus)

Preparation: Place the herbs into an appropriate vessel, pour 1½ pints of boiling hot water over them, cover tightly and steep for 15 minutes; strain, sweeten to taste, allow to cool; bottle and keep in a cool place.

Dosage: 2 fluid ounces 3 to 4 times daily.

Amenorrhea (suppressed menstruation), female weakness

4 ounces Motherwort herb (Leonurus cardiaca)
3 ounces Camomile flowers (Chamaemelum nobile; Anthemis nobilis)
2 ounces Blue cohosh root (Caulophyllum thalictroides)
1/2 ounce Golden seal root (Hydrastis Canadensis)
1/4 ounce Ginger root (Zingiber officinalis)

Preparation: Simmer 1 teaspoonful to the cup 5 minutes slowly, covered well.

Dosage: 1/4 cup 3 to 4 times a day.

Gastrointestinal tonic

1 ounce Motherwort herb (Leonurus cardiaca)
1 ounce Dandelion root (Taraxacum officinale)
1/2 ounce Golden seal root (Hydrastis Canadensis)
1/2 ounce European century herb (Erythraea centaurium)
1/4 ounce Ginger root (Zingiber officinalis)

Preparation: Simmer the herbs in 3 pints of water and reduce down to 1 quart; strain, sweeten to taste, allow to cool; bottle and keep in a cool place.

Dosage: 3 tablespoonfuls 3 to 4 times daily.

Growth characteristics:
Perennial root-stock; native of Europe, naturalized and found extensively in many parts of the United States; in fields and pastures, on banks and under hedges in a gravelly or calcareous soil (it is very hardy, and needs no special soil); blossoms in June-September. Motherwort propagates itself very readily by scattering its seeds, and the roots continue for many years.

Allied plants:
Hawthorn berry or May blossom (Crataegus laevigata; C. oxyacantha; ROSACEAE); fresh or dried haws or fruits, flowers; specific for organic and functional heart disorders (dyspnea, rapid and feeble heart action, hypertrophy, valvular insufficiency, heart oppression), sore throats, dropsy, kidney troubles; the wood used as fuel is said to make the hottest fire known (better than oak), and the root stock is excellent for grafting several garden fruits (such as pear, medlar, etc.).

LIFE ROOT or GOLDEN RAGWORT or SQUAW WEED
(Senecio aureus; COMPOSITAE)

Common names:
Life root, ragwort, squaw weed, golden senecio, golden groundsel, golden ragwort, false valerian, female regulator, coughweed, cocash weed, uncum root, waw weed, uncum. Note: This herb is not to be confused with another "ragwort" (Senecio jacobaea) belonging to the same family.

Identifying characteristics:

Stem	Erect, slender, fluted or grooved, near smooth, branched, cottony, 1 to 2 feet high, sparingly clothed with small leaves.
Leaves	Radical; roundish, kidney-shaped or cordate, long petioles, up to 6 inches long, 2-3 inches broad, crenate-dentate, stem; decrease in size upward on the stem, incise (cut into as far as the mid-rib), lyrately pinnate, then pinnatifid, upper ones are sessile. Powder: dark green.
Flowers	Heads, few in number, golden yellow, loosely arranged corymb at summit, disk, 10 rays (outer ray florets slightly reflexed), 2/3-1 inch broad, white hairy pappus.
Fruit	Glabrous achene.
Rhizome	1-2 inches long (resembles arnica in size), numerous roots, herb bark, blackish surface, internally a large dark-colored pith surrounded by a ring of short white wood bundles.
Taste	Bitter, astringent, slightly acrid, pungent.
Odor	Slight, characteristically aromatic.

Parts used:
Herb, root.

Therapeutic action:
Emmenagogue, diuretic, pectoral, tonic, astringent, stimulant, vulnerary, expectorant, febrifuge, diaphoretic.

This herb is used by the American Indians. In the first stages of consumption it is often used, as its tonic properties, combined with the pectoral, have a very beneficial effect. It is very effective in regenerating the renal and urinary areas. It will also be found most useful for all types of pulmonary complaints, fevers, etc.

Medicinal uses:
Amenorrhea (suppressed menstruation), leucorrhea, dysmenorrhea, uterine atony, physical debility, consumption, tuberculosis, gravel, urinary complaints, pulmonary problems, fevers, diarrhea, etc.

Preparations:
Decoction, fluid extract, infusion, powder, solid extract, tincture.

Dosage:

Decoction	(root) 1/2-2 fluid ounces 3 to 4 times daily.
Fluid extract	1/2-1 fluid teaspoon.
Infusion	(herb) 2-6 fluid ounces 3 to 4 times daily.
Powder	1/2-1 teaspoon.
Solid extract	325-650 milligrams.
Tincture	5-40 drops.

ADMINISTRATION

Oral

Amenorrhea: Make 1/2 ounce of powder or fluid extract to 1 pint of water, and take 2 fluid ounces 4 times daily until the desired effect is obtained.

Pulmonary complaints: Use the fluid extract or tea form.

Vaginal

Leucorrhea (aggravated cases): Combine with white pond lily; use as a vaginal douche and drink in tea form.

FORMULAS

Asthmatic spasms (inhalant)

1 ounce	Life root herb or root (Senecio aureus)
1 ounce	Mouse ear or cud weed herb (Gnaphalium obtusifolium)
1 ounce	Wormwood herb (Artemisia absinthium)

Preparation: Simmer the herbs for 10 minutes in 1 quart of water, pour the whole into a vessel which can be covered with an inverted funnel.

Administration: Inhale the steam as warm as convenient for 1/2 hour 3 times daily. Take a vapor bath 2 times weekly, if the vapor bath cannot be given or when a severe attack comes on, placing the feet in hot mustard will help.

Growth characteristics:
Perennial; native of Virginia and Canada, also found in the northern and western parts of Europe; grows best on low marshy grounds or on the banks of creeks (where there is ample moisture); flowers May-June.

SOUTHERNWOOD or OLD MAN or LAD'S LOVE
(Artemisia abrotanum; COMPOSITAE)

Common names:
Southernwood, old man, lad's love, boy's love, appleringie; Garderobe (Fr.).

Identifying characteristics:

Stem	Ornamental shrub (can be trimmed to shape), branched.
Leaves	Grayish-green, bipinnatifid (feathery), hairy (covered with minute white pubescence), soft, finely-divided segments are very slender, linear, pointed.
Flowers	Inconspicuous, yellow-white, in loose panicles, terminal.
Taste	Bitterish, aromatic.
Odor	Characteristic, sweet, pungent, peculiarly lemony (said to be disagreeable and repellent to insects).

Parts used:
Herb, oil.

Therapeutic action:
Stimulant, emmenagogue, tonic, antiseptic, detergent, astringent, anthelmintic, deobstruent, aromatic, nervine, vulnerary, condiment.

Southern wood has proven to be a valuable remedy for menstrual problems, and it is effective for worms in children. It is a good stimulant tonic and possesses some nervine properties. It is extraordinary externally for easing pain, dispersing swellings, and arresting gangrenous conditions. And it has useful drawing properties for extracting splinters, thorns, etc. from the skin.

Medicinal uses:
Amenorrhea, dysmenorrhea, menorrhagia, worms, sciatica, moth and insect repellent, cramps, convulsions, ague, inflammation of eyes, old ulcers, pain,

swellings, gangrene, wounds, etc.

Preparations:
Decoction, fluid extract, infusion, oil, powder, tincture. The infusion is generally preferred to the decoction due to the medicinally valuable volatile oil.

Dosage:

Decoction	1 tablespoonful.
Fluid extract	1/2-1 fluid teaspoon.
Infusion	2 fluid ounces 3 to 4 times daily.
Oil	Use externally only.
Powder	1/2-2 grams.
Tincture	5-30 drops.

ADMINISTRATION

Give in smaller and repeated doses for best results.

Oral

Cramps, convulsions, sciatica: Give a warm tea of the bruised seeds.

Worms (children): Give 1 teaspoon of the powder (seed or herb) in molasses morning and evening. A strong decoction is excellent worm medicine, but it is nauseous and bitter.

Menstrual obstruction (amenorrhea, dysmenorrhea): See "FORMULAS."

Skin

Inflammation of eye: Mix the oil in a few crumbs of bread and apply to eye.

Pimples: Place the oil into heated barley meal and apply to the affected area.

Splinters, thorns, etc.: Apply the bruised herb to the affected part.

Fits of ague, fevers: Massage the oil onto the backbone.

FORMULAS

Menstrual obstruction (amenorrhea, dysmenorrhea)

1 part	Southernwood herb, bruised (Artemisia abrotanum)
1 part	Pennyroyal herb (Mentha pulegium; Hedeoma pulegioides)
1 part	Mugwort leaves (Artemisia vulgaris)

Preparation: Use 1 ounce of the combination to 1 pint of boiling hot water, cover tightly and steep for 10-15 minutes; strain, sweeten to taste, allow to cool; bottle and keep in a cool place.

Dosage: 2 fluid ounces 3 to 4 times daily.

Sciatica (fomentation)

2 ounces	Southernwood herb (Artemisia abrotanum)
2 ounces	Mugwort leaves (Artemisia vulgaris)
2 ounces	Wormwood herb (Artemisia absinthium)
1 quart	Apple cider vinegar.

Preparation: Place the herbs into the apple cider vinegar and 2 quarts of water, cover tightly and simmer for 20 minutes.

Administration: Foment the affected parts for 1 hour 2 to 3 times daily; keep warm in bed. Note: Do not add any stimulating liniment such as prickly ash or cayenne to the area, as this will be quite discomforting.

Growth characteristics:
Perennial; native of southern Europe (indigenous to Spain and Italy), and a favorite in old castle and monastery gardens of medieval Europe; it grows in average soil in full sun; it is an excellent border plant because of its upright and dense growth, and it is readily propagated by cuttings which root easily (space 5 feet apart for the mature plant).

Collection:
Gather the herb when it is in flower or in August (if it does not flower).

Drying and preservation:
Follow the same instructions as for wormwood, see page 118.

Sister plants:
-Mugwort or Felon Herb (Artemisia vulgaris; COMPOSITAE); leaves, root; menstrual obstruction (amenorrhea), inflammatory swellings, gravel, epilepsy, fevers, gout, bruises, abscesses, carbuncles, rheumatism, cramps, cold, palsy, hysteria; stem: angular, purplish, 3 feet or more high; leaves: smooth and dark green above, dense cottony hairs beneath, alternate, pinnate lobed, lanceolate, acute, sharply serrate; flowers: reddish or pale yellow oval heads with cottony rosettes arranged in long terminal panicles; it has no essential oil.
-Field Southernwood (Artemisia campestris; COMPOSITAE); herb, similar to Southernwood but less potent; common in most parts of Europe.

For alternative emmenagogue herbs which can be used when the foregoing are not available, please see Chapter 17.

CHAPTER 9

THE EXPECTORANT AND DEMULCENT HERBS

Many of the demulcents, and especially the expectorants, are also anti-catarrhal, and these are particularly valuable to purify and cleanse the system. "It has often been said," wrote Dr. Shook, "that catarrh is the greatest curse of mankind." It may be a big problem to many people, but we are not prepared to say that it is the greatest curse. In fact, it may be one of the greatest blessings, for the annoyance it causes calls our attention to the need to cleanse our body. Catarrh is nature's warning signal that a thorough cleansing is needed.

Excess mucus in the body often results from partial decomposition of blood plasma, due to a nutritional shortage of potassium chloride, the element that enables fibrin to remain in solution in the blood. Dr. Shook explains further:

> In all inflammatory processes, there is an exudation or sweating out of fibrin from the blood into the surrounding tissue. This exuded fibrin becomes non-functional and insoluble. No new fibrin can be formed without the aid of potassium chloride. When the exudation of fibrin is from the mucous membrane, it is called catarrh. Advanced stages of fibrinous exudation in different organs and tissues is variously named cystitis, cysts, adhesions, etc. When the exudation of fibrin is excessive, the chemical balance of the blood is upset, and nature calls for potassium and chlorine. If potassium chloride is not available, the body will take these two elements from any other compound containing them, such as potassium phosphate (thus robbing the nerves) or calcium chloride (which robs the heart muscle) and so on and on until a whole series of unbalanced conditions are created which are given fancy names and made profoundly mysterious, because we consume so much sodium chloride and so little potassium chloride. Nature provides an abundance of potash and chlorine in food and herbs.

Dr. Shook includes the following herbs as sources for potassium chloride: bladder wrack, Irish moss, greater celandine, elecampane, gravel root, wild yam, couchgrass, stinging nettle, pleurisy root, gum plant, wild cherry bark, apple (fruit, bark, apple cider vinegar), etc.

The anticatarrhal herbs contain a good deal of potassium chloride, which enables the fibrin to become soluble again, restoring the balance to the blood, and thereby eliminating further exudations. There are over 100 botanicals that facilitate expectoration of mucus (expectorants), and the same number that possess soothing, mucilaginous and inflammation-relieving properties (demulcents). These two classes are considered together because so often both properties are possessed by the same herb.

The right herb for your particular problem.
We often fall into the pattern of only using a certain herb for a particular complaint. We want to use it on everybody—just as penicillin and sulfa drugs were prescribed by medical doctors as the "cure-all" for everyone and for everything. This does not always work, even with our greatest herbs, because people are different. Knowing the properties of herbs is not sufficient for the work of natural healing; we must also seek inspiration to select the right remedy for a particular problem.

Expectorants act upon the broncho-pulmonary membrane, altering the quality and increasing the quantity of its secretions and facilitating discharge of the fluid or semi-fluid mucus from the trachea or lungs or bronchi, through coughing and spitting. These may be further classified as *nauseating expectorants* and *stimulant expectorants*. Nauseating expectorants act mechanically when given in large doses, expelling mucus in the act of vomiting. When given in small doses, they increase osmosis from the inflamed mucous membrane. Stimulant expectorants largely eliminate through the bronchial mucous membrane, which they stimulate (diminishing the secretion and increasing the blood-pressure) while facilitating expectoration.

Demulcents soothe, soften and allay irritation of mucous membranes. These have slippery, mucilaginous or oleaginous properties which, in solution, will coat, shield, lubricate and soothe the inflamed, abraded mucous membrane surfaces, or other tissues, from irritating substances. They protect against irritation if there should be some harmful substance on the mucous membranes, relieve the pain from inflammations, and provide nourishment for healing to take place.

These herbs are suitable carriers, used to suspend other insoluble herbs in mixtures or emulsions so that they can be taken orally. The term "demulcent" generally refers to agents employed internally for the mucous membranes, and the term "emollient" refers to similar agents used externally on the skin. Most demulcents are emollient when applied externally, and in poultices they retain warmth and moisture, while absorbing pus from sores, boils, abscesses, etc. through the skin.

COMFREY
(Symphytum officinale; BORAGINACEAE)

Common names:
Comfrey, knitbone, healing herb, bruisewort, consound, blackwort, wallwort, gum plant, black root, slippery root, nipbone, knitback; yalluc (Saxon); Schwarzwurz (Ger.); consuelda, sinfito (Span.).

Identifying characteristics:

Stem	Very hairy, 2-3 feet high, freely branched at the joints, rough, angular, and hollowed.
Leaves	Ovate to lanceolate, upper leaves are smaller, fewer and hug the stem, the lower leaves are very large, and many are on long petioles (the ones lying on the ground are so hairy and prickly that they will cause any tender part of the hands, face and body to itch when touched), green, with wavy margins.
Flowers	Pale whitish or pale purple, terminal to the many branches, somewhat long and hollow like the finger of a glove.
Seed	Small, and black.
Root	Spindle-shaped, thick and brownish-black bark, gray and horny wood, branched and penetrates deeply into the earth, deeply wrinkled, short fracture, short wood bundles and broad medullary rays.
Taste	Sweetish, mucilaginous, and faintly astringent.
Odor	None.

Part used:
Root (externally) and leaves.

Therapeutic action:
Demulcent, cell proliferant, pectoral, astringent, nutritive, tonic, expectorant, hemostatic, alterative, vulnerary, mucilage, and styptic.

Dr. Shook wrote the following on comfrey:

> It does not seem to matter much which part of the body is broken, either internally or externally; comfrey will heal it quickly. It is a great cell proliferant or new cell grower, it grows new flesh and bone alike, stops hemorrhage, and is wonderful for coughs, soothing and healing the inflamed tissues in a most remarkable manner.

Comfrey is one of the finest healers for the respiratory system, especially in hemorrhage of the lungs; it has saved thousands of lives. The root has been used as both a tonic and a vulnerary from very ancient times up to the present. The root and young leaves contain a toxic alkaloid which, according to some modern research, may cause liver damage if taken in large amounts (more than the liver can process and eliminate). If the liver is congested or weak, it is better to use the mature leaf for internal use, avoiding the root and young leaf if possible. Generally, very large amounts are required to produce any harmful effect, so just be wise in your use of the root and young leaves.

The root and young leaves are most beneficial as a poultice in healing any obstinate or ulcerous wound. Comfrey is an ingredient in many herbal preparations, and it may be given wherever a mucilaginous or demulcent medicine is required. The chief healing element in comfrey is allantoin, a cell proliferant which promotes the granulation and formation of epithelial cells.

Medicinal uses:
Cough, ulcerated and inflamed lung conditions, bronchitis, hemorrhage, asthma (excessive expectoration), tuberculosis, pleurisy, pneumonia, inflamed stomach or bowels, ulcerated kidneys, gravel, bloody urine, diarrhea, dysentery, bruises, sprains, swellings, fractures, cancer, torn ligaments, ruptures, broken bones, cuts, gout, gangrene, heart problems, ulcerous wounds, hemoptysis, catarrh, scrofula, anemia, leukorrhea, female debility, boils, gum boils, sinusitis, burns, and insect bites.

Preparations:
Decoction, fluid extract, infusion, powder, and tincture. The comfrey root contains a large amount of mucilage that is best extracted by water.

Decoction: (root) Put 1/2-1 ounce of the root in 1 quart of water. For bowel problems, use milk, which has a glue-like action in attaching the herb to the inflamed membranes.

Dosage:

Decoction	2 fluid ounces 3 times daily.
Fluid extract	1/2-2 teaspoonfuls.
Infusion	1 cupful, 3 times daily.
Mucilage	See "FORMULAS."
Powder	2 #00 capsules or 1 teaspoonful.
Tincture	1/2-1 teaspoonful (fluid teaspoon).

ADMINISTRATION

Comfrey may be used in all combinations of fomenting.

Oral

Diarrhea, dysentery, and cough (delicate children): Give the mucilage sweetened with honey in teaspoonful doses frequently; it strengthens, nourishes, soothes and heals.

Inflamed kidneys: Combine comfrey root with gravel root (Eupatorium purpureum) in a decoction.

Hemorrhage of the lungs: Give the mucilage of comfrey often, in large doses (give 6-8 ounces of the decoction or mucilage 1 mouthful at a time, mixing well with saliva). Rest 1 hour, then repeat until all soreness is gone and there is no blood in the sputum. If the patient sleeps, awaken and continue with the same dosage for two hours and administer every three hours thereafter. Do not give food for at least twelve hours.

Tuberculosis or consumption: Combine comfrey with garlic, 1 tablespoon of fresh garlic juice to every pint of mucilage of comfrey, and stir well. This is the best remedy ever discovered for this problem, according to Dr. Shook.

Ulcerated stomach, intestines, larynx, mouth, tonsils, etc.: Combine comfrey with burdock root (Arctium lappa).

Scrofula, anemia, dysentery, diarrhea, leukorrhea, female debility, internal pains and bruises: Give a tea of comfrey decoction or infusion.

Skin

Inflammation, bruises, sprains, swellings, suppuration of boils: Apply a fomentation made from the comfrey root or leaves.

Wounds, bruises, burns, varicose veins, ulcers, boils, etc.: Paint the part with pure olive oil to prevent sticking, then saturate a thick layer of cotton with comfrey mucilage and apply to the affected parts. Cover with plastic or waxed paper, bandage, and leave on until nearly dry. Make a fresh application by following the same procedure. If pus is present, paint the part with oil of garlic instead of olive oil and take 1 teaspoonful of the oil internally. This will prevent or stop putrefaction and pus formation. Use fomentation wrung out of a strong decoction.

Ruptures, burns, bruises, sores, ulcers, white swellings, fresh wounds, sore breasts, fractures, sprains, etc.: Apply a comfrey poultice of the fresh, bruised leaves. It relieves pain in an hour.

Boils: A comfrey fomentation or fresh poultice is much better than cutting and draining. The fomentation will draw and drain the boil.

Skin lotion: Juice or decoction mixed in equal parts with glycerine is an excellent skin lotion and beauty aid to tone, soften, and rejuvenate.

FORMULAS

Mucilage of comfrey root

2 ounces	Comfrey root, cut (Symphytum officinale)
1 quart	Distilled or d-cell water
6 ounces	Honey
2 ounces	Glycerine

Preparation: Soak the root in water for 12 hours. Bring to a boil, cover and simmer for 30 minutes. Strain, then filter and squeeze through muslin or linen cloth. Return liquid to the clean pot, add the honey and glycerine, simmer for 5 minutes and set aside to cool. Place in a wide-mouthed bottle and keep in a cool place.

Dosage: Coughs, raw or sore throat, slight hemorrhage: 2 fluid ounces every hour until tissues are healed and coughing stops. Hemorrhage of the lungs: see "ADMINISTRATION." Note: Do not give food for at least 12 hours during this treatment so that the mucilage will reach the blood and lungs without interference and loss of energy; it is very nutritive itself.

Lung tonic

1/2 ounce	Comfrey root (Symphytum officinale)
1/2 ounce	Horehound (Marrubium vulgare)
1/2 ounce	Elecampane root (Inula helenium)
1/2 ounce	Ground ivy (Glechoma hederacea)
1/2 ounce	Ginger root (Zingiber officinalis)
1/2 ounce	Cayenne (Capsicum frutescens; C. minimum)
2 teaspoons	Nutmeg (Myristica fragrans)

1½ pounds Yellow D sugar (or 1/2 pound of honey)

Preparation: Simmer the first 4 herbs slowly in 3 pints of water for 20 minutes. Add the nutmeg, cover and simmer 4 minutes longer. Strain over the ginger and cayenne and add the sugar while hot. Allow to cool and bottle.
Dosage: 1-2 tablespoons every 2 hours.

Nervine cough syrup

1 ounce	Comfrey root (Symphytum officinale)
1 ounce	Turkey rhubarb (Rheum palmatum)
1 ounce	Spikenard (Aralia racemosa)
1 ounce	Skunk cabbage (Symplocarpus foetidus)
1 ounce	Horehound (Marrubium vulgare)
2 pounds	Yellow D sugar (honey may be substituted to taste)

Preparation: Boil the herbs slowly in 5 pints of water for 30 minutes; add the sugar or honey while hot (and for preserving for any length of time, add 1 ounce of grain alcohol or glycerine).

Dosage: 2 teaspoons, 3 to 4 times daily.

Tuberculosis or consumption remedy

1 pint	Mucilage of comfrey (Symphytum officinale)
1 tablespoon	Garlic, fresh juice (Allium sativum)

Preparation: Stir well or shake together.

Dosage: 2-6 fluid ounces, every 4 hours.

Anemia

1 ounce	Comfrey root (Symphytum officinale)
1 tablespoon	Garlic, fresh juice (Allium sativum)

Preparation: Simmer the mixture slowly for 20 minutes in 1 quart of water. Strain, bottle and keep in a cool place.

Dosage: 2 fluid ounces, every 4 hours.

Asthma

1 ounce	Comfrey root (Symphytum officinale)
1 ounce	Elecampane (Inula helenium)
1 ounce	European angelica (Angelica archangelica)

1 ounce	Spikenard (Aralia racemosa)
1 ounce	Horehound (Marrubium vulgare)

Preparation: Bruise and steep the herbs in 1 pint of honey for 6-8 hours at 125° F. until the mixture is in liquid form.

Dosage: 1 tablespoonful taken every few minutes until relieved and then several times daily.

Bronchitis

1/2 ounce	Comfrey root (Symphytum officinale)
1/2 ounce	Horehound (Marrubium vulgare)
1/2 ounce	Boneset (Eupatorium perfoliatum)
1/2 ounce	Coltsfoot (Tussilago farfara)
1/4 ounce	Elecampane root (Inula helenium)
1 teaspoon	Ginger (Zingiber officinalis)
1 teaspoon	Acid tincture of Lobelia (Lobelia inflata) see page 400

Preparation: Simmer the first 5 herbs for 20 minutes in 1 quart of water, strain hot over the ginger and cover closely until cool. This can be made more palatable by adding up to 1 pound of honey to the decoction of the 5 herbs, bring to a simmer (remove scum), then pour over the ginger and cover closely. Add the acid tincture of lobelia when cool; this will help in removing mucus.

Dosage: 2 tablespoonfuls, every 2 to 3 hours.

Debility

4 ounces	Comfrey root (Symphytum officinale)
2 ounces	Elecampane (Inula helenium)
1 ounce	Horehound (Marrubium vulgare)
1/2 ounce	Bethroot (Trillium erectum, T. pendulum)

Preparation: Simmer the herbs slowly for 20 minutes in 3 quarts of water. Strain, sweeten, bottle and keep in a cool place. The mixture may be preserved with glycerine or with 1 pint of honey.

Dosage: 1 tablespoon, 3 times a day or more.

Burn paste
(burn, sprains, wounds, etc.)

3 parts	Comfrey leaves and flowers, fresh (Symphytum officinale)
1 part	Lobelia, powder (Lobelia inflata)
Sufficient	Honey and wheat germ oil (equal parts) for base

Preparation: Mix the honey and wheat germ oil in the blender, gradually adding first the comfrey, then the lobelia until reaching a paste consistency. Cover and keep cool. The paste may be preserved by adding a little glycerine but better results are obtained when freshly-made.

Administration: Apply the burn paste externally on the afflicted area. Internally drink a tea of comfrey or pineapple and comfrey.

Pleurisy

1 ounce	Comfrey root (Symphytum officinale)
1 ounce	Vervain (Verbena officinalis, V. hastata)
1 ounce	Pleurisy root (Asclepias tuberosa)
1/2 ounce	Hyssop (Hyssopus officinalis)
1 teaspoon	Cayenne (Capsicum frutescens; C. minimum)

Preparation: Boil the first 4 herbs slowly in 3 pints of water down to 1½ pints. Strain over the cayenne, set aside to cool, bottle and keep in cool place.

Dosage: 3 tablespoonfuls every 2 to 3 hours.

Administration: Give slippery elm gruel and also a strong nettle tea (Urtica dioica) freely. Relieve any constipation with a catnip (Nepeta cataria) enema.

Pneumonia

1 ounce	Comfrey root (Symphytum officinale)
1/2 ounce	Pleurisy root (Asclepias tuberosa)
1/2 ounce	Horehound (Marrubium vulgare)
1/4 teaspoon	Cayenne (Capsicum frutescens; C. minimum)

Preparation: Simmer the first 3 herbs for 20 minutes in 1 quart water. Strain the mixture over the cayenne, cover until cool, bottle and keep in a cool place.

Dosage: 2 fluid ounces, 4 times daily.

Administration: This formula may be used with a vapor bath or cayenne, elder and peppermint tea.

Sprains, swellings (fomentation)

4 ounces	Comfrey powdered root (Symphytum officinale)
2 quarts	Distilled water

Preparation: Boil slowly for 15 minutes in water, strain.

Administration: Soak a natural fiber cloth in the preparation, wring out excess to keep from dripping and apply to the area as warm as possible. Foment for 1 hour 2 to 3 times daily.

Tuberculosis or consumption with hemorrhage remedy (good for those with antipathy for garlic)

1 pint	Mucilage of comfrey (Symphytum officinale)
4 ounces	Elecampane root, cut (Inula helenium)
1 tablespoon	Garlic juice (Allium sativum)
1/2 pints	Distilled or d-cell water

Preparation: Boil the elecampane root vigorously in the water for 15 minutes. Strain, press and set aside to cool. Mix the cooled elecampane root with the comfrey mucilage and garlic juice (shake well together) and sweeten with honey.

Dosage: 1 teacupful (6 fluid ounces), 3 to 4 times daily.

General nutrient, emollient, healing formula (ulcers, cancer, syphilis, skin diseases)

1 pint	Mucilage of comfrey (Symphytum officinale)
4 ounces	Burdock root (Arctium lappa)
1 quart	Distilled or d-cell water.

Preparation: Boil the burdock root briskly for 15 minutes in the water. Strain, then simmer and reduce to 1 pint. Set aside to cool and add the comfrey mucilage. Sweeten with honey. Shake well before using.

Dosage: 2-3 fluid ounces, 3 to 4 times daily.

External application (cancer, syphilis, skin diseases, etc.)

Saturate lint or cotton with the comfrey healing formula above and apply to the affected parts. Keep moist and change often (do not allow to dry before removing).

Congenial combinations:
For ulcerated conditions (internally and externally) comfrey root in combination with burdock root (Arctium lappa) is most beneficial. For an inflamed kidney or urinary condition, comfrey in combination with gravel root (Eupatorium purpureum) will relieve the inflamed kidney or urinary condition.

Growth characteristics:
Perennial root; native of Europe and naturalized to the United States. Comfrey

grows in low grass, moist places (damp fields, ditches, river banks, waste places), and it may be cultivated in your herb garden or potted and grown indoors. It is hardy and easy to grow and flowers all summer. It grows prolifically from root cuttings and belongs in every medicinal garden.

Allied plants:
Marshmallow (Althaea officinalis; MALVACEAE) Action very similar to comfrey.

MULLEIN
(Verbascum thapsus; SCROPHULARIACEAE)

Common names:
Mullein, great mullein, white mullein, blanket herb, mullein dock, velvet dock, torches, old ladies flannel, velvet plant, woolen, bullock's lungwort, flannel flower, rag paper, candlewick plant, clown's lungwort, Aaron's rod leaf, Jupiter's staff, shepherd's club, hare's bear, pig taper, cow's lungwort, flannel leaf, wood blade, torch weed, lungwort, Jacob's staff, Peter's staff, shepherd's staff, beggar's stalk, beggar's blanket, Adam's flannel, Cuddie's lungs, feltwort, fluff weed, old man's flannel, duffle, Hag's taper; Wollkraut (Ger.); gordolobo (Span.).

Identifying characteristics:

Stem — Stout, straight, simple (unbranched), 1-4 feet high and woolly (with branched hairs).

Leaves — Large, thick, flannel-like (velvety/hairy), pale green, rough on both sides, lower ones are lanceolate-oblong and in a rosette on the ground, upper ones are alternate and strongly clasp the stem becoming recurrent, smooth and more ovate in shape, 6-8 inches long, and 2-2½ inches broad. It is distinguished from *Verbascum nigrum* and other mulleins in that the leaves narrow at the base into two wings which pass down the step. Powder: dark green.

Flowers — 5 golden-yellow rounded petals (corolla), about 1 inch across, cup-shaped, densely packed on a thick, wool spike that is 1 or more feet long, thick, tough (moist), brittle (dry), 1 pistil and 5 anther bearing stamens (3 upper ones are short and wooly).

Fruit — Capsule or pod.

Taste — Bitterish and somewhat albuminous.

Odor — Faint and rather pleasant (flowers).

Part used:
Leaves, flowers, root, and fruit.

Therapeutic action:
Demulcent, astringent, emollient, pectoral, nutritive, absorbent, diuretic, antisep-

tic, hemostatic, anodyne, narcotic, anti-asthmatic, anticatarrhal, antispasmodic, vulnerary, germicide, and anthelmintic (vermicide).

Mullein has a special affinity for the respiratory organs, valuable for all pulmonary complaints. It is the only herb known to man that has remarkable narcotic properties without being poisonous and harmful. It is a great herbal pain killer and nervous soporific, calming and quieting all inflamed and irritated nerves. In wasting disorders (such as tuberculosis or consumption), the weight steadily increases, expectoration becomes easy, cough calms, and the general condition is improved. Mullein soothes and strengthens the bowels and renal system, and is one of the most important for the glands and the serous and mucous membranes. It stops the escape of fluids from ruptured vessels, and eliminates toxins.

Medicinal uses:
Pulmonary disease, catarrhal cough, tuberculosis, hemorrhage of lungs, dysentery, diarrhea, glandular swellings, thickening of lung tissue, phthisis, asthma, hay fever, pleuritic effusion (pleurisy), cellular dropsy, synovial dropsy, scrofula, chronic abscesses, bronchitis, cramps, spasms, ear diseases, croup, dyspnea, sinusitis, sciatica, inflammatory rheumatism, toothache, open sores, pain, warts, inflamed hemorrhoids (piles), ulcers, tumors, mumps, tonsillitis, malignant sore throat, swollen joints, dysentery, diarrhea, bleeding bowels, swollen testicle or scrotum, nasal congestion or catarrh, scrofula, sprains, and mastitis (gathered breasts).

Preparations:
Decoction, fluid extract, infusion, powder, and tincture.

Dosage:

Decoction	1 tablespoonful 3 to 4 times daily (may be taken in much larger doses, but it is 4 times the strength of the infusion more astringent and anodyne).
Fluid extract	1/2-1 teaspoonful (fluid teaspoon).
Infusion	2-3 fluid ounces or more 3 to 4 times daily.
Powder	2 #00 capsules 3 times a day.
Tincture	1/2-1 teaspoonful.

ADMINISTRATION

When the disease is advanced, use the strong decoction of leaves and flowers singly, or in combination with comfrey root (Symphytum officinale) and garlic juice (Allium sativum).

Anal

Hemorrhoids: Apply mullein ointment and take the tea internally.

Inflamed piles, ulcers, etc.: Apply fomentation or wash from a hot infusion or decoction made from the leaves.

Oral

Cough, phthisis or tuberculosis, pulmonary diseases, hemorrhage, asthma, bronchitis, croup, hay fever, etc.: Drink the strong decoction of leaves and flowers, or combine with comfrey root and garlic juice.

Diarrhea, dysentery, and bleeding of the bowels: Boil 1 ounce of mullein in 1 pint of milk for a few minutes, strain and give in 1/2 cupful doses after each bowel evacuation (in this case, milk from an animal source is used like a glue to adhere the mullein to the lining of the bowel).

Glandular swellings: See "FORMULAS."

Induce sleep, relieve pain, and laxative (large doses): Drink the infusion made from the flowers.

Skin

Vermicide and parasiticide: Take 1 teaspoonful of mullein oil 3 to 4 times daily.

Appendix inflammation: Apply hot mullein leaf poultice with lobelia herb and ginger. Take lady's slipper formula internally.

Earache and inflammation of inner ear: Use warm mullein oil, 2-3 drops in the ear 2 to 3 times daily. Apple cider vinegar is also a healing agent.

Burns: Apply juice of mullein leaves mixed with apple cider vinegar.

Glandular swellings: See "FORMULAS."

Mumps: Apply a fomentation as hot as possible on the swollen glands, wrung out of a tea made from mullein leaves; also the fresh leaves soaked in apple cider vinegar may be applied.

Neuralgia, sore throat, pleurisy, pneumonia, bruises, sores, wounds, lacerations, swollen joints, torn ligaments, purulent ophthalmia, appendicitis, skin diseases: Rub mullein oil in well, or apply on saturated cotton and cover.

Bronchitis and croup cough: See "FORMULAS."

Arthritis, painful and swollen joints: Cover a small quantity of mullein with boiling hot vinegar, cover tightly and simmer for 20-30 minutes. Strain and add a little tincture of cayenne, a powerful stimulant and rubefacient, and a tincture or fluid extract of lobelia as a relaxant. Foment (cover the area with a natural fiber cloth saturated with the vinegar infusion) this on affected area.

FORMULAS

Infusion of Mullein

1 ounce	Mullein leaves, cut (Verbascum thapsus)
1/2 pint	Distilled or d-cell water

Preparation: Pour the boiling hot water over the leaves, cover and steep in a warm place for 15 minutes. Strain through muslin (to filter out the hairs), sweeten with honey to taste or add 1 ounce glycerine to preserve. Cool, bottle and keep in a cool place.

Dosage: 2-3 fluid ounces or more 3 to 4 times a day.

Strong decoction
(inflamed tissues, tuberculosis,
chronic diarrhea, dysentery, pulmonary complaints)

4 ounces	Mullein leaves and flowers (equal parts) cut (Verbascum thapsus)
3 pints	Distilled or d-cell water
4 ounces	Glycerine

Preparation: Place the herb in the water, bring to a boil and simmer slowly for 15 minutes. Strain, press, and then return the liquid to a clean pot and reduce to 1 pint. Add the glycerine while hot, allow to cool, bottle and keep cool.

Dosage: 1 tablespoon 3 to 4 times daily (may be taken in much larger doses). Children: 1 teaspoon doses. Note: This decoction is 4 times the strength of the infusion and is more astringent and anodyne.

Bronchitis, croup, cough, rheumatism, stiff joints, mumps, glandular swellings, and dropsy, (fomentation)

2 ounces	Mullein (Verbascum thapsus)
1/2 ounce	Lobelia, herb powder (Lobelia inflata)
1 teaspoonful	Cayenne (Capsicum frutescens; C. minimum)

Preparation: Simmer in 2 quarts of apple cider vinegar, closely cover for 15 minutes and then strain.

Administration: Foment as warm as is convenient over the lungs, or over the affected part.

Glandular swellings (fomentation)

1 ounce Mullein leaves (Verbascum thapsus)
1 ounce Wood Sanicle, herb (Sanicula europaea)
1/2 ounce Lobelia, herb (Lobelia inflata)

Preparation: Simmer slowly in 2 quarts of water for 15 minutes and then strain.

Administration: Foment as hot as possible for 1 hour 3 times daily.

Glandular swellings (to be given in combination with the above fomentation)

1 ounce Wood sanicle (Sanicula europaea)
1 ounce Red clover (Trifolium pratense)
1/2 ounce Sarsaparilla root (Smilax officinalis)
1/2 ounce Elder flowers (Sambucus canadensis)

Preparation: Simmer in 2 quarts of water down to 1 quart; strain.

Dosage: 2 fluid ounces (3-4 tablespoonfuls), 5 to 6 times daily.

Mullein oil (a specific cure for ear diseases)

2 ounces Mullein flowers (Verbascum thapsus) dried.
Sufficient Olive oil (Olea europaea).

Preparation: Place the mullein flowers into a jar or wide-mouthed bottle, add sufficient pure olive oil to show 1 inch of oil above the flowers, stopper and shake well. Place in a warm place or expose to the sun for 7 to 14 days, macerating or shaking well every day. Pour off and press out the oil and bottle; do not cap or cork tightly when cold, then allow to heat or else the expanding air will break the bottle. Note: If using fresh mullein flowers; after the daily maceration, replace the stopper (cap) with several layers of cheese cloth to allow moisture to escape. Secure cloth tightly with rubber band.

Dosage: 2-6 drops of the warmed oil in the ear, 2 to 3 times daily or rub on any affected part that is swollen or irritated.

Asthma

3 grams Mullein (Verbascum thapsus)
3 grams Sage (Salvia officinalis)
3 grams Plantain (Plantago major, P. lanceolate)

Preparation: Steep for 15 minutes in 1 pint of water; strain and sweeten with honey. Bottle and keep in a cool place.

Dosage: 1 tablespoonful every hour.

Colds

1 part	Mullein (Verbascum thapsus)
1 part	Boneset (Eupatorium perfoliatum)
1 part	Pennyroyal (Mentha pulegium)
1 part	Hops (Humulus lupulus)
1 part	Chestnut leaves (Castanea sativa; C. dentata)
1 part	Catnip (Nepeta cataria)
1 part	Cudweed or Mouse ear (Gnaphalium obtusifolium)
1 part	Wintergreen (Gaultheria procumbens)
1 part	Peppermint (Mentha piperita)
1 part	Bloodroot (Sanguinaria canadensis)
1 part	Coltsfoot (Tussilago farfara)

Preparation: Of the mixed herbs, use 1 teaspoonful to each cup of boiling hot water; infuse and keep in a hot place for 15 minutes. When cool use 1 tablespoonful each hour or more when needed.

Diphtheria (fomentation)

1 ounce	Mullein (Verbascum thapsus)
1 ounce	Cudweed or mouse ear (Gnaphalium obtusifolium)
1 ounce	Ragwort (Senecio jacobaea)

Preparation: Simmer for 20 minutes in 1 quart of water.

Administration: Remove the herbs and apply as a poultice as warm as possible to the throat, wrap the poultice well and leave until cold. Reheat the herbs in the liquid they were prepared in.

Diphtheria (decoction)

1/2 ounce	Mullein (Verbascum thapsus)
1/2 ounce	Raspberry leaves (Rubus idaeus)
1/2 ounce	Agrimony (Agrimonia eupatoria)
1/4 ounce	Bayberry bark (Myrica cerifera)
1/4 teaspoon	Cayenne (Capsicum frutescens; C. minimum)
1/2 ounce	Myrrh, tincture (Commiphora myrrha, var. molmol)

Preparation: Simmer the first 4 herbs slowly for 20 minutes in 1 quart of water; strain hot over the cayenne and add the myrrh tincture when cold.

Dosage: 1-2 teaspoons every hour until relieved and then 4 to 5 times daily.
Administration: See that the bowels are functioning properly (use the lower bowel tonic and, if necessary, a catnip enema). Undiluted and unsweetened lemon juice is excellent for all types of sore throats, or fresh pineapple juice may be given freely.

Potter's emollient

1 part Mullein flowers (Verbascum thapsus)
1 part Marshmallow flowers (Althaea officinale)
1 part Mallow flowers, high (Malva sylvestris) or low (M. rotundifolia)
1 part Pellitory-of-the-wall (Parietaria officinalis)

Preparation: Infuse the herbs for 15 minutes in a proportionate quantity of water and keep well-covered; strain.

Dosage: 1 tablespoon per hour, more or less as needed.

Mumps (poultice)

2 ounces Mullein powder (Verbascum thapsus)
2 ounces Camomile flowers pwd. (Chamaemelum nobile; Anthemis nobilis)

Preparation: Mix with hot distilled water to form paste, spread on cloth and apply to entire area.

Administration: Apply as warm as possible without inconvenience, cover well and change the application when cool. Repeat until the swelling is relieved. Give the patient tea of raspberry leaves (Rubus idaeus) or bayberry bark (Myrica cerifera) which will cleanse the stomach and remove canker from the digestive tract.

Piles and hemorrhoids

1 part Mullein leaves (Verbascum thapsus)
2 parts Yarrow (Achillea millefolium)

Preparation: Infuse and cover well for 15 minutes in a proportionate amount of water; strain, sweeten, cool, bottle and keep in a cool place.

Dosage: 1 cupful, 2 to 3 times daily.

Congenial combinations:
Mullein combines well with black cohosh (Cimicifuga racemosa) and lobelia (Lobelia inflata) in liniments. In advanced cases of disease, mullein is very beneficial in combination with comfrey root (Symphytum officinale) and garlic juice (Allium sativum).

Growth characteristics:
Biennial, common in the United States and probably introduced from Europe. Grows on banks, by roadsides, waste ground, slovenly fields, in gravel, sandy or chalky soil. Flowers in July and August. It grows freely in certain low mountain locations, and can easily be propagated in most medicinal gardens; be sure that the soil is not too rich.

Drying and preservation:
Do not use the flowers that have turned brown.

Sister plants:
Clasping-leaved mullein (Verbascum phlomoides; V. thapsiforme; SCROPHULARIACEAE); this plant is medicinally similar to mullein (Verbascum thapsus).

CHICKWEED
(Stellaria media; CARYOPHYLLACEAE)

Common names:
Chickweed, star weed, star chickweed, stitchwort, scarwort, satin flower, adder's mouth, Indian chickweed, Huehnerbiss; Vogelmiere (Ger.); Alsine, pamplina de canarios, and hierba pajarera (Span.).

Identifying characteristics:
Stem — Prostate, weak, brittle, straggling, leafy, freely branched, 4-6 inches long, line or hairy fringe of white hairs along one side only, and changing direction each pair of leaves.
Leaves — Small, opposite, ovate-cordate, sessile above, lower ones on flat and hairy petioles and upper ones seated on stem.
Flowers — White, very small, deeply-cleft or two-parted petal singly on slender pedicels from the axis of the upper leaves, and in terminal clusters.

Part used:
Herb.

Therapeutic action:
Demulcent, emollient, nutritive, resolvent, pectoral, alterative, refrigerant, mucilage and discutient.

Chickweed is an excellent remedy for pulmonary complaints, any form of internal or external inflammation of the membranes or skin, and weakness of the stomach and bowels, especially bleeding of the bowels or lungs. It is excellent for external applications to wounds, skin diseases, inflamed surface, etc. It is a very nutritious food, eaten raw in salads or steamed as an ordinary vegetable, with the water used as a soothing and healing medicine either internally or externally. It is well-thought of as a weight-loss aid.

Medicinal uses:
Asthma, bronchitis, swollen testicles, inflamed surfaces, skin eruptions, erysipelas, boils, scalds, burns, inflamed or sore eyes, tumors, hemorrhoids, cancer, ulcerated throat and mouth, deafness, wounds, blood poisoning, constipation, burning and itching genitals, scurvy, blood disorders, pleurisy, coughs, colds, hoarseness, rheumatism, peritonitis and appendicitis.

Preparations:
Decoction, fluid extract, infusion, ointment, powder, and tincture.

Dosage:

Decoction	2 fluid ounces 3 to 4 times daily (or every 2 to 3 hours when necessary).
Fluid extract	1/2-1 teaspoonful.
Infusion	3-4 cupfuls daily between meals; sip a swallow at a time, mixing well with the saliva.
Powder	1 teaspoonful 3 or 4 times a day or more as needed.
Tincture	1/2 teaspoonful as needed.

ADMINISTRATION

Anal

Inflamed or ruptured appendix: Give a cool small enema of chickweed infusion or decoction (stronger and more effective), at the same time drink the tea and apply fomentation as hot as possible over the affected area.

Inflammation or weakness of the bowels: Give injection of chickweed decoction or infusion 1 to 2 times daily.

Hemorrhoids and rectal cancer: Bathe the area 2 to 3 times daily with the decoction, infusion, or diluted tincture (as warm as possible), then apply chickweed ointment or Dr. Christopher's healing ointment.

Oral

Chest troubles (asthma, bronchitis, peritonitis, stomach and bowel weakness, etc.): Boil the fresh herb, eat the vegetable and drink the water freely. Drink the decoction, and apply hot fomentation of the decoction over the chest area.

Blood poisoning: Drink the decoction internally and apply a chickweed poultice externally over the affected part.

Constipation: Take 1 cup of the warm decoction every 3 hours until bowels are regulated.

Skin

Chickweed ointment should be applied after bathing any external part with the tea.

Inflamed surfaces, skin diseases, skin eruptions, cancerous sores, itching dermatitis, and hives: Drink burdock seed tea as a diaphoretic to open skin pores and glands from the inside, and wash the affected parts with a strong decoction 2 or more times daily (more often for local eruptions). Apply chickweed ointment; a chickweed bath is also excellent.

Erysipelas: No matter how bad the pain and swelling, make a decoction from a handful or two of fresh chickweed. Bathe the surface every 1/2 hour and apply chickweed ointment. The pain and swelling will be gone in a few hours.

Swollen testicles, burning and itching genitals: Bathe the area with a strong decoction and apply chickweed ointment.

Boils, scalds, burns, inflamed or sore eyes, ulcerations, mouth or throat, deafness, wounds, etc.: Use the decoction warm as a wash and apply the ointment, which may be used externally and internally.

Nasal

Inflamed or abraded surfaces: Apply the chickweed ointment or Dr. Christopher's healing ointment.

FORMULAS

Chickweed ointment

1 pound	Chickweed, fresh green (Stellaria media)
16 ounces	Olive oil
2 ounces	Beeswax

Preparation: Cut up the chickweed and place all the ingredients in a stainless steel pot. Cover and place into an oven for 3 hours at 200 degrees F., stir, strain through fine wire, pour into jar and cool. Note: When using fresh herb, the ointment will contain water which will greatly decrease its shelf life. Store in refrigerator or freezer for longer-term storage.

Administration: Apply as needed. Note: This ointment should be available in every household. The base may be used to make any kind of ointment.

Dr. Christopher's black healing ointment

3 quarts	Liquid mutton tallow (1 quart for each 4 ounces of dry herbs or for each 10 ounces of fresh herbs which is approximately 6 pounds of very clean mutton tallow and is obtainable from the butcher)
2 ounces	Chickweed herb (Stellaria media) dried (5 oz. fresh)
2 ounces	Comfrey root (Symphytum officinale) dried (5 oz. fresh)
2 ounces	Marshmallow root (Althaea officinalis) dried (5 oz. fresh)
2 ounces	Golden seal root (Hydrastis Canadensis) dried (5 oz. fresh)
2 ounces	Lobelia herb with seed (Lobelia inflata) dried (5 oz. fresh)
2 ounces	Kino (Pterocarpus marsupium), (when possible)
1 ounce	Poke root (Phytolacca americana) dried or fresh
2 pounds	Beeswax
6 ounces	Olive oil (Olea Europæa)
2 ounces	Wheat germ oil (if not available substitute more olive oil)
1 pint	Pine tar (Pinus sylvestris) can be obtained from a nursery

Preparation: Cut up the mutton tallow, place it into a stainless steel pan (never use iron or aluminum, but you can use Pyrex or enamel if it is not chipped), cover and render in oven at 170° F. Pour off the tallow as it renders, press out the remainder and throw away the crackling. Place the tallow back into the pan and warm up to a liquid. Place all the herbs into the liquefied tallow base (acts as a catalyst and draws the medicinal virtues of the herbs into the fat) and place into oven for 4 to 8 hours. Remove and strain through a fine wire strainer, add beeswax and put back into oven to warm to a liquid again. Add the olive oil, wheat germ oil, and pine tar (do not cook it after the pine tar is added or it will curdle), use a beater (hand or electric) to homogenize or whip while hot and then pour it into an ointment or wide-mouthed jar to set. Do not try to move the jars until cool enough to be firm or there will be a nasty mess to clean up.

Administration: Apply externally or internally as needed. Note: This particular ointment has been on the market for many years. According to reports sent in it has been used successfully to cure various complaints, including skin cancer.

Extra strength "black" drawing and healing ointment

To the herbs in the recipe above add the following:

2 ounces	Red clover blossoms (Trifolium pratense)
2 ounces	Mullein (Verbascum thapsus)
4 ounces	Plantain (Plantago major)
4 ounces	Chaparral (Larrea tridentata)
Sufficient	Additional mutton tallow to contain all the herbs (if necessary)
Sufficient	Additional olive oil and beeswax to achieve desired consistency

Preparation: Follow the guidelines above.

**Erysipelas (St. Anthony's fire)
and all skin diseases**

A few handfuls	Chickweed (Stellaria media)
Sufficient	Distilled water

Preparation: Make a strong decoction by simmering 15 minutes.

Administration: Bathe the affected parts often with the warm tea. In case the blisters are ulcerating, use the slippery elm poultice and then apply chickweed ointment. Give the tea combination internally (see "FORMULAS" under red raspberry on page 158.) Use a decoction of elder flowers (simmer 2 ounces for 10 minutes in 1 quart of water) to bathe the affected area freely.

Congenial combinations:
For inflamed surfaces, skin eruptions and diseases, etc.; Chickweed should be used in combination with burdock seed (Arctium lappa), which opens the pores and acts upon the setaceous or oil glands.

Growth characteristics:
It is an annual or biennial and a common plant of Europe and North America. It grows in fields, waste places, roadsides, around dwellings and especially in moist and shady places. It flowers from the beginning of spring until the last of autumn. Chickweed is considered to be a curse by many gardeners because of its creeping and twining among other plants. Nevertheless, it is an excellent addition to your home medicinal garden; try to collect the seeds as they mature to sow in the spring for the next year's crop.

Collection:
It is best used fresh; but chickweed may be gathered and dried at the flowering stage.

MARSHMALLOW
(Althaea officinalis; MALVACEAE)

Common names:
Marshmallow, althea, marshmallow root, mortification root, mallards, sweet weed, cheese plant, wymote, mauls, guimauve, schloss tea, white mallow; Racine de Guimauve, (Fr.); Radix Althaeae, Althee, Eibischwurzel, gemeiner Eibisch (Ger.); Malvavisco (Span.).

Identifying characteristics:

Stem	Several woolly stems, 2-4 feet high, erect, round, bushy and leafy. It is distinguished from common mallow by the velvety down covering

of the stem and leaves.

Leaves — Soft velvety (dense covering of stellate hairs on both sides), 1-3 inches long, 1¼ inch broad, cordate, ovate, pointed, irregularly serrate at margins, 5-lobed below and 3-lobed above, grayish-green, and brittle when dry.

Flowers — Large (1-2 inches in diameter), pink, pinkish-blue or purple, luxuriant maxillary panicles, stamens unite into a tube and anthers are kidney-shaped.

Root — Slender, tapering, 6-12 inches long, 2/5-4/5 inch thick, fleshy externally, yellowish-brown (unscraped), grayish-white (scraped), internally yellowish-white and fibrous. It has accentuated longitudinal furrows when spirally twisted and covered with somewhat loosened bast-fibers. The bark has a fibrous fracture. Wood fractures short and granular. Powder: whitish.

Taste — Sweetish and mucilaginous.

Odor — Faint and aromatic.

Part used:
Root (greater potency), leaves, and flowers.

Therapeutic action:
Demulcent, emollient, mucilage, nutritive, vulnerary, absorbent, laxative, diuretic, and protective.

Marshmallow is high in lime and calcium. The root is especially high in oxygen and pectin. When the powdered root is applied to moist surfaces, it will draw and absorb all moisture. Marshmallow is very soothing and healing to inflamed respiratory, alimentary, intestinal, and genito-urinary areas.

Its diuretic and demulcent qualities are especially useful for urinary problems because it has no astringent action and is somewhat relaxing. The powdered or crushed fresh roots make a first-rate poultice, and the leaves are excellent as a fomentation for inflammation. Its power in the decoction form for arresting gangrene (historically called mortification), or putrefaction has been so great that it has been popularly-called "mortification root." Marshmallow is one of the best mucilage agents, giving off about 35% each of vegetable mucus and starch. It is soothing and healing to the mucous membrane and agreeable to the taste. The powdered root is very absorbent. It is used in pharmacies to harden pills, troches, electuaries, etc.

Medicinal uses:
Cough, pharyngitis, laryngitis, pulmonary complaints (chronic, acute), diabetes, renal hemorrhage, diarrhea, dysentery, inflammation (organ or surfaces), infections, burns (fire, acid, etc), inflamed or swollen joints and muscles, chronic constipation, gravel, kidney and bladder inflammation, malnutrition, rickets, weak digestion, inflamed or sore eyes, bronchitis, gonorrhea, cystitis, colds, hoarse-

ness, vaginal irritation, catarrh, vaginal douche, pneumonia, strangury, all kidney diseases, skin eruptions, psoriasis, rectal irritation (enema), gout, Bright's disease, abscesses, sores, mastitis, gum boils, and neuralgia.

Preparations:
Decoction, fluid extract, infusion, syrup, powder, and tincture.

Dosage:

Decoction	1 teacupful (6 fluid ounces), 3 times daily (regular).
Fluid extract	1/2-2 teaspoonfuls.
Infusion	1 teacupful 3 to 4 times daily.
Powder	2 #00 capsules each hour till pain leaves, then decrease as needed.
Syrup	(root) 1/2-2 teaspoons.
Tincture	1/2-1 teaspoonful.

ADMINISTRATION

Oral

Pulmonary complaints: Combine with other expectorant and demulcent remedies.

Hemorrhage of the urinary organs, diarrhea, dysentery, and to enrich mother's milk: Boil the powdered root in soymilk (tofu-milk) and drink freely.

Spasmodic asthma: Use the whooping cough formula below, adding 1/2 ounce lobelia herb (Lobelia inflata), with slightly more water added; but finishing with 1 pint of liquid.

Whooping cough (specific): See "FORMULAS."

Skin

Inflamed or sore eyes: Infuse marshmallow leaves and bathe eyes frequently; in severe cases, bind saturated cotton on loosely and apply, leave on for 15 minutes and then make a fresh application.

Obstinate inflammation and threatened mortification (gangrene): Apply a poultice of the powdered or fresh crushed roots on the affected area as hot as possible and renew it before it dries. This is even more effective with the addition of slippery elm (Ulmus rubra; U. fulva).

Eyewash for inflammation: See "FORMULAS."

Gathered breasts (mastitis), gum-boil, and neuralgia: See "FORMULAS."

FORMULAS

Decoction of Marshmallow root

2 ounces	Marshmallow root, cut or granulated (Althaea officinalis)
3 pints	Distilled or d-cell water

Preparation: Soak the herb for 1 hour in the water, bring to a boil and simmer slowly down to 1½ pints; strain, press and bottle.

Dosage: 1 teacupful (6 fluid ounces) 3 times daily (taken warm), sweeten to taste if desired.

Eyewash for inflammation

1 ounce	Marshmallow root (Althaea officinalis)
1/4 ounce	Raspberry leaves (Rubus idaeus)
1½ pints	Distilled water

Preparation: Simmer slowly (low heat) in the distilled water down to 1 pint; strain, and cool.

Administration: Bathe the eyes with the cold tea about 6 times daily.

Whooping cough (specific)

2 ounces	Marshmallow root (Althaea officinalis)
2 ounces	Thyme (Thymes vulgaris)
2 pounds	Yellow D sugar (or 1 pound honey)
1 quart	Distilled or d-cell water

Preparation: Simmer the herbs slowly, while covered, down to 1 pint, strain, press and return the liquid to the clean pot. Add the sugar, bring to a boil and simmer slowly for 5 minutes (skimming as is necessary), cool, bottle, and keep in a cool place.

Dosage: 1 tablespoonful every 2 to 3 hours; Children: 1-3 teaspoonfuls (according to age).

Administration: Feed the child fruit juices, especially pineapple, and keep off starchy, greasy, and mucus-forming foods. Improve the diet to accelerate healing and to prevent the condition from recurring.

Gathered breast (mastitis), gum-boils, neuralgia

1 part	Marshmallow root (Althaea officinalis)
1 part	Camomile flowers (Chamaemelum nobile; Anthemis nobilis)
1 part	Poppy heads, dried (Papaver somniferum)

Preparation: Mix with enough boiling water to poultice consistency.

Administration: Apply as hot fomentation (repeatedly) to the affected area.

Flatulent colic (stomach distension, rumbling bowels, griping pains, and constipation)

1/2 ounce	Marshmallow root (Althaea officinalis)
1 ounce	Sweet flag root (Acorus calamus)
1/2 ounce	Fennel seeds (Foeniculum vulgare)
1/2 ounce	Dandelion root (Taraxacum officinale)
1 teaspoon	Cayenne (Capsicum frutescens; C. minimum)
1 teaspoon	Ginger (Zingiber officinalis)

Preparation: Simmer the first 4 herbs (well-covered) for 30 minutes in 1 quart of water, strain hot over the cayenne and ginger, cover and allow to cool.

Dosage: 3 tablespoonfuls or more every 1/2 hour until relieved; then 4 times daily.

Administration: Clear the bowels with a catnip (Nepeta cataria) enema. Place hot flannel packs or a hot bran bag over the stomach or abdomen to give comfort and ease. Regulate the bowels with the lower bowel tonic. This condition is often caused by poor digestion, which should be treated with digestive tonics.

Cough, bronchial affections

2 ounces	Marshmallow (Althaea officinalis)
2 ounces	Licorice (Glycyrrhiza glabra)
2 ounces	Elecampane (Inula helenium)

Preparation: Simmer 1 teaspoonful of mixture to a cup of water for 15 minutes or more, then steep and set aside until cool.

Dosage: 1 tablespoonful each hour or at periods of spasms.

Cough and bronchitis, etc.

1/4 teaspoon	Marshmallow (Althaea officinalis)

1/2 teaspoon Coltsfoot (Tussilago farfara)
1/2 teaspoon Ground ivy (Glechoma hederacea)
1/2 teaspoon Licorice (Glycyrrhiza glabra)
1/2 teaspoon Elder flowers (Sambucus canadensis)

Preparation: Infuse the herbs for 15 minutes in 1 pint of hot water, cover and let stand until cool. Strain, sweeten with honey, bottle and keep cool.

Dosage: Use a tablespoonful or more as needed during coughing for irritation of the throat and use each hour thereafter.

Potter's diaphoretic

8 parts Marshmallow root (Althaea officinalis)
4 parts Licorice (Glycyrrhiza glabra)
4 parts Spanish iris or Orris root (Iris florentina)
4 parts Ground ivy (Glechoma hederacea)
1 part Aniseed (Pimpinella anisum)
4 parts Coltsfoot leaves (Tussilago farfara)
2 parts Red poppy flowers, dried (Papaver somniferum)
2 parts Mullein (Verbascum thapsus)

Preparation: Mix and use 1 teaspoonful of herbs to each cup of boiling water simmer 15 or 20 minutes, then steep and set aside until cool enough to drink.

Dosage: Use 1/2 cupful or more every 2 hours, or more frequently if needed, keeping the patient well covered with a hot water bottle on the feet with a vinegar-soaked towel surrounding the feet.

Potter's diuretic, #2

1 part Marshmallow root (Althaea officinalis)
1 part Asparagus root (Asparagus officinalis)
1 part Licorice root (Glycyrrhiza glabra)
1 part Strawberry root (Fragaria vesca)
1 part Couchgrass root (Agropyron repens)

Preparation: Simmer 1 teaspoonful to the cup of mixed herbs slowly for 15 minutes.

Dosage: 2 fluid ounces each hour.

Marshmallow ointment
(inflammatory eruptions, facial sores, wounds, ulcers, etc.)

8 ounces Marshmallow leaves, fresh (Althaea officinalis)

8 ounces Elder flowers, fresh (Sambucus canadensis)
1 pound Leaf lard
1/2 pound Beeswax

Preparation: Bruise the herbs and place them with the lard and beeswax into an appropriate container; cover, and simmer in the oven (150° F.) until the herbs are crisp. Strain through a wire strainer and stir until cold. If stronger salve is required, place a second batch of herbs into the product and simmer as before, etc.

Note: This salve will cleanse, digest and heal sores, wounds, ulcers, etc.

Inflammation of the kidneys

1/2 ounce Marshmallow root (Althaea officinalis)
1/2 ounce Dandelion root (Taraxacum officinale)
1/2 ounce Uva ursi (Arctostaphylos uva-ursi)
1/2 ounce Wild carrot (Daucus carota)
1/2 ounce White poplar or quaking aspen bark (Populus tremuloides)
1/2 ounce Pellitory-of-the-Wall (Parietaria officinalis)
1/2 teaspoon Cayenne (Capsicum frutescens; C. minimum)

Preparation: Boil the first 6 herbs slowly in 1 quart of water down to 1 pint; strain hot over the cayenne.

Dosage: 3 tablespoons every hour until the pain is eased, then every 2 hours.

Administration: Place pieces of flannel in hot water, wring them out and at the same time apply across the kidneys and lumbar region.

Nephritis (fomentation)

4 ounces Marshmallow herb or root (Althaea officinalis)
4 ounces Wormwood (Artemisia absinthium)
4 ounces Southernwood (Artemisia abrotanum)

Preparation: Simmer for 30 minutes in 1 gallon of water.

Administration: Place a piece of flannel in the liquid, wring it out and apply as hot as conveniently possible over the kidneys. Cover with a thick piece of blanket and change the application when it begins to cool. Repeat for 1 hour and at the same time give an appropriate tea internally.

Potter's Pectoral, #1 (flowers)

1 part Marshmallow flowers (Althaea officinalis)
1 part Mallow flowers (cheeses) (Malva sylvestris; M. rotundifolia)

1 part	Coltsfoot flowers (Tussilago farfara)
1 part	Violet or blue violet flowers (Viola odorata)
1 part	Mullein flowers (Verbascum thapsus)
1 part	Red poppy flowers, dried (Papaver somniferum)
1 part	Ground ivy (Glechoma hederacea; Nepeta glechoma)

Preparation: While covered, infuse the herbs 10 to 15 minutes in an proportionate amount of warmed, distilled water (1 teaspoonful of herbs to a cup), strain and sip the clear liquid.

Dosage: Use from 1 tablespoonful to 2 fluid ounces as often as needed or whenever cough or irritation requires.

Potter's Pectoral, #2

10 parts	Marshmallow root (Althaea officinalis)
20 parts	John's bread (Ceratonia siliqua)
1 part	Mallow flowers (cheeses) (Malva sylvestris; M. rotundifolia)
12 parts	Licorice root (Glycyrrhiza glabra)
2 parts	Ground ivy (Glechoma hederacea; Nepeta glechoma)
2 parts	Maidenhair (Adiantum pedatum; A. Capillus-Veneris)
2 parts	Hyssop (Hyssopus officinalis)
2 parts	Liverwort (Anemone hepatica; Hepatica Americana)
2 parts	Balm (Melissa officinalis)
4 parts	Mullein flowers (Verbascum thapsus)
6 parts	Jujube berries (Ziziphus jujuba; Z. vulgaris)
2 parts	Red poppy flowers, dry (Papaver somniferum)
6 parts	Currants
6 parts	Raisins
20 parts	Figs
24 parts	Barley (Hordeum vulgare)

Preparation: Combine all ingredients as best as possible and make an infusion using 1 oz. of the combination to a pint of water, simmer slowly 20 minutes.

Dosage: 1 tablespoon each hour or as needed.

Potter's Pectoral
"Brust Thee (burst tea)", #3

8 parts	Marshmallow root (Althaea officinalis)
4 parts	Coltsfoot leaves (Tussilago farfara)
3 parts	Licorice root (Glycyrrhiza glabra)
2 parts	Mullein flowers (Verbascum thapsus)
2 parts	Aniseed (Pimpinella anisum)
1 part	Spanish iris or Orris root (Iris florentina)

Preparation: Infuse 1 teaspoonful to a cup of water.

Dosage: 2 tablespoonfuls each hour until phlegm is loose, then a tablespoonful each hour as needed.

Sprains, and bruises (fomentation)

2 ounces Marshmallow root or leaves (Althaea officinalis)
2 ounces Camomile flowers (Chamaemelum nobile; Anthemis nobilis)

Preparation: Boil the herbs for 10 minutes in 2 quarts of water.

Dosage: 2 tablespoonfuls each hour until phlegm is loose, then a tablespoonful each hour as needed.

Administration: Foment the affected parts for 1 hour, 2 to 3 times daily, then bind up the affected part firmly. Comfrey root is also excellent when used alone or added to the above combination.

Breast tea

8 parts Marshmallow root (Althaea officinalis)
4 parts Coltsfoot (Tussilago farfara)
4 parts Elder flowers (Sambucus canadensis)
3 parts Licorice (Glycyrrhiza glabra)
4 parts Plantain (Plantago major; P. lanceolate)
3 parts Hyssop (Hyssopus officinalis)
2 parts Aniseed (Pimpinella anisum)
2 parts Mullein (Verbascum thapsus)
4 parts Ground ivy (Glechoma hederacea)
4 parts Veronica or speed well (Veronica officinalis)
1 part Spanish iris or orris root (Iris florentina)

Preparation: Mix the herbs well; use 1 teaspoonful of the herbs to each cup of water; steep 10 to 15 minutes.

Dosage: 1 teacupful 3 to 4 times daily.

Congenial combinations:
For obstinate inflammation, slippery elm will accentuate the healing action.

CASE HISTORY

Gangrenous limb.
Dr. Christopher treated a case where a man had injured his leg and gangrene had

set in. He went to a medical doctor, who insisted that it should be amputated. He refused to do that so he came to Dr. Christopher. Dr. Christopher dug up a large quantity of marshmallow root in the yard, sufficient to make enough decoction to completely submerge the leg in the liquid and after just a number of hours, the tissue returned to normal. This is the plant that people keep trying to weed out of their yards. It has big, deep roots which gather generous amounts of minerals and nutrients.

Pitchfork wound.
In another Christopher case, a man ran a pitchfork into his foot, but went back to work even though it was painful. By afternoon his condition worsened and his boss sent him to the hospital, The medical doctor said that tetanus shots would be a must or else he might risk amputation. The man hesitated and said that he was too busy and would have to put it off. The doctor warned that he might not be living the next day. After he left the doctor, he came to Dr. Christopher.

Dr. Christopher told him to gather some comfrey and marshmallow root, which were growing abundantly on the farm, and to pack the foot with five pounds each of onion and salt as a drawing poultice for four hours, then to apply the comfrey and marshmallow as a poultice. By the next noon, the swelling had completely subsided and there was only soreness at the place where the pitch fork had punctured his foot. He continued using the poultice until in a very short period it was healed. This treatment has not only saved limbs, but it has also saved lives. In a case where no drawing herbs are available, copious amounts of honey on the area will cause a drawing, as well as soothing and healing, or soak the injured part in cayenne tea.

Growth characteristics:
Perennial; found in almost all tropical areas (in the United States, it is found in the salt marshes from the Massachusetts coast to New York), and sub-tropical parts of the world (in moist, marshy or swampy places). The first two years produce only a tap-root, which will soon become tough, woody, branched, and not of much value medicinally. Marshmallow flowers between July and September. What is used and referred to elsewhere as "marshmallow" (with similar therapeutic value and properties) is the low mallow plant (Malva rotundifolia) which is also known as "Malva."

Collection:
The root is generally gathered late in autumn, peeled (but this is not necessary), and dried carefully. The tap-root of the first and second year growth (prior to branching) is reported to yield greater medicinal potency.

Sister plants:
-Malva or Low Malva (Malva rotundifolia; MALVACEAE) called "marshmallow" in many parts, and is medicinally similar; but it does not yield as much mucilage, about one half as much as marshmallow (Althaea officinalis). It is

biennial; procumbent (prostrate) and has spreading stems. The leaves are orbicular up to 3¼ inches broad, cordate (heart-shaped), 5-7 lobed, less pubescent (hairy), and on petioles up to 8 inches in length.
-High Mallow (Malva sylvestris; MALVACEAE), medicinally similar to marshmallow (Althaea officinalis), with less, though plentiful mucilage. It is biennial, the stem is erect, and 3 feet high. The leaves are orbicular, reniform (kidney-shaped), cordate (heart-shaped), 4-4½ inches long, 6-8 inches broad, 3-7 lobed, petioles up to 4 inches in length, pale, crenate-dentate, and pubescent (hairy).
-Holly hock (Alcea rosea; MALVACEAE); similar medicinal properties, see page 390.
-Cotton (Gossypium herbaceum; MALVACEAE); the root, the hairs, and the oil are useful in place of the drug ergot. Cotton is a parturient to hasten birth and is used for female problems, uterine tumors and hemorrhages.

SLIPPERY ELM
(Ulmus rubra; U. fulva; ULMACEAE)

Common names:
Slippery elm, red elm, elm bark, moose elm, Indian elm, rock elm, sweet elm, American elm; Cortex Ulmi Interior (Br.); Ecorce d'Orme (fauve) (Fr.); Ulmenrinde, Ruesterrinde (Ger.); Olmo (Span.).

Identifying characteristics:

Stem	Large tree, 50-60 feet high, 1-4 feet thick, reddish-brown bark and wood. Bark is deeply furrowed (strait perpendicularly), very rough and scaly. Innermost layer next to wood is buff white, tough and fibrous texture and mealy fracture. Branches and twigs are rough, grayish and hairy. Powder: light brown (fawn).
Leaves	Large, 4-8 inches long, 2-3 inches broad, oblong, acuminate (tapering to a slender point), rough on both sides, petiolate, pubescent (hairy), unequally serrate, unequal at subcordate base, deep yellowish, olive green above, lighter and sometimes rusty- downy beneath. Buds are covered with a dense russet down.
Flowers	Small, appearing before leaves (March-April), sessile (attached directly by the base), no stalk or petiole in cluster, downy calyx and corolla wanting.
Fruit	Samara, long, flat, broadly oblong (nearly round in outline), 1/2-3/4 inch long, entire, notched, 1-celled, yellow wing, silky with short fulvous (dull yellow) hairs with ripening in the spring at intervals of 2 to 4 years.
Taste	Distinctively "slimy" or mucilaginous.
Odor	Strong and characteristic.

Part used:
Inner bark.

Therapeutic action:
Emollient, demulcent, pectoral, nutritive, expectorant, diuretic, slightly astringent, and tonic.

The slippery elm is one of the most valuable medicines in the herbal world. This was an important botanical medicine and food for both the American Indians and pioneers. It possesses an abundant mucilage which will soothe irritation, disperse inflammation, draw out impurities, heal rapidly, and greatly strengthen. It is especially soothing and healing to irritated and inflamed surfaces, the various mucous membranes internally, or wounds, burns, chapped skin, etc. Externally it is most beneficial for inflammatory conditions of the stomach, lungs, intestines and urinary organs.

The powder made into a mucilage beverage or gruel is a bland and nutritive food for babies, thus an excellent weaning food. It is also wonderful for the elderly or convalescents; it possesses as much nutrition as oatmeal, though it is much easier on the system, and is an excellent sustaining food. The gruel is a valuable remedy in all cases of weakness, pulmonary complaints, stomach inflammation, lung hemorrhage, etc. It is especially efficient in absorbing noxious gases and neutralizing any acidity in the stomach. Because of its mucilaginous nature, it is easy to assimilate and eliminate. Its action is so gentle that it can be retained by delicate stomachs when other substances are rejected. It is wonderful for checking infant diarrhea.

As a poultice, slippery elm is one of the greatest remedies for soothing injured or inflamed parts, and also provides the elements for speedy healing and strengthening of the tissue.

Medicinal uses:
Consumption or tuberculosis, asthma, bronchitis, pneumonia, gastritis, nephritis, gastric ulcers, pyloric inflammation or ulceration, calculi, scalding urine, croup, diphtheria, inflammation of the bowels, skin eruptions, sores, ulcerated stomach, stomach weakness, boils, carbuncles, abscesses, chilblains, purulent ophthalmia, wounds, burns, diarrhea, coughs, dysentery, pleurisy, sore throat, poison ivy, female problems, leukorrhea, tumors, vaginal irritation, etc.

Preparations:
Decoction, infusion, mucilage, powder, pessaries, suppositories and tincture.

Dosage:

Decoction	2 fluid ounces 3 to 4 times daily.
Infusion	1 teacupful 3 to 4 times daily.
Powder	1 teaspoon or more in capsule 3 times or more per day.

Tincture	5-40 drops 2 to 3 times.
Mucilage or Gruel	1/2-1 pint (warm) 1 to 3 times daily (more if needed).

ADMINISTRATION

Anal

Inflammation of bowels: While stirring, slowly pour 1 pint of boiling hot water over 1 ounce of powdered bark to make an infusion. Allow it to stand until the proper enema temperature is reached. Strain off clear liquid and inject into the bowels.

Oral

Asthma, bronchitis, chronic cough (especially whooping cough), lung trouble, cystitis, catarrh of bladder, poison ivy, burns, tuberculosis: See "FORMULAS" under "Asthma remedy."

Heartburn or sore throat: Chew the bark.

Tuberculosis: Use the "Asthma remedy" formula, adding 1 teaspoon of garlic juice; take 1 teaspoonful frequently, according to the severity of the case.

Ulcerated stomach: Use slippery elm gruel.

Weak stomach and vomiting, pneumonia, nephritis, inflammation, ulceration: A gruel of slippery elm is often well-received when all food is ejected. See "FORMULAS."

Soothing nutritive for weaning babies: Boil a small portion or lump of whole slippery elm bark, pour off clear liquid and sweeten. It soothes colic pains at the same time.

Skin

Drawing and healing poultice (inflamed surfaces, ulcers, wounds, burns, boils, skin diseases, purulent ophthalmia, chilblains, etc.): Add water to the powder to make a thick poultice and place on the affected part. You might add other herbs as needed. Stripping the bark straight from the tree and binding the inner side to a bad wound will work.

Poison ivy and burns: Apply the "Asthma remedy" formula below as a fomentation locally to the affected parts and allow to remain 1 hour. Wash off with biodegradable soapy water and rinse. Reapply until all itch and symptoms disappear.

Skin eruptions and sores: Wash with slippery elm tea.

Boils, carbuncles, abscesses: See "Slippery elm poultice" below.

Vaginal

Pessaries and suppositories (base) for inflammation of the vagina, ovarian inflammation, uterine weakness, impurities, leucorrhea, growths, and tumors: As a medicinal base, powdered slippery elm bark can be easily formed into suppositories and moistened as needed to insert into the female genito-urinary organs. Use the "Slippery elm pack" formula.

FORMULAS

Slippery elm mucilage #1

6 grams	Slippery elm, bruised (Ulmus rubra; U. fulva)
3 ounces	Water

Preparation: Place the herb into the boiling water, cover well and keep on low heat for one hour. Strain through a fine wire strainer.

Administration: Use alone or for emulsions and mixtures.

Slippery elm mucilage #2
(for the mucous membranes of the stomach and intestines)

1 teaspoon	Slippery elm, powder (Ulmus rubra; U. fulva)
1 pint	Distilled or d-cell water

Preparation: Mix the slippery elm with sufficient cold water to make a smooth paste. When thoroughly mixed, pour over the boiling hot water while stirring steadily and flavor with cinnamon, nutmeg, grated lemon rind, lemon oil, etc.

Dosage: 1/2 pint (warm) 1 to 4 times daily.

Slippery elm gruel
(strengthening, soothing and healing of inflamed surfaces)

3 ounces	Slippery elm, powder (Ulmus rubra; U. fulva)
8 ounces	Distilled water (adjust to desired consistency)
1 teaspoon	Honey (adjust to desired taste)
dash	Cinnamon or nutmeg, powdered

Preparation: Make a paste by adding water, a little at a time, to the slippery elm powder while stirring; add honey and seasonings to your desired flavor. Can be made with hot or cold water.

Dosage: Drink warm 1/2-1 pint, 1 to 3 times daily.

Slippery elm poultice

Mix the slippery elm powder into a proper consistency with hot or boiling water (a sufficient amount should be used to make a fairly thick covering), and apply as hot as is convenient. Change as often as required, or from every 3 hours to 2 times daily.

For an obstinate boil
or any other external problems

3 parts Slippery elm powder (Ulmus rubra; U. fulva)
1 part Lobelia powder (Lobelia inflata)

Preparation: Make a poultice as directed above and use over the affected area which will relax and hasten suppuration.

Asthma syrup
(bronchitis, croup, whooping cough, etc.)

1 ounce Slippery elm (Ulmus rubra; U. fulva)
1 ounce Boneset (Eupatorium perfoliatum)
1 ounce Licorice (Glycyrrhiza glabra)
1 ounce Flaxseed or linseed (Linum usitatissimum)
1 pint Blackstrap molasses

Preparation: Simmer the herbs for 20 minutes in 1 quart of water, strain and stir in the molasses while hot and sweeten with honey.

Dosage: 1 tablespoonful as required.

Bruises (poultice)

1 pound Slippery elm powder (Ulmus rubra; U. fulva)
1 pound Wild indigo powder (Baptisia tinctoria)
1/2 pound Myrrh gum (Commiphora myrrha, var. molmol)
1/4 pound Prickly ash, powder (Zanthoxylum americanum)

Preparation: Wet and mix to paste consistency with good brewer's yeast.

Administration: Apply over the affected area and cover.

Bronchitis, croup, whooping cough, etc.

1 ounce	Slippery elm (Ulmus rubra; U. fulva)
1 ounce	Boneset (Eupatorium perfoliatum)
1 ounce	Flaxseed or linseed (Linum usitatissimum)
1 stick	Licorice (Glycyrrhiza glabra)

Preparation: Simmer the herbs for 20 minutes in 1 quart of water. Strain, add 1 pint of apple cider vinegar, sweeten with sugar and when cool, bottle and keep in a cool place.

Dosage: 1 tablespoonful 2 to 3 times daily. Note: For bronchial catarrh, either the apple cider vinegar may be used or 1 pint of black strap molasses.

Burns and scalds (after skin is broken)

1 part	Slippery elm, powder (Ulmus rubra; U. fulva)
1 part	White pond lily (Nymphaea odorata)
Sufficient	Olive oil or raw linseed (flax seed) oil

Preparation: Mix to paste consistency.

Administration: Apply as a poultice. This will soothe and draw out all inflammatory pains and swellings. However, the "burn paste" under "comfrey" is preferred for this condition. Use cold water applications for several hours, and take cayenne, composition powder (see page 147-148), or strong peppermint tea internally; thereafter, apply this poultice.

Gastritis (inflammation of the stomach)

1 ounce	Slippery elm (Ulmus rubra; U. fulva)
1 ounce	Raspberry leaves (Rubus idaeus)
1/2 ounce	Marshmallow root (Althaea officinalis)
1/2 ounce	Agrimony (Agrimonia eupatoria)
1 teaspoon	Cayenne (Capsicum frutescens; C. minimum)

Preparation: Simmer the first 4 herbs for 20 minutes in 1 quart of water and strain hot over the cayenne.

Dosage: 2 fluid ounces every hour, or more frequently if the case requires.

Administration: Always use slippery elm gruel for this condition, and give cayenne. Where there is persistent vomiting, cleanse the stomach with an emetic of lobelia. A cayenne fomentation on the abdomen will ease bad pains, the lower bowel tonic will regulate. A catnip enema relieves the bowels.

Sores (hasten suppuration)
and gangrenous wounds (will arrest gangrene)

sufficient Slippery elm powder (Ulmus rubra; U. fulva)
sufficient Brewing yeast
sufficient Raw milk

Preparation: Mix the herb and yeast with hot milk. If the brewing yeast is not available, dissolve a yeast cake in warm water and mix.

Administration: Apply over the affected area and cover.

Offensive gangrenous wounds or sores
(antiseptic poultice)

1 part Slippery elm, powder (Ulmus rubra; U. fulva)
1 part Vegetable charcoal, powder (activated charcoal)

Preparation: Mix with hot water or with infusion of wormwood (Artemisia absinthium) to paste consistency.

Administration: Apply over the affected area and cover.

Slippery elm
(nutritive for infants, convalescent, etc)

1 ounce Slippery elm powder (Ulmus rubra; U. fulva)
1 teaspoon Maple syrup, yellow D sugar or fructose (fruit sugar)

Preparation: Mix the ingredients together, then add 1 pint of boiling hot water slowly, mixing as it is poured on. Flavor with cinnamon or nutmeg to suit taste.

Administration: Serve as a nutritive food.

Asthma remedy
(also for bronchitis, chronic cough, whooping cough, lung trouble, cystitis, catarrh of bladder, poison ivy, burns, and tuberculosis)

2 ounces Slippery elm bark, powder (Ulmus rubra; U. fulva)
1 ounce Horehound, cut (Marrubium vulgare)
1 ounce Garden thyme, cut (Thymes vulgaris)
1 ounce Red clover tops, cut (Trifolium pratense)
1 ounce Yerba santa, cut (Eriodictyon californicum)
1 ounce Lobelia herb, cut (Lobelia inflata)
1 ounce Resin weed leaves, cut (Grindelia robusta)
1 teaspoon Cayenne, powder (Capsicum frutescens; C. minimum)

1½ pounds Blackstrap molasses
1/2 pint Glycerine

Preparation: Soak the herbs for 2 hours in 2 quarts of distilled or d-cell water and bring to a boil (well-covered). Simmer slowly for 30 minutes; strain and press. Return the liquid to the clean pot and reduce to 1 pint; add the blackstrap molasses and glycerine. Bring to a boil and simmer very slowly for 5 minutes; cool and bottle. *Note:* Slippery elm mixes more uniformly with the other ingredients when first made into a paste and stirred into the water.

Dosage: 1 tablespoon every hour until relief and relaxation is obtained; thereafter, 1 tablespoon 3 to 4 times daily.

Slippery elm pack
(female genito-urinary problems, growths, tumors, etc.)

Preparation: Add sufficient water to slippery elm to make a bolus (soft mass). Knead until it is quite stiff, 3 inches long, and the size (diameter) of the patient's middle finger. Cut into 3 pieces, each 1 inch long.

Onto a fine sea sponge, sew a piece of silk thread firmly, leaving 3-4 inches of the thread extra. Smear the sponge with equal parts of Vaseline and glycerine and set aside for use.

Administration: Dip 1 piece of the slippery elm bolus into hot water and insert as far as possible into the vagina. Follow with the second and third pieces. Next, insert the smeared sponge into the vaginal opening, which will hold the bolus in place, and leave for 2 days. Remove the sponge by pulling down on the silk thread, syringe (rinse) thoroughly with a cleansing agent such as an infusion of yellow dock (Rumex-crispus) or Dr. Christopher's Vaginal Douche (yellow dock combination), and repeat the pack.

CASE HISTORY

A time to live and a time to die.
A Dr. Christopher case history in his own words: We once had a case of an eight-year-old boy who was like a skeleton. He could not eat any food or drink any water. He'd lain in the hospital so long that he had developed very bad bed sores. His spine was open with the bones protruding, as was his hip bone, which also protruded through the flesh. The hospital physician sent him home from the hospital as a hopeless case. There was nothing more they could do for him.

He was put on slippery elm gruel, one teaspoon at a time. Poultices of slippery elm were placed on his hips and spine. Within weeks, he was back to normal weight, his flesh was restored, and he looked like a perfect specimen of health, but he lacked energy. Nothing we gave him would give him strength. It was suggested that our healing ministrations could be contrary to the Lord's will concerning this boy. With this change, it was believed his time had come, and the only thing the parents could do was to administer to him and dedicate him to the Lord. This was done with the boy's approval, and as soon as the "Amen" was said, the little boy looked up and smiled. He then said, "Good-bye Daddy, good-bye Doc," and he was gone with a smile on his face.

Growth characteristics:
Perennial; grows extensively in North and South America, flourishes in high open places and in firm, dry soil.

Collection:
For best results, the ten-year-old bark is used. The best quality of slippery elm bark can be folded lengthwise without breaking, while inferior grades are brittle. The bark should be collected in the spring and the epidermis should be removed and dried.

Drying and preservation:
The powder should be grayish or fawn colored. The dark or reddish powder should be rejected.

Sister plants:
-English elm or European elm (Ulmus campestris; ULMACEAE); thinner bark, cinnamon color, mucilaginous, bitterish, astringent with similar therapeutic properties and uses.
-Black elm (Ulmus effusa; ULMACEAE); The bark is therapeutically very similar.

ELECAMPANE
(Inula helenium COMPOSITAE)

Common names:
Elecampane, scabwort, elf dock, yellow starwort, wild sunflower, horse heal, velvet dock; Aunee (Fr.); Alantwurzel (Ger.); enula campana, helopia (Span.).

Identifying characteristics:

Stem	Thick, solid, striate (furrowed), villous (pubescent, hairy, downy) above, 2-6 feet high, usually unbranched, and the plant similar in appearance to the horseradish.
Leaves	Large, 10-18 inches long, 4-8 inches broad, ovate (broadly oblong and pointed), alternate, dark green above, serrate (saw-edged), rough above, pubescent woolly beneath, fleshy midrib, and long petioled (some with heart-shaped, clasping bases).
Flowers	Large, usually solitary, 2-4 inches across, brilliantly golden-yellow,

	on long stout peduncles (stems).
Root	Rhizome with roots, similar in color and appearance to belladonna, grayish-brown, hard, up to 3 inches long, 1 inches thick, longitudinally wrinkled (horny) with occasional buds or stem-scars, short fracture, internally light brown, many oleoresin canals, fibrinous near the cambium zone, roots are cylindrical, tapering, curved, curled, up to 5¼ inches long, 3/5 inch thick, radiant transverse structure and numerous dark cells. Powder: light brown.
Taste	Acrid, bitter, pungent.
Odor	Aromatic and camphoraceous.

Part used:
Rhizome and roots.

Therapeutic action:
Expectorant, carminative, diaphoretic, tonic, diuretic, alterative, antiseptic, astringent, gently stimulant, stomachic, emmenagogue, antispasmodic, anti-asthmatic, antiscorbutic, vulnerary, antivenomous, and emetic (large doses.)

Elecampane helps with all pulmonary and catarrhal problems. Its sodium phosphate cleans the liver and digestive organs, the potassium chloride dissolves the fibrinous exudations and mucoid matter, and its calcium chlorine supports, feeds, and tones the heart muscles.

It is a stimulant, relaxant, and tonic to the mucous membrane, a warming, strengthening, cleansing and toning agent to the gastric, alvine and pulmonary membranes. Because of its efficient expectoration of pulmonary mucus, some herbalists have considered elecampane a specific for consumption and pulmonary disorders. It promptly clears up old chronic diseases of the lungs and chest. It is a rich source of inulin, a polysaccharide (carbohydrate).

Medicinal uses:
Cough, asthma, bronchitis, all pulmonary complaints, dyspepsia, acute catarrhal affection, tuberculosis, snake bites, dyspnea or shortness of breath, wheezing, cystitis, skin diseases, inflammations (all forms), putrid sores and cankers, rash (skin and face), tooth decay, whooping cough, dropsy, diphtheria, kidney and bladder stones, retention of urine, delayed menstruation (amenorrhea), phthisis (tuberculosis of the lungs), vesical catarrh, sluggish liver, kidney problems, bowel problems, ulcers, malnutrition, rickets, glandular insufficiency, nervous debility, and muscular weakness.

Preparations:
Decoction, fluid extract, powder and tincture.

Dosage:

Decoction	1 tablespoonful to 2 fluid ounces, between meals in an equal

	amount of water, 3 to 4 times daily.
Fluid extract	1/2-1 teaspoonful (30-60 drops).
Powder	1/2-1 teaspoon.
Tincture	1/2-1 teaspoonful (fluid teaspoon).

ADMINISTRATION

Elecampane is seldom given alone, but usually in a compound with medicines of a similar nature.

Oral

Chronic lung troubles: Use the decoction up to 1 teacupful (6 oz.) made fresh each day, omitting the glycerine. To increase the tonic quality and to obtain a slight laxative action, add 1 teaspoonful of mandrake (Podophyllum peltatum) to the dosage, at the time of administration.

Diaphoretic: Make the decoction without glycerine, and while the patient is well-covered in bed, administer as hot as can be taken in 1/2 teacupful doses until a free perspiration is obtained.

Dyspepsia: Give in small and repeated doses.

Diphtheria: Take the "General body nutritive" formula internally, and apply externally as a fomentation. See "FORMULAS".

Malnutrition, rickets, glandular insufficiency, nervous disability, weakly children, poor digestive powers, muscular weakness, and convalescence: Give the "General body nutritive" formula. See "FORMULAS".

Tooth decay: Chew the root; this preserves the teeth from putrefaction.

Tuberculosis: Use the decoction alone, or combine with echinacea. The "General body nutritive" formula can also be used. See "FORMULAS".

Whooping cough: Give the decoction of the root alone, sweetened with honey or give the "General body nutritive" formula. See "FORMULAS".

Skin

Putrid sores, cankers, and rash: Apply the agent externally as a fomentation poultice, ointment, or wash.

FORMULAS

Decoction of elecampane root

2 ounces	Elecampane root, cut or powder (Inula helenium)
1 quart	Distilled or d-cell water
4 ounces	Glycerine

Preparation: Soak the root for 2 hours in the water and bring to a boil. Simmer slowly while closely covered for 30 minutes, strain and return the liquid to the clean pot. Reduce to 3/4 pint, add the glycerine while hot and strain. Let cool, bottle, and keep in a cool place.

Dosage: 1 tablespoon in 2 fluid ounces of water, 3 to 4 times daily.

General body nutritive, flesh builder, tuberculosis, whooping cough, etc.

2 ounces	Elecampane root, cut (Inula helenium)
1 pint	Sweet almond oil (Prunus dulcis, var. dulcis; Amygdalus dulcis)
1 quart	Comfrey mucilage (Symphytum officinale)

Preparation: Place the root into the sweet almond oil, and put in a warm place, but do not boil, a double boiler with hot water is excellent. Let the mixture stand closely covered for 4 hours, stirring thoroughly every hour. Next boil the water underneath for 10 minutes, then filter the oil through a fine cotton cloth and let drip until cool enough to handle. Squeeze the oil from the cloth and let stand until cool. Add the comfrey mucilage and shake together well until the oil is uniformly suspended in the mucilage.

Dosage: 1 tablespoonful to 2 fluid ounces (according to the patient's ability to digest), sweetened with honey. Shake the bottle well immediately before pouring each dosage. Note: This formula is a wonderful substitute for cod liver oil. Dr. Shook asserts that it is far more nourishing, emollient and healing than cod liver oil or any other food extract or concentrate ever discovered or compounded by man. It is stomachic, antiseptic and germicidal.

Asthma

1/2 ounce	Elecampane (Inula helenium)
1/2 ounce	Horehound (Marrubium vulgare)
1/2 ounce	Hyssop (Hyssopus officinalis)
1/2 ounce	Vervain (Verbena officinalis)
1/2 ounce	Wild cherry (Prunus serotina; P. virginiana)
1/2 ounce	Skunk cabbage root (Symplocarpus foetidus)
1/2 teaspoon	Cayenne (Capsicum frutescens; C. minimum)
2 fluid ounces	Acid tincture of Lobelia (Lobelia inflata) see page 400 or "anti-spasmodic tincture"

Preparation: Simmer the first 6 herbs for 20 minutes in 3 parts of water. Strain while hot over the cayenne; when cool, add the lobelia and stir well.

Dosage: 2 fluid ounces (3-4 tablespoonfuls) every 3 to 4 hours.

Administration: If the bowels need attention, you may clear them with a catnip enema, or regulate them with the lower bowel tonic (also 1/4 ounce of bayberry bark (Berberis vulgaris) added to the formula will act as a cathartic).

Asthma

1/2 ounce Elecampane root (Inula helenium)
1/2 ounce Comfrey root (Symphytum officinale)
1/2 ounce Horehound (Marrubium vulgare)
1/2 ounce Black cohosh (Cimicifuga racemosa)
1/2 ounce Spikenard (Aralia racemosa)
1/2 ounce Skunk cabbage (Symplocarpus foetidus)

Preparation: Pour 3 pints of boiling hot water over the herbs and steep for 1 hour; strain and sweeten with honey.

Dosage: 2 fluid ounces every 3 to 4 hours.

Bronchitis

1 part Elecampane root (Inula helenium)
1 part Comfrey root (Symphytum officinale)
1 part Horehound (Marrubium vulgare)
1 part Wild cherry bark (Prunus serotina; P. virginiana)
1 part Spikenard (Aralia racemosa)

Preparation: Steep a heaping teaspoonful of the mixture for 30 minutes in a cup of hot water and sweeten with honey.

Dosage: 1 cupful 2 to 3 times daily.

Administration: Strain or simply drink the clear liquor.

Coughs, asthma, bronchitis, etc.

1 ounce Elecampane root, powder (Inula helenium)
1 ounce Skunk cabbage, powder (Symplocarpus foetidus)
1 ounce Aniseed, powder (Pimpinella anisum)
1 ounce Pleurisy root, powder (Asclepias tuberosa)
1/2 ounce Licorice root, powder (Glycyrrhiza glabra)
1/4 ounce Lobelia herb, powder (Lobelia inflata)

1/2 ounce	Ginger, powder (Zingiber officinalis)
1/4 ounce	Cayenne, powder (Capsicum frutescens; C. minimum)

Preparation: Mix the herb powders (all should be fine) together well, use 1 teaspoonful to each cup of hot water (1 ounce to a pint of water) and sweeten with honey or molasses.

Dosage: 2 fluid ounces to 1/2 cupful, 3 to 4 times daily.

Cough syrup

2 ounces	Elecampane root (Inula helenium)
4 ounces	Spikenard root (Aralia racemosa)
4 ounces	Marshmallow root (Althaea officinalis)
2 ounces	Blood root (Sanguinaria canadensis)
2 ounces	Coltsfoot (Tussilago farfara)
2 ounces	Boneset (Eupatorium perfoliatum)
1 ounce	White poplar or quaking aspen bark (Populus tremuloides)
2 ounces	Slippery elm bark (Ulmus rubra; U. fulva)
1/2 ounce	Senega (Polygala senega)
1/2 ounce	Lobelia herb (Lobelia inflata)

Preparation: Place the herbs in 3 pints of grain alcohol (vodka) and let stand for 14 days out of sunlight (shake occasionally), strain and add sufficient honey to make a syrup.

Dosage: 1 tablespoonful occasionally in mucilage of slippery elm.

Tuberculosis, with severe hemorrhage

1 ounce	Elecampane root (Inula helenium)
3 ounces	Comfrey root (Symphytum officinale)
1 ounce	Horehound (Marrubium vulgare)
1 ounce	Licorice root (Glycyrrhiza glabra)
1 ounce	Iceland moss (Cetraria islandica)
1/2 ounce	Peruvian bark (Cinchona calisaya)
1/4 ounce	Composition powder (see page 147-148)
1/4 teaspoon	Cayenne (Capsicum frutescens; C. minimum)
3 ounces	Acacia or gum Arabic (Acacia Senegal)
1 pound	Yellow D sugar (or 1/2 pound of honey)
1 ounce	Queen's delight, tincture (Stillingia sylvatica)
1 ounce	Antispasmodic tincture (see page 399)

Preparation: Simmer the first 7 herbs in 3 quarts of water down to 2 quarts; strain hot over the cayenne and dissolve in the sugar (or honey) and acacia. To each 14 fluid ounces add the given amount of queen's delight and antispasmodic tincture.

Dosage: (first week) 2 fluid ounces 5 to 6 times daily; (second and third weeks) increase gradually to 8 times daily.

Administration: Along with the formula, give a 1/2 pint slippery elm gruel morning and evening, also slippery elm and fresh lemon drink. Be sure to stay on the regenerative diet.

Congenial combinations:
Elecampane root combines well with echinacea root (Echinacea angustifolia; E. purpurea). Mandrake root or May apple (Podophyllum peltatum) combines well with elecampane root to increase its tonic qualities and make it slightly laxative Note: Large amounts of Podophyllum peltatum can be dangerous.

Growth characteristics:
Perennial; found mostly from Nova Scotia to the Carolinas, and westward to Minnesota and Missouri, and is common in Europe. It grows in pastures, along roadsides, and blossoms from July to September.

Sister plants:
-Fleawort or fleabane (Pulicaria dysenterica; Inula dysenterica (LINN.). Its properties and uses are similar to elecampane and is common in Europe.
-Carline Thistle (Carlina acaulis; Radix Carlinae). Properties and uses similar to elecampane; typhoid, impotence, amenorrhea, and paralysis of the tongue. It is common in Europe.

HOREHOUND
(Marrubium vulgare; LABIATAE)

Common names:
Horehound, hoarhound, white horehound, common horehound, marrubium; marrubio (Span.).

Identifying characteristics:

Stem	Square, covered with white and woolly hair (tomentose), spreading branches, numerous stems, 1-2 feet high, bushy and leafy.
Leaves	Cordate (heart-shaped) and roundish-ovate, opposite, 3/5-2 inches long, coarsely crenate, crinkly, gray-green, blunt-toothed, rough (strongly rugose-veined), power petioled, upper sessile, and white-hairy.
Flowers	Small and whitish or cream-colored, tubular, in dense maxillary whorls just above the upper leaves, 10-toothed, calyx-erect spreading and pungent.

Root	Fibrous, shot root stock and exudes a persistent bitter acid.
Taste	Aromatic and bitter, but pleasant.
Odor	Characteristic (distinct).

Part used:
Herb.

Therapeutic action:
Expectorant, tonic, stomachic, diaphoretic, bitter, slightly diuretic, emmenagogue, pectoral, aromatic, hepatic, resolvent, stimulant, cathartic (large doses), anthelmintic (vermifuge), and culinary.

Horehound is probably the most popular of the herbal remedies to the respiratory system. It is taken most frequently in the lozenge or cough drop form. It is quite effective for all pulmonary complaints as an expectorant, tonic and diaphoretic. As a mild diaphoretic, horehound will promote profuse perspiration and will relieve the hyperemic conditions of the lungs and other congestions by promoting a gentle outward flow of the blood. It has been highly valued as a soothing expectorant for at least 350 years. Culpepper wrote that "it helpeth to expectorate tough phlegm from the chest."

As an emmenagogue agent, in case of abnormal absence or suppression of the menstrual discharge (amenorrhea), it will regulate the flow and in parturition, it will assist the expulsion of after-birth.

Medicinal uses:
Hoarseness, coughs, asthma, pulmonary troubles, amenorrhea, croup, chest colds, congestion, dyspepsia, jaundice, hysteria, expelling of worms, chronic sore throat, tuberculosis, dyspnea or difficult breathing, constipation, suppressed urine, chronic rheumatism, colic, stomach ache, intermittent fever, pneumonia, chronic hepatitis, tuberculosis of the lungs, cachexia, and catarrh.

Preparations:
Concentrate, fluid extract, infusion, powder, solid extract, syrup, and tincture.

Dosage:

Concentrate	1/2-1 teaspoon.
Fluid extract	1/2-1 fluid teaspoon.
Infusion	2 fluid ounces 3 to 4 times daily.
Powder	1/4-1/2 teaspoon.
Solid extract	325 mg.-1 gram.
Syrup	1/2-1 teaspoonful.
Tincture	10-60 drops (1/6-1 teaspoon).

ADMINISTRATION

Oral

Children's cough, croup, and chest colds: Make a syrup of the infusion or concentrate and honey (as much as desired) or take the warm infusion freely.

Obstructed menstrual flow (from recent cold): Use the warm infusion with a little ginger (Zingiber officinalis) sweetened with honey.

Laxative: Take in larger doses.

Dyspepsia, jaundice, asthma, hysteria, expelling of worms: Take cold.

Asthma, dyspnea or difficult breathing: Use horehounds syrup.

FORMULAS

Biliousness

1 ounce	Horehound (Marrubium vulgare)
1 ounce	Dandelion (Taraxacum officinale)
1/2 ounce	Sweet flag (Acorus calamus)
1/4 ounce	Mountain flax (Linum catharticum)

Preparation: Simmer the herbs in 3 pints of water down to 1/2 pint, strain and let stand until cool. Bottle and keep in a cool place.

Dosage: 2 fluid ounces after meals.

Bronchial affections

1 ounce	Horehound (Marrubium vulgare)
1 ounce	Coltsfoot (Tussilago farfara)
1/2 ounce	Marshmallow root (Althaea officinalis)
1/2 ounce	Valerian (Valeriana officinalis)
1/2 ounce	Pleurisy root (Asclepias tuberosa)

Preparation: Simmer the herbs for 10 minutes in 3 pints of water, strain and sweeten. Cool, bottle and keep in a cool place.

Dosage: 2 fluid ounces 4 times daily.

Common cough

1 ounce	Horehound (Marrubium vulgare)
1/2 ounce	Hyssop (Hyssopus officinalis)
1/2 ounce	Comfrey root (Symphytum officinale)

1 ounce Licorice (Glycyrrhiza glabra)

Preparation: Simmer the herbs in 1 quart of water down to 1 pint, strain and sweeten with 6 ounces of honey. Cool, bottle and keep in a cool place.

Dosage: 1 tablespoonful as often as needed, every hour or two. Note: If the cough is excessive and the phlegm is difficult to loosen, add 1 teaspoonful of lobelia herb (Lobelia inflata) to the formula, or 1/2 ounce of the acid tincture of lobelia (see page 400) to the product.

Horehound candy

2 ounces	Horehound herb, dried (Marrubium vulgare)
1½ pints	Distilled or d-cell water
3½ pounds	Yellow D sugar

Preparation: Make a decoction of the herb by simmering down to 1 pint, add the sugar, simmer down to a due consistency of hardness, stirring occasionally. Pour into an appropriate, greased and flattened vessel. Mark into sticks or squares with a knife as it becomes hard enough to retain its shape.

Administration: Give as needed.

Growth characteristics:
Perennial; native of Europe and naturalized to the United States, where it has spread rapidly almost throughout the entire country through its abundant seeding and spreading of roots. It grows on dry, sandy fields, waste places, and roadsides. Horehound flowers from June-September. It is best to start horehound from seed.

Collection:
Gather the herb when it is just beginning to bloom.

***Sister plants*:**
Black horehound (Ballota nigra; LABIATAE). An herb with similar uses as horehound or white horehound. Some herbalists claim that it is superior for gravel, amenorrhea, menorrhagia, dysmenorrhea, dropsy, cough, hoarseness, bronchitis, consumption, stomach weakness, biliousness, bilious colic, vomiting, sour stomach, tonic to mucous membranes, and as a corrective for acrid discharges.

For lung and respiratory complaints, combine with agents such as marshmallow (Althaea officinalis), hyssop (Hyssopus officinalis), lobelia (Lobelia inflata), elecampane (Inula helenium). For parturition, toning up the uterine membranes, and reestablishing equilibrium to the parts, combine with motherwort (Leonurus cardiaca).

WILD CHERRY

(Prunus serotina; P. virginiana; P. rubra; P. obova;
Cerasus serotina; C. virginiana; ROSACEAE or DRUPACEAE)

Common names:

Wild cherry bark, choke cherry, rum cherry, wild black cherry, black cherry, Virginia prune, black choke, rub cherry, cabinet cherry, whiskey cherry; Pruni Virginianae Cortex, Virginian Prune Bark (Br.); Ecorce de Cerisier de Virginie (Fr.); Wildkirschenrinde (Ger.).

Identifying characteristics:

Stem	Large tree, 30-80 feet high (P. serotina) or 8-10 feet high, (P. virginiana or choke cherry) straight trunk, blackish and rugged outside bark. Branches on the young trees are hard, blossomy, and greenish-brown or purple. The older trees are rust brown. The bark (unrossed) has transversely elongated lenticels (cortical pores), light brown inner surface with delicate reticula (netted) striations, numerous minute fissures with short and granular fracture. Powder: light brown, with fragments of yellow brown cork and stone cells.
Leaves	Thick, oval, 2-5 inches long, smooth (glabrous), shining, bright green above and somewhat hairy on the veins beneath, serrate, glandular teeth, petiolate (stalked) and 2 small glands on the margin at the base (the leaves of the choke cherry are more sharply-toothed).
Flowers	Small and white racemes (clusters) at the ends of leafy branches, somewhat drooping, appear after the leaves (May-June).
Fruit	Drupe, very dart purple, black, (P. serotina) dark red or crimson (P. virginiana or choke) about the size of a pea, globular, pulpy, sweet and has an astringent taste that puckers the mouth. It ripens between August and September. The seed is sub-globular, bitter almond flavor, containing a bland, fixed oil.
Taste	Astringent, aromatic, agreeable bitter.
Odor	Characteristic (distinct): resembles bitter almond when macerated in water.

Part used:

Dried inner bark.

Therapeutic action:

Expectorant, tonic, astringent, pectoral, nervine, sedative, aromatic, bitter and stimulant (to digestive tract).

The wild cherry is an excellent tonic for convalescence and is a valuable remedy for all catarrhal affections. Its tonic action is mild, soothing and slightly astringent to the mucous membranes (especially those of the respiratory organs and the alvine canal). It has a volatile oil (similar to cascarilla, Virginia snake root, etc.) which acts as a local stimulant in the alimentary canal which increases the appetite and aids in digestion. When prepared in cold water, it yields hydrocyanic acid to the solution, which acts as nervine sedative, quieting nervousness, irritability and relieving heart excitement.

Medicinal uses:
Cough, consumption, bronchitis, nervous excitement, gastritis, atonic conditions of digestive organs (weakened stomach and bowels), whooping cough, dyspepsia, catarrh, fevers, scrofula, palpitation, spasms, colds, influenza, high blood pressure, diarrhea (children), asthma, hectic fever phthisis (febrile tuberculosis of the lungs), and ophthalmia (inflammation of the eye).

Preparations:
Decoction, fluid extract, infusion (volatile oil), powder, solid extract, syrup and tincture. The dried inner bark is used from all portions of the tree, but that from the root is the strongest in potency (as it deteriorates very rapidly, only the freshly-dried part should be used).

Dosage:

Decoction	2 fluid ounces 3 to 4 times daily between meals.
Fluid extract	1/2-1 teaspoonful.
Infusion	1 teacupful 3 to 4 times daily between meals.
Powder	1/4-1/2 teaspoon.
Solid extract	50-200 milligrams.
Syrup	1/2-2 teaspoonfuls.
Tincture	1/2-1 teaspoonful.

ADMINISTRATION

Oral

Cough: The syrup form is very soothing and beneficial in loosening phlegm, lessening irritability to the membranes, and quieting the nerves.

Nervine sedative: Large doses will decrease the action of the heart. It is best to combine a diffuse stimulant, such as ginger (Zingiber officinalis).

Hectic fevers: Use the warm infusion (it is much inferior to Peruvian bark).

Skin

Ophthalmia or inflammation of the eyes: Use the cold infusion.

FORMULAS

Decoction of wild cherry bark

2 ounces	Wild cherry bark, cut (Prunus serotina; P. virginiana)
12 ounces	Distilled or d-cell water

Preparation: Soak the bark 6 hours in cold water. Bring to a boil and simmer 30 minutes. Strain and cool, bottle and keep in a cool place.

Dosage: 2 fluid ounces, 3 to 4 times daily.

Bronchitis

1 ounce	Wild cherry bark (Prunus serotina; P. virginiana)
1 ounce	Wahoo (Euonymus atropurpureus)
3 teaspoons	Blood root (Sanguinaria canadensis)
1 ounce	Elecampane root (Inula helenium)
1 ounce	Comfrey root (Symphytum officinale)
1 ounce	Golden seal (Hydrastis Canadensis)

Preparation: Combine all the herbs and simmer 20 minutes slowly, using 1 teaspoonful of the combination to a cup of water.

Dosage: 1 teaspoon of the infusion each 1/2 hour, more or less as needed.

Dr. Nowell's cough syrup
(common cough, asthma, bronchitis, etc.)

1 ounce	Wild cherry bark (Prunus serotina; P. virginiana)
1 ounce	Horehound (Marrubium vulgare)
1 ounce	Aniseed (Pimpinella anisum)
1/2 ounce	Elecampane root (Inula helenium)
1/4 ounce	Lobelia root (Lobelia inflata)
1 pound	Honey

Preparation: Place the honey in 1½ pints of water, bring to a simmer and remove any scum. Add the herbs and simmer well-covered for 15 minutes; strain (the produce should be 2½ pints) and add 1 pint raspberry vinegar.

Dosage: 1 tablespoonful every 1 to 3 hours, adult; 2 teaspoons for children 12 years and younger.

Cough syrup

4 ounces	Wild cherry bark (Prunus serotina; P. virginiana)
1 ounce	Elecampane root (Inula helenium)
1 ounce	Spikenard root (Aralia racemosa)

1 ounce Lippia (Lippia dulcis)
1/4 ounce Lobelia herb (Lobelia inflata)

Preparation: Make a syrup of 1 pound of honey in 1½ pints of water (as given in the foregoing formula), add the herbs, cool and simmer for 20 minutes. Strain, bottle, and keep in a cool place.

Dosage: Tablespoonful doses as needed.

Pulmonary, chest, bronchial and catarrhal affections

4 parts Wild cherry bark, cut (Prunus serotina; P. virginiana)
3 parts Yerba santa leaves, cut (Eriodictyon californicum)
9 parts Cascarilla bark, cut (Croton eleuteria)
2 parts Irish moss, cut (Chondrus crispus)
2 parts Hyssop, cut (Hyssopus officinalis)
6 parts Elecampane root, cut (Inula helenium)
1 part Asthma weed, cut (Euphorbia pilulifera; E. hirta)
2 parts Aniseed (Pimpinella anisum)

Preparation: Mix the herbs well; use 1 teaspoon of the mixture to each cup of water and place in an appropriate vessel. Simmer 3 to 4 minutes, then steep for 10 minutes; strain, sweeten with honey, keep it cool place.

Dosage: 1 cupful before and/or after meals, and upon retiring at night.

Congenial combinations:
Wild cherry combines well with alimentary stimulants such as Virginia snake root (Aristolochia serpentaria) and cascarilla (Croton eleuteria).

Growth characteristics:
Perennial; ranges generally throughout the United States, growing in the woods and open places. P. serotina grows in fertile soil in fields, woods, along fences, and seldom in clusters (the wood is valuable for furniture, being hard, red, fine-grained, and easily polished).

Collection:
Best gathered in autumn, immediately rossed (deprived of the outside layer by scraping or shaving the outer bark and exposing green phelloderm). The young, thin bark is best, and that of very large or small branches should be rejected. Be sure bark is rossed and not mixed with old stems.

Drying and preservation:
The bark should be kept dry and in tightly-closed containers. The inner bark of the root deteriorates quite rapidly, so it needs to be used fresh or recently dried.

***Sister plants*:**
Cherry; fruit and bark; pulmonary complaints, cough, bronchitis, tuberculosis, heart troubles, stomach troubles, dyspepsia, fever, high blood pressure.

LICORICE
(Glycyrrhiza glabra; G. glandulifera; G. echinata; G. lepidota; LEGUMINOSAE (subfamily FABOIDEAE)

Common names:
Licorice root, liquorice root, sweetwood, Spanish juice root, lick weed, Italian juice root; Glycyrrhizae Radix (Br.); Reglisse, Bois de Reglisse-doux, Racine douce (Fr.); Radix Liquiritis Suessholz, Spanisches Seussholz, Lakritzenholz (Ger.); regiliz (Span.).

Identifying characteristics:

Stem	2-5 feet high erect, striated, few branches, several arising from the thick rhizome (crown). G. glabra (G. glandulifera or Russian variety): somewhat pubescent (hairy).
Leaves	Imparipinnate, leaflets in pairs of 4-7, ovate, entire, smooth, dark green and glutinous (gluey) beneath. G. glabra (Russian): hairy and glandular beneath.
Flowers	Purplish or yellowish-white, pea-shaped, in racemes (elongated axis bearing flowers on short stems in succession toward the apex).
Root	G. glabra (Spanish): Nearly cylindrical, upper portion, somewhat knotty 6-8 inches long, 1/5-4/5 inch thick, yellowish-brown to dark brown, wrinkled longitudinally, coarsely fibrous fracture, internally yellow, porous wood, prominent alternate buds on thinner rhizomes and distinct corky patches on thicker rhizomes. Powder: brownish-yellow with reddish-brown cork cells. G. glabra (Russian): nearly cylindrical, somewhat tapering, sometimes split longitudinally, 6-12 inches long, 2/5-2 inches thick pale yellow when outer cork layer removed, coarsely fibrous fracture and radially cleft wood. Powder: yellow without cork cells.
Taste	Spanish: Sweetish and slightly acrid. Russian: less sweet.
Odor	Characteristic.

Part used:
Dried rhizome and root.

Therapeutic action:
Demulcent, expectorant, emollient, flavoring, pectoral, aperient, slightly stimulant and sialogogue.

Licorice is very soothing and softens the mucous membranes, and at the same time, it is cleansing of catarrhal affections, especially of the respiratory tract. It has an agreeable taste and increases the flow of saliva and mucus when slowly chewed or sucked; the increased secretions act as emollients to the throat. Licorice is one of the oldest, mildest and yet most efficient laxatives (aperients), and is especially safe and effective for delicate or constipated children, or for adults having stomach weakness who are unable to take the stronger laxatives (cathartics). It softens, soothes, lubricates, and nourishes the intestinal tract.

It soothes and heals any inflamed mucous membranes and catarrhal conditions. It is a corrective agent for other stronger herbal laxatives (strong cathartics and purgatives), modifying their action. It is excellent to cover the taste of agrimony or other bitters in herbal preparations (such as senega, guaiacum, senna, etc.), and the powdered extract or root is excellent as an excipient (substance used to give preparations a suitable form or consistency) in pills and demulcent troches or lozenges. The chief active principle in licorice is a substance known as glycyrrhizin or glycyrrhizic acid, which is 50 times sweeter than sugar cane and while other sweets will increase the thirst, licorice will alleviate thirst. It also contains phytosterols that facilitate estrogen production (female hormone).

Medicinal uses:
Cough, sore throat, hoarseness, wheezing, dyspnea, chest and lung complaints, febrile catarrhal conditions, bronchitis, hemorrhoids, bowel and urinary affections, inflammation of mucous membrane and skin, and gastric ulcers. It acts as a medicinal excipient, cover for bitter herbs, and a coating for pills.

Preparations:
Decoction, elixir, fluid extract, infusion, powder, syrup and tincture. The black, dry, very brittle licorice, with a shiny fracture is the best grade to use.

Dosage:

Decoction	1 teaspoonful to 1 tablespoonful as required.
Fluid extract	1/2 teaspoonful.
Infusion	2 fluid ounces, 3 to 4 times daily.
Powder	1/2-1 teaspoon.
Syrup	1 teaspoonful to 1 tablespoonful or more as required.
Tincture	1/2-1 teaspoonful

ADMINISTRATION

Licorice is generally used in combination with other aids.

Oral

Cough, hoarseness, sore throat, etc.: Use the syrup (see “FORMULAS”).

Laxative, hemorrhoids: Licorice powder when taken internally will in 10 to 15 hours (3 to 6 hours on an empty stomach) free and soften stools without griping. It is especially valuable for persons suffering from hemorrhoids, as the softer or fluid stools resulting from licorice powder lessens the pain produced by normal movement of the bowels. It is best given at bedtime.

Skin

Inflamed surface: Licorice as a syrup, wash, etc. is soothing and protecting.

FORMULAS

Syrup of licorice

4 ounces	Licorice root, cut or powdered (Glycyrrhiza glabra)
1 quart	Distilled or d-cell water
1½ pounds	Yellow D sugar (or 3/4 pound of honey)

Preparation: Stir the herb into the water while cold; cover and soak for 2 hours, stir, and slowly bring to the boiling point. Boil slowly for 15 minutes; strain and return to a clean vessel. Bring to boiling point again, stir in the sugar (or honey), continue stirring until dissolved; remove from heat and allow to cool while stirring occasionally.

Dosage: 1 tablespoonful or more 3 to 4 times daily (regulate dosage according to bowel movements). Children: 1 teaspoonful to 1 tablespoonful 2 to 3 times daily (according to condition).

Cough syrup
(asthma, bronchitis, croup, whooping cough, etc.)

1 ounce	Licorice (Glycyrrhiza glabra)
1 ounce	Slippery elm (Ulmus rubra; U. fulva)
1 ounce	Boneset (Eupatorium perfoliatum)
1 ounce	Flaxseed or linseed (Linum usitatissimum)
1 pint	Molasses
1/2 pound	Yellow D sugar

Preparation: Simmer the herbs for 20 minutes in 1 quart of water. Strain and add the molasses and sugar, stirring the mixture thoroughly, and bottle.

Dosage: 1 tablespoonful as needed.

Persistent and irritated cough
(chest complaints)

1 ounce	Licorice root, cut or powdered (Glycyrrhiza glabra)

1/2 cupful	Flaxseed or linseed whole or crushed (Linum usitatissimum)
1 teaspoon	Lemon juice (Citrus limon)

Preparation: Simmer the first 2 ingredients in 1 quart of water to syrup consistency; strain and add the lemon juice.

Dosage: Give freely warm or cold. Children: up to 1 teacupful.

Growth characteristics:
Perennial; root penetrates deeply into the ground. Indigenous to Spain, southern Italy, Greece, Asia Minor, Syria, Iraq, Russia and northern China (similar latitudes as the lemon and orange). Licorice is cultivated in many parts of the world and planted by cuttings in rows 4 feet apart. Large quantities of the root are imported from Europe (Alicante, Tortosa, Hamburg) for medicines, beverages, foods, etc. and even greater quantities of the fluid extract are imported (principally from Spain).

Collection:
Commercially. In the autumn of the fourth year the roots are dug when they are the sweetest (before the plants have borne fruit, which exhausts sweetness in the sap) by removing 2 to 3 feet of earth. This exposes the subterranean portion of the herb and allows the whole plant to be easily uprooted, where the roots are severed, cleaned, washed, trimmed, assorted, cut and marketed in bundles, bales and bags.

Drying and preservation:
The Spanish variety is usually unpeeled, but there is bitterness and acidity in the bark, which constitutes only about 1/10 of the world consumption. The Russian variety is usually peeled, larger, richer in glycyrrhizin and active principles, and is in greater demand.

Sister plants:
-Rest Harrow (Ononis spinosa); root; odor and taste similar to licorice.
-Indian or Wild Licorice (Abrus precatorius); root; cultivated in India and Brazil; a substitute for licorice.

HOLLYHOCK
(Alcea rosea; Althaea rosea; MALVACEAE)

Common names:
Hollyhock, common hollyhock, garden hollyhock, Althaea rose, malva flowers, bysmallow, hollyhock-holler, hollek, hollinhocke, holyhoke; Passe-ro-Rose tremiere (Fr.); Stockrosen (Ger.); Alcea rossa, Malva rosa, Rosa di mare (Ital.); Malva arborea, Mal Roca, Malva real, Malva rosea (Span.).

Identifying characteristics:

Stem	Tall, simple, and hairy.
Flowers	Large, 3-5 inches broad, on very short peduncles (nearly sessile) and forming a long spike, 5 petals (corolla) are all shades of purple, rose white, or yellow (usually purple), tomentose (fine, matted hair) calyx, petals and stamens unite to form a tube.

Part used:
Flowers, leaves and roots.

***Therapeutic action*:**
Emollient, demulcent, and diuretic

Hollyhock has a therapeutic action and use similar to marshmallow (Althaea officinalis), but it is not quite as mucilaginous. It is very beneficial in chest and bronchial complaints, and it is especially soothing to the mucous membrane. It has a marked influence on the kidneys, bladder and urinary organs.

***Medicinal uses*:**
Bronchial troubles, inflammation of the bladder, etc.

Preparations:
Fluid extract, infusion, powder, and tincture.

Dosage:
Use the same as marshmallow root.

Fluid extract	1/2-2 teaspoonfuls.
Infusion	1 teacupful, 3 to 4 times daily.
Powder	2 #00 capsules each hour until pain leaves, then as needed.
Tincture	1/2-1 teaspoonful.

ADMINISTRATION

Refer to page 355 on marshmallow.

FORMULAS

See pages 358-363 using hollyhock in place of the marshmallow.

Congenial combinations:
Hollyhock combines with comfrey (Symphytum officinale) and is more beneficial when used with other remedies. For inflammations, the adding of slippery elm will assist healing action.

***Sister plants*:**
Marshmallow (Althaea officinalis; MALVACEAE); root, see page 355.

See Chapter 17 for expectorant and demulcent herbs to be used when the forego-ing are not available.

CHAPTER 10

LOBELIA

The herbalist Samuel Thomson is famous for promoting Lobelia during the nineteenth century. He discovered the herb when only a child, although the Native Americans had been using it for many years previous.

> Sometime in the summer, after I was four years old [1773], being out in the fields in search of the cows, I discovered a plant which had a singular branch and pods that I had never seen before. I had the curiosity to pick some of the pods and chew them. The taste and operation produced was so remarkable that I never forgot it. Afterwards, I used to induce other boys to chew it, merely by way of sport, to see them vomit. I tried this herb in this way for nearly twenty years, without knowing anything of its medicinal virtues.
>
> I had at that time [8 years old] a very good knowledge of the principal roots and herbs to be found in that part of the country, with their names and medicinal uses. The neighbors were in the habit of getting me to go with them to show them such roots and herbs as the doctors ordered to be made use of in sickness for syrups, etc. and by way of sport they used to call me doctor. While in the field at work, I often used to find the herb, which I tasted when four years old, and gave it to those who worked with me, to see them spit and vomit, but I never observed any bad effects produced by it, which simple experiments eventually led me to observe the value of it in disease.
>
> The herb which I had discovered when four years old, I had often met with; but it had never occurred to me that it was of any value as a medicine, until about this time [1791-1794]—when mowing in a field with a number of men one day, I cut a sprig of it, and gave it to the man next to me, who ate it; when we got to the end of the piece, which was about six rods, he said he believed what I had given him would kill him, for he never felt this way before. I looked at him and saw that he was in a most profuse perspiration, being as wet all over as he could be; he trembled very much, and there was no more color in him than a corpse. I told him to go to the spring and drink some water; he attempted to go and got as far as the wall, but was unable to get over it, and laid down on the ground and vomited several times. He said he thought he threw off his stomach two quarts. I then helped him into the house, and in about two hours he ate a very hearty dinner and in the afternoon was able to do a good half day's labor. He afterwards told me that he never had anything do him so much good in his life; his appetite was remarkably good, and he felt better than he had felt for a long time. This cir-

cumstance gave me the first idea of the medicinal virtues of this valuable plant; which I have since found, by twenty years' experience, (in which time I have made use of it in every disease I have met with, to great advantage), to be a discovery of the greatest importance. (*Narrative of the Life of Samuel Thomson*, pp. 17, 19, 30-31).

LOBELIA
(Lobelia inflata; LOBELIACEAE)

Common names:
Lobelia, puke weed, emetic herb, emetic weed, Indian tobacco, asthma weed, gag root, vomitwort, eyebright, wild tobacco, or bladderpod.

Identifying characteristics:

Stem	Cylindrical and angular, hairy, 6 inches to 3 feet high. It has a yellowish-green color.
Leaves	Alternate, ovate-lanceolate (oblong), serrate, veiny, hairy, and pale green in color.
Flowers	Numerous, small and pale blue in color, positioned on long, loose racemes with short pedicels.
Fruit	Inflated, two-celled oval capsule, containing a number of small (1/2 to 1/3 inch long), ovate-oblong, light brown seeds. These are coarsely reticulated on the outer surface.
Odor	Slight and irritating.
Taste	Strongly acrid, resembling tobacco.

Part used:
Herb and seeds (the latter are much stronger).

Therapeutic action:
Antispasmodic, emetic, stimulant (in small doses), relaxant (in larger doses); nervine (sedative), expectorant, anti-venomous, counter-irritant, emmenagogue, diaphoretic, diuretic, cathartic, astringent, and a nauseant.

Lobelia is one of the greatest herbs ever given to the world. If the herb is used skillfully, we concur with Dr. Thomson that "there is no vegetable which the earth produces more harmless in its effect on the human system, and none more powerful in removing disease and promoting health than lobelia." Lobelia is a general corrector of the whole system, as it is easily diffused and able to influence the entire body. Lobelia is an efficient relaxant, and is believed to be the best counter-irritant known to mankind. Its action is felt immediately on the serous, mucous, muscular and nervous systems, especially the sympathetic nervous system. As a powerful antispasmodic, lobelia causes immediate relaxation and expansion of any contracted parts of the respiratory system, such as bronchial tubes, esophagus, glottis and larynx. This allows the "breath of life" (oxygenized blood) to flow freely to the tissues. Lobelia is especially important in removing obstruction and congestion within the body, especially the blood vessels. If there is depression through the vasomotor system, it corrects this, and strengthens the muscular action of the vessel walls which propel the blood, thus being a key to health throughout the body.

Lobelia is a selective herb. When a fetus is dead, or in an extremely weakened condition, lobelia will cause it to abort. However, if the fetus is well and healthy, and the mother is weak, it will cause the mother to heal and strengthen, enabling her to carry the child until the proper time of delivery. Lobelia accurately and intelligently selects which way it is to go. It is truly a "thinking" herb.

Throughout the years of Dr. Christopher's practice, lobelia was administered many times, with numerous miraculous healings. Time after time, lobelia has helped the very young to the very old, with positive results when used correctly. As for lobelia being a poison, this myth has been promulgated by allopaths to dissuade potential patients from using this God-given herb and being healed. Once Dr. Christopher quickly swallowed as much as four tablespoons of honey-sweetened tincture of lobelia at one time, mistaking it for apple cider vinegar. After retching and vomiting profusely from the emetic properties of the herb, he felt nothing but improvement, and suffered no damage whatsoever, only a good cleaning out!

The belief that lobelia is a dangerous poison (including the statement in Joseph Meyer's *The Herbalist,* that "lobelia is too dangerous for internal use by the unskilled") began with Dr. Samuel Thomson's amazing success as a country herbal doctor. His achievements exposed the inadequacy of then-current orthodox inorganic theories and practices. This incited professional jealousy, because patients chose Thomson's herbal cures over the orthodox physicians, losing them prestige and money. When Dr. Thomson could not be easily removed from the scene by the usual maneuver of filing "malpractice" charges, the medical profession organized to legislate their craft as the only legal medical practice.

Dr. Nowell said this concerning the misclassification of lobelia as a "poison:"

> So successfully did he (Dr. Thomson) use it, that the regulars of his day classed it a poison, as some writers said only a poison could bring about the speedy results that Dr. Thomson obtained by its use. If the student goes to buy a one-ounce package of the herb from the drug store, he will find it labelled poison, and in practically all the official works such as B.P., the C.P., the U.S.P. and the American Dispensatory, etc. It is classed as a poison.

That it has no poisonous properties we very definitely affirm. Dr. H. Nowell used it for nearly thirty years, in all manner of cases, and at all ages. We have friends who have likewise used it freely, and if half that is said against it by the medical world were true, thousands should have been dead from its use. It is a very powerful herb, however, and, like other powerful herbs, must be used wisely.

Throughout all the nineteenth-century prosecutions, there was never been a single instance of harm resulting from the use of lobelia. Even back in Thomson's day there were studies showing its safety. Prof. W. (William) Tully of Yale College, wrote to Dr. H. Lee of Middletown, Conn., March 22nd, 1838:

> Lobelia inflata is entirely destitute of any narcotic powers. I have been in the habit of employing this article for twenty-seven years, in large quantities and for a long period, without the least trace of any narcotic effect. I have used the very best official tincture in the quantity of three fluid ounces in twenty-four hours, and for four and seven days in succession, and I have likewise given three large tablespoonfuls of it within half an hour, without the least indication of any narcotic operation.
>
> I have known four and five tobacco pipes full of it smoked in immediate succession and without any narcosis, and I have also known it to be given by enema with the same result. . . .Dr. Bigelow, of Boston, was the first person who ascribed narcotic powers to this agent, and he did this in 1817, but not from his own observation. I am confident (the old women's stories in the books are to the contrary notwithstanding) that Lobelia inflata is a valuable, a safe, and a sufficiently gentle article of medicine, and I think the time will come when it will be much better appreciated.

The final absurdity of this whole issue is the alternative—the truly poisonous, inorganic antidotes that are offered by orthodoxy in most official publications as "remedies" against purported lobelia "poisoning." The following is an example:

> Place in recumbent position, empty stomach if vomiting has not been free, give tannin, cardiac and respiratory stimulants, strychnine, thebaine, alcohol, atropine or belladonna, digitalis, morphine, artificial heat, ergot or castor oil.

Medicinal uses:
Abscesses, adynamia (weakness), angina pectoris (heart excitability), asthma, blood poisoning, blood circulation problems, boils, bronchial problems, bruises, catarrh, chicken pox, cold sweats, colds, colic, congestion, constipation, convulsions, cough, cramps, croup, digestive disturbances (nervous dyspepsia, acute indigestion, etc.), drowning, dyspnea, diphtheria, earache, eczema, epilepsy, fainting, febrile troubles (fevers), felons, female problems, heart weakness, hepatitis, hydrophobia (mad dog bites), hysteria, inflammations, insect stings and bites, laryngitis, measles, meningitis, nephritis, nervousness, palpitation, peritonitis, periostitis, phrenitis, pleurisy, pneumonia, poison ivy, poison oak, rheuma-

tism, ringworm, scarlet fever, smallpox, spasms (spine, muscles, chest, or genital organs), sprains, stomach irritation (small doses), tetanus (lock jaw), vomiting (small doses), whooping cough, and zymotic diseases.

Lobelia will allay and regulate violent pains in the loins during labor, which are due to the rigidity of the passages.

Thomson writes:

> In cases where the spasms are so violent that they are stiff, and the jaws become set, by pouring some of this liquid into the mouth between the cheek and teeth, as soon as it touches the glands roots of the tongue, the spasms will relax, and the jaw will become loosened so that the mouth will open; then give a dose of it, and as soon as the spasms have abated, repeat it. After this, administer appropriate restorative or tonic herbs.

Preparations:
Decoction, fluid extract, infusion, pills, poultice, powder, syrup, and tincture. Do not use lobelia tincture from drug stores, as it is extracted with an etheric menstruum.

Infusion:	The seed is best used when crushed.
Powder:	Use the leaves, stems, flowers and/or pods.
Tincture:	Use the green or dried herb.

Dosage:
With prudence, lobelia may be given in either small or large doses, at shorter or longer intervals.

Decoction	1/2 cupful.
Fluid Extract	10 to 30 drops.
Infusion	1 cupful.
Powder	200-650 milligrams.
Solid Extract	100-300 milligrams.
Syrup	1 to 4 teaspoons.
Tincture	1/2 to 1 teaspoonful, or 10 to 30 drops.

ADMINISTRATION

Lobelia rapidly influences all parts of the body. However, due to its highly diffusible nature, it should always be used with a more permanent stimulant such as cayenne or peppermint.

Anal

For fevers, pneumonia, pleurisy, nephritis, hepatitis, meningitis, etc.: Add lobelia to a catnip enema.

Oral

Asthma: Lobelia tincture is excellent as an emetic to free breathing and promote healing.

Hepatitis: See "FORMULAS."

Hydrophobia: Steep 1 tablespoonful of lobelia in 1 pint of boiling water and drink as much as possible to induce vomiting and cleansing of the stomach. Follow this mixture with a high enema of lobelia and catnip.

Pleurisy: Give lobelia and pleurisy root in an infusion.

Typhoid, typhus, spotted fever, scarlet fever, etc.: Give 1 teaspoonful of Antispasmodic tincture (see "FORMULAS") in a little warm water every 1/2 hour. Wash the body daily, with 2 parts of hot water and 1 part apple cider vinegar. Change bedclothes and sheets daily, and give the patient warm water every 2 hours.

Baby convulsions: Place a drop or two of the Antispasmodic tincture on the tip of the finger and put it into the baby's mouth. This will stop the problem immediately.

Painful cramps and spasms: Give one teaspoonful of Antispasmodic tincture in 1/2 cup of sweetened warm water. This action will take about 15 seconds.

Skin

Earache: Place a few drops of warm lobelia tincture in the ear and plug it with cotton.

Mucus and spasmodic congestion (especially babies): Rub lobelia tincture into the neck, chest, and between the shoulders.

For any external problems: Apply a poultice consisting of 1 part lobelia and 2 parts slippery elm.

Swellings, pneumonia, pleurisy, boils, etc.: Make a compress or plaster of lobelia, of hops, bran, or lard.

Rheumatic fever: Rub the whole body from the neck to the toes with Antispasmodic tincture. In bad cases (where the patient cannot sit up or move the arms or legs), give 1 teaspoonful of Antispasmodic tincture in a little hot water every 1/2 hour until the patient perspires freely. Keep the patient in bed and allow him to cool down; then wash him with apple cider vinegar and hot water. Give the patient 1 teaspoonful of Antispasmodic tincture in hot water every 2 hours during the first day, and every 3 hours for a few days thereafter. When the case demands, rub some Antispasmodic tincture externally at the base of the skull and neck and along the sternum, and be sure to sponge the patient with apple cider vinegar and hot water.

FORMULAS

Antispasmodic tincture
(epilepsy, convulsions, lockjaw, delirium, tremors, fainting, hysteria, cramps, suspended animation, etc.)

1 ounce	Lobelia seed, crushed (Lobelia inflata)
1 ounce	Skullcap (Scutellaria lateriflora)
1 ounce	Skunk cabbage (Symplocarpus foetidus)
1 ounce	Gum myrrh (Commiphora myrrha, var. molmol)
1 ounce	Black cohosh (Cimicifuga racemosa)
1/2 ounce	Cayenne (Capsicum frutescens; C. minimum)

Preparation: Macerate in at least 1 pint of grain alcohol (use enough alcohol to cover all the herbs) in a tightly capped vessel, and shake well at least once a day. After 10 to 14 days, strain, squeeze or press out the liquid.

Dosage: 1 to several drops.

Liver problems, jaundiced skin

1 part	Lobelia (Lobelia inflata)
1 part	Pleurisy root (Asclepias tuberosa)
1 part	Catnip (Nepeta cataria)
1 part	Bitter root (Apocynum androsaemifolium)

Preparation: Mix the herbs well and steep 1 teaspoon of this combination in 1 cup of boiling water for 15 to 20 minutes; strain.

Dosage: 2 tablespoonfuls every 2 hours, hot.

Tincture of lobelia

2 ounces	Lobelia herb, stem, flowers, and leaves (Lobelia inflata)
2 ounces	Crushed lobelia seed (Lobelia inflata)
1 pint	Apple cider vinegar

Preparation: Macerate in a tightly capped bottle for 10 to 14 days. Shake every time you walk by it, or at least once a day. Strain off the liquid, and bottle it for use. When making a simple tincture of lobelia, vinegar is the menstruum of choice over alcohol.

Acid tincture of lobelia

2 ounces	Crushed lobelia seed (Lobelia inflata)
1/2 ounce	Lobelia herb (stems, flowers, and leaves)
1 teaspoonful	Cayenne (Capsicum frutescens; C. minimum)
1 pint	Apple cider vinegar

Preparation: Same as tincture of lobelia.

Syrup of lobelia

2½ ounces	Lobelia herb (Lobelia inflata)
2 pints	Distilled or d-cell water

Preparation: Simmer this mixture down to 1 pint. Strain and dissolve 2 pounds of raw sugar or 1 pound of honey into it.

Dosage: 1 teaspoonful (for coughs); 1/2 to 1 cupful as an emetic.

Puerperal convulsions

2 teaspoons	Lobelia fluid extract (Lobelia inflata)
4 teaspoons	Ladies slipper fluid extract (Cypripedium calceolus)
1/2 teaspoon	Cayenne tincture (Capsicum frutescens; C. minimum)
6 ounces	Honey water or simple syrup

Dosage: 1 teaspoonful every 1/2 hour.

Compound lobelia capsules (dyspepsia, rheumatism, inflammation, asthma, consumption, chills, jaundice and fevers)

1 ounce	Lobelia herb powder (Lobelia inflata)
1 ounce	Lobelia seed powder (Lobelia inflata)
1 ounce	Cayenne powder (Capsicum frutescens; C. minimum)
2 ounces	Acacia vera or Gum Arabic powder (Acacia Senegal)
1 ounce	Anise seed, powdered (Pimpinella anisum)

Preparation: Mix and fill into #0 capsules.

Dosage: 2 to 6 capsules per day, as the case requires.

Congenial combinations:
During labor, lobelia allays pain and regulates the muscular action of the uterus. For menstrual disorders, when lobelia is used with agents such as pennyroyal, the pain and contraction are relieved and normalcy is established. As a general rule,

lobelia should always be preceded by or given in combination with a stimulant. When used as a relaxant, do not combine with cayenne or golden seal, but with a more diffusive agent, such as ginger. When used as an emetic, lobelia should be preceded with a stimulating tea such as peppermint or cayenne.

CASE HISTORY

The great healing and relieving agent.
Many individuals have learned the great value of lobelia. Students at Dr. Christopher's school, suffering from some injury, such as hitting a finger with a hammer, have immediately soaked the injured part in tincture of lobelia. This removed the pain at once.

Lobelia, in combination with other herbs, quickly draws out both pain and congested blood. Just a few drops of tincture of lobelia in the ear speedily relieves earache. Convulsing babies have been instantly calmed by rubbing a few drops of lobelia into the gums or mouth. Terrific pain from muscle over-exertion has been abated by massaging lobelia into the affected muscles. This relief has been so quick, patients have called it "blessed." Tincture of lobelia is also very useful in combating blood poisoning.

Many births have been markedly eased by the use of lobelia, despite the mother's past history of difficult deliveries. With the use of lobelia, a dead fetus will be passed in abortion, rather than remaining inside the mother's body. People writhing in pain and rolling on the floor have been immediately calmed with the administering of one half-teaspoonful of tincture of lobelia. There are so many cases of miraculous healings with the use of lobelia that it would take pages to cite the details. There is truly no end to the ways in which lobelia may be used to heal and regenerate the body.

Be wise when using lobelia. There have been cases of respiratory arrest when a person took too much lobelia, particularly without an accompanying stimulant. One mother massaged her colicky baby's back with the tincture, without apparent results. She then gave the baby a drop of the tincture on his tongue. He vomited, and then passed out. The poison control center was contacted, and she was told just to hold the baby and wait till the effects of the herb passed through the system (poison control has no record of any harm caused by lobelia). After about an hour, the baby recovered. The mother, having seen the powerful potential of lobelia was more cautious after that. As you use lobelia, be aware of how powerful it can be.

A specific for asthma.
A Dr. Christopher case history told is his own words: Lobelia is well known for its great value in curing asthma. I had an interesting experience during my practice in Evanston, Wyoming more than twenty years ago. One night, after getting up for night calls and finally retiring at 2 a.m., I heard a knock at the door. There

stood two young fellows carrying a wizened little gentleman between them. They asked, "Can you help Dad? We can't reach his regular doctor, who has cared for him all these years, and he needs help." We brought him in and gave him a cup of peppermint tea. He had to sit up, because he had not been able to lie in bed for over twenty years. He had suffered severe asthma attacks for twenty-six years, and for twenty of those years had been propped up at night and could sleep for only short spells of thirty minutes or so. He had been under heavy medication during all that time, with no hope of ever getting well. After the peppermint tea had been down fifteen minutes or so, I gave him a teaspoonful of tincture of lobelia, followed ten minutes later with a second teaspoonful. He started to throw up phlegm from his lungs. During the time that the emetic principle was working and bringing up phlegm from his lungs and bronchial cavities, he ejected over a cupful of varicolored materials, ranging from light to dark, plus other liquids. At five o'clock, we released him, and the boys took him home. Two days later, I heard the results. Instead of being propped up as usual in the chair, he said to his boys: "I'm going to lie in a bed; I can sleep tonight." For the first time in twenty years, he slept the full night in a bed, and he has slept in a bed from that day on. As a result of his asthma, he had never been able to hold a job for over twenty years; but that same week he went out and got a job as a gardener.

Growth characteristics:
Lobelia is an annual plant in warm latitudes and a biennial in moderate and northern latitudes. Lobelia is found in meadows, pastures, woods, and grassy places in nearly all parts of the United States. It flowers from July to September. Thomson writes:

> The emetic herb may be found in the first stages of its growth at all times through the summer. It ranges from the size of a six-cent piece to that of a dollar and larger, lying flat on the ground in a round form, like a rose pressed flat. This is to bear the weight of the snow which covers it during the winter, as it is subject to be winterkilled, like wheat. In the spring, it appears yellow and pale, like other things suffering from wet and cold; but when the returning summer spreads enlivening rays upon it, it lifts up its leaves and shoots forth a stalk to the height of twelve to fifteen inches, with a number of branches carrying its leaves with its growth. In July, it puts forth small, pointed, pale blue blossoms, which are followed by small pods about the size of a white bean. These contain numerous very small seeds. This pod exactly resembles the human stomach, having an inlet and outlet higher than the middle; from the inlet, it receives nourishment, and by the outlet, it discharges the seeds.
>
> This plant is common in all parts of this country, wherever the land is fertile enough to yield support for its inhabitants. It is found on every variety of soil which is used for cultivation; from the highest mountains, to the lowest valleys. In hot and wet seasons, it is most plentiful on dry and warm lands; in hot and dry seasons, on clayey and heavy lands.

> When the season is cold (either wet or dry), it rarely makes its appearance; and if the summer and fall are very dry, the seeds do not come up, and of course, there will be very little of this herb to be found the next season. In season when the herb is plentiful, it may be found growing in highways and pastures; by the sides of old turnpikes, and in stubble land; particularly when it has been laid down to grass the year before. When grass is scarce, it is eaten by cattle, and it is hard to be found when full grown. It is a wild plant and a native of this country; but there is no doubt of its being common to other countries. It may he transplanted and cultivated in gardens, and it will be much larger and more vigorous than when growing wild. If some stalks are left, it sows itself, and probably may be produced from the seed.

Collection:
The whole lobelia plant is active, and should be gathered from the last part of July to the middle of October. Thomson writes:

> It comes to maturity about the first of September, when the leaves and pods turn a little yellow; this is the best time to gather it. . . . I have been in search of this herb from Boston to Canada, and was not able to collect more than two pounds; and in some seasons, I have not been able to collect any. I mention this to show the uncertainty of its growth, and to warn people to be careful and lay up a good stock of it when plenty. In the year 1807, if I had offered a reward of a thousand dollars for a pound of this herb, I should not have been able to have obtained it. I have seen times that I would have given two dollars for an ounce of the powder, but there was none to be had, and this necessity taught me to lay up all I could obtain when it was plenty.
>
> This plant is different in one very important particular from all others that I have a knowledge of; that is, the same quantity will produce the same effect in all stages of its growth, from the first appearance till it comes to maturity; but the best time for gathering it, as before mentioned, is when the leaves and pods begin to turn yellow; for then the seeds are ripe, and you have all there can be of it. It should then be cut and kept clean, and spread in a chamber or loft to dry, where it can be open to the air in the day time, and shut from the damp air during the night.

Drying and preserving:
The best form in which to preserve lobelia is the tincture form. It should not be stored in paper, as both the herb and the seeds contain a volatile oil that can be readily absorbed and lost.

CHAPTER 11

THE NERVINE AND ANTISPASMODIC HERBS

Thomas Deschauer writes concerning the nervous system:

> The nerves are like a network of electrical wires in a city. Here electricity or power is carried to every home and factory to supply light and to run machinery, street cars, etc. Small wires are used where little power is in demand, while heavy loads are carried over cables. The proper wire is important. If a wire is too light or too fragile for the current, it might give way, and we would have a breakdown in the electrical system.

Instead of electricity, our *nerve network* carries nerve fluid. This fluid behaves in the same manner as electricity; it runs like the chemical apparatus of our bodies, and instigates and keeps up the flow of the different secretions of the various organs of the body. We have a large nerve-wire and a mass of fine lines that radiate from it. The nerve wires are only as strong as their fiber, and fiber is built and wasted every day. It all depends on you, on how strong or how weak you keep these fibers, for the nerves, like all parts of the body, depend upon the health of the blood and on the daily habits of your life for strength and efficiency.

Never use drugs to stimulate the nerves, as this will do more harm than good. Don't use chemical sedatives or stimulants, but remove the causes of nervousness by avoiding incorrect habits of eating and drinking, and by avoiding worry. Unhealthy eating habits poison the system, filling it up with acids which irritate the nerve fibers and cause inflammation of the nerves, sciatica, etc. Avoid excessive eating and drinking, and especially avoid sexual excesses. Proper rest is also important. Excesses result in inadequate nerve fluid and eventual nervous prostration. The entire body will suffer, and not a single organ will escape damage.

Nervine herbs act as nerve tonics. Their function is to feed, regulate, strengthen, and rehabilitate the nerve cells. They act as either stimulants or sedatives, lessening the aberration, irritability, or pain of the nervous system. These should not be confused with the inorganic narcotics or opiates used by orthodox physicians, which are eventually debilitating, and damage life in the fibers and tissues.

Antispasmodics prevent or relieve excessive contractions (spasms) of the voluntary or involuntary muscles in any part of the body. Many function by stimulating the higher nervous, coordinating, and power centers (the nervines); others by depressing all of the vital functions (lobelia, American hellebore, etc.); and a number stimulate the muscular fibers of the intestines to expel gaseous accumulations (asafetida, valerian, wild yam, cajuput, etc.). The majority of these herbs heal damaged or overworked nerves, and relieve nervous tension and irritability caused by irregular and painful action of the muscles. These herbs are most effective in cases of suspended animation or locked joints, so they are especially useful as anti-tetanus agents.

LOBELIA
(Lobelia inflata; LOBELIACEAE)

Lobelia is the best antispasmodic herb and is a powerful nervine as well. Lobelia is such a useful herb that it deserves and has been given its own chapter (see CHAPTER 10).

SCULLCAP or SKULLCAP
(Scutellaria lateriflora; LABIATAE)

Common names:
Scullcap, skullcap, blue scullcap, pimpernel, helmet-flower, mad-dog skullcap, mad dogweed, madweed, mad-dog, hood wort, hooded willow herb, side-flowering scullcap, American scullcap, blue pimpernel; Pimpernelle (Ger.); marajes (Span.).

Identifying characteristics:

Stem	Square, small, smooth, erect, leafy, branched, and 1 to 2 feet high.
Leaves	Opposite, ovate-lanceolate, 1 to 3 inches long (growing gradually smaller toward the top of the stem), coarsely serrated (toothed), thin, rounded at the base and acuminate or pointed at the apex, and on slender petioles or pedicles about 1 inch long. Powder: dark green.
Flowers	One-sided axillary, leafy and spike-like racemes (other species have terminal racemes); several or many, 1/4 inch long, pale blue, bilabiate (two-lipped) calyx (the upper lip has a helmet-like protuberance), 4 stamens that are in pairs under the upper lip, and an unequally cleft pistil.
Fruit	4 nutlets.
Taste	Slightly bitter, but not nauseating.
Odor	Slight.

Part used:
Dried herb.

Therapeutic action:
Nervine tonic, antispasmodic, diuretic, calmative, antivenomous, and an astringent.

Scullcap is one of nature's best nervine agents. It is as stimulating to the nerves as quinine, but lacks the harmful side- and after-effects. It is especially calming and nutritive in neurasthenic conditions (characterized by emotional conflict, worry, disturbances of digestion and circulation, etc.). It is an excellent antispasmodic agent for restlessness, tremors, spasms, twitching of the muscles, and hyper-sensitivity.

Dr. Nowell asserts:

> It will influence the spinal cord and the sympathetic nervous system (supplying the various involuntary organs and blood vessels) as well as the brain, bringing to all a tonic influence which is quite permanent. . . It tones and soothes the nervous system and, without any narcotic properties, quiets the patient and often brings about quiet, natural sleep.

Dr. Shook said, "Scullcap is a slow-working but sure remedy for practically all nervous affections, but it must be taken regularly for a long period of time to be of permanent benefit."

Medicinal uses:
Nervous sleeplessness (insomnia), hysterical fits, convulsions, spinal meningitis, chorea (St. Vitus Dance), epilepsy, delirium, nervous headache, facial neuralgia, insanity, hydrophobia (mad dog bites), poisonous insect and snake bites, cranial and uterine neuralgia, seminal (generative) weakness, general nervousness, nervous exhaustion, tremors, spasms, muscular twitching, hyperesthesia, neuralgia, intermittent fevers, palsy, rheumatism, suppression of excessive sexual desire, aches, pain, rickets, convalescence from fevers, and incontinence of urine.

Preparations:
Fluid extract, infusion, powder, solid extract, and tincture.

Dosage:
Scullcap is quite harmless and may be taken in larger doses for severe cases.

Fluid extract	1/2-1 teaspoon.
Infusion	2 fluid ounces 3 to 4 times daily, and 1/2-1 glassful at night upon retiring.
Powder	1/4-1/2 teaspoon (1/2-1 gram) or a #00 capsule, 2 to 3 or more times daily.
Solid extract	300-650 milligrams.
Tincture	1/2-1 teaspoonful.

ADMINISTRATION

Anal

Hysteria: When scullcap tea cannot be taken orally, a small quantity may be given rectally every 30 minutes to 1 hour.

Epilepsy: A stronger infusion of scullcap should be made for adults. This is 2 to 3 ounces to each pint of distilled or D-cell water, covered and steeped for 30 minutes in a hot place. Adults should take 2 fluid ounces (or 1 cupful diluted) 3 to 4 times daily. Continue the treatment several weeks or longer, if necessary.

Heart weakness: Scullcap combined with cayenne and golden seal cannot be surpassed.

Hydrophobia, poisonous insect or snake bites: Take 1 teaspoonful of warm scullcap infusion or 1/2 teacupful of the strong infusion diluted with water every hour until the symptoms subside.

Insanity: After the patient is under the influence of lobelia and lady slipper, scullcap may be given freely with good effect.

Insomnia: 1 teacupful of warm scullcap infusion nightly upon retiring.

Nervous exhaustion: Scullcap infusion must be taken over a period of time in order to receive permanent effect.

Neuralgia: Drink 2 fluid ounces of scullcap infusion every 1 to 2 hours and 1 cupful upon retiring. 1 pint during a single evening would not be harmful.

Spasms, tremors, chorea, etc.: A strong infusion is the quickest and most effective form for adults.

FORMULAS

Dr. Coffin's antispasmodic powder

2 ounces	Scullcap powder (Scutellaria lateriflora)
2 ounces	Stomach bitters powder (see bayberry formulas page 146)
1 ounce	Valerian root powder (Valeriana officinalis)
1/4 ounce	Lobelia powder (Lobelia inflata)
1/4 ounce	Cinnamon powder (Cinnamomum zeylanicum)
1/4 ounce	Cayenne powder (Capsicum frutescens; C. minimum)

Preparation: Mix and sift the herbs.

Dosage: 1 teaspoonful in a cup of hot water, every hour if necessary.

Chickenpox

1 ounce	Scullcap (Scutellaria lateriflora)
1/2 ounce	Pleurisy root (Asclepias tuberosa)

Preparation: Infuse for 20 minutes in 1 quart of boiling hot water, strain, sweeten and take warm.

Dosage: 2 fluid ounces 3 to 4 times daily.

Administration: For itching skin, bathe with a combination of 1 ounce tincture of lobelia and 7 ounces of witch hazel fluid extract.

Chlorosis, green sickness

1 ounce	Scullcap (Scutellaria lateriflora)
1 ounce	Blue cohosh (Caulophyllum thalictroides)
1/2 ounce	Golden seal (Hydrastis Canadensis)

1/2 ounce Coriander seed (Coriandrum sativum)
1/4 ounce Orange peel (Citrus Aurantium or C. sinensis)

Preparation: Steep the herbs for 20 minutes in 1 quart of boiled, distilled water; strain and add up to 1 pound of honey and 2 ounces of glycerine.

Dosage: 2 fluid ounces 3 to 4 times daily.

Debility

1 part Scullcap (Scutellaria lateriflora)
1 part Camomile (Chamaemelum nobile; Anthemis nobilis)
1 part Gravel root (Eupatorium purpureum)

Preparation: Steep 1 teaspoonful of the mixed powders for 20 minutes in 1 pint of water; strain, sweeten, bottle, and keep in a cool place.

Dosage: 2 fluid ounces every 2 to 3 hours during the day.

Epilepsy

1/2 ounce Scullcap (Scutellaria lateriflora)
1/2 ounce Wood betony (Stachys officinalis)
1/4 ounce Valerian root (Valeriana officinalis)
1/2 ounce Pennyroyal (Mentha pulegium)
1/2 ounce Centaury (Erythraea centaurium)
1/2 teaspoon Cayenne (Capsicum frutescens; C. minimum)
1/2 teaspoon Bayberry bark (Myrica cerifera)

Preparation: Infuse the first 5 herbs in 1 quart of water. Cover closely, and keep warm in the oven for 1 hour, then strain over the cayenne and bayberry. Sweeten, bottle, and keep in a cool place.

Dosage: 2 tablespoonfuls 6 times daily.

Epilepsy

1/2 teaspoon Scullcap (Scutellaria lateriflora)
1/2 teaspoon Lobelia (Lobelia inflata)
1/2 teaspoon Cayenne (Capsicum frutescens; C. minimum)

Preparation: Infuse the herbs for a few minutes in 1/2 pint of boiling water. Sweeten with honey or yellow D sugar.

Dosage: 2 tablespoonfuls every 30 minutes, until the patient perspires. Then give the formula for epilepsy under Valerian (see page 415), the one which contains wood betony.

Administration: For a few minutes, place the patient's feet in hot mustard and water. Put the patient in bed with a hot water bottle at his feet. This bottle should be wrapped in flannel which has been wrung out with apple cider vinegar. The formula may then be administered.

Dr. Nowell's general nervine tonic; hysteria

1 part Scullcap herb powder (Scutellaria lateriflora)
1 part Hops powder (Humulus lupulus)
1 part Valerian root powder (Valeriana officinalis)
1 part Gum asafetida powder (Ferula assa-foetida)
1 part Gentian root (Gentiana lutea)

Preparation: Mix the herbs thoroughly and sift (if necessary) through a fine sieve. Fill #0 capsules with the mixture, or use 1 teaspoonful of the mixture to a cup of hot water.

Dosage: 2 to 6 capsules daily as required; or 1/2 cupful of the infusion (warm), 3 to 4 times daily. *Note:* For constipation, add a little cascara sagrada bark (Rhamnus purshiana) to the mixture, or give some senna tea (Cassia angustifolia; C. senna).

Dr. Shook's infusion of scullcap

1½ ounces Scullcap herb, cut (Scutellaria lateriflora)
1¼ pints Distilled or D-cell water

Preparation: Bring the water to a boil and pour over the herb, then cover and let steep for 20 to 30 minutes in a hot place. Strain and sweeten with honey, bottle when cool and keep in cool place.

Dosage: 2 fluid ounces 3 to 4 times daily, and 1 dose before retiring to bed. Children: 2 teaspoons to 1 tablespoonful, 3 to 4 times daily, between meals.

Insomnia
(sleeplessness, especially morphine addict)

1 part Scullcap (Scutellaria lateriflora)
1 part Lady slipper (Cypripedium calceolus var. pubescens)
1 part Hops (Humulus lupulus)
1 part Catnip (Nepeta cataria)
1 part Black cohosh (Cimicifuga racemosa)

Preparation: Mix the herbs together. Use 1 heaping teaspoonful of the mixed herbs to a cupful of hot water, cover and steep for 15 to 20 minutes.

Dosage: Sip the warm, clear tea before retiring.

Nerve tonic

2 parts	Scullcap (Scutellaria lateriflora)
1 part	Blue cohosh (Caulophyllum thalictroides)
1 part	Golden seal (Hydrastis Canadensis)
1/16 part	Cayenne (Capsicum frutescens; C. minimum)

Preparation: Use as an infusion or syrup.

Dosage: 2 teaspoonfuls after meals and at bedtime (syrup); 3 tablespoonfuls after meals (infusion).

Dr. Shook's nervine tonic

2 ounces	Scullcap herb, cut (Scutellaria lateriflora)
2 ounces	Vervain herb, cut (Verbena officinalis)
2 ounces	Damiana leaves, cut (Turnera aphrodisiaca)

Preparation: Soak the herbs in 2 quarts of distilled water. Simmer slowly for 20 minutes in an appropriate open vessel; strain, and return the liquid to the clean vessel. Slowly boil down to 3 pints. Strain, and then add 1 pint glycerine and 1 pint of honey. Stir well until mixed, let cool, bottle, and keep in a cool place.

Dosage: 1 tablespoonful in 1/2-1 cup of water, 3 to 4 times daily (preferably this should be 1 hour before meals). Children: 1-2 teaspoons in water, 3 to 4 times daily.

St. Vitus dance (chorea)

1/2 ounce	Scullcap (Scutellaria lateriflora)
1/2 ounce	Feverfew (Chrysanthemum parthenium)
1/2 ounce	Lady slipper (Cypripedium calceolus var. pubescens)

Preparation: Infuse the herbs in 1 quart of boiling water and steep for 2 hours; strain, sweeten, bottle, and keep in a cool place.

Dosage: 2 fluid ounces 3 to 4 times daily.

CASE HISTORY

Cured of epilepsy.
A 15-year-old boy had been afflicted with epilepsy since birth. His family was

quite wealthy and had spent a great deal of money trying to give him the best medical care, before coming to herbs. With 9 months of herbal treatment from Dr. Christopher, the boy was able to go to school as a normal child. He was a brilliant youngster, and caught up with his grade within 1½ years.

Growth characteristics:
Scullcap is a perennial plant which is indigenous to America. It grows best in wet and shady ground and is found in meadows, by ditches and sides of ponds. Flowers from July to September.

Collection:
Scullcap should be gathered while in bloom each year. It deteriorates rapidly with age.

Drying and preservation:
Care should be taken to dry scullcap in the shade, and then to store it in air-tight containers. This is because the herb deteriorates rapidly from age and heat. It is best preserved in tincture form.

Sister plants:
-Western scullcap or larger scullcap or Hyssop Skullcap (Scutellaria integrifolia). An herb with terminal racemes, hairy stems, and possessing similar therapeutic properties to Scutellaria lateriflora.
-European Scullcap (Scutellaria galericulata). A nearly smooth herb with single and axillary flowers and similar therapeutic properties to Scutellaria lateriflora.
-(Scutellaria pilosa); an herb with terminal racemes, a hairy stem, and leaves in distinct pairs. It, too, has similar therapeutic properties to Scutellaria lateriflora.

VALERIAN
(Valeriana officinalis; VALERIANACEAE)

Common names:
Valerian, English valerian, all-heal, great wild valerian, German valerian, fragrant valerian, wild valerian, common valerian, cat's valerian, Vermont or American-English valerian, setwall, vandal root, amantilla, capon's tail; Radix Valerianae Minoris, Valerianae Rhozoma (Br.); Valeriane officinale, Racine de Valeriane (Fr.); Radix Valeriane, Baldrian (wilde), Baldrianwurzel (Ger.).

Identifying characteristics:

Stem — It is a large, handsome plant, 2 to 4 feet high. The stem is round, fluted and channeled (groove, furrowed), smooth, hollow, thick, pale green in color, and branched at the top.

Leaves — Pinnate (4 to 10 pairs along a clasping petiole), opposite leaflets 1 to 2½ inches long, lanceolate and dentate (coarsely serrated).

Flowers	White or pink, small, with terminal corymbs (large tufts at the stalk head). They are agreeably fragrant, sessile (attached directly by the base), tubular, with 5 lobed corolla (petals) and 3 stamens.
Fruit	Capsule, pale brown, compressed (flattened laterally), plano-convex, oblong-ovate, 4-ribbed, and 1-seeded.
Roots	Rhizome, roots and rootlets; upright rootstock (rhizome) 4/5 to 1 inches long, 2/5 to 4/5 inches thick. The upper portion (crown) often shows leaf scales of stem bases, and is yellowish brown or grayish in color. It is many-fibered, with numerous short lateral (horizontal) branches or stolons; hard, cylindrical, and tuberous (roundish swellings) with numerous, slender, brittle, thread-like roots, short and horny fracture. It is internally light brown or pale grayish-brown in color, with thick bark and central woody cylinder. Old roots are often hollow. The powder is grayish-brown.
Taste	Sweetish, disagreeable, camphoraceous, somewhat bitter, and nauseous.
Odor	Characteristic of valeric acid, becoming stronger and disagreeably fetid upon aging; it is highly attractive to cats (the odor excites the sexual appetite) and possibly to rats also.

Parts used:
Rhizome and roots; also the herb.

Therapeutic action:
Stimulating antispasmodic, tonic, nervine (sedative), anodyne, cathartic, diaphoretic, anti-thermic, diuretic (lithotriptic), aromatic, carminative.

Valerian is powerfully antispasmodic in its effect upon the system. It is gently stimulating, very soothing and quieting to the nervous system. Valerian is an effective calmative. It influences circulation by slowing the action of the heart, while increasing its force; therefore it has been very beneficial in cases of cardiac (heart) palpitation.

Potter's Cyclopaedia states that valerian "may be given in all cases to allay pain and promote sleep. It is strongly nervine without any narcotic effects, and enters into various herbal nervine and antispasmodic compounds." Valerian produces an exhilarating sensation, and is especially useful for women of all ages who may have emotional swings during their menstrual cycles. Besides acting upon the circulatory system, it stimulates secretion and peristalsis of the stomach and intestines. Valerian is an excellent anti-flatulent for infants. It is very useful for hysterical and hypochondriacal subjects. It heals ulcerated stomachs and is powerful in preventing digestive fermentation.

Medicinal uses:
Nervous debility, weakness or irritation, hysteria, restlessness in measles and scarlet fever, convulsions in infants due to worms, colic, cramps, insomnia, neu-

ralgia, dysmenorrhea, hypochondria, flatulence, whooping cough, diabetes, delirium with vital depression, cholera, epilepsy, hemicrania, nervous coughs, delirium tremens, typhoid, vertigo, low fevers, colds, gravel, palpitation of the heart, stomach ulcers, digestive fermentations, sores, pimples, and dyspnea.

Preparations:
Elixir, fluid extract, infusion, powder, solid extract, and tincture. Never boil the root; much of its therapeutic value is in the volatile oils. Valerian may be preserved with glycerine.

Dosage:

Elixir	1/2 to 1 teaspoon.
Fluid extract	5 to 15 drops.
Infusion	2 fluid ounces 3 times daily, before meals, and before retiring to bed at night.
Powder	300 mg.-1 gram.
Solid extract	300-650 milligrams.
Tincture	1 to 2 fluid teaspoons.

ADMINISTRATION

Valerian is potent, so be careful to give it in the prescribed dosages only.

Oral

Cough, dyspnea (shortness of breath), and expectorant: Strain a hot decoction of licorice (Glycyrrhiza glabra), anise seed (Pimpinella anisum) and raisins over valerian. Steep, allow to cool, strain.

Dysmenorrhea (difficult or painful menstruation): When taken hot, valerian will promote menstruation.

Hysteria, convulsion, colic, cramps, dysmenorrhea, etc.: (See "FORMULAS").

Palpitation of the heart: Administer hot valerian with cayenne pepper (Capsicum frutescens; C. minimum).

Restlessness in measles and scarlet fever, etc. (children, infantile convulsions): Give small doses of valerian infusion 2 to 3 times daily. A sound sleep will generally result.

Skin

Sores and pimples: Apply valerian root or herb externally, and drink valerian tea at the same time.

FORMULAS

Antispasmodic powder (fits, convulsions, hysteria, cramps, etc.)

1 ounce	Valerian root powder (Valeriana officinalis)
1 ounce	Scullcap powder (Scutellaria lateriflora)
1 ounce	Skunk cabbage powder (Symplocarpus foetidus)
1/4 ounce	Lobelia powder (Lobelia inflata)
1/4 ounce	Cinnamon powder (Cinnamomum zeylanicum)
1/4 ounce	Cayenne powder (Capsicum frutescens; C. minimum)

Preparation: Mix thoroughly and sieve. Use 1/2 teaspoonful in 3-4 ounces of sweetened hot water.

Dosage: 3-4 ounces (warm) every 2 hours; children in proportion.

Convulsions, hysteria, colic, cramps, and dysmenorrhea

1 ounce	Valerian fluid extract (Valeriana officinalis)
1 ounce	Wild yam fluid extract (Dioscorea villosa)
1 ounce	Blue cohosh fluid extract (Caulophyllum thalictroides)
1 ounce	Anise seed essence (Pimpinella anisum)
6 ounces	Ginger syrup (Zingiber officinalis) see page 544

Preparation: Mix thoroughly and stir 1-3 teaspoons into a cup of water.

Dosage: 3-4 fluid ounces (warm) every 2 hours; children in proportion.

Dizziness

3 grams	Valerian (Valeriana officinalis)
2 grams	Tansy (Tanacetum vulgare)
2 grams	Caraway (Carum carvi)
1 gram	Rue (Ruta graveolens)

Preparation: Infuse the herbs 15 to 20 minutes in 1 pint of water. Strain, sweeten, bottle and keep in a cool place.

Dosage: 2 fluid ounces, 3 to 4 times daily.

Epilepsy

1 ounce	Valerian (Valeriana officinalis)
1 ounce	Catnip (Nepeta cataria)

1 ounce	Horehound (Marrubium vulgare)
1 ounce	Pellitory-of-the-wall (Parietaria officinalis)
1 ounce	Peony root (Paeonia officinalis)
1 ounce	Wood betony (Stachys officinalis)
1 ounce	Scullcap (Scutellaria lateriflora)

Preparation: Infuse the herbs for 1 hour in 2 quarts of hot water, cover tightly, and keep warm. Allow to cool, and then strain.

Dosage: 2 tablespoonfuls every 2 hours (adding 10 drops of antispasmodic tincture to each dose).

Administration: Make the patient perspire with the epilepsy formula (scullcap, lobelia, cayenne) found under Scullcap and then give the following formula:

Epilepsy

2 parts	Valerian (Valeriana officinalis)
3 parts	Mistletoe (Viscum album)
3 parts	Shavegrass (Equisetum hyemale)
1 part	Yellow or ladies' bedstraw (Galium verum)
1 part	Wormwood (Artemisia absinthium)

Preparation: Use 1 teaspoonful of the mixture to each cupful of water.

Dosage: 1 teacupful, 2 to 3 times daily.

Dr. Shook's high blood pressure compound

3 teaspoons	Valerian root, cut (Valeriana officinalis)
3 teaspoons	Licorice root, cut (Glycyrrhiza glabra)
6 teaspoons	Buckthorn bark, cut (Rhamnus Frangula)
4 teaspoons	Speedwell or Culver's root, cut (Veronicastrum virginicum)
3 teaspoons	Linden flowers, cut (Tilia europaea)
1 teaspoon	Rue herb, cut (Ruta graveolens)
1 teaspoon	Goldenrod (Solidago virgaurea)

Preparation: Mix well, divide into 20 (1 teaspoon) doses. For a tea, use 1 dose to 3 cups of boiling water, cover and simmer 2 to 3 minutes. Steep for 10 minutes, or steep in hot water for 1/2 hour, strain and sweeten to suit taste. For powder, divide 1 dose into 3 parts (1/3 teaspoon).

Dosage: For tea, take 1 cupful 3 times daily before or after meals. For powder, take 1/3 dose 3 times daily before or after meals, which may be mixed with honey, mucilage, etc.

Insomnia
(sleeplessness, caused by nervousness)

1 part	Valerian (Valeriana officinalis)
1 part	Vervain (Verbena officinalis, V. hastata)
1 part	Scullcap (Scutellaria lateriflora)
1 part	Wood betony (Stachys officinalis)

Preparation: Infuse the herbs for 20 minutes. Mix 1 teaspoonful of the herbs to each cupful of boiling hot water; cover tightly. Strain and sweeten.

Dosage: 1 teacupful, 2 to 3 times daily, and taken warm upon retiring.

Nerve tonic

1 ounce	Valerian (Valeriana officinalis)
1 ounce	Scullcap (Scutellaria lateriflora)
1/2 ounce	Catnip (Nepeta cataria)
1 teaspoon	Coriander (Coriandrum sativum)
1/2 teaspoon	Cayenne (Capsicum frutescens; C. minimum)

Preparation: Infuse the first 4 herbs for 15 to 20 minutes in 1 quart of boiling hot water and cover tightly. Strain hot over cayenne, cover and allow to cool. Sweeten to suit taste, bottle and keep in a cool place.

Dosage: 2 fluid ounces 3 times daily. Take warm upon retiring.

Restlessness, insomnia, hysteria, neuralgia

1/2 ounce	Valerian (Valeriana officinalis)
1/2 ounce	Scullcap (Scutellaria lateriflora)
1/2 ounce	Mistletoe (Viscum album)

Preparation: Infuse the herbs in 1½ pints of boiling hot water. Cover tightly, and let stand for 2 hours. Strain and sweeten to taste.

Dosage: 2 to 4 tablespoonfuls, 4 times daily.

Growth characteristics:
Valerian is a perennial plant. It is found in damp places, such as low-lying woods and meadows, along banks of rivers and lakes; generally, in marshy and swampy ground, but it also flourishes equally well in dry places. This has resulted in a variety of characteristics which suggests the existence of four types of valerian, yet they are one and the same, and yield identical constituents. Very little of the wild variety (indigenous to Europe) is used commercially, though it is smaller and more potent. The cultivated types are produced in England (the best), Germany,

Netherlands, and the English-American variety in the states of New Hampshire, Vermont and New York. It flowers from June to August. The tops are generally cut off in the spring to keep the medicinal strength from dissipating into the plant and to strengthen the root.

Collection:
The rhizome and roots are gathered in the autumn from the dry soil plants, after the leaves have begun to decay. The dry soil plants are more developed, but others should not be overlooked. The roots and rhizomes should be dug carefully, as there are many of them and they are spreading and brittle. They should be cleaned. There is no specific odor at this time.

Drying and preservation:
Dry the entire plant, or split it as soon after digging as possible. Care should be taken to preserve the volatile oils. Pack tightly and keep dry to prevent deterioration.

Sister plants:
-Indian valerian (Valeriana wallichii; Valeriana Indicae Rhizoma (Br.), VALERIANACEAE). The rhizome is practically identical and therapeutically equivalent to the official European variety. It is 2 inches long, 2/5 inches thick, brown and curves, with many root scars and a few thick roots. It grows in the Himalayas.
-(Valeriana phu; VALERIANACEAE). The rhizome is tall, perennial, found in western Asia and southern Europe and yields valeric acid. The odor and taste are weaker than the official.
-(Radix Valerianae Majoris; VALERIANACEAE). The rhizome is 4 to 6 inches long, 1/2 inch thick, annulated (ringed), brown and yields valeric acid. The odor and taste are weaker than the official.
-(Valeriana mexicana; V. toluccana, VALERIANACEAE). The rhizome is indigenous to Mexico and yields valeric acid. The odor and taste are weaker than the official variety.

LADY'S SLIPPER or NERVE ROOT
(Cypripedium calceolus var. pubescens; C. reginae; ORCHIDACEAE)

Common names:
Lady slipper, lady's slipper, cypripedium, nerve root, American valerian, moccasin plant, large yellow lady's slipper, yellow moccasin flower, whippoorwill's shoe, umbel, Noah's ark; Frauenschuh (Ger.); chapin, zapatilla de señorita (Span.).

Identifying characteristics:
Stem There are several stems arising from the fleshy rhizome which are round, leafy, 1 to 2 feet tall, and hairy. This hairiness is irritating and

	causes skin eruptions.
Leaves	Oval or elliptical and pointed at the apex (acuminate). They are 3 to 6 inches long, and 2 to 3 inches broad; alternate (generally the same number on each side), sheathed, pubescent (hairy) and parallel-nerved.
Flower	Solitary, large, and resembles a slipper or moccasin. It is pale yellow in color and is born at the top of a leafy stem.
Roots	The curved fleshy rhizomes are orange-brown or brownish in color, 1 to 4 inches long, 1/12 to 1/4 inches thick, with many cup-shaped scars on the top surface. The roots are numerous, thickly-matted, wavy, fibrous, and unbranched, and are 1 to 6 inches long. The fracture is short and white and the powder is yellowish brown.
Taste	Sweetish-bitter, pungent or acrid and aromatic.
Odor	Distinct, heavy and slightly valerianic.

Part used:
Rhizome and roots.

Therapeutic action:
Antispasmodic, nervine, tonic, relaxant, stimulant, antiperiodic, diaphoretic, and diuretic.

Lady's slipper is almost a pure nervine and relaxant. Its action is slow, yet it influences the entire nervous system. A common name for lady's slipper is "American Valerian" because of the generic properties it shares with valerian. Lady's slipper is an excellent pain reliever, is beneficial in female weaknesses, induces sleep, and relieves hysteria and most nervous disorders, including any enfeebled nerve condition. Its efficiency is increased when combined with tonic herbs.

Medicinal uses:
Nervous sleeplessness, nervous headache, hysteria, convulsions, nervous exhaustion (overworked and worried conditions), flatulence, indigestion, chorea (St. Vitus' Dance), weakness and trembling of limbs, nervous irritability, nervousness, cholera, epilepsy, hypochondriasis, neuralgia, female weaknesses, rigid os uteri, recent cold or fever, and inflamed appendix.

Preparations:
Decoction, fluid extract, infusion, powder, solid extract, and tincture. Lady slipper may be preserved in glycerine.

Dosage:
Lady slipper is non-poisonous and perfectly safe. It may be taken in larger doses when needed.

Decoction	(strong) 1 tablespoonful in 2 fluid ounces of water 3 to 4 times daily (this is 3½ times stronger than the infusion).
Fluid extract	1/2 to 1 teaspoonful.

Infusion	2 fluid ounces 3 to 4 times daily, 1 hour before meals. Children: 2 teaspoons to 1 tablespoonful, according to age.
Powder	1 teaspoon.
Solid extract	300 mg.-1 gram.
Tincture	15 to 30 drops (1/4 to 1/2 teaspoonful).

ADMINISTRATION

Anal

Insomnia: Give an injection (enema) upon retiring (for nymphomania, add some lobelia). Prevent seminal emissions.

Oral

Congestions with nerve irritation, delirium of typhoid: Combine lady slipper with a positive stimulant such as cayenne or golden seal.

Children's colds and fevers: Administer 1/4 to 1/2 the adult dose of the strong decoction, hot.

Break up recent colds or fevers: Cover the patient closely and give 2 tablespoonfuls of the strong decoction in 1 teacupful of very hot water.

Epilepsy: "See "FORMULAS."

General nerve troubles and sleeplessness: Give 1 tablespoonful of the strong decoction in warm water.

Hysteria and convulsions: See "FORMULAS."

Nervous and weakly children (especially with symptoms of contortions or twitching muscles; St. Vitus' Dance): 2 teaspoons to 1 tablespoonful given in a copious amount of honey (to avoid nausea or objection).

Parturition (tired nervous system, rigid os uteri, nervous irritability, colic and after-pains): See "FORMULAS."

Nervous exhaustion (overworked and worried conditions): Give small and frequent doses of the infusion or decoction.

Neuritis: See "FORMULAS."

Neuralgia (children): See "FORMULAS."

FORMULAS

Infusion of lady's slipper

1 ounce	Lady's slipper root, cut (Cypripedium calceolus var. pubescens)
1¼ pints	Distilled or d-cell water

Preparation: Bring the water to a boil and pour it over the herb. Cover and steep for 15 minutes; strain and sweeten to taste.

Dosage: 2 fluid ounces 3 to 4 times daily, preferably before meals. Children: 2 teaspoons to 1 tablespoonful, according to age and condition.

Strong decoction of lady's slipper

4 ounces	Lady's slipper, root, cut (Cypripedium calceolus var. pubescens)
1 quart	Distilled or d-cell water
8 ounces	Glycerine

Preparation: Soak the herb in the cold water for 2 hours. Bring to a boil and simmer for 15 minutes; strain and return the liquid to the clean vessel. Reduce by slow boiling to 3/4 pint. Remove from the heat and add the glycerine while hot, mixing thoroughly. Cool, bottle and keep in a cool place.

Appendix inflammation

1 teaspoon	Lady's slipper root (Cypripedium calceolus var. pubescens)
1/2 teaspoon	Lobelia herb (Lobelia inflata)

Preparation: Mix herbs in powder form and place in 1 cupful of boiling hot water, cover with a saucer and steep for a few minutes.

Dosage: 1 cupful every 1/2 hour.

Administration: Do not take cathartics at the same time. Apply a mullein leaf poultice with lobelia and ginger externally over the affected area.

Convulsions, fits

1/2 ounce	Lady's slipper root (Cypripedium calceolus var. pubescens)
1/4 ounce	Scullcap herb (Scutellaria lateriflora)
1/4 ounce	Rue herb (Ruta graveolens)
4 ounces	Yellow D sugar
1/2 ounce	Antispasmodic tincture (see page 399)

Preparation: Infuse the first three herbs in 1 pint of boiling hot water; cover tightly and let stand until cool. Strain, add the sugar, and simmer. Remove scum, cool, and add the antispasmodic tincture.

Dosage: 1 teaspoonful every 3 hours.

Administration: Attend to the bowels (lower bowel tonic), strengthen the stomach with tonics, and exercise care in the diet (the regenerative diet).

Delirium of fevers and nervous tension

2 parts Lady's slipper (Cypripedium calceolus var. pubescens)
1 part Lobelia (Lobelia inflata)

Preparation: Infuse for 15 minutes covered tight. Strain and sweeten to taste.

Dosage: 2 teaspoons occasionally.

Epilepsy

1/4 ounce Lady's slipper root powder (Cypripedium calceolus var. pubescens)
1/4 ounce Golden seal root powder (Hydrastis Canadensis)
1/4 ounce Lobelia seed powder (Lobelia inflata)
1/4 ounce Cayenne (Capsicum frutescens; C. minimum)

Preparation: Mix together in a mortar, or rub the powders together with the back of a spoon. Fill #4 (much smaller than #0) capsules with this mixture.

Dosage: 1 capsule every 3 hours if the fits are frequent; otherwise, give 1 capsule night and morning.

Administration: This formula should follow the one given under "scullcap" (scullcap, lobelia, cayenne). Follow this with the other formula (see page 409) given under "scullcap" (scullcap, wood betony, etc.).

Epilepsy

1 part Lady's slipper root (Cypripedium calceolus var. pubescens)
1 part Peony root (Paeonia officinalis)
1 part Virginia snake root (Aristolochia serpentaria)
1 part Peruvian bark or Cinchona (Cinchona calisaya)

Preparation: Mix thoroughly. Use 1 teaspoonful of this mixture to one cup of water. Simmer slowly 10 or 15 minutes and sweeten.

Dosage: 1 teaspoonful to 1 tablespoonful every 2 hours.

Hysteria
(relax nerve tension, soothe and tone nerves)

1 ounce	Lady's slipper root (Cypripedium calceolus var. pubescens)
1/2 ounce	Scullcap herb (Scutellaria lateriflora)
1/4 ounce	Ginger (Zingiber officinalis)
1/4 ounce	Raspberry leaves (Rubus idaeus)

Preparation: Infuse the herbs in 1½ pints of boiling hot water, cover tightly, and allow to cool. Strain, and sweeten to taste.

Dosage: 2 fluid ounces, 4 to 5 times daily.

Administration: Prevent all excitement and allow the patient to rest comfortably. Make the surroundings as cheerful as possible. Give the nervine formula as a calmative, or use the nervine capsules given under "scullcap" (see page 310) and tone up the digestive tract with the formula given under "raspberry" (see page 161).

Hysteria with convulsions

1 ounce	Lady's slipper root (Cypripedium calceolus var. pubescens)
1/2 ounce	Asafetida gum (Ferula assa-foetida)
1/4 ounce	Ginger (Zingiber officinalis)
1/4 ounce	Lobelia herb (Lobelia inflata)

Preparation: Infuse the herbs in 1½ pints of boiling hot water. Cover tightly, and allow to cool. Strain and sweeten to taste.

Dosage: 2 fluid ounces 4 to 5 times daily.

Nervous headache

1/2 ounce	Lady's slipper root (Cypripedium calceolus var. pubescens)
1/2 ounce	Catnip herb (Nepeta cataria)
1/2 ounce	Scullcap herb (Scutellaria lateriflora)

Preparation: Infuse the herbs in 1½ pints of boiling hot water. Cover tightly, and allow to cool. Strain, and sweeten to taste.

Dosage: 1 to 2 warm cupfuls daily.

Insomnia (nervous sleeplessness)

1 ounce	Lady's slipper root, fluid extract (Cypripedium calceolus)
1 ounce	Pleurisy root, fluid extract (Asclepias tuberosa)

1 ounce Skunk cabbage root, fluid extract (Symplocarpus foetidus)
1 ounce Scullcap herb, fluid extract (Scutellaria lateriflora)

Preparation: Mix the fluid extracts thoroughly.

Dosage: 1/2 to 1 teaspoonful, 3 times daily.

Neuritis (nerve inflammation)

1 ounce Lady's slipper root (Cypripedium calceolus var. pubescens)
1 ounce Scullcap herb (Scutellaria lateriflora)
1/2 ounce Damiana (Turnera aphrodisiaca)
1/2 ounce Wild Yam (Dioscorea villosa)
1/2 ounce Ginger (Zingiber officinalis)

Preparation: Pour 1 quart of boiling hot water over the herbs, cover tightly, and let stand until cool. Strain and sweeten to taste.

Dosage: 2 fluid ounces every 3 to 4 hours.

Administration: A vapor bath or ginger bath will give soothing relief. Give external applications of stimulating liniments (such as cayenne and prickly ash tinctures), and apply a poultice of camomile flowers and poppy heads, or a heated hops bag to the affected area. Nervine capsules assist in many cases.

Parturition or child-birth
(colic and after-pains)

3 parts Lady slipper root (Cypripedium calceolus var. pubescens)
2 parts Wild yam (Dioscorea villosa)
1 part Ginger (Zingiber officinalis)

Preparation: Infuse 1 ounce of the herb compound for 20 minutes in 1 pint of boiling water (covered tightly). Strain, and sweeten to taste.

Dosage: Administer doses of 2 fluid ounces as the case requires.

Soothing syrup for children,
(neuralgia mixture)

2 ounces Lady's slipper, fluid extract (Cypripedium calceolus var. pubescens)
1 ounce Scullcap, fluid extract (Scutellaria lateriflora)
1 ounce Pleurisy root, fluid extract (Asclepias tuberosa)
1 ounce Prickly ash, fluid extract (Zanthoxylum americanum)
1 ounce Lobelia, tincture (Lobelia inflata)
1 ounce Anise seed, essence (Pimpinella anisum)

Preparation: Mix thoroughly.

Dosage: 1/4 to 1 teaspoonful in warm, sweetened water or in a little warm catnip tea.

Growth characteristics:
Lady's slipper is a perennial plant which grows best in damp, boggy woods, thickets, and hilly ground from Nova Scotia to the mid-west. It flowers from may to July, and may be cultivated in the herb garden.

Collection:
Dig in August or September.

Sister plants:
Small Yellow Lady's Slipper (Cypripedium parviflorum; ORCHIDACEAE). The root is therapeutically equivalent to the larger variety. This plant has a bright yellow pouch with occasional purplish sepals and petals, and has a delicately fragrant flower about one-half the size of its big sister. Both varieties usually grow in the same locale and have the same blooming season. The smaller, fairer and sweeter variety roams westward to Washington.

MISTLETOE

(Viscum album; V. flavescens; Arceuthobium pusillum;
Phoradendron flavescens; LORANTHACEAE)

Common names:
European mistletoe (V. album), all heal, American mistletoe (V. flavescens; Phoradendron flavescens), birdlime mistletoe, golden bough, devil's fugue; Mistel (Ger.); muerdago, caballera, and visco (Span.).

Identifying characteristics:

Stem	Evergreen parasite, smooth-jointed, copiously branched, and one foot or more high.
Leaves	European: opposite, heathery, rather tough, oblong-lanceolate, and about 2 inches long, with entire margins, and rounded apex. It is sessile and has 4 to 5 longitudinal veins. The American plant has similar characteristics, but has shorter, more pubescent leaves which are more yellowish-green in color.
Roots	Penetrate through the bark into the wood.
Flowers	Yellowish heads.
Fruit	White berries.
Taste	Insipid (tasteless).
Odor	None.

Part used:
Leaves, ripe berries, and young twigs.

Therapeutic action:
Nervine, antispasmodic, tonic, slight narcotic, diuretic, emmenagogue, emetic.

Mistletoe is highly valued for its nervine and antispasmodic properties, used in any trouble caused by weakness or a disordered state of the nervous system. It will quiet, soothe, and tone the nerves, lessening cerebral excitement and influencing febrile conditions. It is useful in female weakness of the generative organs and will incite uterine contractions. It gives tone in cardiac (heart) affections, because it possesses non-injurious properties that can be used instead of the powerful whipping action of digitalis or bromides.

Medicinal uses:
Hysteria, epilepsy, uterine hemorrhages, amenorrhea, dysmenorrhea, heart troubles (especially in typhoid fever), blood pressure, convulsions, delirium, nervous debility, fits, nervousness, chorea (St. Vitus' Dance), cardiac dropsy, and cholera.

Preparations:
Decoction, fluid extract, infusion, powder, and tincture.

Dosage:

Decoction	1 teaspoonful to 3 tablespoonfuls every 1 to 3 hours.
Fluid extract	1/4 to 1 fluid teaspoon.
Infusion	3-4 fluid ounces 2 to 3 times daily.
Powder	(leaves) 1/2 to 2 teaspoons.
Tincture	1/2 to 1 fluid teaspoon.

ADMINISTRATION

Oral

Chorea, epilepsy, nervousness, hysteria, delirium, etc.: Use the mistletoe decoction or infusion according to need.

FORMULAS

Chorea (St. Vitus' Dance)

1 ounce	Mistletoe (Viscum album; V. flavescens)
1/4 ounce	Cramp bark (Viburnum trilobum; V. opulus)
1/4 ounce	Hops (Humulus lupulus)
flavoring	Peppermint or anise essence (or very small amount of oil)

Preparation: Simmer the first 3 herbs for 5 minutes, or infuse in 1 pint of boiling hot water and steep for 1 hour. Strain and add 1/2 pound of yellow D sugar (or 1/4 pound honey), simmer, and skim off scum. Remove from heat, allow to cool and add flavoring. Sugar may be omitted and the tea used fresh.

Dosage: 2 teaspoons 3 times daily (6 years old), 1 tablespoonful 4 times daily (10 years old). Give the dosage according to age and condition.

Administration: The involuntary twitching and contraction of muscles is most common before the age of puberty and parents should avoid drawing attention to the problem. A vapor bath, followed by a sponging with equal parts of apple cider vinegar and cold water is helpful prior to administering formula.

Convulsions and epileptic fits

6 fluid teaspoons	Mistletoe, tincture (Viscum album; V. flavescens)
6 fluid teaspoons	Lady's slipper, tincture (Cypripedium calceolus)
4 fluid teaspoons	Valerian, tincture (Valeriana officinalis)
4 fluid teaspoons	Scullcap, extract (Scutellaria lateriflora)
4 fluid teaspoons	Horse nettle or bull nettle, extract (Solanum carolinense)

Preparation: Add distilled water to the herbs to make 24 ounces of fluid (1 ounce water per fluid teaspoon herb tincture).

Dosage: 1 tablespoonful every 4 hours. Children: in proportion.

General remedy for many nervous troubles

1/2 ounce	Mistletoe (Viscum album; V. flavescens)
1/2 ounce	Valerian root (Valeriana officinalis)
1/2 ounce	Vervain herbs (Verbena hastata)

Preparation: Simmer the herbs for 10 minutes in 1½ pints of water. Strain and sweeten to taste. For weak digestive organs, add a little cayenne.

Dosage: 2 tablespoonfuls 3 times daily.

Growth characteristics:
This plant is a true parasite since it does not draw nourishment from soil or the dead debris in trees but from the life blood of the tree it grows on. It can be grown from seed which is rubbed onto the underside of the branches of Apple, Hawthorn, Ash, and other trees. The species most generally used grows throughout Europe.

WOOD BETONY

(Stachys officinalis; S. Betonica; Betonica officinalis; LABIATAE)

Common names:
Wood betony, bishopswort, herb Christopher, betony, beefsteak plant, high heal-all; betonica (Span.).

Identifying characteristics:

Stem	Clustered, simple, slender, square, pubescent (hairy) and 6 to 18 inches high.
Leaves	Distant pairs, rough, hairy, oblong-lanceolate. They are 2 to 3 inches long, 3/4 to 1 inch broad, mostly radical (basal), pinnately lobed and with crenate margins (rounded scallops).
Flowers	Greenish-yellow and purplish-red in color. Labiate, with smooth calyx; short, dense, oval, and with a terminal spike.
Roots	White and thready.
Taste	Bitter.
Odor	Slight and pleasant.

Part used:
Herb.

Therapeutic action:
Nervine, tonic, antiscorbutic, aromatic, carminative, astringent, alterative, stomachic, aperient, anthelmintic, and antivenomous.

Wood betony is an excellent remedy for all head and face pains, and for nervous troubles. It is a tonic for general digestive disorders, and is an efficient alterative in cleansing impurities from the blood (as in scrofula, rheumatism, jaundice). It will open obstructions of the liver and spleen, mildly stimulate the heart, and expel worms from the system.

Medicinal uses:
Pain of the head and face, neuralgia, hysteria, dizziness, dyspepsia, impure blood, rheumatism, scrofula, jaundice, biliousness, nervous troubles, heartburn, stomach cramps, colic pains, insanity, headache, pain, convulsions, colds, dropsy, gout, influenza, consumption, worms, poisonous snake and insect bites and delirium.

Preparations:
Fluid extract, infusion, powder and tincture.

Dosage:

Fluid extract	1/2 to 1 fluid teaspoon.
Infusion	2 fluid ounces, 3 to 4 times daily.
Powder	1-3 grams.
Tincture	1/2 to 1 fluid teaspoon.

ADMINISTRATION

Wood betony may be used alone, or combined with other botanical remedies.

FORMULAS

Biliousness, nervous troubles, heartburn, stomach cramps, colic pains

1 ounce Wood betony (Stachys officinalis)
1/2 ounce Rosemary herb (Rosmarinus officinalis)
1/2 ounce Scullcap herb (Scutellaria lateriflora)
1/2 ounce Yarrow herb (Achillea millefolium)

Preparation: Infuse the herbs for 20 minutes in 1 quart of water, keeping the mixture tightly covered. Strain and sweeten to taste.

Dosage: 2 fluid ounces, 4 times daily.

Nervine, stomachic, tonic, antivenomous compound

2 parts Wood Betony (Stachys officinalis)
1 part Scullcap (Scutellaria lateriflora)
1 part Sweet flag or calamus root (Acorus calamus)

Preparation: Add 1 teaspoonful of the compound to each cup of water. Cover tightly and steep for 20 minutes; strain and sweeten to taste.

Dosage: 2 fluid ounces, 3 to 4 times daily.

Nervous headache

1 ounce Wood betony (Stachys officinalis)
1 ounce Rosemary herb (Rosmarinus officinalis)
1 ounce Peppermint (Mentha piperita)

Preparation: Pour 1 quart of boiling hot water over the herbs and cover closely until cool. Strain and sweeten to taste.

Dosage: 3 tablespoonfuls every 2 hours until relieved, and then 4 times daily.

Administration: Nervine capsules are good for this problem, or a simple infusion of scullcap.

Dr. Rudgley's formula for paralysis

4 handfuls	Wood betony (Stachys officinalis)
1 handful	Rosemary (Rosmarinus officinalis)
1 handful	Sage (Salvia officinalis)
2 pounds	Juniper berries (Juniperus communis)
24 grams	Senna powder (Cassia angustifolia; C. acutifolia)
24 grams	Ginger (Zingiber officinalis)
15 grams	Cubeb (Piper Cubeba)
2 pounds	Yellow D sugar
15 grams	Sweet flag or calamus (Acorus calamus)

Preparation: Simmer the first 3 herbs slowly in 1 gallon of water down to 1/2 gallon. Strain, add the sugar, bring to a boil and remove the scum. Strain hot over the remaining herbs, cover tightly until cool and then strain.

Dosage: 1 tablespoonful morning and night.

Growth characteristics:
Wood Betony grows in thickets, shady waysides and dry, open woods from Nova Scotia to the Rocky Mountains. It flowers from July to August, and may be grown in an herb garden.

CRAMP BARK or HIGH CRANBERRY
(Viburnum trilobum; V. Opulus; CAPRIFOLIACEAE)

Common names:
Cramp bark, high cranberry, guelder rose, snowball tree, cranberry tree, white dogwood, marsh elder, water elder, squaw bush; mundillo, sauquillo (Span.).

Identifying characteristics:

Stem	It is a handsome upright shrub, 4 to 12 feet high with several nearly smooth and branched stems coming from the same root.
Bark	Thin 1/50-1/8 inch thick quills, light gray in color with brownish stripes. It has curved and chip-like fragments, lenticels (warts or corky growths), fissures (faintly longitudinal cracks) and thin scales. The inner surface is pale yellowish brown in color, tough, with flat splinters, and fractures into 2 layers. The powder is light grayish to brown in color.
Leaves	Three-lobed, three-veined, dentate and broadly wedge-shaped.
Flowers	Very showy, large white, greenish-white or reddish-white cymes.
Fruit	Red, ovoid, resembling and used as a substitute for the common cranberry. The fruit succeeds the flowers; it ripens late and remains on the bush after the leaves have fallen. It is very acid.

Taste	Peculiar, but not unpleasant. It is bitterish and mildly astringent.
Odor	Slight and characteristic.

Part used:
Dried stem bark.

Therapeutic action:
Antispasmodic, nervine, tonic, relaxant, diuretic, expectorant, astringent, sedative and emmenagogue.

Cramp bark is highly regarded as an antispasmodic agent. It is considered one of the best female regulators and relaxants of the ovaries and uterus, and is highly effective in preventing abortions caused by nervous affections (stress) during pregnancy. Cramp bark will speedily quiet the uneasiness and relieve the pains of uterine and abdominal cramps and is a remedy for nervous disorders and spasms of all kinds.

Medicinal uses:
Nervous conditions of pregnancy, abortive prevention, dysmenorrhea, menorrhagia, ovarian irritation, asthma, hysteria, cramps, spasms, flatulent stomach, fits, convulsions, fainting, neuralgia and lockjaw.

Preparations:
Decoction, fluid extract, infusion, powder, and tincture.

Dosage:

Decoction	(strong) 1 tablespoonful 3 to 4 times daily.
Fluid extract	1/2 to 2 fluid teaspoons.
Infusion	2 fluid ounces, 3 to 4 times daily.
Tincture	1/2 to 1 fluid teaspoon.

ADMINISTRATION

Oral

Cramps, vomiting in pregnancy, nervous indigestion, delayed menstruation, hysteria, congestion and hardening of the liver, enuresis, cystitis, prevent abortion, epilepsy, St. Vitus' Dance: See "FORMULAS."

Cramps of pregnancy, uterine pains, or any nervous trouble during pregnancy: Give the decoction of cramp bark alone, or combine with other appropriate agents. See "FORMULAS."

FORMULAS

Strong decoction of cramp bark

2 ounces Cramp bark (Viburnum trilobum; V. opulus)
1 quart Distilled or D-cell water

Preparation: Boil slowly in a closed vessel for 20 minutes, strain and return to clean vessel. Reduce to 3/4 pints, add 4 ounces glycerine or 3 ounces yellow D sugar. Boil slowly 5 minutes, cool and bottle.

Dosage: 1 tablespoonful 3 to 4 times daily. Children: 1 teaspoonful or more.

Asthma

5 teaspoonfuls Cramp bark, fluid extract (Viburnum trilobum; V. opulus)
5 teaspoonfuls Lobelia, tincture (Lobelia inflata)
1 teaspoonful Ginger, essence or tincture (Zingiber officinalis)

Preparation: Mix thoroughly.

Dosage: 5 drops in warm water every 10 minutes until relieved. If nausea and emesis follow, these will only hasten relief.

Cramps from pregnancy, uterine pains, or any nervous troubles during pregnancy

2 parts Cramp bark (Viburnum trilobum; V. opulus)
1 part Squaw vine (Mitchella repens)
1 part Wild yam (Dioscorea villosa)
1 part Blue cohosh (Caulophyllum thalictroides)

Preparation: Mix the herbs thoroughly, and use 1 ounce of the herbs in 1 quart of boiled, distilled water. Infuse for 20 minutes tightly covered; strain, and sweeten to taste.

Dosage: 2 fluid ounces, 3 to 4 times daily.

Cramps, nerve tonic

1 ounce Cramp bark (Viburnum trilobum; V. opulus)
1/2 ounce Skunk cabbage (Symplocarpus foetidus)
1/2 ounce Scullcap (Scutellaria lateriflora)
2 teaspoons Cardamon seeds (Elettaria Cardamomum)
2 teaspoons Cayenne (Capsicum frutescens; C. minimum)

Preparation: Use as a strong infusion, or make into a tincture by macerating the herbs 4 days in 1 pint of a good wine or brandy. Strain, press and bottle.

Dosage: 1 tablespoonful 4 times daily.

Dr. Shook's compound nervine, hepatic and female regulator
(see "ADMINISTRATION" for uses)

1 ounce	Cramp bark, cut (Viburnum trilobum; V. opulus)
1 ounce	Wild yam, cut (Dioscorea villosa)
1 ounce	Vervain (Verbena officinalis; V. hastata)
1 ounce	Scullcap (Scutellaria lateriflora)
1 ounce	Cloves (Syzygium aromaticum; Eugenia aromatica)
12 ounces	Glycerine

Preparation: Dissolve 8 ounces of the glycerine into 2 quarts of distilled water; put the mixed herbs into the cold water and soak for 12 hours. Bring the mixture to a boil, and simmer slowly for 30 minutes. Strain, return the liquid to the clean vessel and reduce by simmering to 1 pint. Add 4 ounces of glycerine; cool, bottle, and keep in a cool place.

Dosage: 1 teaspoonful to 2 teaspoons in warm water. Children's dosage is proportionate to age and condition.

Dysmenorrhea
(difficult or painful menstruation)

1 ounce	Cramp bark (Viburnum trilobum; V. opulus)
1 ounce	Squaw vine (Mitchella repens)
1 ounce	White poplar or quaking aspen bark (Populus tremuloides)
1/2 ounce	Unicorn root (Aletris farinosa)
1/2 ounce	Bethroot (Trillium erectum; T. pendulum)
1/2 ounce	Blue cohosh (Caulophyllum thalictroides)
1/2 ounce	Pennyroyal (Mentha pulegium; Hedeoma pulegioides)
1/2 ounce	Sacred bark (Rhamnus purshiana)
1/2 ounce	Allspice or pimento berries (Pimento officinalis)

Preparation: Place the herbs in 1 quart of water; cover tightly. Steep for 20 minutes, then strain and sweeten with honey. Add 2 tablespoonfuls of glycerine.

Dosage: 1 tablespoonful before meals and at bedtime.

Growth characteristics:
Cramp bark is perennial and is found in northern and western United States. It grows in low rich lands, foothills, the woods, and the borders of fields. Cramp bark flowers in June and is a very showy plant.

Sister plants:
Black Haw or Stagbush or Sweet Viburnum or American Sloe (Viburnum pruni-

folium; RUBIACEAE) The root bark is used in threatened abortion, after-pains, dysmenorrhea, nervous diseases of pregnancy, menorrhagia, asthma and hysteria. See *The Herbalist* for a description.

HOPS

(Humulus lupulus; H. americanus; CANNABACEAE)

Common names:

Hops and humulus.

Identifying characteristics:

Stem	Herbaceous twiner (left to right), with several rough angular and flexible stems. It is up to 20 feet long and will twist around any adjacent support.
Leaves	Opposite, deep green, very rough, cordate (heart-shaped), venate or nerved (veined), stalked, serrated and 3 or 5 lobed.
Flowers	Dioecious (male and female plants), with numerous greenish pistil cone-like spikes, which produce the fruit.
Fruit	Strobiles or catkins. Ovoid-cylindrical (roundish), 1¼ inches long, with numerous yellow-green membranous scales that curve over each other. The fruit is reticulate-veined (network), with numerous brownish glandular hairs at the base of each scale and enclosing a glandular achene.
Taste	Aromatic, slightly astringent, and exceedingly bitter.
Odor	Strong, characteristic, and somewhat agreeable. With heavy processing, the odor becomes disagreeable, resembling that of valerian.

Part used:

Fruit or strobiles (cones, catkins).

Therapeutic action:

Nervine (sedative), tonic, anodyne, cholagogue, diuretic (lithotriptic), stimulant, anthelmintic, stomachic, febrifuge, aperient, alterative, feeble hypnotic, somewhat diaphoretic, astringent and anaphrodisiac.

Hops is a powerful, stimulating and relaxing nerve tonic. It increases heart action and capillary circulation, yet will produce soothing slumber in nervous and excited cerebral conditions. Hops is beneficial in affections of the throat, bronchi, and chest. Its stomachic tonic effects are due to an 11% crystalline bitter principle and *lupulin* acid (lupulite); the primary stimulant and secondary sedative effects are due to a 2% content of volatile oil and lupulin.

Hops increase the flow of urine and dissolves calculi, and with certain liver problems (such as jaundice), its alterative property relieves the secreting glands by increasing the flow of bile and toning up the organ. Hops has a relaxing influence upon the liver and gall ducts, and is aperient to the bowels. Hops is able to reduce inflammation and relieve accompanying pain.

Medicinal uses:
Nervous conditions, sleeplessness, chorea, dyspepsia, debility, atony, worms, tremors of delirium, hysteria, calculi, irritable bladder, bronchitis, liver problems, excessive sexual desires, nymphomania, painful erection in gonorrhea, rheumatism, inflammation, neuralgia, gathered breasts (mastitis), boils, abscesses, tumors, ulcers, toothache, and earache.

Preparations:
Fluid extract, infusion, powder, and tincture.

Dosage:

Fluid extract	1/2-1 fluid teaspoon.
Infusion	1-2 fluid teaspoons.
Powder	325 mg.-1 gram.
Tincture	1/2-1 fluid teaspoon.
Lupulin	130-325 milligrams.

ADMINISTRATION

Oral

Bronchitis: Combine the hops with a little lobelia (Lobelia inflata).

General tonic and sedative: Take the infusion (1 ounce of hops to 1 pint of water) in doses of 2 fluid ounces.

Sleeplessness, nervous troubles, delirium, etc: Take the infusion in 2 to 3 tablespoonful doses every 1 to 3 hours as needed.

Cholagogue (liver), diuretic, anaphrodisiac and gonorrhea: Simmer 1 tablespoonful of hops for 10 minutes in 1 pint of water and drink 1/2 pint morning and evening.

Insomnia, nervous irritation: Take 2 to 3 cupfuls of hot hops infusion or stuff a pillow with hops (sprinkled with alcohol if desired) to sleep on.

Tremors of delirium: Combine tincture of hops with tincture of cayenne and take in 1/2 to 1 teaspoonful doses.

Worms: Take 1/2 to 1 pint of hops decoction (1 ounce of hops to 1 pint of water, simmered 10 minutes) in the morning on an empty stomach.

Skin

Inflammation, rheumatism, neuralgia, boils, gatherings: Use hops poultice and fomentation.

Toothache, earache, neuralgia: Apply a flannel bag of hops, and moist heat over the affected area.

FORMULAS

Chorea (St. Vitus' Dance)

1 part	Hops (Humulus lupulus)
1 part	Cramp bark (Viburnum trilobum; V. opulus)
1 part	Black cohosh (Cimicifuga racemosa)

Preparation: Infuse 1 teaspoonful of the herb compound for 20 minutes in 1 pint of hot, distilled water and cover tightly. Strain and sweeten to taste.

Dosage: 2 fluid ounces, 3 to 4 times daily.

Neuralgia

1 part	Hops (Humulus lupulus)
1 part	Black cohosh (Cimicifuga racemosa)
1 part	Camomile (Chamaemelum nobile; Anthemis nobilis)
1 part	Yarrow (Achillea millefolium)
1 part	Sage (Salvia officinalis)
1 part	Peppermint (Mentha piperita)

Preparation: Combine 1 teaspoonful of the herbs with 1 cup of water. Infuse (do not boil), and steep 20 minutes.

Dosage: 1 to 2 tablespoonfuls each hour. Use a fomentation or poultice, with 3 parts mullein and 1 part lobelia.

Hops tonic

1 ounce	Hops (Humulus lupulus)
1 ounce	Dandelion root (Taraxacum officinale)
1 ounce	Buchu leaves (Agathosma betulina; A. crenulata)
1 teaspoonful	Ginger (Zingiber officinalis)

Preparation: Boil the first 2 herbs slowly for 30 minutes in 1 gallon of water. Add 1 pound of yellow D sugar, and bring to a second boil; skim off the impurities. Pour the hot mixture over the buchu and ginger, cover tightly, and steep until cool. Optionally, yeast may be added when lukewarm and left to work overnight. Strain, bottle, and keep in a cool place.

Dosage: 1 tablespoonful before meals.

Growth characteristics:
Annual stems, perennial root; found in the northern temperate zones of North America, Europe and Asia. It grows in hedges and open woods. Hops are largely cultivated in the United States and England for the purpose of alcoholic drinks (beer, ale, porter).

Collection:
Gather when mature, usually in the late summer and early fall.

Drying and preservation:
Care should be taken to preserve the volatile oils of the lupulin. Lupulin is the slightly transparent, golden, kidney shaped grains or powder which constitutes 1/7 of hops. The hops, and especially the lupulin should be kept dark and in tightly-covered containers. When the hops turn dark-reddish with a valerian-like odor from aging, it should be discarded.

BLACK COHOSH or BLACK-SNAKE ROOT
(Cimicifuga racemosa (Nutt.); Actaea racemosa (Linn.); Macrotys racemosa (Eaton); M. actaeoides (Raf.); RANUNCULACEAE)

Common names:
Black cohosh, black snake root, squaw root, rattle root, bugbane, cimicifuga, macrotys, tall bugbane, bugwort, rattleweed, rattlesnake, rattlesnake root, rich weed; Cimicifuga Rhizoma, Actaeae Racemosae Radix (Br.); Racine d'Actee a Grappes (Fr.); Schwarze, Schlangenwurzel (Ger.).

Identifying characteristics:

Stem	Simple (unbranched), slender, smooth, furrowed, 3 to 8 feet high and leafy.
Leaves	Alternate, with long petioles and thrice compounded leaflets (1 to 2 inches long) that are oblong and incised (deeply toothed or cleft). The leaflet ends are often compounded.
Flowers	Numerous, feathery, white, small and regular, in an elongated wand-like raceme (simple inflorescence in which the elongated axis bears flowers on short stems in succession toward the apex). The flowers are 8 to 20 inches long, fetid, with petal-like sepals that fall early, numerous 2-cleft stamens with long filaments, and 1 to 2 sessile pistils with broad stigmas.
Fruit	Dry oval pods with seeds in 2 rows.

Rhizome	Horizontal, large (4/5 to 6 inches long, 2/5 to 1 inch thick), hard and knotty. The rhizomes are slightly annulate, with circular scars of bud scale leaves, and an upper surface with numerous hard, erect, curved branches terminated by deep cup-shaped scars showing a radiate structure. They are dark brown or grayish-black in color, and the lower and lateral surfaces have numerous root- scars, a few short roots, and a horny fracture. Internally, the rhizome is whitish and mealy or dark brown and waxy. The bark is distinctly radiate wood with a central pith of the same thickness. The roots are cylindrical, obtusely quadrangular, 1/23 to 1/8 inch thick, and 1¼ to 4 inches long, brownish or blackish in color and longitudinally wrinkled, with a short fracture. The internal cortex is thin, brownish and has yellowish wood with 4 to 6 rays. Powder: light brown.
Taste	Bitter, pungent and astringent.
Odor	Slight and nauseous.

Part used:
Rhizome and roots.

Therapeutic action:
Antispasmodic, alterative, emmenagogue, diuretic, astringent, expectorant, diaphoretic, arterial and nervine sedative, cardiac stimulant, stomachic-tonic, antiseptic, antivenomous.

As a cardiac stimulant, black cohosh root slightly depresses the heart rate while it increases the force of the pulse and equalizes circulation. It is a valuable emmenagogue in pelvic disturbances and uterine troubles as it effectively contracts the uterus and increases the menstrual flow. Black cohosh has a strong effect on the muscular system, and is used for various forms of rheumatism, arthritis, and neuralgia. It is a viable expectorant for acute chronic pulmonary and bronchial affections. Black cohosh exerts a tonic influence over the mucous and serous tissues, stimulating the secretions of the liver, kidneys and lymph. It also aids digestion. In parturition, black cohosh is helpful in initiating uterine contractions, checking hemorrhage, and allaying the nervousness and afterpains of delivery.

Medicinal uses:
Insomnia, headache (back of the head, at the base of the brain), rheumatism, chorea, amenorrhea, dysmenorrhea, subinvolution, spinal irritation, pelvic disturbances, uterine troubles, apoplexy, eruptive diseases (smallpox, etc.), whooping cough, cholera, periodical convulsive fits, epilepsy, nervous excitability, asthma, tremors of delirium, spasmodic affections, consumption, cough, scrofula, neuralgia, hysteria, fatty heat, acute and chronic bronchitis, phthisis (tuberculosis of the lungs), dyspepsia, uterine hemorrhage, rheumatoid arthritis, lumbago, peritonitis, seminal emissions, nerve inflammation, ulcers, dropsy, spinal meningitis, liver and kidney troubles, poisonous insect and snake bites.

Preparations:
Fluid extract, infusion, powder, solid extract, syrup, and tincture. Alcohol is the best menstruum to extract the antispasmodic properties.

Dosage:
Black cohosh is a very potent agent, and an overdose will produce nausea and vomiting.

Fluid extract	5 to 30 drops.
Infusion	1 teaspoonful every 30 minutes to 3 tablespoonfuls every 3 hours, according to need.
Powder	325 milligrams 3 times daily.
Solid extract	50-200 milligrams.
Syrup	2 teaspoons to 1 tablespoonful 3 to 4 times daily.
Tincture	1/2 to 1 fluid teaspoon.

ADMINISTRATION

The black cohosh syrup can be used as a base for alterative compounds.

Oral

Apoplexy: See "FORMULAS."

Cough, whooping cough, liver and kidney troubles: Give the syrup form.

Dysmenorrhea, amenorrhea: Give a warm infusion of equal parts of black cohosh and blue cohosh (Caulophyllum thalictroides).

Colic, convulsions, nerve troubles: Give the syrup form; see "FORMULAS."

Insomnia, headache, indigestion, bronchitis, etc.: Give black cohosh infusion in small doses.

High blood pressure, heart palpitation, hemorrhage, uterine contractions, etc.: Give a full dose of black cohosh infusion.

FORMULAS

Apoplexy

1 ounce	Black cohosh, fluid extract (Cimicifuga racemosa)
1 ounce	Wood betony, fluid extract (Stachys officinalis)
1 teaspoon	Cayenne, tincture (Capsicum frutescens; C. minimum)

Preparation: Mix thoroughly.

Dosage: 1 teaspoonful every 30 minutes until patient improves and then every 1 to 2 hours as condition warrants.

Administration: Give the patient a foot bath in hot water with mustard and cayenne. Soak a piece of flannel in apple cider vinegar and wring it out. Wrap this around a hot water bottle, and place it on the feet. Give an injection (enema) made up of about 1/4 teaspoonful each of tinctures of lobelia (Lobelia inflata), scullcap (Scutellaria lateriflora), and cayenne (Capsicum frutescens; C. minimum) in 3/4 pint of warm water to help equalize the circulation and remove pressure from the brain. If the injection does not evacuate the bowels, repeat it. The patient should perspire freely.

Colic, convulsions and spasmodic nerve troubles (children's syrup)

2 ounces	Black cohosh (Cimicifuga racemosa)
1¼ pints	Distilled or D-cell water
4 ounces	Glycerine
1 pound	Yellow D sugar

Preparation: Place the herb and glycerine in the water, cover well, and let stand for 4 hours, stirring from time to time. Bring the mixture to a boil and simmer for 15 minutes; strain and return it to the clean vessel. Stir in the sugar, simmer for a few minutes, and skim if scum arises. Allow to stand until cool, bottle, and keep in a cool place.

Dosage: 2 teaspoons to 1 tablespoonful, 3 to 4 times daily. 1/4 to 1/2 teaspoonful for young children, 1 teaspoonful for children 5 years of age, and 1½ to 2 teaspoonfuls, 3 times daily for children 3 to 15 years old.

Dr. Christopher's glandular balance formula

1 part	Black cohosh (Cimicifuga racemosa)
1 part	Licorice root (Glycyrrhiza glabra) for adrenal glands
1 part	Bladderwrack (Fucus vesiculosus) for thyroid (or substitute kelp)
1 part	Golden seal (Hydrastis Canadensis)
1 part	Lobelia (Lobelia inflata) for all glands
1/2 part	Ginger (Zingiber officinalis)
1/4 part	Cayenne (Capsicum frutescens; C. minimum)

Preparation: Use in fine powder form. Mix the herbs together thoroughly and place in #0 capsules, which are equivalent to 1/4 teaspoonful.

Dosage: 1 to 2 capsules before noon (1/4 to 1/2 teaspoonful).

Epilepsy, chorea (St. Vitus' Dance)

1 ounce Black cohosh powdered (Cimicifuga racemosa)
1 ounce Blue cohosh powdered (Caulophyllum thalictroides)
1 ounce Vervain powdered (Verbena officinalis, V. hastata)

Preparation: Place the herbs into 1¼ pints of 90 proof alcohol (vodka or good whiskey). Cap tightly, shake well and set in a moderately warm place. Shake well each day for 14 days, being careful to open the bottle each time before shaking and close. Filter and bottle.

Dosage: 1 teaspoonful in 1 ounce of water (sweetened with honey) 3 to 4 times daily. Do not administer this preparation to children under 5 years of age. Place 5 drops in 1 tablespoonful of honey water for children 5 to 7 years old, 10 drops in honey water for those 8 to 12 years of age, 1/2 to 1 teaspoonful in 2 fluid ounces of honey water for children 13 to 16 years old. *Note:* Do not give an overdose. If it produces nausea or vomiting, reduce the dosage 1/4 to 1/2 by diluting well with honey water.

Lung hemorrhage

1 part Black cohosh; tincture (Cimicifuga racemosa)
1 part Blood root, tincture (Sanguinaria canadensis)

Preparation: 1 teaspoonful of tincture in 1/4 cup of water.

Dosage: 1 teaspoonful every 3 hours.

Whooping cough

1 ounce Black cohosh, tincture (Cimicifuga racemosa)
2 ounces Red root, tincture (Ceanothus americanus)
1 ounce Blood root, tincture (Sanguinaria canadensis)
1/2 ounce Lobelia, tincture (Lobelia inflata)

Preparation: Mix and shake well before using.

Dosage: 15 to 20 drops in honey water.

Congenial combinations:
Black cohosh combines well with blue cohosh (Caulophyllum thalictroides) in uterine problems.

Growth characteristics:
Black cohosh is perennial and is found mainly from Canada to Georgia and east of the Mississippi River. It grows best in shady and rocky places such as rich

woods, woodland borders, and hillsides. Black cohosh flowers from June to August.

Collection:
The rhizome and roots should be gathered in the autumn, when they are most active.

Drying and preservation:
The rhizome deteriorates with age and should be used shortly after gathering. It also may be preserved in the tincture form.

WILD YAM or COLIC ROOT
(Dioscorea villosa; DIOSCOREACEAE)

Common names:
Wild yam, colic root, china root, yuma, rheumatism root, wild yamwurzel, liver root, devil's bones and dioscorea.

Identifying characteristics:

Stem	Delicate and slender vine, twining climber, wooly, and reddish-brown in color. 1/5 inch in diameter, and 5 to 18 feet long.
Leaves	Ovate (2-4 inches in length and 3/4 of the length in width) cordate (heart-shaped), acute and glabrous or smooth on the upper surface with soft hairs on the lower.
Flowers	Very small and pale green in color with panicles.
Fruit	Triangular winged capsules with 1 to 2 flat seeds in each cell.
Rhizome	A long, branched, woody cylindrical tube, crooked (often compressed, bent and nodular) and 1/4 to 4/5 inch thick. The stem is scaly above with slender tough roots beneath, and pale brown in color. The fracture is scaly to short, yellowish internally with scattered wood bundles. The powder is whitish.
Taste	Starchy and insipid, and afterwards acrid.
Odor	None.

Part used:
Rhizome or root.

Therapeutic action:
Antispasmodic, relaxant (sedative), stimulant, antibilious, diaphoretic, expectorant, diuretic, hepatic, cholagogue, stomachic, tonic, anti-emetic, antirheumatic, anti-asthmatic and emetic (large doses).

Wild yam is considered one of the best anticatarrhal agents. It has been proven very valuable in pulmonary and catarrhal conditions. As a stimulant, relaxant, and antispasmodic, it is beneficial in all cases of nervous excitability. Wild yam relaxes the muscular fibers, soothes the nerves, and gives positive relief from pains, especially those associated with bilious colic, gall stones, and uterus. It is of great value in nervousness, restlessness, nausea, and pains that are common to pregnancy. Wild yam has a potent tonic effect on the uterus when taken throughout the period of pregnancy. It is excellent for relieving the trying cramps during pregnancy (especially during the latter stages), and will greatly assist in preventing a miscarriage. Wild yam relieves flatulence of the stomach and bowels, and soothes any abdominal and intestinal irritations and spasms.

Medicinal uses:
Bilious colic, rheumatism, jaundice, stomach catarrh, hardening and blocking of the liver, nausea of pregnancy, cholera morbus, neuralgic affections, spasmodic hiccough, whooping cough, spasmodic asthma, bronchitis, dysmenorrhea, flatulence, gall stone pains, nervousness, restlessness, uterine cramps, miscarriage preventative, hysteria, vomiting, abdominal and intestinal irritation.

Preparations:
Decoction, fluid extract, powder and tincture.

Dosage:

Decoction	(strong) 2 teaspoons to 2 fluid ounces in water 3 to 4 times daily, between meals.
Fluid extract	1/2-1 fluid teaspoon.
Powder	300-650 milligrams.
Tincture	5-20 drops.

ADMINISTRATION

Oral

Dysmenorrhea: Give wild yam decoction with a small quantity of ginger (Zingiber officinalis) as a diffusive stimulant.

Emesis: Take wild yam decoction in large doses.

Colic (all forms), abdominal and intestinal irritation, spasms, spasmodic asthma, vomiting and hepatic congestion: Take 1 tablespoonful of the warm decoction every 30 minutes until relieved.

Liver affections, rheumatic pains, spasms: Take 1 to 3 cupfuls of cold wild yam decoction during the day. Mix this well with saliva, one mouthful at a time.

Rheumatism, bronchitis, spasms, asthma, whooping cough, liver congestion, nausea of pregnancy, jaundice, bilious colic, etc.: Use the strong decoction; see "FORMULAS."

Uterine tonic, prevent miscarriage, and to ease pains: See "FORMULAS."

FORMULAS

You may use another form of the formula (i.e. decoction instead of fluid extract, etc.) by keeping the ingredient quantities proportionate.

Strong decoction of wild yam
(Bilious colic, rheumatism, bronchitis, spasmodic asthma, vomiting, hepatic congestion, nausea of pregnancy, jaundice, etc.)

2 ounces	Wild yam, cut (Dioscorea villosa)
1 quart	Distilled or D-cell water
4 ounces	Glycerine

Preparation: Put the herb and water in an appropriate vessel and boil slowly for 20 minutes. Strain, return to the clean vessel and reduce by simmering to 3/4 pint. Remove the mixture from the heat and add the glycerine. Let stand until cool, bottle, and keep in a cool place. The sweetening may be added while hot, or the dosage may be taken plain or in honey water.

Dosage: 2 teaspoons to 1 tablespoonful in water 3 to 4 times daily, between meals. 2 fluid ounces may be taken in severe cases. Children: 1 teaspoonful or more, according to age and condition.

Biliousness, colic

2 ounces	Wild yam, fluid extract (Dioscorea villosa)
1 ounce	Pleurisy root, fluid extract (Asclepias tuberosa)

Preparation: Mix thoroughly.

Dosage: 1 teaspoonful as often as is required.

Children's colic

2 teaspoonfuls	Wild yam, fluid extract (Dioscorea villosa)
2 teaspoonfuls	Pleurisy root, fluid extract (Asclepias tuberosa)
10 drops	Cinnamon, essence (Cinnamomum zeylanicum)
10 drops	Anise, essence (Pimpinella anisum)

Preparation: Mix the herbs thoroughly. Four ounces of simple syrup may be added, or the mixture may be taken with honey water.

Dosage: 1/2 teaspoonful in water every 15 minutes or as often as required.

Uterine tonic, to prevent miscarriage, ease cramps and pains

1 ounce	Wild yam (Dioscorea villosa)
1 ounce	Squaw vine (Mitchella repens)
1 ounce	False unicorn (Chamaelirium luteum)
1/2 ounce	Cramp bark (Viburnum trilobum; V. opulus)

Preparation: Simmer for 20 minutes in 1 quart or water, strain and sweeten to taste.

Dosage: 2 fluid ounces every 3 to 4 hours.

Congenial combinations:
Wild yam combines well with other uterine agents and acts as a uterine tonic and antispasmodic during pregnancy. When using wild yam as a uterine agent, combine it with ginger (Zingiber officinalis). For the pulmonary and stomach areas, combine with cayenne (Capsicum frutescens; C. minimum) and golden seal (Hydrastis Canadensis), etc.

Growth characteristics:
Wild yam is a perennial root and an annual vine, found throughout the United States. It thrives best in moist places, running over bushes and fences and twining about the growth in thickets and hedges. Wild yam flowers from June to July.

For alternate nervine and antispasmodic herbs to be used when the foregoing are not available, please see chapter 17.

CHAPTER 12

THE STIMULANT HERBS

Stimulants quicken, excite and increase nervous sensibility, thereby stimulating energy in the body and enhancing its function. These herbs stimulate naturally, in contrast with unnatural drugs and alcohol, which irritate and debilitate the system, and in the case of alcohol, depress it. Stimulants increase the power of the pulse and carry the blood to all parts of the body, equalizing and restoring the circulation in all parts.

CAYENNE
(Capsicum frutescens; C. minimum; C. annuum; SOLANACEAE)

Common names:
African pepper, African red pepper, American red pepper, bird pepper, capsicum, cayenne pepper, Spanish pepper; Capsique or Poivre de Cayenne (Fr.); Spanisher Pfeffer, Schlotenpfeffer (Ger.).

Identifying characteristics:
The varieties of fruit may vary greatly in size color and pungency. The most pungent is the yellowish red fruit of Sierra Leone; the African birdseye cayenne (Capsicum fastigiatum) are small (1/3 to 1/2 inch long, 1/8 to 1/6 inch thick), pungent, bright pods and retain the heat in the body longer than any other variety. Zanzibar chilies often have the stalks attached. The African varieties grow on shrub-size plants and the fruit is small and pungent, while the American varieties are herb-size plants, the fruit being larger and heart-shaped.

Part used:
Fruit (oil is in the seeds).

Therapeutic action:
Stimulant, tonic, carminative, sialagogue, stomachic, rubefacient, pungent, alterative, astringent, antispasmodic, sudorific, emetic, antiseptic, condiment, antirheumatic.

Cayenne is the purest and most certain stimulant, used medicinally and also as a condiment. This herb is a great food for the circulatory system. It feeds elements that may be lacking into the cell structure of the arteries, veins and capillaries to give them the elasticity of youth again, as the blood pressure adjusts itself to normal. When the venous structure becomes loaded with sticky mucus, the blood has a harder time circulating; therefore, higher pressure forces the liquid through. Cayenne regulates the flow of blood from the head to the feet so that it is equalized. Cayenne (as a stimulant) is an activator, carrier, and accentuator.

Cayenne influences the heart immediately, then gradually extends its effects to the arteries, capillaries, and nerves. The frequency of the pulse is not increased, but it is given more power. In equalizing the blood circulation, cayenne produces natural warmth, and in stimulating the peristaltic motion of the intestines, it aids in assimilation and elimination. It rebuilds the tissue in the stomach. It also heals stomach and intestinal ulcers.

Medicinal uses:
Apoplexy, arrest gangrene or mortification, arthritis, asthma, asthmatic asphyxia, atonic gout, bleeding, bleeding of the lungs, chilblains, chills, colds, cold extremities, congestion, constipation, cough, cramps, debility, delirium tremens, diphtheria, dyspepsia, emesis (strong dose), functional sluggishness, fatigue, heart trouble and heart attacks, hemorrhage, hemorrhoids, high and low blood pressure, indigestion, inflammation, kidney and related problems, lethargy, low fevers, lumbago, menorrhagia, neuralgia, offensive breath, pains in the stomach and bowels, palpitation, pleurisy, profound shock, quinsy, rheumatism, scarlet fever, strokes, tonsillitis, toothache (oil), typhoid fever, ulcers, vomiting, wounds, yellow fever.

Preparations:
Cayenne is prepared as a decoction, infusion, ointment, powder, and tincture.

Cayenne is seldom used in the vagina as a bolus. It could be, but it is too uncomfortable. Very seldom is it used as a decoction, because some value is lost when cayenne is simmered for any length of time. In using cayenne, the most common form of preparation is an infusion, made by pouring water over the cayenne and letting it sit. The infusion can be used with absolute safety.

We use cayenne in a liniment quite frequently, in a proportion of 1/8 or 1/16 part to other oils, etc. Use very little oil at a time, as it is very potent. With the ointments, cayenne is used in approximately 1/8 proportion to other herbs. There are cayenne ointments and gels specifically for external use.

Cayenne is used in nearly all fomentation, plasters, and poultices where speed is necessary, or where quick relief (as in arthritis, rheumatism, bursitis, sore muscles and those types of cases) is desired. Externally, it is used dry (on wounds), and the powder is used in formulas mixed with many other types of herbs. In using the powder in poultices, plasters, suppositories, enemas, etc. the cayenne is used 1/8 part in proportion to the other herbs that are used, according to the case.

The liquid extract or tincture is easily kept and very valuable to have on hand. Use this moderately, as it is many times stronger than the infusion. The extract or tincture is invaluable for emergency use.

Dosage:

Infusion	1/4 teaspoonful 3 times daily; then after three days, increase 1/2 teaspoonful 3 times daily; then add 1/4 teaspoonful each day thereafter until the minimum recommended dosage of 1 teaspoonful 3 times daily is reached. Heart palpitation: In acute stages, repeated dosages of one to two teaspoonfuls every 1/2 hour (more frequently when required). Hemorrhage: 1 teaspoonful of powder in 1 cup of hot water. Inflammation: 1 teaspoonful every hour until pain ceases. Pains in the stomach and bowels, constipation: 1/2 to 1 teaspoonful of powder in 1 cupful of very warm water.
Oil	Less than 5 milligrams.
Powder	See "Infusion," (300 mg.-1 gram).

ADMINISTRATION

Cayenne is an old standby and is used in modern medicine yet today in counter-irritant ointments for sore muscles, arthritis, etc.; in liniments, sports rubs and in many other ways. You will see it listed as capsicum in the ingredients. Cayenne can be used on any part of the body, the fastest-acting being the liquid form.

Anal

Ointment: Cayenne may be applied on hemorrhoids for it does bring relief and healing, but the patient should be warned of its potency.

Oral

Take cayenne in the powdered or cold infusion. During the first few days of taking cayenne, it will be hot going in, and hot going out. You can soon become accustomed to it, so that soon you will feel that it gives a lovely glow and warmth. But each time you stop using it for a period of time, and then start again, the same reaction occurs.

Baby: We have given cayenne tea by an eye dropper to a six-week-old baby that was born with chronic asthma, making it possible for him to breathe again.

Capsules: A lot of people use cayenne in capsules. Dr. Christopher was taught in school to use it in capsules, but he found that it always gives an excuse not to take cayenne when we run out of capsules or when we haven't had time to fill them. It's all right to use capsules because they melt when they get into the stomach. But when you take it straight, right out of the container, you can always have it at hand. Some people mix it with peanut butter first, but if a person needs the healing effects of cayenne in a hurry, cayenne should be taken in water so it will go into the tissues right away. If coated with oil, it won't have as speedy an effect.

Heart attack: Prop up the patient and pour hot cayenne tea down, and the attack will stop immediately. Dr. Christopher was called in the middle of the night so many times for heart attack, and this was the remedy he used. A teaspoon of cayenne in hot water should bring the patient out of the heart attack. In case you have no cayenne in an emergency of a heart attack, use black pepper, tripling the dosage.

Hemorrhage: A hemorrhage may occur in the lungs, stomach, uterus, or nose—flowing fast. Just take a teaspoonful of cayenne in a glass of extra-warm water, drink it down, and by the count of ten the bleeding will stop. Instead of all the pressure being centralized, it is equalized, and the clotting becomes more rapid. Whether the bleeding is internal or external, a teaspoon of cayenne taken orally in a glass of hot water will stop the bleeding quickly. For the lungs, a vapor bath, along with the warm cayenne infusion, will be very beneficial.

Skin

Toothache: Clean the cavity and place cotton saturated with cayenne oil into the cavity.

External bleeding: For external bleeding, the cayenne powder or tea may be taken internally, or the powder placed directly on the wound.

Diphtheria and quinsy: Apply tincture of cayenne around the neck, then cover with a flannel fomentation of cayenne infusion, and drink cayenne internally.

Eyes: Use cayenne as an eyewash, in combination with other herbs.

Liniments and Ointments: Cayenne ointment is extremely valuable because it is so powerful in bringing out toxic poisons, and it is also used as a counter-irritant. Even many famous commercial ointments, such as those from Rawleighs, Watkins and others, are high in cayenne. It can be used alone without burning or blistering.

Plaster: Cayenne can be used in the plaster form, like mustard, although we find that the ointment form is much easier to use.

Wounds: Even with severe wounds, so deep that they may be exposed to the bone, you can fill them with cayenne pepper (and if cayenne is not available, black pepper) to stop the bleeding and bring quick healing. Many people, when they see the skin reddened by the cayenne, believe that the skin is irritated; but cayenne is a counter-irritant; there is no itching involved with it. Cayenne actually brings the blood to the surface to take away any toxic poisons, or to start the healing; so the redness comes to the skin from the blood that has rushed to the surface to carry off wastes.

Cold feet: Sprinkle a few grains in the shoes or socks (but too much here will produce too much heat and give a burning sensation).

Vaginal

Cayenne should not be used directly in the vagina without mixing it with something else.

Nasal

The mucus membrane of the nose is very delicate and cayenne is generally not used in that area.

FORMULAS

Apoplexy

1/2 teaspoon Cayenne powder (Capsicum frutescens; C. minimum)
1/2 teaspoon Mustard powder (Brassica nigra; B. hirta)

Preparation: Place the powder in hot bath water.

Administration: Soak in bath water as hot as possible until the patient sweats profusely. Watch apoplexy patients so that they do not faint and allow the head to slip down into the water.

Coughs, consumption, tuberculosis

1 teaspoonful	Cayenne powder (Capsicum frutescens; C. minimum)
1-2 ounces	Slippery elm bark powder (Ulmus rubra), cut to match thickness of cayenne powder
1 slice	Lemon (Citrus limon)
2 tablespoons	Honey

Preparation: Infuse in 1 pint of boiling water; steep and bottle unstrained.

Dosage: Use from a teaspoon to a tablespoon, according to age, as often as needed.

Liniment for lung congestion, sprains, etc.

1 tablespoon	Cayenne powder (Capsicum frutescens; C. minimum)
1 pint	Apple cider vinegar

Preparation: Simmer for 10 minutes in closed container; bottle while hot and unstrained.

Administration: Apply over the area where needed without too much massage.

Liniment for wounds, bruises, burns, pyorrhea, etc.

1 ounce	Cayenne powder (Capsicum frutescens; C. minimum)
1 ounce	Golden seal (Hydrastis Canadensis)
2 ounces	Myrrh gum (Commiphora myrrha, var. molmol)

Preparation: Place into 1 quart of rubbing alcohol or apple cider vinegar; macerate (shake well) 3 times daily for 10 days; strain and store in colored bottle.

Administration: Apply freely on area when needed.

Liniment for sprains, bruises, rheumatism and neuralgia

2 ounces	Cayenne tincture (Capsicum frutescens; C. minimum)
2 ounces	Lobelia fluid extract (Lobelia inflata)
1 teaspoon	Oil of Wormwood (Artemisia absinthium)
1 teaspoon	Oil of Rosemary (Rosmarinus officinalis)
1 teaspoon	Oil of Spearmint (Mentha spicata)

Preparation: Mix ingredients thoroughly.

Administration: Apply as much as can be absorbed; and then to speed the action use hot fomentation with a hot water bottle on the troubled area, if possible.

Sore throat

1 teaspoon	Cayenne powder (Capsicum frutescens; C. minimum)
1/2 pint	Red (Garden) Sage tea (Salvia officinalis)
2 tablespoons	Apple cider vinegar
2 tablespoons	Sea salt
2 tablespoons	Honey

Preparation: Steep the cayenne with the sage tea; then mix the remaining ingredients.

Dosage: Mouthful, gargle 4 to 12 times daily. Take a tablespoonful or two orally after the gargle has been spit out. Take it orally as often as needed, but at least after gargling.

Congenial combinations:
Cayenne can be used with almost any other herb. It can be used by itself, as it would be in healing *stomach ulcers;* it can be used alone to stop *hemorrhaging;* it can be used alone as a daily food. And if you are brave, you can use it as an enema for *obstinate constipation.*

Cayenne is used with bayberry or pleurisy root to increase perspiration, and with tonics to reduce perspiration. It will take uterine agents such as holy thistle directly to the uterus; although ginger will carry all the herbs to the reproductive organs and abdominal area even faster than cayenne.

-For uterine hemorrhage, combine cayenne with bayberry and take orally.
-It always follows the use of lobelia in order to activate the secretions.
-For gastro-flatulence and indigestion, cayenne combines with lobelia.
-A strong dose of cayenne powder will excite vomiting; also use in combination with other emetics.

CASE HISTORY

Hunzas.
Cayenne is one of the main foods of the Hunza, who live in a high isolated mountainous area in Asia Minor. They live over a hundred years of age in good health. They eat sparingly, generally a mono-diet; apricots, fresh or dried are their mainstay, with cayenne as the supplement. They play polo at 100 years and older and they do not die of diseases, but generally from falls and accidents.

High blood pressure, hemorrhoids.
A Dr. Christopher case history in his own words: I traveled with a man younger than myself several years ago all over the western part of the United States on business. He marveled at the stamina that an older man could have on long drives without displaying the usual fatigue. Each morning I would get up and have my cayenne and my wheat germ oil (I don't pay attention to anyone else, I just take them, regardless). Finally he got curious and said, "What's that stuff?" So I gave him an illustrative lecture, and he responded, "Well, I have hemorrhoids; my mother died of high blood pressure, and I have high blood pressure; and with the hemorrhoids I have to wear a belt, as you probably noticed, to keep my hemorrhoids up in place. Do you think that (meaning cayenne) will help?" "Not unless you take it," I replied. "Well, I will start taking it." Then I added, "I don't think you're man enough; I don't think you are brave enough," and I turned and walked away.

Now, he was well-proportioned and a weight lifter, so after I left, he went over and got into my can and started using the cayenne along with the wheat germ oil, and by spring he did not have to wear a belt any longer as his hemorrhoids were cleared. Then he had an amazing surprise when he went to his doctor for a regular check-up; the doctor took his blood pressure three or four times and said, "This is supposed to be progressively worse. I don't know what has happened; your systolic and diastolic are near perfect. You don't need to come back any longer. I don't know what happened!" Well, he did not have to go back, and today this gentleman who lives in the Salt Lake City area has no high blood pressure, for he has continued taking his cayenne.

Growth characteristics:
Native of South and Central America; introduced into Africa and East Indies; cultivated in U.S.

Collection:
Gather the fruit when ripe, and expose it to the sun until dried, but do not wash.

Drying and preservation:
Oil of cayenne will keep indefinitely if it is tightly capped. The length of time the powder itself will keep depends upon the storage conditions. We have kept cayenne in the powdered form for up to a year, but it was stored in a fairly cool place. To keep cayenne as a powder, hermetically seal or wax the can (as a honey can). Don't ever put cayenne in a paper sack, for a paper takes the precious oils out of it. A carton box that has been waxed on the inside is all right, and it will keep well in cellophane and plastics.

Bugs: To keep weevils and worms out of cayenne, use elder leaves (any elder leaves that become powdered and mix into the cayenne will do no harm, but be beneficial). *Refrigeration:* Do not refrigerate it. As a powder at room temperature, kept sealed, it should keep well six months to a year; and hermetically sealed, it should keep two to three years.

For longer preservation of cayenne, you need to make it into a tincture. Tincture will keep indefinitely as long as it is in a dark place (we use 3-4 ounce colored-glass bottles) and it is well-stoppered (i.e., capped or corked). We have had tinctures that after twenty years storage, were as good as new.

JAMAICA GINGER
(Zingiber officinalis; ZINGIBERACEAE)

Common names:
Jamaica ginger, black ginger, race ginger, African ginger; Ginembre (Fr.); Rhizoma (Radix) Zingiberis, Ingwer (Ger.).

Identifying characteristics:
Reed-like plant with horizontal rhizome segments, light brown, depressed stem-scars, starchy, resinous, internally yellowish, agreeable aromatic odor, pungent taste (Jamaica is the least pungent and most delicate ginger).

Part used:
The dried rhizome or root (with the outer cortical layers partially or completely removed).

Therapeutic action:
Diffusive stimulant, antispasmodic, carminative, diaphoretic (hot), aromatic, sternutatory, rubefacient, anodyne, sialagogue, pungent, condiment, aphrodisiac. Ginger is a milder stimulant; it goes from the capillaries, through the venous structure, to the heart and back again. It is more diffusive than cayenne, but may be used as a substitute for it when it is unavailable.

Medicinal uses:
Boils, bronchitis (chronic), cholera, colds, colic, congestion, diarrhea, dyspepsia (atonic), flatulence (suppressed gas), flu, gout (atonic), griping, headache, hemorrhage of lungs, menstruation, nausea, neuralgia, paralysis of tongue, reproductive problems, rheumatism, sore throat, toothache.

Preparations:
Generally use ginger in infusion. Once in a while it is decocted with other herbs. It is good in many forms: bolus, essence, infusion, liniment, liquid extract, plaster, poultice, tincture, syrup.

Dosage:
Fluid extract 15-60 drops.
Infusion 2 fluid ounces or 1 teacupful at a time.

Oil	2-3 drops in a cupful of water.
Powder	500 milligrams.
Tincture	5-20 drops.

ADMINISTRATION

It combines with almost all herbs.

Anal

Ginger is often used alone or combined with other herbs in an injection of no more than a cup (so that it can be retained); it gives its influence to the whole system.

Oral

Ginger can be administered in teas, capsules, pills, or any way you wish; the fresh root of ginger is chewed for cases of paralysis of the throat.

Babies: For babies, make the ginger tea in the same proportions (a teaspoonful to the cup) and give less of it (with an eye dropper). For very small babies, use distilled water and dilute it.

Reproductive problems: Ginger tea is excellent for trouble in the genital-reproductive organs. Use ginger alone for menstrual cramps; you may be amazed at how effective it is. In nearly all cases, it's used in capsule or tea form, generally in equal parts with other herbs.

Flatulence: See "FORMULAS."

Carrier: Ginger is generally combined with herbs for the abdominal area, because it is a carrier. Ginger accentuates most of the herbs for the lower abdominal and colon areas.

Hemorrhage of lungs and salivary glands: Chew rhizome or root.

Skin

Muscle spasms and irritations: Use in a liniment or plaster.

Fevers: Ginger can be put into the bath water (1 teaspoonful or by the pound) to take the burning off dermatitis.

Nasal

Very seldom is ginger used in the nose.

FORMULAS

Flatulence

1 teaspoonful	Ginger (Zingiber officinalis)
1 teaspoonful	Baking soda

Preparation: Place ingredients in 1 glass of warm to hot water; stir until the water clears.

Dosage: Drink 1 glassful as needed.

Maturation poultice for boils

1 part	Ginger (Zingiber officinalis)
1 part	Flour (Cornmeal or flax seed meal)

Preparation: Mix ingredients with small amount of water to make a thick paste.

Administration: Apply amply over affected area; then cover with plastic and bandage.

Mild laxative

1/4 teaspoon	Ginger powder (Zingiber officinalis)
20 leaves	Senna (Cassia angustifolia)
1 slice	Lemon (Citrus limon)

Preparation: Place in cup; steep with 1/3 cup of boiling water (be sure to cover); sweeten to taste with honey.

Dosage: Drink the clear liquid from 1 cup.

CASE HISTORY

Stomach pains.
Dr. Chriostpher recalled this case: I remember when a lady called from Salt Lake to my residence in Cottonwood at three o'clock in the morning. Her daughter was screaming in the background with terrible stomach pain. I was tired, as I had been out on night calls and had just barely retired to bed, and I said, "Take some ginger and baking soda. The pain will stop; and go back to bed. I'll call in the morning." She begged, "Oh, you've got to come." So I said, "All right." I pulled on my clothes and set out. It was eight or ten miles, so before I got there, the pains grew so acute that she finally decided to do what I told her to do. And when I arrived, the daughter met me at the door—all smiles—no pain.

Growth characteristics:
Perennial herb; native of India and Hindustan; cultivated in West Indies and Africa. It thrives best on new forest soil producing when one or more years old (the younger rhizomes are best); but with some skill, it can be grown in your own herb garden.

Collection:
Dig rhizomes or roots in January or February after the stems have withered; clean carefully to avoid bruising.

Drying and preservation:
Dry as rapidly as possible, while conserving the volatile oils and resins. In fact, in some of the cases, if bottled tightly in dark bottles, ginger powder will last far longer than the original whole herb would as a dry herb. Ginger is best kept hermetically sealed in the powder form or in tincture. A liquid extract is also good.

Jamaica ginger is best: Please be careful that you get the right kind of ginger; Jamaica ginger is best. Some dealers adulterate ginger and put fillers in, as with a lot of foods, so that more profits can be made. Get your ginger right from the health store, herb store, or a reliable source, so that it will be a good product. If possible grow your own, and pound the rhizome with a mortar and pestle; then you will be certain of the value.

VIRGINIA SNAKE ROOT
(Aristolochia serpentaria; ARISTOLOCHIACEAE)

Common names:
Serpentari, snake weed, sangrel, suagrel, sangree root, pelican flower, birthwort; Couleuvree de Virginie, Serpentarie (Viperine) de Virginie (Fr.); Virginische schlangenwurzel (Ger.).

Identifying characteristics:
Rhizome or root is more or less curved (2/5 to 1¼ inches long, 1/25 to 1/12 inch thick), short stem bases on upper portion, thin, nearly straight, yellowish-brown roots extending from lower portion internally the wood is yellowish-white; it has a bitter taste, and an aromatic, camphoraceous odor.

Part used:
Dried rhizome and roots.

Therapeutic action:
Diuretic, emmenagogue, aphrodisiac, antiperiodic, stomachic, cardiac stimulant, expectorant, exanthema, anodyne, febrifuge, diffusive stimulant, tonic, diaphoretic, antispasmodic, nervine.

It influences the circulation, skin, and kidneys. It is quite stimulating to the gastric membrane, is an excellent digestive aid, activates the secretive organs and increases the power of other herbal agents.

Medicinal uses:
Dyspepsia, diphtheria, poison ivy rash, fevers (especially typhoid). Since it is a stimulant, it is also a remedy for rheumatism. It is also good for nettle rash, poison ivy, poison snake bite, etc. Snake root generally is used as a tonic inside the body. This is not a genital or rectal medicine.

Preparations:
Concentrate, infusion, liquid extract, tincture, plasters. Boiling the root will slightly damage the value, so use the infusion. Plasters for acute congestion, pleurisy, pneumonia: combine with lobelia and bran (or hops).

Dosage:
In gastric problems, strong doses may cause nausea, vomiting and purging, so use small dose.

Infusion	1 tablespoonful 4 to 6 times daily.
Decoction	1 cupful during the day.
Fluid extract	30 drops.
Powder	1/2-2 grams.
Tincture	5-20 drops.

ADMINISTRATION

Skin

Nettle rash or poison ivy: Apply a wash of fluid extract.

Oral

Nettle rash or poison ivy: Give infusions as freely as the patient can take it for a few hours, then stop. Keep patient off of any mucus-forming foods.

Congenial combinations:
It is acceptable to the digestive organs when Peruvian Bark cannot be taken. Has good effect where childbirth is slow, the extremities are cold, pains inefficient, and will prevent possible hemorrhaging.

Growth characteristics:
Perennial herb; native to U.S.; grows in rich, shady and hilly woods (W. Pennsylvania to Indiana).

PEPPERMINT
(Mentha piperita; LABIATAE)

Common names:
Balm mint, brandy mint, curled mint, lamb mint, peppermint; Menthe poivree (Fr.); Pfefferminz (Ger.).

Identifying characteristics:
This is the most pungent of all the mints. Do not confuse spearmint with peppermint, however, as the spearmint grows along ditch banks and has dull leaves whereas the peppermint has shiny leaves and requires special growing conditions. Spearmint multiplies by a creeping root stock, producing long and numerous suckers 2-4 feet high; the stem is square and purplish; the leaves are a light green (with purplish-brown mixture), and sharply serrate, and slightly hairy.

Part used:
Whole herb, oil.

Therapeutic action:
Stimulant, sudorific, carminative, emmenagogue, aromatic, stomachic, antispasmodic, nervine, sedative, febrifuge, and rubefacient (oil). It is one of the great stimulant herbs, and also acts as a marvelous antispasmodic. It also strengthens the nerves and heart muscles, assists in digestion, cleanses and gives tone to the entire body. Peppermint is a soothing sedative for nervous and restless people of all ages, promoting relaxation and sleep. The oil is an excellent stomach aid.

Medicinal uses:
Cholera morbus, colic, colon trouble, convulsions (children, babies), diarrhea, dizziness, dysentery, dysmenorrhea, earache, fainting, fevers (all types), flatulence (stomach, bowels), flavoring agent, griping, flu, hiccough, inflammation, menstrual obstructions, nausea, nervous headache, nervousness, neuralgia, palpitation of the heart, restlessness, rheumatism, seasickness (prevent), sleeplessness, spasms (stomach, bowels), toothache, vomiting.

Oil: Burns, cholera morbus, colic, diarrhea, dysentery, dysmenorrhea, flatulence, heart palpitation, hiccough, inflammation, nausea, nervous headache, neuralgia, rheumatism, spasmodic pains, toothache, vomiting.

Preparations:
Never boil the herb itself, as the medicinal principles are extremely volatile and contain much of the medicinal potency. The peppermint infusion is made by pouring boiling water over the mint; then cover and keep in a warm place for ten minutes; strain, sweeten and drink hot.

Dosage:
Essence A few drops in water.

Extract	1-2 fluid teaspoons.
Infusion	1-2 cupfuls daily between meals. For children, take 1/4 to 1/2 the adult dose (1 teaspoonful to 1 tablespoonful diluted with equal parts of boiling water.)
Tincture	1/2-1 fluid teaspoon.

ADMINISTRATION

This is the most extensively used medicinal herb in the world.

Anal

Enema: This form of administration is excellent for cholera, colon problems, and for convulsions and spasms in children.

Oral

Fainting or dizzy spells: Take a hot, strong peppermint tea.

Fevers: Take in dose of 1 pint as hot as can be taken; this is even better when combined with elder flowers.

Flu: For one of the greatest flu remedies there is, see "FORMULAS."

Griping: It will soothe the gastrointestinal area from irritating foods and unripe fruits.

Headache: Drink a cupful of hot peppermint tea; then lie down and relax.

Indigestion: See "Congenial Combinations."

Inflammation: See "FORMULAS."

Menstrual obstructions: See "FORMULAS."

Stomach problems: See "FORMULAS."

Vomiting: See "Congenial Combinations."

Skin

Oil: Apply externally on the affected area for rheumatism, neuralgia, and headache.

FORMULAS

Flu remedy, fevers, inflammation

1 ounce Peppermint leaves (Mentha piperita)
1 ounce Elder flowers (Sambucus canadensis)

Preparation: Place in appropriate vessel and pour 1/2 pint of boiling water over the herb; cover tightly and keep warm on stove for 15 minutes; strain and cover immediately and keep warm.

Dosage: 1 teacupful every 30 to 45 minutes until the patient perspires; then 2 tablespoonfuls every 1 to 2 hours.

Administration: This tea taken hot will break down congestions, equalize circulation, and restore a functional equilibrium. Keep patient well covered in bed overnight; then sponge the body in the morning with equal parts of apple cider vinegar and water (this will act as a tonic and cleanse waste matter from the pores). For children: Give smaller doses and sweeten.

Menstrual obstructions
(For a highly nervous or hysterical person)

1 part Peppermint herb (Mentha piperita)
1 part Wood Betony herb (Stachys officinalis)

Preparation: Make infusion (cover well).

Dosage: 2 fluid ounces every three hours.

Stomach tonic

3 grams Peppermint leaves (Mentha piperita)
3 grams Fennel seed (Foeniculum vulgare)
1 gram Turkey rhubarb (Rheum palmatum)

Preparation: Infuse in 1 pint of water.

Dosage: 2 fluid ounces 3 times daily, or more (according to need).

CASE HISTORY

Always before an emetic.
Peppermint has so many wonderful uses, but one in particular that is a must is to use it always before an emetic. We have had actual cases where people have thrown up (using lobelia as an emetic) for as much as three hours, but by preceding it with peppermint tea, there has been no soreness in the stomach or bowel areas.

Growth characteristics:
Perennial herb; grows wild in low, wet ground; but it may be cultivated in your herb garden (out of the sun) or indoors (under 65° F.) from a transplanted start of roots or cuttings (these root rapidly in a glass of water). Starts can be potted in heavy soil and must be kept well-soaked. Peppermint should be left outdoors until after the first frost. Be very careful to keep the different mints apart, as they tend to cross.

Collection:
Collect when in bloom, during dry weather (August to September) for drying. It can be used fresh any time.

CLOVES

(Syzygium aromaticum; Eugenia aromatica; E. caryophyllata; Caryophyllus aromaticus; MYRTACEAE)

Common names:
Cloves, mother cloves, clavos; Girofle, Clous (aromatiques) de Girofle (Fr.); Gewurznelken, Naegelein (Ger.).

Identifying characteristics:
This is a handsome evergreen tree that grows 30 to 40 feet high, has extensive branching, yellowish bark, leaves that are 4 inches long and 2 inches wide, rose-colored flowers, berry-like fruit. The flower buds or cloves are tack-shaped, 2/5 to 3/4 inch long and dark brown when dried. The lower portion of the clove consists of the calyx tube enclosing (in its upper half) the ovary filled with minute ovules; and the upper portion has four calyx teeth, surrounded by the unopened globular corolla of four concave overlapped petals. The taste is hot, pungent, and spicy, and upon pressing the calyx tube with a finger nail, oil should exude.

Part used:
Dried, unexpanded flower buds.

Therapeutic action:
Stimulant, stomachic, aromatic, carminative, expectorant, anti-emetic, antispasmodic, astringent, rubefacient, antiseptic, digestive, condiment.

This herb increases circulation, promotes digestion and nutrition, raises the body temperature, stimulates the excretory organs, and stimulates and disinfects the kidneys, skin, liver and bronchial mucous membrane. It is the most powerful of the aromatic and carminative herbs.

Medicinal uses:
Ague, bad breath, bronchial catarrh, cholera morbus, cold extremities, colic,

condiment, convulsions (infantile), corrective, diarrhea, dysentery, dyspepsia, epilepsy, flatulence, griping, indigestion, low blood pressure, mucus, colitis, nausea, neuralgia, palsy, poor circulation, phthisis, rheumatism, sour stomach, toothache (oil), twitching, vomiting (pregnancy), zygotic diseases.

Preparations:
Used chiefly in combination with other aids.

Dosage:

Fluid extract	5-30 drops.
Infusion	1/2-1 fluid ounce three times a day.
Oil	1-5 drops.
Powder	130-200 milligrams.
Tincture	3-4 drops three times daily.

ADMINISTRATION

Use oil of cloves in toothache; use in liniments; use as a cover for strong-tasting herbs.

Oral

Cholera morbus: See "FORMULAS."

Griping: See "FORMULAS."

Indigestion, poor digestion, bad breath: Carry cloves in pocket and chew on them, but go into the cause.

Nausea: See "FORMULAS."

Stomach problems: See "FORMULAS."

Toothache: Rub oil of cloves and oil of peppermint on gums.

Vomiting (pregnancy): See "FORMULAS."

Skin

Infantile convulsions: Place poultice on nape of neck.

Colic, flatulence: Place poultice over stomach.

FORMULAS

Infusion of cloves

1 teaspoonful Cloves, whole or powdered (Syzygium aromaticum)
1 pint Distilled water.

Preparation: Boil the water; and pour over the cloves and steep for 20 minutes in a closed stainless steel container over a very low flame. (The residue of the first infusion may be used a second time to make another infusion.)

Cholera morbus

2-3 tablespoons Cloves (Syzygium aromaticum; Eugenia aromatica)
1/2 pint Soymilk (tofu-milk)

Preparation: Simmer in soymilk 5 minutes.

Dosage: 1 tablespoonful hot every 15 minutes.

Nausea, vomiting in pregnancy #1

1 teaspoonful Cloves (Syzygium aromaticum; Eugenia aromatica)
1 teaspoonful Turkey rhubarb powder (Rheum palmatum)
1 teaspoonful Cinnamon (Cinnamomum zeylanicum)
1 ounce Spearmint (Mentha spicata)

Preparation: Simmer the first three herbs in 1 pint of water for 5 minutes; pour this decoction over the spearmint; put the lid on tightly and let this infuse until cool; strain.

Dosage: 2 tablespoonfuls to 1/4 cupful every 1/2 hour until the nauseated condition subsides.

Nausea or vomiting in pregnancy #2

1 part Cloves powder (Syzygium aromaticum; Eugenia aromatica)
1 part White poplar, Quaking aspen bark powder (Populus tremuloides)

Preparation: Use about 1 gram of powder or fill a #00 capsule.

Dosage: Take powder or capsule at onset of nausea or vomiting, as needed.

Growth characteristics:
Perennial tree; native to the Mulucca Islands of Asia and Southern Philippines; cultivated in Asia, Africa, South America, West Indies. Trees yield when six years old, reach their peak at twelve years, then decline and perish at twenty years.

Collection:
Collect just before ripe; the clove is white at first, then turns green, pink, and bright red; it is gathered at the pink stage by hand-picking on ladders and platforms or beating the trees with bamboos and catching the falling buds on outstretched cloths.

Drying and preservation:
The clove contains aromatic and volatile oil, so drying should be done quickly and without exposure to bad weather.

HORSERADISH
(Armoracia rusticana; Cochlearia Armoracia; Rorippa Armoracia; CRUCIFERAE)

Common names:
Great raifort, horseradish, mountain radish, red cole.

Identifying characteristics:
The plant grows 2 to 3 feet high, with leaves 8 to 12 inches long and 4 to 5 inches wide; it has white flowers and a two-celled fruit pod. The root is 12 inches long and 1/2 to 1 inch thick, tapering, conical-shaped, yellowish, scaly, warty, white and fleshy inside with many stones and a central pith; it has a pungent mustard-like odor when the root is scraped or bruised (irritating to the nostrils) and has a sharp, acrid, mustard-like taste.

Part used:
Fresh or dried root.

Therapeutic action:
Stimulant, aperient, rubefacient, pungent, condiment, diaphoretic, diuretic.

Horseradish is one of the most prolific stimulant herbs there is, especially to the digestive organs (dried root), kidneys, skin and circulation. It will give pleasant warmth in the stomach, relieve the gall ducts, stimulate alvine (intestinal) action, and increase the flow of urine. **Caution: do not use this herb during pregnancy.**

Medicinal uses:
Bile, bronchitis, catarrh (gastric, intestinal), constipation (atonic), coughs, dropsy, dyspepsia (atonic), hoarseness, indigestion, jaundice, low blood pressure, malnutrition, neuralgia (local), palsy, paralysis, poor circulation, pulmonary complaints, rheumatism, sciatica, scrofula, scurvy, sinus trouble (breaks mucus, cleanses), sluggish liver and stomach, urine (aid), vomiting, weak chest, wheezing, whooping cough, worms.

Preparations:
Take a fresh root (which is far more powerful than the dried) and grate it fine (horseradish can be difficult to grate because it is so stringy), mix it with a small amount of lemon juice or apple cider vinegar (lemon juice is preferable when fresh and used within a few days) and then refrigerate.

Dosage:
We recommend that horseradish be taken in much the same way as cayenne: start with a small amount, then work up to one teaspoonful three times a day.

ADMINISTRATION

Oral

Start with 1/4 teaspoonful and hold it in your mouth until it is nothing but sawdust (i.e., until the fragrance is gone). It will immediately start cutting the mucus loose from the frontal and sphenoidal sinuses and will start draining down the throat.

FORMULAS

Torpid (numb or lacking energy) stomach and liver, with constipation

1/2 ounce	Horseradish, fluid extract (Armoracia rusticana)
1/2 ounce	Gentian, tincture (Gentiana lutea)
1/2 ounce	Dandelion, fluid extract (Taraxacum officinale)
6 ounces	Syrup of orange (Citrus aurantium)

Preparation: Mix thoroughly.

Dosage: 1 teaspoonful at meal times.

Dropsy # 1

4 ounces	Horseradish root, freshly scraped (Armoracia rusticana)
1 quart	Apple cider vinegar
4 ounces	Vegetable glycerine

Preparation: Put root in cider and let stand 12 hours in fairly hot place. Loosen cap occasionally, tighten and reshake. After 12 hours of steeping, remove to cool place and steep another 12 hours. Strain and add glycerine.

Dosage: 1 tablespoonful to the cup of water 3 to 4 times daily (before meals and one dose at night).

Dropsy #2

1 ounce Horseradish (Armoracia rusticana; Cochlearia Armoracia)
1/2 ounce Mustard, crushed seed (Brassica nigra; B. hirta)

Preparation: Pour 1 pint of boiling water over the herbs; cover and steep until cool; strain.

Dosage: 2-3 tablespoonfuls three times daily.

Growth characteristics:
Perennial herb; native of Europe, it can be cultivated and grown in your herb garden.

Collection:
Fresh roots from cultivated plants.

Drying and preservation:
The root can be dried, but it would be better preserved (because of the valuable volatile oils) in fluid extracts or tincture form.

BLACK PEPPER
(Piper nigrum; PIPERACEAE)

Common names:
Black pepper, pepper.

Identifying characteristics:
The leaves are ovate, smooth, dark green, and 4 to 6 inches long and 1/7 to 1/4 inch wide; the flowers are whitish; the berry-like fruit is green at first, then red, and is yellow when ripe; and the fruit has an aromatic odor and pungent taste.

Part used:
Dried fruit (berries and powder). The unripe fruit is black; the ripe is white.

Therapeutic action:
Stimulant, tonic, antiperiodic, diaphoretic, carminative, aromatic, rubefacient, pungent, condiment, febrifuge.

This is an active stimulant, especially to the gastrointestinal tract. It may be used as a substitute for cayenne.

Medicinal uses:
Cholera morbus, colic, condiment, fevers (periodic, intermittent), flatulence,

gums, indigestion, rheumatism (plaster), sore throat (gargle).

Preparations:
Do not boil or heat black pepper. When heated, the molecular structure changes very quickly from organic to inorganic, making it an irritant to the kidney, liver and gall bladder areas. This should always be used fresh. Much of that which is purchased in grocery stores has had dangerous preservatives added to keep vermin out, so please try to use the whole pepper or peppercorn and grind it fresh in a small pepper mill (which is relatively inexpensive).

Dosage:
Oleoresin 30 milligrams.
Powder 100 mg. to 1 gram.

ADMINISTRATION

Oral

As a diaphoretic: Make the fresh pepper into a tea and drink large amounts hot. This will cause the patient to sweat; and if done in combination with a hot bath, so much the better.

Sore throat: Mix the powder in a small amount of water and gargle a mouthful.

Skin

Rheumatism: Use in plaster form.

FORMULAS

Cholera morbus

4 teaspoons	Black pepper powder (Piper nigrum)
3-4 tablespoon	Sea salt
3 ounces	Apple cider vinegar

Preparation: Mix in 3 ounces of warm water

Dosage: 1 tablespoonful three times daily.

Growth characteristics:
Perennial; woody evergreen climber; native of East Indies, Java, Sumatra; cultivated elsewhere.

Collection:
The berries are most potent when gathered before they are ripe (the black is the

unripe berry), as they contain a valuable oleoresin. The white (ripe) pepper is less pungent, but may be used after the berry is soaked in water and the external coat is peeled off.

PRICKLY ASH
(Zanthoxylum americanum, Z. clava-Herculis, Z. faxineum; RUTACEAE)

Common names:
Northern prickly ash, pellitory bark, prickly ash, suterberry, toothache bark, toothache bush, yellow wood.

Identifying characteristics:
This is a deciduous shrub that grows 10 to 15 feet high, branches alternately and is covered with prickly, conical spines on the bark (4/5 to 6 inches long, 1/5 to 1/2 inch wide). The bark is about 1/12 inch thick, is fragmented (the outer part shows green and the inner shows yellow), and has a bitter, acrid and pungent taste that causes salivation, but there is very little odor. The small, blue-black berries (the size of currants) grow in enclosed gray shells that cluster on top of the broaches (these appear before the leaves).

Part used:
Bark and berries (the berries are considered the most effective, as they contain a volatile oil).

Therapeutic action:
General stimulant, cardiac stimulant, tonic, alterative, pungent, deobstruent, diuretic, antiseptic, diaphoretic, sialogogue, nervine.

The action of this general stimulant is slower than cayenne, but its effects are more permanent, and it will remove obstructions in every part of the body. Berries: these possess volatile oils that are stimulant, antispasmodic, and carminative, and act principally upon the mucous membranes.

Medicinal uses:
Asthma, cholera, cold extremities, colds, colic, diarrhea, dropsy, dyspepsia (atonic), female problems (chronic), flatulence, liver (hepatic) problems, lumbago, paralysis, paralysis of tongue, pharyngitis, syphilis, rheumatism (chronic), scrofula, skin diseases, sluggish circulation, sores in mouth, toothache, ulcers, wounds.

Preparations:
Fluid extract, elixir, infusion, syrup.

Dosage:

Fluid extract	1/2-1 teaspoon (bark), 10-30 drops (berries)
Infusion	1 tablespoon four times daily; or 1 cupful cold during the day.
Powder	1/2-2 grams.
Solid extract	100-300 milligrams.
Tincture	5-20 drops.

ADMINISTRATION

Oral

Sores in mouth, toothache: Chew the bark or berries.

FORMULAS

Infusion of Prickly ash

1/2 ounce	Prickly ash berries (Zanthoxylum americanum; Z. Clava-Herculis), or crushed powdered bark
1 pint	Distilled, boiling water

Preparation: Steep in covered vessel two hours before use.

Blood purifier, improve blood circulation

1/2 ounce	Prickly ash bark (Zanthoxylum americanum; Z. Clava-Herculis)
1/2 ounce	Guaiac resin (Guaiacum officinale; G. sanctum)
1/2 ounce	Buckbean herb (Menyanthes trifoliata)
6 pods	Cayenne pepper (Capsicum frutescens; C. minimum)

Preparation: Simmer for 15 minutes, but keep tightly covered until cool (so that the valuable volatile oils do not escape).

Dosage: 2 fluid ounces three times daily.

Liniment for rheumatism

1 ounce	Prickly ash bark powder (Zanthoxylum americanum)
4 ounces	Olive oil, heated (Olea europaea)

Preparation: Mix ingredients thoroughly.

Administration: Massage in liniment night and morning.

Rheumatism

1/2 ounce	Prickly ash bark (Zanthoxylum americanum; Z. Clara-Herculis)
1/2 ounce	Buckbean or Bogbean (Menyanthes trifoliata)
1/2 ounce	Guaiacum chips or raspings (Guaiacum officinale, G. sanctum)
1/3 tspn.	Cayenne powder (Capsicum frutescens; C. minimum)

Preparation: Boil 15 minutes in 1/2 pint of water; strain.

Dosage: 2 fluid ounces 3 to 4 times daily.

Growth characteristics:
Perennial tree; native to North America and grows east of the Mississippi River from Canada to Florida, in moist places (woods, thickets, river banks); it flowers in April and May.

For alternate stimulant herbs to be used when the foregoing are unavailable, please see chapter 17.

CHAPTER 13

THE TONIC HERBS

Tonics permanently increase tone throughout the entire system and give increased vigor, energy, and strength, stimulating assimilation of nutrients. These herbs are invigorating, refreshing and permanently strengthening to every body organ. They work primarily within the digestive system, yet all body organs are positively influenced. They produce normal tone to the tissues of an organ, resulting in healthier muscles and function. These herbs sharpen the appetite, promote better waste elimination, aid in digestion, soothe the stomach, and gradually build up strength, energy, and health. As a rule, the tonic herbs are bitter, usually given during convalescence from disease or in any run-down condition. Be sure that the patient is past the acute stage of the disease before you administer tonics.

BARBERRY
(Berberis vulgaris; Berberis dumetorum; BERBERIDACEAE)

Common names:
Barberry, bearberry, berbery, berberidis, pepperidge bush, gouan, barbaryn, barboranne, berber, guild, jaundice berry, maiden barber, piperidge(s), piprage, piperidge tree, rults, woodsore, woodsour; epine vinette, vinettier (Fr.); Berberize, Gemeiner Sauerdorn (Ger.); Berberi, berbero, crespino, uvetta, scotanella (Ital.).

Identifying characteristics:
This is an erect, many-branched, spreading, and deciduous shrub that grows 3 to 8 feet tall (but can reach to 10 or 12 feet). The stem bark is thin, yellowish-gray on the outer surface, with an orange-yellow inner bark that separates into thin layers. The wood is yellow; the branches are armed with sharp three-pronged spines; the leaves are oval, toothed and spiny (soft bristles); and the small, yellow flowers (having a disagreeable odor) cluster on racemes but are hardly noticeable when the small flowers come out in May-June. The root bark is dark brown externally and fractures short when broken. The bark is very bitter. The scarlet or bright-red oblong berries are very acid, and make a very picturesque sight in September when the twigs are weighted down with this beautiful fruit.

Part used:
Bark, root bark (this is the most active); berries.

Therapeutic action:
Tonic, laxative (mild), antiseptic, refrigerant, bitter astringent, antacid, diuretic, resolvent, stomachic, cholagogue, purgative (large dose). Berries: refrigerant, astringent, antiscorbutic (contains citric and malic acids).

This is one of nature's most valuable herbs, a famous Indian remedy. It is one of the best medicines to correct liver secretions because it causes the bile to flow more freely and it removes waste matter from the stomach and bowels. It is an excellent tonic for delicate and weak people (particularly for children), building from anemia and general malnutrition to complete recovery in just a few weeks. It regulates the digestive system, lessens the size of the spleen, and removes obstructions in the intestinal tract.

Medicinal uses:
Loss of appetite, bilious conditions, catarrh, constipation, general debility, diabetes, chronic diarrhea, weak digestion, dropsy, dysentery, dyspepsia, fevers, gall bladder problems, sluggish intestinal action, jaundice, liver complaints, skin problems, enlarged spleen.

Preparations:
Decoction, fluid extract, infusion, powder, preserve (see page 542), pills, solid extract, syrup, tincture.

Dosage:
This is perfectly harmless in large doses, but should not be given to the point of producing diarrhea.

Concentrate	2 teaspoons to 1 tablespoonful 3 times daily. Children: 1/2 to 1 teaspoonful in honey water three times daily until the bowels move freely, then reduce dose.
Infusion	2 fluid ounces (2-3 tablespoons) 3 to 4 times daily.
Fluid extract	1/2 to 1 teaspoon.
Powder (Bark)	1/4 teaspoonful 3 to 4 times daily.
Solid extract	325-650 milligrams.
Tincture	1/2-1 fluid teaspoon.

ADMINISTRATION

Oral

Colds, promote perspiration: Just before retiring to bed, put 1 tablespoonful or more of barberry jelly (made from the ripe berries) in 6-8 ounces of hot water and drink hot.

Fevers, convalescence from fevers: Stir 1 tablespoonful of barberry jelly in 6-8 ounces of very cold water and drink cold.

Gargle, mouthwash: Use proper dilution in water.

Sore throat: Take 1 teaspoonful of barberry jelly frequently.

FORMULAS

Bilious Colic

1/2 ounce	Barberry bark (Berberis vulgaris)
1/2 ounce	Dandelion root (Taraxacum officinale)
1/2 ounce	Agrimony (Agrimonia eupatoria)
1/2 ounce	Centaury (Erythraea centaurium)
1/4 ounce	Composition powder (see page 147-148)

1/4 teaspoon Cayenne (Capsicum frutescens; C. minimum)

Preparation: Simmer first five ingredients of the compound in 1 quart of water down to 1/4 pint (decoction), strain hot over the Cayenne (infusion).

Dosage: 2 fluid ounces 4 to 6 times daily.

Biliousness, digestive tonic (tincture)

4 ounces Barberry bark (Berberis vulgaris)
4 ounces White poplar or Quaking aspen bark (Populus tremuloides)
4 ounces Wild cherry bark (Prunus serotina)
1 gallon Apple cider vinegar

Preparation: Crush and macerate the herbs and soak for 1 week in apple cider vinegar; strain, bottle.

Dosage: 1 tablespoonful 3 or more times daily.

Concentrate of Barberry

4 ounces Barberry bark, cut (Berberis vulgaris)
3 pints Water (distilled when possible)
8 ounces Glycerine (vegetable)

Preparation: Soak the bark one hour in the water; boil the bark slowly in one pint of water until the water barely covers the bark; strain this liquid through a cloth and set aside; return the herb to the vessel and cover with one quart of water and boil for 15 to 20 minutes; strain and mix the two quantities of liquid together; place in a clean pot and simmer the liquid down into a concentrate of 1 pint; take this off the heat, add the glycerine, cool and bottle.

Infusion of Barberry

1 ounce Barberry bark, cut (Berberis vulgaris)
1/4 pint Water (distilled is always better than ordinary water)

Preparation: Boil the water and pour over the herbs while boiling; cover and steep for 15 minutes in a hot place, strain, bottle and keep in a cool place.

Jaundice

1/2 ounce Barberry bark (Berberis vulgaris)
1/2 ounce Raspberry leaves (Rubus idaeus)
1/2 ounce Agrimony (Agrimonia eupatoria)
1/2 ounce Cleavers (Galium aparine)

1/4 ounce	Mountain flax (Linum catharticum or use L. usitatissimum)
1/4 teaspoon	Cayenne (Capsicum frutescens; C. minimum)

Preparation: Simmer the first five ingredients of the compound for 15 minutes in one quart of water, strain over the cayenne.

Dosage: 2 fluid ounces 3 times daily.

Laxative, germicide, pinworms in children

4 ounces	Barberry bark, cut (Berberis vulgaris)
1 heaping teaspoon	Mandrake root or May apple, cut (Podophyllum peltatum)
4 ounces	Glycerine

Preparation: Simmer the herbs slowly for 15 minutes in about 1½ pints of water, strain and set aside; cover the herbs (1 inch above the top of the herbs) with water and simmer until the water is level with the herbs, strain; place both quantities of liquid in a clean pot and simmer down to 8 ounces; take this concentrate off the heat, stir in the glycerine; let stand until cool, bottle and keep in a cool place.

Dosage: 1 tablespoonful night and morning until the bowels move freely. Children: 1/2-l teaspoonful.

***Growth characteristics*:**
This bush/shrub is found widely in the temperate zones of America and Europe, and parts of Asia. It grows in thickets, woods, or hedges, by roadsides, in dry or hard, gravelly soil, and many species thrive well in cultivated gardens, especially gardens that are shady, rocky, and well watered. It grows wild mainly in New England and the Middle states, and less often in Canada and the West but it is occasionally found here on rich soil. When barberry is grown in dry, gravelly or rocky conditions, many of the leaves and twigs become modified into thorns (these diminish the water loss through evaporation and act as a natural protection); but in well-watered garden soil, much of this thorny armor turns into an abundance of leafy rosettes and numerous twigs. It can be grown in your medicinal garden.

Sister plants:
Oregon Grape (Mahonia aquifolium; M. repens; Berberis aquifolium). This is a sister plant to barberry and is very similar in chemical composition and therapeutic action, but barberry is slightly superior in its slightly higher percentage of berberine. But where barberry acts with greater speed and effectiveness upon the liver, stomach and digestive organs, the wild Oregon grape acts more favorably and is more reliable in scorbutic and syphilitic problems.

CALUMBA

(Jateorhiza palmata; J. calumba; Cocculus palmatus; MENISPERMACEAE)

Common names:
Calumb, colombo, colombo root, foreign colombo, jateorhiza, koamwa, kalumb; Calumbae Radix, Menispermum palmatum, (Br.); Colombo, Racine de Colombo, Racine de Valumbe (Fr.); Radix Colombo, Kolombowurzel (Ger.).

Identifying characteristics:
This is a climbing vine strongly resembling yellow parilla (Menispermum canadense); the rhizome is short, thick, irregular, and branching. The extending roots have a thin, grayish-brown skin that is marked with transverse warts. The male plant has a single stem of about 1 inch thickness proceeding from the root, while the female has two. The leaves are large (10 inches long, 14 inches wide), petiolate (stalked), hairy and palmately-lobed (3 to 7 lobes); and the flowers are small and inconspicuous (borne in pendulous maxillary panicles). The roots coming from the rhizome are many, fleshy, fusiform (tapering at each end, spindle-shaped), and resemble parsnips (but they are larger, more cylindrical, and grow in clusters). These are sold commercially in oval disks 1½ to 4 inches wide and 1/4-4/5 inch thick, with biconcave centers, which are roughly wrinkled and internally yellowish (grayish-yellow or yellowish-brown), and the external bark is grayish-brown. These sections show vascular bundles in radiating lines, are mealy and fracture short; they have a slight odor, and an aromatic, mucilaginous and very bitter taste.

Part used:
Root.

Therapeutic action:
Tonic, febrifuge, stomachic, anti-emetic, digestive stimulant (stimulates the nerves of the digestive tract, which dilate the gastric vessels and augment secretion), sialagogue, antiseptic, disinfectant, anthelmintic, cathartic (large doses), mild laxative (small doses), and slightly demulcent.

This bitter tonic, without astringency or aroma, is one of the most effective, and purest tonic strengtheners for patients that are worn out to the point of indolence (especially in hot, swampy climates), promoting digestion, toxic elimination, tone and nourishment to the whole body system. Calumba is a good substitute for Peruvian bark when it is unavailable. It is excellent to use before confinement to increase energy and endurance. It resembles golden seal as a gastric tonic, but not a nervous system tonic.

Medicinal uses:
Bed wetting, cholera infantum, cholera morbus, colon trouble, constipation, convalescence from fevers, debility, diarrhea (chronic), dysentery, dyspepsia (atonic), fevers (remittent and intermittent), flatulence (bowel), indigestion, liver torpor

(inactivity), mucus colitis, pinworms (children), prolapsed uterus, phthisis (tuberculosis), pulmonary consumption, rheumatism, sea-sickness, stomach problems, vomiting in pregnancy.

Preparations:
Decoction (see "FORMULAS"), infusion (place 1 ounce of the herb in 1 pint of cold water, bring to a simmer for thirty minutes or more.

Dosage:

Concentrate	1/2-1 teaspoon.
Decoction	1 tablespoonful 3 to 4 times daily between meals. Children: 1-2 teaspoonfuls in honey water 2 times daily.
Fluid extract	10-30 drops.
Infusion	2 tablespoonfuls 3 to 4 times daily.
Powder	(root) 1/2-2 grams.
Solid extract	100-300 milligrams.
Tincture	1-10 drops.

ADMINISTRATION

This herb is given orally, or by anal injection in extreme cases.

FORMULAS

Decoction of calumba

1 ounce	(2 tablespoonfuls) Calumba root, cut (Jateorhiza palmata)
1 pint	Water
2 ounces	Glycerine

Preparation: Boil the water and pour this over the root; place this on very low heat (not boiling) for 30 minutes; strain and add the glycerine; cool, bottle and keep in a cool place.

Flatulence (intestinal)

1/2 ounce	(1 tablespoon) Calumba powder (Jateorhiza palmata)
1/2 ounce	Ginger powder (Zingiber officinalis)
1 teaspoon	Senna powder (Cassia angustifolia)

Preparation: Make an infusion by pouring 1 pint of boiling water over the above ingredients; cover tightly and steep for one hour. Strain and sweeten to taste (if desired).

Dosage: 2 fluid ounces 3 times daily.

Weak and Impaired digestion

1 ounce	Calumba root (Jateorhiza palmata)
1 ounce	White poplar or Quaking aspen bark (Populus tremuloides)
1 ounce	Raspberry leaves (Rubus idaeus)
1/2 ounce	Horehound herb (Marrubium vulgare)
1/2 teaspoon	Cayenne (Capsicum frutescens; C. minimum)

Preparation: Simmer the first four herbs about 15 minutes in one quart of water; strain while hot over the cayenne.

Dosage: 1 fluid ounce 3 to 4 times daily.

Growth characteristics:
Perennial root; this plant is a native of the southeastern forests of Africa in and near Mozambique (lower Zambezi River), and is cultivated in Africa and the East India Islands.

Note: Beware of adulterated calumba.
Calumba is sometimes adulterated with white bryony root (Bryonia alba) which is a hydragogue cathartic—large doses are *dangerous*. It may be adulterated with American columbo (Frasera caroliniensis), which has different therapeutic action from calumba (see below). These adulterations are dyed yellow with turmeric or safflower and made bitter with columbo or quassia (giving a near physical resemblance to the African calumba root). These adulterations can be recognized by the following simple tests: (1) the color will be slightly lighter, (2) they are not mucilaginous, (3) they lack the dark cambium zone and radiating lines of the true root, and (4) they redden litmus paper. Other more technical tests can be made, such as: the adulterations precipitate with iron salts, evolve ammonia with fixed alkalies, and contain no starch.

AMERICAN COLUMBO
(Frasera caroliniensis; F. Walteri; F. canadensis; GENTIANACEAE)

Common names:
Colombo, Columbo, American colombo.

Identifying characteristics:
The herb grows 3 to 8 feet tall, has a dark purple stem 1 to 2 inches thick, with leaves that are in whorls of 4 to 6. The root comes in pieces 3 to 4 inches long and 1/2 to 1 inch thick, has a thick bark that is pale brownish-gray; and the transverse section is yellowish-brown. The root fractures short, is spongy, and the taste is sweetish, then bitter, with a flavor resembling Gentian.

Part used:
Root.

Therapeutic action:
Tonic, mild stimulant, moderately bitter. This herb is a gentle stimulant, a general tonic, especially promoting appetite and aiding in digestion.

Medicinal uses:
Obstinate constipation, diarrhea (children), weak digestion (children), dyspepsia, gangrene (internally and externally), leucorrhea, miscarriage prevention, prolapsed uterus, vaginal ulceration.

Preparations:
Decoction, infusion powder, and tincture.

Dosage:

Infusion	2 fluid ounces 3 to 4 times daily.
Powder	1-4 grams (1/3 to 1 teaspoon).

FORMULAS

Dyspepsia

1 ounce	American columbo, tincture (Frasera caroliniensis)
1 ounce	Golden seal, tincture (Hydrastis Canadensis)
1 ounce	Leptandra or Culver's Root, tincture (Veronicastrum virginicum)

Preparation: Mix thoroughly.

Dosage: 2 teaspoonfuls after meals.

Tendency to miscarriage, foul leucorrhea

3 ounces	American columbo (Frasera caroliniensis)
2 ounces	Unicorn root (Aletris farinosa)
1 ounce	Golden seal root (Hydrastis Canadensis)
1 ounce	Squaw vine (Mitchella repens)
1	Orange peel (Citrus aurantium)

Preparation: Simmer 1/2 hour in 3 quarts of water, strain.

Dosage: 2 fluid ounces (2-3 tablespoonfuls) 3 to 4 times daily.

Congenial combinations:
This herb combines beneficially with uterine agents and vaginal tonics, especially where there is prolapsed uterus, uterine and vaginal ulcerations, etc.

Growth characteristics:
Perennial herb; native to the United States; bears large, yellow and purple dotted flowers in July.

GOLDEN SEAL
(Hydrastis Canadensis; RANUNCULACEAE)

Common names:
Golden seal, yellow root, hydrastis, orange root, ground raspberry, yellow puccoon, yellow paint root, Indian paint, Indian plant root, turmeric root, jaundice root, Ohio Curcuma, Indian turmeric, eye balm root, eye root, yellow eye; Hydrastis rhizome (Br.); Racine Orange Scau d'Or (Fr.); Hydrastisrhizom, Canadische Gelbwurzel (Ger.).

Identifying characteristics:
The plant grows 6 to 24 inches high, bearing 2-3 large, unequal, alternate, terminal leaves which are slightly hairy and palmate (having 3 to 5 lobes each). The stems above the ground are purplish and hairy, and are yellow below. The flower is solitary, small, white or rose-colored with a fruit resembling a raspberry. The fresh root or rhizome is short (about 2 inches long, 3/4 inch thick), having an abundance of rootlets a foot or more in length; the fracture is greenish-yellow, with broad medullary rays radiating from the woody center of the transverse section. The herb tastes very bitter, and the odor is strong and disagreeable.

Part used:
Dried rhizome and roots. The price of this root has always been unusually high, but if you require golden seal for a particular malady, do not attempt to substitute other herbs; they will not achieve the same results. Always use the herbs you need, no matter what the price! Never use the commercial colorless fluid extract, however, as it does not contain the needed therapeutic values of the herb.

Therapeutic action:
Tonic, laxative, alterative (mucous membranes), detergent, ophthalmic, antiperiodic, aperient, diuretic, antiseptic, deobstruent (glandular system), cholagogue, anti-emetic, nervine, hemostatic (uterine).

This is a powerful tonic for problems with assimilation; it effectively tones debilitated mucus membranes and any other tissues it contacts, increases gastric secretions and flow of bile, improves the appetite, and aids in digestion. In some cases, it is laxative, but without astringency. It is a particularly effective uterine hemostatic, and it is one of the very few herbs that will tone and sustain venous circulation. It is considered to be one of the best general medicinal aids in the entire herbal kingdom. Its therapeutic action ranks somewhere between Turkey rhubarb and bloodroot. Golden seal was named by the Thomsonians, who employed it extensively during the early part of the nineteenth century in the United States.

Medicinal uses:
Chronic alcoholism, acute alimentary inflammation, biliousness, bladder problems, bronchitis, cancer, canker sores, catarrh in alimentary and excretory channels, catarrh of mucous membranes, chronic dyspepsia, colds, chronic constipation (from sluggish liver and intestinal secretions), cystitis, general debility, digestive disorders, dysmenorrhea, eczema, erysipelas, external cleansing agent, eye affections, intermittent fevers, fistulas, flu, gastric disorders (irritability, ulceration), glandular inflammation, gonorrhea, hemorrhage (including slight bleeding in the pelvic tissues), hemorrhoids (internal and external), jaundice, leucorrhea, liver troubles, lotion, malaria, menorrhagia, nasal catarrh, nausea in pregnancy (small doses), cracked and abraded nipples, pharyngitis, pyorrhea, rectal fissures and prolapse, ringworm, scarlet fever, secretion deficiencies, skin diseases, open sores, spinal meningitis, stomach troubles, syphilitic sores, enlarged tonsils (tonsillitis), typhoid fever, ulcers, uterine ulceration and erosion, vaginal douche.

Preparations:
Decoction, elixir, fluid extract, infusion, powder, solid extract, tincture, douche.
Note: People with hypoglycemia sometimes experience a drop in blood sugar when using golden seal; if this is the case, do not use. **If hypoglycemic, heal the pancreas before attempting to use golden seal.**

Dosage:
Generally give small and frequent doses.

Elixir	1/2-1 teaspoon (30-60 drops).
Fluid extract	5-30 drops.
Infusion	1-2 teaspoonful 3 to 6 times daily.
Powder	1/2-2 grams.
Solid extract	50-100 milligrams.
Tincture	1/2-2 teaspoonfuls.

ADMINISTRATION

Anal

Chronic gonorrhea, gleet: Use injection (see “FORMULAS”).

Nasal

Congestion or pulmonary catarrh: Snuff powder into nostrils.

Oral

Indigestion: Use infusion or tincture combination (see “FORMULAS”).

Pyorrhea: Dip the toothbrush into the powder and brush teeth.

Sore throat: Use as gargle (see “FORMULAS”).

Ulcers in mouth: Use the infusion as a wash.

Dyspepsia: 650 milligrams of the powdered root or a tablespoonful of decoction 3 times daily or 1-2 teaspoonfuls of tincture 3 times daily.

Ringworm: 1 level teaspoonful of powder in 1/2 cupful of warm water, sweeten to taste (dilute for children).

Skin

The local application of golden seal will yield results that are superior to most other herbal agents.

Skin lotion: 1 teaspoonful of powder in 1 pint of boiling water, dissolve and let stand until cool.

Eruptive diseases (smallpox, measles, scarlatina, etc.), itching, burning of skin: Use as wash (see “FORMULAS”).

Erysipelas, eczema: Use as wash (see “FORMULAS”).

Inflamed or sore eyes: Use the infusion as an eye wash.

Ringworm: Use a local application of the decoction, fluid extract, tincture, etc.

Vaginal

Leucorrhea: Use injection (see “FORMULAS”).

Vaginal douche: 1 teaspoonful of powder in 1 pint of boiling water; dissolve and let stand until cool.

FORMULAS

Biliousness

4 ounces	Golden seal (Hydrastis Canadensis)
4 ounces	Balmony (Chelone glabra)
4 ounces	Dwarf elder (Sambucus Ebulus)
2 ounces	Gentian (Gentiana lutea)
2 ounces	Prickly ash bark (Zanthoxylum americanum; Z. clava-Herculis)
2 ounces	Wahoo (Euonymus atropurpureus)

Preparation: Make 2 quarts of syrup.

Dosage: 2 tablespoonfuls after meals.

Offensive catarrh (snuff)

1 ounce	Golden seal powder (Hydrastis Canadensis)
2 teaspoons	Bayberry bark powder (Myrica cerifera)
2 teaspoons	Raspberry leaves powder (Rubus idaeus)

Preparation: Rub thoroughly in a mortar and place through a fine sieve.

Administration: Use several times daily as a snuff.

Chapped hands

1 part	Golden seal (Hydrastis Canadensis)
1 part	Goldthread (Coptis trifolia)
1 part	Elder bark (Sambucus canadensis)

Preparation: Steep in warm olive oil; harden with beeswax if desired.

Administration: Apply freely as needed.

Itching, burning of skin, eruptive diseases (smallpox, measles, scarlatina, etc.)

1 ounce	Golden seal (Hydrastis Canadensis)
9 ounces	Linseed oil (Linum usitatissimum)

Preparation: Mix thoroughly.

Administration: Apply freely as needed.

Erysipelas and skin diseases (liniment)

1 ounce	Golden seal, tincture (Hydrastis Canadensis)
1/2 ounce	Myrrh, tincture (Commiphora myrrha, var. molmol)
1/2 ounce	Echinacea, tincture (Echinacea angustifolia)

Preparation: Mix thoroughly.

Administration: Apply as needed.

Eyewash for inflamed eyes

1 teaspoon   Golden seal, tincture (Hydrastis Canadensis)
2 ounce   Boiling distilled water

Preparation: Mix thoroughly and let sit till cool enough to use (the hot water will dissipate the alcohol in the tincture).

Administration: Use as an eyewash.

Gleet, chronic gonorrhea, leucorrhea

2 parts Golden seal (Hydrastis Canadensis)
1 part Wild Geranium or Cranesbill (Geranium maculatum)

Preparation: Infuse in 1 pint of boiling water, cover tightly until cool, strain.

Administration: Apply 2 to 3 times daily with a fine camel hair brush.

Indigestion

1 part Golden seal, tincture (Hydrastis Canadensis)
1 part Balmony, tincture (Chelone glabra)
1 part Cayenne, tincture (Capsicum frutescens; C. minimum)

Preparation: Mix combination thoroughly.

Dosage: 25-30 drops in 3 tablespoons of water 3 times daily before meals. Children: The cayenne may be omitted; 5-10 drops in sweetened water.

Kidneys

1 part Golden seal (Hydrastis Canadensis)
1 part Gravel root (Eupatorium purpureum)

Preparation: Mix thoroughly. Place 4 teaspoons of mixed herbs in pot with 1 quart boiling water. Simmer for twenty minutes. Let cool. Strain.

Snuff for choked nostrils

1 ounce   Golden seal powder (Hydrastis Canadensis)
1 ounce   Lobelia powder (Lobelia inflata)
1 ounce   Raspberry leaves (Rubus idaeus)

Preparation: Sieve or grind finely in mortar; mix the fine powder thoroughly.

Administration: Snuff a small amount into the nose as needed.

Reproductive organs tonic

1 part Golden seal (Hydrastis Canadensis)
1 part Squaw vine (Mitchella repens)

Preparation: Make an infusion. Drink as needed.

Spinal nerves and epilepsy

4 parts Golden seal (Hydrastis Canadensis)
3 parts Hops (Humulus lupulus)
2 parts Scullcap (Scutellaria lateriflora)

Preparation: Mix together and infuse the herbs using 1 teaspoonful of the ingredients to each cupful of boiling water or 2 ounces of herbs in 1½ pints of boiling water; cover tightly until nearly cool, strain; or mix the compound thoroughly in powder form and place into #0 capsules.

Dosage: Infusion: 2 tablespoonfuls to 2 fluid ounces or more, as the case demands, 3 times daily (take it cold so that it will go slowly through the system); Capsules: 1-2 capsules (as the case demands) every 2 hours.

Syphilitic ulcers

4 teaspoons Golden seal powder (Hydrastis Canadensis)
1 teaspoon Myrrh powder (Commiphora myrrha, var. molmol)
325 milligrams Cayenne powder (Capsicum frutescens; C. minimum)

Preparation: Rub up well in mortar.

Administration: Fill the ulcers several times daily.

Congenial combinations:
This herb can be used in almost any preparation where a tonic is needed.

Growth characteristics:
The root is perennial, the stem is annual; the plant is native to eastern North America, from Ontario to Minnesota, and south to Georgia and Kentucky (it is most abundant west of the Allegheny mountains in Ohio, Indiana, West Virginia, Kentucky). The plant grows best in shady woodlands and mountain meadows—in rich, soft, damp soils, having ample shade, with good natural drainage, and ample leaf mold.

Plant propagation is usually done by dividing the root stock, cutting a few roots with each bud, then drying the rest of the root for market or individual use. A single, small, greenish-white flower appears in May or June on a short branch (a continuation of the stem above the upper leaf), which develops into a bright red berry-like fruit (resembling a large raspberry). Usually only one flower head develops, having 10-30 small seeds; the stem and leaves usually die soon after the fruit ripens (but may extend in most seasons until frost); usually two winter buds appear at the base of the stems; but ordinarily only one will activate in the springtime.

Collection:
The roots are dug in the autumn after the tops have died down. Care must be taken to clean the foreign matter lodged in the fibrous root masses, and to remove the root buds for further propagation before drying the remainder of the root stock. Do not use the root before it is 4 years old, as its medicinal value matures only with this period of time.

Drying and preservation:
The cured root is best kept in rather loose masses in a dry, airy place that is free of vermin.

PERUVIAN BARK
(Cinchona calisaya; C. ledgerana; C. officinalis; C. succirubra; RUBIACEAE)

Common names:
Peruvian bark, cinchona bark, Jesuit's bark, countess' powder, jacket bark, crown bark, foso bark. C. calisaya and C. ledgerana: Yellow cinchona, calisaya bark, yellow Peruvian bark, cinchona flava; Cinchonae Flavae Cortex (Br.); Quinguina (C. calisaya), juane (Fr.); China Regia, Kalisayarinde, Koinigschina (Ger.).

Identifying characteristics:
C. calisaya: The quills (a quill is a form of the bark that becomes in-rolled when dried; it is a roll of the dried bark such as a quill of cinnamon, cinchona, etc) are marked with white patches, and broad longitudinal fissures and regular transverse cracks that are 6 to 12 millimeters apart; the outer cork layer frequently exfoliates. This variety has the highest potency in organic quinine.
C. ledgerana: This is considered by some to be a variety of C. calisaya. It has single or double quills which exhibit light gray patches of lichen, with numerous fissures and transverse cracks.
C. officinalis: This has narrow quills, with numerous longitudinal and transverse cracks (giving a characteristic roughness to the back of the bark.)
C. succirubra (C. pubescens): This has two varieties—the South American is flat and the Javan is quilled. The south American variety has red bark and a red inner surface, with longitudinal ridges and bright red warts; the Javan variety has large quills and a reddish-brown outer bark, with wrinkles, reddish warts, and gray

lichens attached.

Part used:
Bark dried from the stems and branches.

Therapeutic action:
Tonic, superior antiperiodic, febrifuge, nervine, astringent (moderate), aperient (moderate), stomachic, antiseptic, sialagogue, anti-pyretic, cardiac stimulant (with large doses it is a cardiac depressant and depressomotor).

This herb is a general tonic that extends its powerful influence through the whole nervous system, to the cerebral-spinal, sympathetic, and even to the peripheral nerves. It will prevent fermentation and putrefaction in the digestive tract. The concentrate is a valuable gargle and throat astringent. Small doses increase the flow of saliva and gastric juices, enhance peristalsis, heart action (stronger and accelerated), cerebral functions and excretion of waste products. Moderate doses diminish the amount of uric and phosphoric acids (but not the flow of urea), and diminish tissue metabolism. Large doses may cause some physical discomfort (vertigo, headache, temporary deafness, etc.); but it will not inflict permanent injury on the patient.

Medicinal uses:
Adynamia, amenorrhea, asthma, bed wetting, chronic bronchitis, acute catarrh, convalescence, general debility, dropsy, drunkenness (liquid extract), atonic dyspepsia, epilepsy, erysipelas, female debility, fevers (all types), flu, gangrene, gastric catarrh, hay fever, indigestion, inflammation, lung problems, malaria, measles, menstrual affections, nervous disorders, neuralgia, pneumonia, acute rheumatism, scarlet fever, scrofula, skin diseases, enlarged spleen, typhus, typhoid, urinary incontinence, variola, whooping cough.

Preparations:
Quinine is commercially obtained from the bark, but this extracted form is inorganic and most dangerous to the health, so we advise to never use it. The natural or organic quinine that is in the bark, however, when used in an infusion or other appropriate form is very beneficial to the body.

Dosage:

Concentrate	1/2-1 teaspoonful.
Decoction	1-2 teaspoonfuls.
Elixir	1/2-1 teaspoonful.
Extract	300 mg.-1 gram.
Fluid extract	1/2-1 teaspoonful.
Infusion #1	1/2-1 teaspoonful before meals when there is poor appetite; otherwise after meals (see “FORMULAS”).
Infusion #2	1/2 cupful (hot or cold) before retiring at night; a mouthful 3 times daily; or 1-2 cupfuls (see “FORMULAS”).

Powder	1/2-1 teaspoonful.
Solid extract	100-500 milligrams.
Tincture	1/4-1/2 fluid teaspoon (teaspoonful).

ADMINISTRATION

This herb is usually given in combination with other herbs, but alone it is also effective. When taken internally, it imparts a warm sensation to the stomach, which gradually spreads over the entire body.

FORMULAS

Infusion #1

1/2 ounce	Peruvian bark, cut (Cinchona calisaya)
1 quart	Cold water

Preparation: Macerate (blend and soak) the bark 24 hours in the water; strain and keep in a cool place.

Infusion 2

Pour a cupful of boiling water over a teaspoonful of the bark or powder; steep for 1/2 hour; strain.

Catarrh (snuff)

2 ounces	Peruvian bark powder (Cinchona calisaya)
2 ounces	Blood root powder (Sanguinaria canadensis)
1/2 ounce	Bayberry root powder (Myrica cerifera)
1/2 ounce	Raspberry leaves powder (Rubus idaeus)

Preparation: Grind these powders very fine in a mortar and sift thoroughly.

Administration: Use a little as needed as a snuff.

Fever tonic #1 (tincture)

2 ounces	Peruvian bark (Cinchona calisaya)
1 ounce	Wild cherry bark (Prunus serotina)
1 teaspoon	Cinnamon (Cinnamomum zeylanicum)
1 teaspoon	Cayenne (Capsicum frutescens; C. minimum)
16 ounces	Brandy

Preparation: Macerate the herbs 1 week (shaking at least 2 to 3 times daily); strain and bottle.

Dosage: 2 fluid ounces every 2 to 3 hours until the fever is broken, then 2 to 3 times per day until the foregoing quantity is used up.

Fever tonic #2 (tincture)

2 ounces	Peruvian bark (Cinchona calisaya)
2 ounces	Wild cherry bark (Prunus serotina)
1 teaspoon	Cinnamon (Cinnamomum zeylanicum)
1 teaspoon	Cloves (Syzygium aromaticum; Eugenia aromatica)
1 teaspoon	Nutmeg (Myristica fragrans)
16 ounces	Brandy

Preparation: Macerate for 10 days (shake vigorously at least 2 times daily).

Dosage: 2 fluid ounces every 2 to 3 hours.

General tonic

1/2 ounce	Peruvian bark (Cinchona calisaya)
1/2 ounce	Gentian root (Gentiana lutea)
1/2 ounce	Orange peel (Citrus aurantium)
1/2 ounce	Calumba root (Jateorhiza palmata)
1/2 ounce	Licorice root (Glycyrrhiza glabra)
1/3 teaspoon	Cayenne (Capsicum frutescens; C. minimum)

Preparation: Simmer in a closely-covered vessel for 15 minutes in 1 quart of water; cool, then strain.

Dosage: 1 teacupful every 3 hours during the day.

***Growth characteristics*:**
Perennial, native of South America. This is an evergreen tree, and grows 20 to 80 feet tall and 4 to 24 inches thick. It is found hugging the mountain sides on the eastern slopes of the Andes chain from Bolivia to Ecuador, and the western Cordilleras chain from Ecuador to Venezuela and the Caribbean Sea. There are 36 species, but only three are official: (1) Red or C. succirubra; (2) Yellow or C. calisaya or C. ledgerana; (3) Pale, crown, loxa, or C. officinalis. The best species thrive where the mean annual temperature is 55° F., with nine months rainy season (heavy rainfall at night, fog and sunshine during the day), with three months of freezing nights and 75° F. temperature during the daytime. The slopes must be well-drained and the best trees grow at 5000 to 8000 feet elevations; but C. succirubra grows well at 2300 feet, and others do well at 11,500 feet. Cinchona is cultivated in several places in the world, but the growing conditions are quite selective. In 1859 the tree was introduced into India, Ceylon, and Java and now 3/4 of the world's commercial bark is grown by cultivation (mostly from hybrids). Java is the chief supplier, while considerable amounts come from India, Ceylon,

and some from Bolivia, Africa, Jamaica, and the Straits Settlements.

Collection:
The bark is best from 6 to 9 year old trees. It becomes more or less worthless when the trees are 15 years old. The yellow bark (C. calisaya, C. ledgerana) contains the richest organic quinine or antiperiodic alkaloids (up to 9%).

HISTORY

Discovery of Cinchona.
The story is told of an Indian who belonged to a tribe in South America who contracted a high fever that was thought by tribal associates to be highly contagious and fatal. As was their custom, this member was cast out from the rest of the tribe to avoid spreading the jungle fever. In a state of delirium, the man crawled on his hands and knees through the dense jungle, trying to find water (his fever had taken him to the point where he was literally dying from thirst). He found a pool of water. A tree had fallen into the pool and the water was very bitter, yet he was thirsty enough that he didn't care and he drank it! He slept and woke to take in more of the glorious tea and slept again and soon the fever left. So he went back to his tribal friends and loved ones, to their great astonishment, and he told them about the miraculous powers in the "healing waters" that had saved his life. These Indians discovered the source of the bitter waters and used the bark thereafter for fevers and other afflictions, and they found it to be marvelously healing. From here, the fame of this great bitter, yet curative herb spread abroad with many other effective cures resulting.

WHITE POPLAR
(Populus tremuloides; SALICACEAE)

Common names:
Poplar, quaking aspen, white poplar, American aspen, quiver leaf, trembling tree, trembling poplar, aspen poplar, abbey, abbey tree, abele tree, abelable, arbeal, arbell, white asp, great aspen, Dutch beech, Dutch arbel, white bark; blanc de Hollande, Peuplier blanc, peuplier grissard, bouillard (Fr.); Weisse pappel, Silberpappel, Abele (Ger.); popolo, biance (Ital.).

Identifying characteristics:
This is a slender tree with thin foliage that grows 30 to 40 feet high; the trunk which is close to the ground reaches 20 inches in diameter, then tapers gradually toward the top; the branches are slender, alternating and scattered; the leaves are broad, heart-shaped, dull-whitish or green with whitish veins. The bark is horizontally marked or scarred on older trees (smooth on younger trees), spotted with whitish and dark patches grayish or rusty green in color). Generally the outer bark is grayish, while the inner surface is smooth and brownish-white (the internal tis-

sue is in alternate buff and white layers); the taste is bitter and there is little odor.

Part used:
Inner bark, leaves, buds.

Therapeutic action:
Tonic, febrifuge, antiperiodic, anti-pyretic, antiseptic, antiferment, diuretic, stimulant, astringent (slight), vermifuge, vulnerary. This herb has long been considered a universal tonic, and may be given freely where a tonic is needed One of the best tonics for old age or when a person is constitutionally weak from disease. It is an effective—some have said superior—substitute for Peruvian Bark or organic quinine, for poplar is often tolerated in a weakened stomach when Peruvian Bark is not. Since it is found everywhere in the mountains of North America, it is available to almost everyone, where Peruvian Bark has to be imported and purchased.

Medicinal uses:
Articular swelling, burns, cancer, cholera infantum, cuts, cystic catarrh, debility, diabetes, diarrhea (sub-acute, chronic), eczema, faintness, flu, gangrene, gleet, gonorrhea, hay fever, hysteria, indigestion, inflammation, intermittent fever, jaundice, kidney complaints, liver problems, neuralgia, purulent ophthalmia, acute rheumatism, strong perspiration, sciatica, syphilitic sores, bad ulcers, urinary complaints and weakness, infected wounds.

Dosage:

Fluid extract	1 teaspoon.
Infusion	1-2 cupfuls (cold) daily, a large mouthful at a time.
Tincture	1/2-1 fluid teaspoon.

ADMINISTRATION

Oral

Gonorrhea: Drink white poplar bark in tea form and use as a wash.

Cancer, bad ulcers, gangrenous wounds, eczema, strong perspiration, burns, syphilitic sores: Use as a wash.

FORMULAS

Cystic catarrh

1 part White poplar bark (Populus tremuloides)
2 parts Uva ursi (Arctostaphylos uva-ursi)

Preparation: Use 1 teaspoon to the cup of boiling water.

Dosage: 1/2 to 1 cupful 3 times a day.

Debility tonic

5 parts	White poplar bark (Populus tremuloides)
1 part	Barberry bark (Myrica cerifera)
1 part	Balmony bark (Chelone glabra)
1/2 part	Golden Seal (Hydrastis Canadensis)
1/2 part	Cloves (Syzygium aromaticum; Eugenia aromatica)
1/4 part	Cayenne (Capsicum frutescens; C. minimum)
Sufficient	Honey or raw sugar

Preparation: Mix herbs well; put 1 heaping tablespoonful of the mixture into 1 quart of boiling, distilled water; cover and steep 15 minutes; strain and sweeten to taste (use up to 8 parts sugar for longer preservation time).

Dosage: 2 fluid ounces 3 times daily before meals, or 1 teaspoonful of powder in a cupful of hot water 1/2 hour before meals.

General tonic
(Dr. Samuel Thompson's spiced bitters)

1 part	White poplar bark powder (Populus tremuloides)
1 part	Barberry bark powder (Berberis vulgaris)
1 part	Balmony powder (Chelone glabra)

Preparation: Mix thoroughly and use 1 teaspoonful of powder to 1 cupful of hot water, sweeten.

Dosage: 1 cupful 3 times daily.

Hysteria

1/2 ounce	White poplar bark (Populus tremuloides)
1/2 ounce	Raspberry leaves (Rubus idaeus)
1/2 ounce	Balmony (Chelone glabra)
1/4 ounce	Calumba root (Jateorhiza palmata)
1/4 teaspoon	Cayenne (Capsicum frutescens; C. minimum)

Preparation: Simmer the first four ingredients of the compound in 1 quart of water down to 1¼ pints; strain over the cayenne and cool.

Dosage: 2-3 tablespoonfuls 3 to 4 times daily.

Dr. Coffins' Bitters
(for biliousness, indigestion, flatulence, general debility)

2 ounces	White poplar bark (Populus tremuloides)
4 ounces	Balmony powder (Chelone glabra)
4 ounces	Bayberry powder (Myrica cerifera)
2 ounces	Ginger powder (Zingiber officinalis)
1/4 ounce	Cayenne powder (Capsicum frutescens; C. minimum)
1/4 ounce	Cloves powder (Syzygium aromaticum; Eugenia aromatica)

Preparation: Mix and sieve thoroughly; take 1 teaspoonful of the mixture and dissolve in 1 cupful of hot water, sweeten.

Dosage: 1 cupful 3 to 4 times daily.

Growth characteristics:
Perennial; native of North America (grows everywhere) and Europe; cultivated.

Collection:
Gather the inner bark from older trees, it is thicker and has more potency.

EUROPEAN CENTAURY
(Erythraea centaurium; GENTIANACEAE)

Common names:
European centaury, centaury, centaurium, century, lesser century, centory, fever-wort, bitter herb, banwort, bloodwort, Christ's ladder, earth gall, feltrike, gall of the earth, hurdreve, sanctuary; Petite herbe a la fievre (Fr.); Tausendgueldenkraut (Ger.); Centaurea minore, biondella (Ital.).

Identifying characteristics:

Stem	Erect and branching 6-20 inches high, narrow base and obtuse apex.
Leaves	Opposite, obovate (oblong and oval-shaped), entire (margins) 3-5 longitudinal ribs.
Flowers	Numerous and star-like, white, yellow, pink, or rose-colored, twisted anthers (the white variety is considered best medicinally).
Odor	Faint and characteristic (disappears when dried).
Taste	Persistently bitter (whole plant).

Part used:
Whole herb (or variously; leaves, top, root).

Therapeutic action:
Tonic, aromatic bitter, stomachic, febrifuge, antiperiodic, and antiseptic.

This herb is an excellent general tonic, a strengthener of the heart; it acts upon the liver in correcting and regulating an over-secretion of bile. Its therapeutic action is similar to gentian (Gentiana lutea) and chiretta (Swertia chirata).

Medicinal uses:
Ague, anemia, debility (delicate and elderly persons), dyspepsia, fevers, freckles, gout, jaundice, liver troubles, stomach problems.

Preparations:
Fluid extract, infusion powder, tincture.

Dosage:

Fluid extract	1/2-1 teaspoonful.
Infusion	2 fluid ounces 3 to 4 times daily.
Powder	325 mg-2 grams.
Tincture	1/2-2 teaspoonfuls.

ADMINISTRATION

Oral

Biliousness: Give 6 ounces of the warm infusion, 1/2 hour before each meal.

Skin

Freckles: Wash the face with a strong infusion four times daily.

FORMULAS

Anemia

3/4 teaspoon	European century (Erythraea centaurium)
1/2 teaspoon	Thyme (Thymus vulgaris)
1/2 teaspoon	Horehound (Marrubium vulgare)
1/2 teaspoon	Hyssop (Hyssopus officinalis)

Preparation: Simmer 5 minutes in one quart distilled water.

Dosage: 1 tablespoonful every 2 hours.

Indigestion
(with no inflammation or gastric ulcer)

1/2 ounce	Centaury herb (Erythraea centaurium)
1/2 ounce	Raspberry leaves (Rubus idaeus)
1/2 ounce	Cleavers (Galium aparine)

1/2 ounce Dandelion root (Taraxacum officinale)
1 teaspoon Ginger (Zingiber officinalis)

Preparation: Simmer the first four ingredients of the compound in 1 quart of water down to 1¼ pints of liquid, strain hot over the ginger, cool.

Dosage: 3 tablespoonfuls (cool) 3 to 4 times daily.

Indigestion, heartburn, flatulence, stomach pains

1/2 ounce Centaury herb (Erythraea centaurium)
1/2 ounce Agrimony (Agrimonia eupatoria)
1/4 ounce Barberry bark (Myrica cerifera)
1/2 ounce Calumba root (Jateorhiza palmata)
1/4 ounce Raspberry leaves (Rubus idaeus)
1 teaspoon Ginger (Zingiber officinalis)

Preparation: Simmer the first five herbs in 1 quart of water down to 1¼ pints of liquid, strain hot over the ginger (adding cinnamon if desired).

Dosage: 2 to 3 tablespoonfuls 3 to 4 times daily.

Stomach tonic

3/4 teaspoon European centaury (Erythraea centaurium)
1/2 teaspoon Buckbean or Bogbean (Menyanthes trifoliata)
1/4 teaspoon Juniper berries (Juniperus communis)

Preparation: Infuse the ingredients in 1 pint of water.

Dosage: One teaspoon in water 1/2 hour before meals.

Growth characteristics:
Annual; a wild plant, difficult to cultivate, found mostly in waste places (barren fields, chalky cliffs, near the sea, etc.), but sometimes in woods; grows from Nova Scotia and Quebec south to Massachusetts, and west to Illinois and Michigan, also in all parts of Europe and North Africa. Its flowers (July to August) open only in fine weather and never in the afternoon.

Collection:
It is best gathered in the flowering season (July to August).

Sister plants:
-Centaury, American (Sabatia angularis; GENTIANACEAE). Also known as rose pink, bitter-bloom, rosy centaury, square-stemmed sabbatia, entire herb: fevers rheumatism, sore throat, dyspepsia; 2 to 3 feet high, sharply 4-angled stem, soli-

tary flowers (July to August) on long peduncles at ends of branches, which are rose-pink in color with a greenish star in the center, found in most parts of the United States in rich, damp soils (moist meadows, high grass, thickets).
-Chirata or Chiretta (Chirayita swertia; Swertia chirata; Ophelia chirata; GENTIANACEAE). Also known as brown chirata; white chiretta, chirayata; entire herb: indigestion, constipation, chronic bronchitis; 3 feet high, yellowish-brown quadrangular stems with separable pith, leaves are opposite, obovate, and entire, simple root; annual plant of the mountains of Northern India.

BLESSED THISTLE or HOLY THISTLE

Cnicus benedictus; Carduus sanctus; C. benedictus; Carbenia benedicta; Centauria benedicta; COMPOSITAE)

Common names:

Blessed thistle, carduus, cardin, St. Benedict Thistle, spotted thistle, bitter thistle, blessed cardus, Our Lady's thistle; Chardon beni (Fr.); Benedicten Distel (Ger.); Cardo beneditto, Cardo santo, Erba turca, Scarline (Ital.).

Identifying characteristics:

Stem	Erect, branched, rather Woolf, round, rough and pliable (they lie flat on the ground).
Leaves	2-3 inches long, grayish-green, brittle, thin and somewhat hairy, oblong and lanceolate, lance-shaped, with wavy-lobed (jagged) and spiny margins (prickles on edges).
Flowers	Yellow, 1 inch long, 1 inches broad, situated on branch ends and almost hidden by upper leaves, surrounded by leathery scales (leaves) tipped with long yellowish-red spines.
Fruit	Long, cylindrical seed, finely-ribbed longitudinally, hairs or beard at top.
Root	White and parted into strings.
Odor	None.
Taste	Very bitter.

Part used:

Whole herb.

Therapeutic action:

Tonic (cold), diaphoretic (hot), emetic (double or triple dosage), emmenagogue, stimulant, febrifuge, antiperiodic, vulnerary.

Blessed thistle is wonderful for nursing mothers, stimulating the production of mother's milk. It is very useful in purifying the blood, aiding circulation, and for all liver problems. As a tonic it strengthens the brain, heart, and stomach.

Medicinal uses:
Biliousness, chronic headaches, colds, dropsy, dyspepsia, emesis, fractured bones (poultice), heart problems, insanity, intermittent fevers, kidneys, liver, loss of appetite, lungs, strengthens memory, menstrual disorders due to colds, painful menstruation, mother's milk, purification of blood.

Preparations:
Fluid extract, infusion, tincture.
When the infusion is made cold it should be steeped several hours.

Dosage:

Fluid extract	1/2-1 teaspoonful.
Infusion	1/2 teacupful 3 times daily.
Tincture	5 to 20 drops (1/3 teaspoonful).

ADMINISTRATION

Oral

Biliousness: Give cold infusion.

Chronic headache: 1 cupful of the infusion twice daily.

Emesis: To cause vomiting, give copious amounts of warm infusion. This will also stimulate the liver and gall ducts; a somewhat loose bowel action will result, with a free discharge of bile.

Mother's milk (Plentiful milk supply): Give cold infusion to nursing mothers. Many herbalists consider blessed thistle to be the best herb for this purpose. Many new mothers have felt blessed indeed to have their milk supply increased with this herb.

FORMULAS

Difficult menstrual period

1 part Blessed thistle (Cnicus benedictus)
1 part Ginger (Zingiber officinalis), this carries the herb to the area.

Preparation: Make a warm infusion.

Dosage: One cup three times a day.

Nursing Mothers

1 part Blessed thistle (Cnicus benedictus)

1 part Raspberry leaves (Rubus idaeus), settles the system.
1 part Marshmallow root (Althaea officinalis)

Preparation: Make a cold infusion.

Dosage: 3 or more cups per day according to need.

Stomach tonic (Potter's)

1 part Blessed thistle (Cnicus benedictus)
1 part Germander (Teucrium chamaedrys)
1 part Centaury (Erythraea centaurium)
1 part Buckbean (Menyanthes trifoliata)

Preparation: Infuse at rate of one teaspoon of combined herbs to a cup of boiling water.

Dosage: One or two tablespoons between meals.

Stomach tonic (tincture)

3 teaspoons Blessed thistle (Cnicus benedictus)
3 teaspoons European centaury (Erythraea centaurium)
3 teaspoons Orange peel (Citrus aurantium)
3 teaspoons Gentian (Gentiana lutea)
3 teaspoons Calamus or Sweet Flag (Acorus calamus)
3 teaspoons Wormwood (Artemisia absinthium)
2 teaspoons Cloves (Syzygium aromaticum; Eugenia aromatica)
2 teaspoons European Avens (Geum urbanum)

Preparation: Macerate for 2 weeks in 1 quart of brandy.

Dosage: 2 tablespoonfuls after meals.

Growth characteristics:
Annual; flowers appear May-August.

Sister plants:
-Common carline thistle (Carlina vulgaris); good both as medicine and as food.
-Common star thistle (Centaurea calcitrapa)
-Dwarf thistle (Carduus acaulis)
-Scotch thistle (Onopordum acanthium)
-Milk or marian thistle (Silybum marianum); seeds and roots; strengthens the memory because of the effect on circulation; excellent for liver congestion and disease; leaves good in salads, peeled stalks can be eaten fresh or baked into pies.
-St. Mary's thistle (Carduus marianus); seeds; hemostatic, emmenagogue, hepat-

ic; uterine hemorrhage, amenorrhea (derangement of portal circulation), liver congestion, jaundice, gall and liver affections.

MYRRH or GUM MYRRH
(Commiphora myrrha, var. molmol; C. molmol; Balsamodendron myrrha; BURSERACEAE)

Common names:
Myrrh, gum myrrh; Herabo myrrha, Resina Balsamodendri, Gummi-resina Myrrha (Somali); Myrrhe (Fr.); Myrrha, Myrrhe (Ger.).

Identifying characteristics:

Trunk	Bush or stunted tree, 8 to 10 feet high, thick trunk, abortive breaching at right angles and terminating with sharp spines.
Bark	Whitish-gray.
Wood	Yellowish-white.
Leaves	Trifoliate, obovate (the central leaf is about 1 inch long, and the sessile leaflets are about 1/2 inch long), stalked on short petioles.
Fruit	About the size of a pea.
Resin	Gum; Rounded, reddish-brown (covered with yellowish dust), irregular tears (or agglutinated masses of tears), waxy fracture, oily and granular, conchoidal, white internal spots or lines, translucent edges, will not dissolve or swell when macerated in water, triturates with water into a brownish-yellow emulsion, yellowish-brown in alcohol tincture solution. There are 3 varieties: (1) Turkey (African), the best and official variety, has about 60% gum (myrrh), 25-40% resin (myrrhin), 4-8% volatile oil (Myrrol). (2) Arabian (called *mur* by Arabs, *mulmul* or *herrabul* by Somalis), resembles the Turkey variety, but is smaller, tougher, without the white internal lines, less resin, has volatile oil and fragrance. (3) Indian (Myrrha indica), commercially known as Opoanax (called *bissabul* by natives, *hebbakhade* by Somalis), resembles a dark myrrh, mushroom-like odor and strong acrid-like taste, contains many impurities, has resin and volatile oil.
Odor	(Turkey, African, or heerabul variety); peculiar, pleasantly agreeable, balsamic aroma.
Taste	Bitter, balsamic and acrid, but not unpleasant.

Therapeutic action:
Tonic, stimulant, powerful antiseptic (mucous membranes), disinfectant (mucous membranes), vulnerary (healing), expectorant, emmenagogue, astringent, carminative, purgative (large doses), emetic (large doses), cardiac stimulant.

Myrrh stimulates the flow of blood to the capillaries and gives a warm and pleasant sensation to the stomach. It increases the number of white blood corpuscles up to four times of the original, when there is a need for fighting infection, and quickens the heart action. It enhances the eliminative function of the mucous membranes in the bronchi and genito-urinary tract, at the same time disinfecting those tissues and reducing mucus discharge from those specific areas. It is an excellent internal tonic for spongy gums, relaxed throat, ulcerated sore throat, ulcers, etc. Topically it makes a good skin tonic and conditioner. It is a good stimulant, disinfectant, and antiseptic on open or ulcerated surfaces, lessens the possibility of infection and speeds healing. It promotes menstruation and expectoration.

Medicinal uses:
Humoral asthma, amenorrhea, anemia, bad breath, bronchial catarrh (bronchitis), caries (teeth), collapse, profound congestion, cough, fresh cuts, cystitis, general debility, chronic diarrhea, diphtheria, atonic dyspepsia, spongy and inflamed gums (tender and bleeding), laryngitis, lung and chest affections, suppressed menstruation, prevent mortification (gangrene), diseased mucous surfaces, sore and abraded nipples, ozena, chronic pharyngitis, prostration, rheumatism (liniment), shock, old sores, sprains, aphthae or sloughy throat, thrush, tuberculosis, ulceration (tongue, mouth, throat), indolent or gangrenous ulcers, umbilical cord protection, chronic uterine and vaginal leucorrhea, wounds.

Preparations:
Decoction, emulsion, fluid extract, infusion, liniment, oil, ointment, pill, plaster, powder, tincture.

Myrrh is only partially soluble in water, so it is preferable to use as an emulsion. If you need to use it in an infusion or decoction, powder it first. The pieces with white streaks have less oil and are best for emulsions and pills, and the pieces without streaks are more oily and are best for tinctures. The undissolved gum in the tincture makes an excellent adhesive substance, similar to acacia (Acacia Senegal).

Dosage:

Infusion	2 fluid ounces 3 to 4 times daily.
Pill	1/2-2 grams.
Powder	325 mg.-1 gram (up to 2 grams may be given).
Tincture	1/2-1 teaspoonful.

ADMINISTRATION

Oral

Bad breath: Take a little internally.

Gums (tender, bleeding, spongy): Apply diluted tincture or use as tooth powder.

Gargle or Mouthwash: Mix 1 teaspoon of powdered myrrh with 2 tablespoons of warm water (make stronger or weaker as desired).

Sore throat, ulceration of tongue, mouth or throat: Use the tincture (diluted freely) as a gargle or mouthwash (for infants or small children, spray into the mouth and down the throat).

Tooth powder: The therapeutic and cleansing properties of myrrh make it a superior tooth powder.

Chronic diarrhea: Mix 1 teaspoon of powdered myrrh with 2 tablespoons of warm water (make stronger or weaker as desired).

Skin

Skin conditioner and protective for tissue atony and debility: After a vapor bath and drying, use partially-diluted tincture as a wash.

Chronic bronchitis, chronic pleurisy, asthma, chronic rheumatism, marasmus: Apply the liniment over entire afflicted region and massage thoroughly.

Ulcerated surfaces (stomatitis), ptyalism, sores, ulcers: Apply diluted tincture or powder form.

Umbilical cord: Apply the powder after severing the cord. This is much milder and nicer to use than the alcohol so often used on new babies; it is antiseptic and helps the cord heal quickly. Put a small package of myrrh powder in the birth kit.

Wounds: Apply diluted tincture or powder form.

FORMULAS

Bad breath

1 teaspoon Myrrh powder (Commiphora myrrha, var. molmol).
1 teaspoon Golden seal powder (Hydrastis Canadensis).

Preparation: Steep 9 minutes in 1 pint of boiling water, pour off clear liquid.

Dosage: 1 teaspoonful 5 to 6 times daily.

Colic, flatulence

4 ounces Myrrh (Commiphora myrrha, var. molmol)
1/2 ounce Nutmeg, ground (Myristica fragrans)
1/2 ounce Cayenne (Capsicum frutescens; C. minimum)

1 quart Brandy

Preparation: Macerate for ten days, then strain and bottle.

Dosage: 1 teaspoonful as needed.

Gargle and mouth wash

1 teaspoon Myrrh powder (Commiphora myrrha, var. molmol)
1 teaspoon Raspberry leaves (Rubus idaeus)

Preparation: Steep in 1 pint of boiling water and let stand 1/2 hour, pour off the clear liquid.

Administration: Use as needed.

Piles, hemorrhoids, sores, ulcers, diphtheria

1 part Myrrh powder (Commiphora myrrha, var. molmol)
1 part Golden seal (Hydrastis Canadensis)

Preparation: For piles and hemorrhoids, mix with hot water sufficient to make a paste; for sores and ulcers and diphtheria, mix the powders thoroughly.

Administration: Apply as needed. For diphtheria, blow a little in the throat.

Shock, collapse, prostration, profound congestions (powerful internal stimulant and antiseptic); externally for rheumatism, neuralgia, sprains, bruises, fresh cuts, indolent ulcers, prevent mortification

1 part Myrrh, tincture (Commiphora myrrha, var. molmol)
1/4 part Cayenne, tincture (Capsicum frutescens; C. minimum)
2 parts Echinacea, tincture (Echinacea angustifolia)

Preparation: Mix thoroughly.

Dosage: 10-15 drops in plenty of water.

Weak Stomach (fermentation)

1 teaspoon Myrrh powder (Commiphora myrrha, var. molmol)
1 teaspoon Golden seal (Hydrastis Canadensis)
1/4 teaspoon Ginger (Zingiber officinalis)

Preparation: Infuse in 1 pint of boiling water, cover closely and steep 10 to 15 minutes, pour off clear liquid.

Dosage: 1 teaspoonful every 2 hours.

Worms

1-1½ ounces	Gum myrrh (Commiphora myrrha, var. molmol)
1/4 teaspoon	Cayenne (Capsicum frutescens; C. minimum)
1/2 pound	Raisins

Preparation: Dissolve the herbs in 1½ pints of hot water, add the raisins and steep for three days.

Dosage: 3 to 4 tablespoonfuls of the liquid while fasting every morning.

Growth characteristics:
Perennial; native to East Africa (Somali country) and Southwest Arabia, and other countries bordering the Red Sea, and is mostly processed in Bombay, India. The trees form an undergrowth in the forests bordering the Red Sea, where the temperatures are high, the vegetation scant, and the water scarce. The Turkey variety comes from East Africa and the Arabian is cultivated in South Arabia, east of Aden.

Collection:
The sap of the myrrh (like the cherry tree) exudes naturally from the pith and bark (or the process is accelerated by artificial incisions through the stem bark); at first being soft and pale yellow, then in drying becoming harder and golden, then dark and reddish.

Sister plants:
-African bdellium (Commiphora africana); resembles myrrh and Indian bdellium, aroma distinct from myrrh and quite bitter.
-Indian bdellium (Commiphora mukul); tears resemble myrrh, yellowish brown color, dusty and translucent, slightly aromatic and not bitter, contains volatile oil, resin, gum.
-Mecca Balsam (Commiphora opobalsamum or Balsamodendron opobalsamum)

Allied plants:
Balm of Gilead (Populous balsamifera; SALICACEAE); a viscid fluid that is opaque, yellowish, and fragrant (contains about 20-30% volatile oil, 70% soft resin, and 12% hard resin.

Cocillana (Guarea rusbyi or Sycocarpus rusby; MELIACEAE) dried bark; expectorant (superior to ipecacuanha, Cephaelis ipecacuanha), laxative, emetic; used in bronchitis, bronchial pneumonia, phthisis; resembles a large apple tree and grows in the river bottoms of Bolivia.

Manila Elemi, or Elemi (Canarium commune); stimulant, irritant; a tall tree growing in the Philippine Islands; oleoresin extracted by artificial incision; becomes soft, yellowish and granular-crystalline; has a strong odor resembling fennel (Foeniculum vulgare) and lemon (Citrus limon); taste is bitter and pungent; used in plasters and ointment.

Marqosa Bark, or Pride of India (Melia Azedarach); bark of root, emetic, anthelmintic; native of China and India, but grown in southern United States; beautiful tree 30 to 40 feet high with quilled bark.

Olibanum, or Frankincense (Boswellia carterii); stimulant, expectorant; grows in E. Africa and S. Arabia; a gum-resin extracted by artificial incision in the bark; tears are yellowish-brown and covered with white dust; balsamic odor and bitter, balsamic taste; only partially soluble in alcohol, and is milky-white in a water emulsion; used in emulsion, fumigation, or plasters.

Note: Watch for the following adulterations which can be found in Myrrh:
-Dark gums that swell or are adhesive with water.
-Vegetable fragments, sand, salt.
-Gum resins of allied species, such as bdellium (African—Commiphora africana; Indian—Commiphora mukul), of which the fracture is more transparent or opaque, and the odor and taste differ.

HISTORY

Historical value of myrrh.
Myrrh is mentioned in the Bible at an early period, where Joseph was sold to a company of Ishmaelite merchants taking a camel caravan "bearing spicery and balm and myrrh" into Egypt (Genesis 37:25). Later, it is mentioned in connection with a purification procedure for women: "for so were the days of their purifications accomplished, to wit, six months with oil of myrrh, and six months with sweet odors, and with other things for the purifying of the women" (Esther 2:12), which undoubtedly had religious implications also, but its beneficial effects alone on the body are well-established. The Hebrews also used myrrh to anoint the tabernacle, ark altar, and sacred vessels. The great value and profound respect placed on myrrh was demonstrated at the birth of Christ; it was one of the gifts selected by the Three Wise men.

BALMONY
(Chelone glabra; SCROPHULARIACEAE)

Common names:
Balmony, bitter herb, turtle-bloom, chelone, snake head, salt rheumy weed, turtle head, shell-tree, cod-head; Chelone, Galane (Fr.); Kahler fuenffaden, Schildblume (Ger.); Galana spicata (Ital.).

Identifying characteristics:

Stem	1-3 feet high, simple, erect, smooth, leafy.
Leaves	Short-stalked, opposite, oblong-lanceolate, acuminate, serrate (saw-edged).
Flowers	Ornamental, odorless, and vary with varieties (white tinged with pink, all white, rose, purple, etc.) about 1 inch long, growing in a dense terminal cluster (spike), two-lipped (the lower lip is spreading and bearded or wooly within, with heart-shaped anthers); the flower head (corolla) is shaped like a tortoise or snake head--hence the names.
Fruit	Capsule or spike, short, ovate, 2-celled, 1/2 inch long; enclosed winged seeds that are nearly circular with dark centers.

Parts used:
Leaves, flowers, or whole herb (fresh).

Therapeutic action:
Tonic, stimulant, antibilious, detergent, anthelmintic, aperient, cholagogue.

This herb was a favorite American Indian remedy, one of the finest tonics for liver malfunction (a specific for the left lobe). It will cleanse the system of morbid bile secretions. The entire digestive tract is toned up by this valuable herb, which stimulates gastric and salivary secretions and increases biliary and fecal elimination. It increases the appetite, and tones the entire system.

Medicinal uses:
Biliousness, constipation, convalescence from febrile and inflammatory sickness, inflamed breasts, debility (digestive organs), dyspepsia, jaundice, liver problems, piles, tumors, painful ulcers, worms (stomach).

Preparations:
Infusion, ointment, powder, tincture.
Alcohol and water are used as the solvents for the flowers.

Dosage:

Fluid extract	1/2-1 teaspoon.
Infusion	1-2 cupfuls daily (or 1/2 cupful before meals).
Powder	325-650 milligrams.
Tincture	1/2-1 teaspoonful (fluid teaspoon).

ADMINISTRATION

Anal

Piles: Use ointment made from fresh leaves.

Oral

Stomach worms: Give the infusion freely in 2 fluid ounce doses.

Skin

Itching, inflamed breasts, tumors, painful ulcers: Apply ointment made from fresh leaves.

FORMULAS

Jaundice

2 parts Balmony (Chelone glabra)
2 parts Golden seal (Hydrastis Canadensis)
2 parts Dwarf elder (Sambucus Ebulus)
1 part Gentian (Gentiana lutea)
1 part Prickly ash (Zanthoxylum americanum; Z. Clava-Hercules)
1 part Wahoo (Euonymus atropurpureus)

Preparation: Combine all herbs and make an infusion using 1 teaspoon of the ingredients to a cup of boiled distilled water. Steep 15 minutes in a warm place; strain and make a syrup by adding (while infusion is warm) 1/2 cup of raw sugar (or 1/4 cup honey) to each cup of liquid; stir and heat until melted.

Dosage: 2 tablespoonfuls after meals.

***Growth characteristics*:**
Perennial; native of eastern United States and Canada, distributed from Newfoundland to Florida on the eastern half of the continent; grows in damp soils, in ditches, in swamps, and beside streams. As a cultivated plant, it does well in crevices in front of a herbaceous border. It flowers July to September.

GENTIAN
(Gentiana lutea; GENTIANACEAE)

***Common names*:**
Gentian, European gentian, yellow gentian, pale gentian, bitter root, bitterwort, felwort, fillwort, balmoney, Radix luteae (or Majoris); Gentianae Radix (Br.); Racine de Gentiane, Gentiane jaune, Grande gentiane (Fr.); Radix Gentianae, Gelberenzianwurzel, Bitterwurzel (Ger.); Genziana, gialla, Genzian maggiore (Ital.).

Identifying characteristics:

Stem	2 to 4 feet high, thick and stout, hollow, erect.
Leaves	Obovate (oblong, ovate), 5-veined, bright yellowish-green.
Flowers	Numerous and in cymes of 20 or more, large and bright orange-yellow (spotted).
Fruit	3-celled obovate capsule, short-stalked, 1/5 inch long, with many winged seeds.
Root	Cylindrical, yellowish-brown (brown external, yellow within when dried—the fresh root is nearly white), long and 1/5 to 3/5 inch thick, tough and flexible when damp, internally spongy, longitudinally wrinkled (lower portion), short fracture.

Part used:
Root.

Therapeutic action:
Tonic, stomachic, febrifuge, emmenagogue, anthelmintic (vermifuge), antiseptic, antispasmodic, cholagogue, emetic (large doses), sialagogue, antibilious, antiperiodic, antivenomous.

Gentian is one of the most valuable bitter tonics and best strengtheners of the human system. It stores vast quantities of condensed oxygen in the roots (the source of its bitterness and exhilarating tonic action), making it one of the most popular revitalizing tonic and stomachic agents for physical exhaustion from chronic ailments, general debility, female weakness, digestive weakness, and lack of appetite. It is intensely bitter, yet it is generally easily received by the stomach, wherein it tones the liver without influencing the secretion of bile. It is powerful, effective and reliable, with action similar to Peruvian bark (Cinchona calisaya).

Medicinal uses:
Atonic gout, amenorrhea, anemia, bites, dog (mad dogs, poisonous insects, snakes, etc.), bruises, cancer (early stages), chills, chronic indigestion, colds, diarrhea, dizziness, dyspepsia, exhaustion, fainting, female weakness, fevers, general debility (especially of digestive organs), hysteria, indigestion, infections, intermittent fevers, jaundice, lameness, liver troubles, malaria, scanty urine, scrofula, side aches, sprains, suppressed menstruation, worms, wounds.

Preparations:
Decoction, fluid extract, infusion, liniment, powder, tincture.

Dosage:
Use in reasonably small doses.

Decoction	See "FORMULAS."
Extract	100-500 milligrams.
Fluid extract	1/2-1 teaspoonful, 3 times daily.
Infusion	See "FORMULAS."

Powder	1/2-2 grams.
Tincture	1/2-1 teaspoonful.

ADMINISTRATION

When possible, combine with some aromatic, such as peppermint.

Oral

Worms (children): As a vermifuge, give a double dose of the infusion without honey 3 to 4 times daily until the worms come out in the stool, then give lesser doses and avoid rich foods and meat (which you should do anyway).

For a vermicide to kill worms and lower organisms in the intestines: Use strong decoction of gentian.

Skin

Liniment for parasitic affections, infected wounds, vermin, sprains, bruises, burns, inflamed joints: Dip gauze or other appropriate material into a strong decoction or diluted tincture; squeeze until the material does not drip; apply to affected area (hot or cold); cover with plastic (or wax paper), and bandage on.

FORMULAS

Decoction #1

4 ounces	Gentian root, cut (Gentiana lutea)
3 pints	Water
4 ounces	Glycerine

Preparation: Steep the cut root for 12 hours in the unheated water; thereafter bring to a boil and simmer 15 minutes in a closely-covered vessel; remove the cover and simmer slowly down to 3/4 pint of liquid (making it a concentrate); remove from heat and add the glycerine; cool, bottle, and keep in a cool place.

Dosage: 1-2 teaspoonfuls in 2 ounces of water, 1 hour before meals. Child: 5-15 drops in honey water.

Decoction #2

1 ounce	Gentian root, cut (Gentiana lutea)
1½ pints	Water

Preparation: Place the herb and the water in an appropriate vessel, bring slowly to a boil, simmer to 1 pint, cool, strain, bottle and place in a cool place.

Dosage: 1/2-1 teaspoonful, 3 times daily.

Infusion #1

1 ounce	Gentian root, cut (Gentiana lutea)
1¼ pints	Water

Preparation: Boil the water and pour over the root; cover and put in a hot place (but not on direct heat), steep for 30 minutes.

Administration: 2 fluid ounces 3 to 4 times daily, preferably 1 hour before meals. Child with weak stomach: 1 to 2 teaspoonfuls 3 to 4 times daily, sweetened with honey. Note: Infusion of gentian is milder-tasting and therefore easier to take for a convalescent, but if you are not getting good results, use decoction.

Infusion #2

1/2 ounce	Gentian root, cut (Gentiana lutea)
1 quart	Water

Preparation: Soak the herb in the unheated water for 24 hours; bring to a boil and remove from the heat; cool, strain, bottle and keep in a cool place.

Dosage: 1/2-1 fluid ounce before meals. Child: smaller dose (proportionate to age, condition, etc.)

Hayfever

5 teaspoons	Gentian root (Gentiana lutea)
5 teaspoons	Bitter orange peel (Citrus aurantium)
1 handful	Tansy (Tanacetum vulgare)
1 handful	Blessed thistle (Cnicus benedictus)
1 handful	Buckbean or bog bean (Menyanthes trifoliata)

Preparation: Simmer for 10 minutes in one quart of water; cool, strain and bottle.

Dosage: 1 tablespoonful with glass of water after dinner and supper.

Gentian-Sweet Flag tonic

4 ounces	Gentian root, cut (Gentiana lutea)
4 ounces	Calamus or Sweet flag root, cut (Acorus calamus)
1 ounce	Orange peel, dried and cut (Citrus aurantium)
1/2 ounce	Cardamon seeds, crushed (Elettaria Cardamomum)
8 ounces	Blackstrap molasses

8 ounces Glycerine

Preparation: Place the first four ingredients in 1 gallon of water and soak for 12 hours in unheated water; bring slowly to a boil, simmer closely-covered for 30 minutes; strain and return to a clean pot; slowly reduce by simmering to 1 quart of liquid; remove from heat and add the blackstrap molasses and glycerine and mix thoroughly; cool, bottle, and keep in a cool place.

Dosage: 1 tablespoonful or less, 1 hour before meals. Child: 1 teaspoonful or less (according to age, constitution, etc.).

Stomach tonic

2 ounces Gentian root, thinly sliced (Gentiana lutea)
1 ounce Bitter orange peel, chopped, dried (Citrus aurantium)
1/2 ounce Cardamon seeds, crushed (Elettaria cardamomum)

Preparation: Macerate in 1 quart of brandy for 12 days, shaking it 1 to 2 times daily (except the last day); strain through 3 to 4 layers cheesecloth.

Dosage: 2 teaspoons 2 hours before meals.

Stimulating tonic

1 ounce Gentian root powder (Gentiana lutea)
2 ounces Coriander seeds, crushed (Coriandrum sativum)
2 ounces Bitter orange peel (Citrus aurantium)
1/4 ounce Cinnamon (Cinnamomum zeylanicum)

Preparation: Mix the above ingredients thoroughly, then infuse 1 ounce of the compound with 1 pint boiling water, steep 10 to 15 minutes, strain.

Dosage: 2-3 tablespoonfuls 3 to 4 times daily.

Tonic

1 ounce Gentian (Gentiana lutea)
1 ounce Peruvian bark (Cinchona calisaya)
1 ounce Dandelion root (Taraxacum officinale)
1 ounce Bitter orange peel (Citrus aurantium)

Preparation: Steep for 1/2 hour in 2 pints of water; strain and add 3 ounces of brandy.

Dosage: 1 teaspoonful after meals.

Growth characteristics:
Perennial; native of alpine and sub-alpine pastures (3000-5000 feet elevation) of southern and central Europe (especially on the Pyrenees and Alps, and in the Balkans; exported largely from Marseilles, France and Germany. Could be cultivated in the home medicinal garden.

Collection:
The rhizome and branching roots are collected when gentian is in flower (after 3 years old, to insure that the plant has produced seed to propagate again.).

Sister plants:
-(Amarella Gentian; GENTIANACEAE), grows in America.
-American Centaury (Erythraea centaurium; GENTIANACEAE).
-American columbo (Frasera caroliniensis; GENTIANACEAE); see page 479.
-Chirata (Swertia chirayata; GENTIANACEAE).
-Willow Gentian (Gentiana asclepiadea; GENTIANACEAE).
-(Gentiana acaulis; GENTIANACEAE).
-(Gentiana macaulyi; GENTIANACEAE).
-(Gentiana saxosa; GENTIANACEAE).
-(Sabbatia campestris): grows in the prairies of America; use similar to Gentian (G. lutea) and European centaury (Erythraea centaurium).
-Blue Gentian or Elliott's gentian (Gentiana catesbaei; Sabbatia elliottii; G. elliottii, GENTIANACEAE): root; grows in grassy swamps of the United States. It is considered to be almost equal in value to Gentian (G. lutea).
-English Gentian (Gentiana campestris; GENTIANACEAE): also known as felwort, baldmoney, field gentian; root, herb; see "Gentian (Gentiana lutea)" for medicinal uses.
-European Centaury (Erythraea centaurium; GENTIANACEAE); see page 494.

Allied plants:
Cornus or Dogwood or American Boxwood (Cornus florida; CORNACEAE)

FALSE UNICORN ROOT or BLAZING STAR or HELONIAS
(Chamaelirium luteum (Gray); Helonias dioica (Pursh.); H. lutea (Ait.); C. Carolinianum (Willd.); Veratrum luteum (Linn.); LILIACEAE)

Common names:
False unicorn root, helonias, starwort, drooping starwort, blazing star.

Identifying characteristics:

Stem	Smooth, angular, 1 to 2 feet high.
Leaves	Rosette of radical leaves that are broad and 4 to 8 inches long spring from the base or root; others are small, acute, and lanceolate.
Flowers	Greenish-white, small and very numerous, clustered in long terminal

	plume-like racemes.
Fruit	Capsule.
Root	(Rhizome) Grayish-brown, large and bulbous, 1/4 to 1 inches long, 3/8 inch thick, roundish (nearly cylindrical) ringed transversely, stem scars on the upper side (bud-scales, leaf bases), wiry root lets on the lower (numerous, yellowish, 2 to 3 inches long), horny fracture, internally grayish-yellow with numerous wood bundles in the center.
Odor	Slight.
Taste	Root (Rhizome and rootlets).

Therapeutic action:
Stimulating tonic, diuretic, anthelmintic (vermifuge, taeniafuge), uterine tonic, emetic (large doses), sialagogue (fresh).

False unicorn is one of the best stimulative tonics for the uterus and ovaries. It can be used to correct almost any problem in the reproductive organs of both male and female and it is also an excellent general tonic. False unicorn is very beneficial to the mucous membranes and can often be tolerated in the stomach where other remedies are not. It is a most valuable regenerative, revitalizing agent in cases of dyspepsia and weakness in the reproductive organs. Do not, however, use this herb for a weakened female where pregnancy is undesirable, for it will increase the possibility of conception.

Be sure to distinguish false unicorn from true unicorn (Aletris farinosa), or else you will not get the therapeutic results you desire. The powder or fluid extract is generally very readily obtained, but few stores ever carry the root itself.

Medicinal uses:
Loss of appetite, Bright's disease, colic, diabetes, digestive disorders, dropsy, dyspepsia, enuresis, gastric-intestinal weakness (mucous membranes), genital-urinary atony (mucous membranes), kidney atony, nausea, prevent miscarriage, prostate problems, tape-worm, uterine problems (barrenness, hemorrhage, leucorrhea, menorrhagia, miscarriage, uterine atony, uterine prolapses, etc.), sterility, relaxed vagina, spermatorrhea.

Preparations:
Decoction, elixir, fluid extract, powder, tincture.

Dosage:

Decoction	2-8 fluid ounces.
Fluid extract	1/2 to 1 teaspoonful.
Powder	1/2-2 grams, 3 to 4 times daily.
Tincture	5-20 drops.

ADMINISTRATION

False unicorn root is generally combined with other agents, but it may be used alone.

Oral

Loss of appetite, worms: Take 500 mg.-1 gram of powder.

Danger of miscarriage, uterine hemorrhage: Give infusion copiously, by the quart. It is usually combined with Lobelia inflata for this purpose, and given in tincture or extract form.

Pre-delivery, preventative in miscarriage: Drink 1 cupful every 1/2 hour.

Skin

Vermicide for insects, bugs, lice, etc.: Use strong decoction as spray or wash.

CASE HISTORY

Saved both babies.
In our offices in Evanston, Wyoming, a few years ago, we had two cases at the same time from different sides of town. In each of these cases, the women still had a long time before delivery, and they were both hemorrhaging. We administered false unicorn, and saved both babies. In one of these cases, the problem was so serious that the doctor said he would scrape the uterus in the morning, for (according to his training) the baby could not live. When he came the next morning, the woman was all right, and the baby was delivered a couple of months later.

***Growth characteristics*:**
Perennial; native of the United States and grows abundantly in some Western States; grows in moist soils, in meadows and woodlands; flowers in June and July.

Sister plants:
American Hellebore (Veratrum viride; LILIACEAE); rhizome, root: sedative, cardiac-depressant, emetic, diaphoretic, errhine, reduce arterial excitement, spinal spasms, pneumonia, cardiac diseases, typhoid fever; perennial herb, 2 to 7 feet high, grows from Canada to Georgia in rich, wet woods and swamps.

For alternate tonic herbs which can be used when the foregoing are unavailable, please see Chapter 17.

CHAPTER 14

THE FIELD OF HERBS

COLLECTION OF HERBS FROM FIELD OR GARDEN

Although each herb is different and some may require unique handling, the following general principles can be used for gathering herbs. More specific instructions accompany the information on each herb.

For a number of good reasons you should gather your own herbs. First, you are assured of their freshness and potency. You also know for certain the source of the herbs; you know they are clean, pure and wholesome. You will save yourself money and gain invaluable self-sufficiency. In the long run, you will build an increasing knowledge of plants and their medicinal uses; in the case of famine or long term emergency you would be able to secure medicine for your family. In such situations, sickness abounds and you would be able to take care of your own family as well as to help others.

Don't expect to be able to recognize every herb you wish to use immediately, however. To learn more about medicinal plants, look for herb walks and other types of classes in your area. Look in your local health food store for resources such as LeArta Moulton's *The Herb Walk* and *Nature's Medicine Chest* for clear pictures and descriptions of many medicinal plants. You can also obtain from your State Extension services a copy of *Weeds of the West* or *Weeds of California*, or whatever state. Field guides such as *Nature Bound* or *Peterson's* or *The Audubon Society* are very helpful. Note: <u>when in doubt, do not use an herb.</u> Some plants which resemble medicinal herbs are poisonous.

Generally, wild plants contain greater medicinal potency than cultivated plants, as wild herbs grow in the select habitats compatible with their botanical virtues. Plants that grow in higher locations and dry soil are exposed to clean air and plenty of sunshine and will generally contain greater potency than the cultivated varieties. They will also have greater potency than those which grow in low, moist, shady or confined places. This is just a rule of thumb; some plants grow best with moisture, and are equally valuable. Some herbs must be cultivated to obtain any sizeable quantity, and though the wild herbs may possess greater potency, do not hesitate to use cultivated variety when the wild types are unavailable. The cultivated varieties are still very valuable medicinally.

PLANT TYPES

Herbs are generally gathered according to their particular growth cycle: annuals, biennials, or perennials.

Annuals

These plants have one growing season—the seed germinates, the plant flowers and bears fruit, and then dies.

Biennials

These plants germinate and establish a good root system during the first year, flower and bear fruit at the end of the second year, and then die. A good example of this would be burdock, wherein the first year a very powerful root is developed, but no blossom or seed. During the second year, the blossoms come and the seeds are gathered, but the root is pithy and almost worthless.

Perennials

These plants live and bear fruit a number of years before they die.

GENERAL GATHERING RULES

The medicinal value of an herb is affected by the time, weather, place and method of collection.

Weather

Herbs must be gathered in dry weather, as those collected in moist or rainy periods are generally weaker and more apt to spoil; soaking herbs in water would have the same effect.

Time of day

Gather in the cool of the morning after the dew has evaporated, or in the evening before the dew forms on the plant. Gather before the sun is high, for the sun causes the leaves to droop, and some of the plant's valuable oils are released into the atmosphere.

Where to gather

Preferably gather wild plants from high, dry soils, exposed to clean air and abundant sunshine.

GATHERING PLANT PARTS

In all cases, gathering must be selective according to the type of plant and the part to be used.

Aromatics

Some examples would be pennyroyal, peppermint, spearmint. Gather after the flower buds are formed and the flower is just about to open. In such plants the extremely volatile medicines will be lost if gathered at the wrong time.

Barks

Or cortices. Gather either in the spring or autumn. Resinous barks, such as cinchona, wild cherry, viburnum, white oak, rubus, pomegranate, cascara sagrada, juglans (hickory, butternut), cinnamon, sassafras, and cascarilla should be gathered in the spring before the flowering season. Other gummy barks: preferably gather in autumn after the foliage has fallen. Generally the barks from younger trees should be used, as their medicinal properties are usually more viable and easily extracted. Take care to separate the decayed parts and impurities from the good barks to be used, and the rougher barks should be rossed (this is scraping or shaving the outer bark), and only the inner bark used.

Buds

(Such as quaking aspen, cloves.) Gather when nicely formed, before the flower expands.

Bulbs

(Such as squills, garlic.) Gather after the leaves of the plant die.

Berries

(Such as buckthorn, elder.) Gather when ripe. Elderberries should be gathered when dark, and do not pick too green. Hawberries of the hawthorn tree should be picked when they are black and almost ready to shatter. Juniper berries and bayberries should be gathered when just ripening but not quite mellow. Juniper berries are usually in two sets of berries on the bush, the green ones and the dark ones. The dark ones are second-year and ripe berries—pick these, but never use the green ones.

Excrescences

(Such as nutgall, oakgall.) Gather when the leaves are matured—after the strength has risen from the roots.

Flowers and petals

(Such as sambucus, lavender, clover, camomile, coltsfoot.) Gather when about to open from the bud (any lengthy delay will result in loss of the essential oils). With larger flowers, the petals should be removed before drying. With some flowers, only the petals are preserved and the colorless claws are cut away, but flowers having an odorless calyx are entirely preserved. When the flowers are too small to pick singly, cut with part of the stalk.

Fruit

(Such as juniper, hops, dill, black pepper, cayenne, cardamon seed.) Gather when succulent and ripe (except when specified to be gathered in the unripe stage, as with cubeb), but before they fall spontaneously.

Gum-Resins

(Such as camphor, copaiba, gamboge.) The gums and resins which come to the surface of barks are easier to collect in the cool of the day (morning and evening) when they are more solidified. A tapping procedure can also be used to extract the saps.

Leaves

(Such as rosemary, eucalyptus, uva ursi, senna, buchu.) Gather as soon as fully matured, before flowering or after maturation of the fruit. The medicinal value shifts in the growing stages from the leaf to the fruit and back again. Take care to gather the leaves when the potency is highest in that particular part.

Take proper care in the harvest. Never totally strip any herb when gathering leaves; avoid damage to the plant. Take a few leaves from this area and from that area, and get ample, but do not rob any bush or tree of all its leaves. The large leaves appearing before the stalk appears usually are more juicy and valuable than those that extend later from the stalk, as the former have the full nourishment of the root, but these often lose their value and die as the stalk begins to rise.

Annuals: Gather when about to flower or in flower.
Aromatic annuals: Gather after the flower buds are formed.
Biennials: Gather the leaves of the second year of growth only (first year leaves do not have their full medicinal value), before the stalk begins to shoot.
Perennials: Gather before flowering (especially if the fibers thereafter become woody).

Leaves with stalks or stems attached should be separated as soon as possible, and all other leaves should be cut close to the root. Leaves should be shaken clean and not washed; they may be wiped.

Herb (whole)

(Such as chondrus, pulsatilla, lobelia, peppermint, catnip, horehounds.) Gather when the heads are formed for flowering, but not yet opened. After the flowers open, the plant begins to lose potency and decay medicinally. If used fresh (e.g., for an infusion), cut only the tops (see "Tops"). *Annuals:* Cut three to four inches above ground to allow a second growth. *Perennials:* Cut the side branches two-thirds down the stalk.

Oleoresins

Similar to gum resins.

Rhizomes or rhizomata

(Such as ginger, calamus, iris, geranium, podophyllum, valerian, arnica, serpentaria, hydrastis.) Similar to roots, (see below).

Roots or radices

(Such as comfrey, sarsaparillas, poke, ginseng.) The roots of annuals and biennials usually have limited value, whereas the roots of perennials possess great virtue, which generally increases in potency over the years. Roots are usually gathered in the early part of spring (last of February, early part of March) when the plant juices are concentrated.

Roots of annuals: Gather before the flowering season and not after, because then the root becomes less active.
Biennial roots: Gather in the autumn of the first year, after the foliage has fallen. The full medicinal strength is concentrated in the first year roots.
Perennial roots: Gather in autumn after the leaves and flowers (or tops) are fully matured and the sap has returned to the roots, or in the springtime before growth period commences and the sap begins to run. If the root is covered by tough bark (such as pareira, ipecac), it should be peeled while fresh, wherein it slips off easily and does not adhere.

Seeds or burrs, pits, etc.

(Such as colchicum, almond, pumpkin, mustard, linseed, nutmeg, burdock, sweet-pit apricot.) There are three kinds of seeds: those with naked heads (fennel, parsley), those in pods (mustard, cresses), and those surrounded by fleshy fruits (melon, cucumbers).

Umbels or naked heads: The heads should be plucked when the seeds are brown and the stalks are dry-looking; they can be separated with slight threshing. Do not wait too long in harvesting or else the seeds will drop. Umbels can be gathered easily by spreading paper in a basket and cutting them directly into it, to prevent the loss of seeds that are ready to fall, take care to thresh very gently the seeds in the finer heads or pods, so as not to bruise the seeds; the umbels can be rubbed between the palms of the hands, with the seeds and chaff being separated through an appropriate sieve which permits passage of the seed, but not the coarser chaff. The chaff may also be separated by holding the seeds high and pouring them slowly in a gentle breeze onto a canvas or other appropriate covering.

Oily seeds from odorous plants and those containing volatile, principles must be gathered every year, as much potency is lost in storage. Other seeds with more permanent and stable properties can be kept several years.

Pods: Seeds in pods should be left on the plant until fully ripe and mature, and plucked after the plant begins drying; and these seeds may be separated (dislodged) from the pods with a strong stroke or two of the plant upon the floor.

Fleshy fruit: The seeds of fleshy fruit must be removed and separated from the surrounding membranes and wet matter, which should be removed after the meat or fruit has become fully ripe and succulent.

Sprouts

Collect before the buds open.

Stalks

Gather in autumn, soon after the flowers decay.

Stem

Herbaceous: Gather after foliage has appeared, before the blossoms develop.
Woody: Gather in autumn after the foliage falls and the leaves decay, and before vegetation occurs in the spring.

Tops

(Such as broom, eternal flower.) Tops are gathered when the whole herbs are to be used fresh, with the tops three to four inches long, but gather only one inch or less when consumed raw.

Tubers or bulbs or corms

(Such as colchicum, India turnip, jalap.) Gather same as roots. Be sure that tubers are not damaged in collection, because many of them lose medicinal potency when cut into too deeply.

Twigs

(Such as dulcamara, scoparius, Dyer's greenwood.) Gather soon after the flowers have decayed.

Woods

(Such as quassia, guaiacum.) Gather when the active principles are most concentrated, which is in the spring or autumn, and preferably from older trees. The albumen (the young soft wood of a dicotyledonous stem, the tissue outside the heart wood and near the cambium) is to be rejected. With resinous woods only the heavier material that will sink in water should be selected.

GENERAL DRYING INSTRUCTIONS

Herbs that grow moldy, smell musty, or become lighter or brown by too much heat or sunlight in the drying process have lost much of their medicinal value. Dry all herbs carefully.

Outdoors

Spread a thin layer of the herb on a drying screen (ordinary window screens covered with cheesecloth, fiberglass screening) mounted on saw horses or legs, placed in racks, propped on chairs, etc. to permit free air circulation both over and under, turning the herb occasionally. Drying should be done in the shade, never in direct sunlight, as quickly as possible so that both the volatile principles and leaf color are retained (three to four days are usually sufficient). Herbs that are dried too slowly (not enough warmth, too much moisture in the air) or with too much heat (direct sunlight), will lose active principles or the volatile particles.

Indoors

Dry in a dust-free room, at mild temperature, and away from direct sunlight (an attic with cross-ventilation is especially good). The herbs may be spread out on a drying screen, or they may be tied in small bundles and hung with the flower heads downward from a line or cord stretched across the room (this is especially good for leafy foliage and when the whole herb is dried). When a drying rack is used, turning the herb occasionally will prevent molding; and in all instances, the herb must be crackly-dry (snap or crumble at slight bending or pressure) before storing, or else the moisture remaining in the herb will cause molding. Those herbs dried on a line or cord should be removed as soon as fully dried, for they will attract dust and insects.

Artificial Heat

Oven drying is generally poor because of the difficulty in accurately regulating the temperature and, if done improperly, the oils evaporate and the herb becomes scorched. But when controlled (under 100° F.), artificial drying is possible and more value will be retained by this quick drying process. The herbs dried quickly will have little odor when they are perfectly dry, but after a period of time some moisture is absorbed again from the atmosphere, and they regain their proper odor. When artificial heat is being used (such as an electric burner or a gas burner), have a fan with an automatic switch, so that whenever the heat is on, the fan is on, and whenever the fan is off, the heat automatically stops. The fan may also be operated by itself. A thermostat would do this automatically.

Separate and label: Be sure to keep all herbs separated and labeled during the drying process as the dried herbs look different from the green plant, and in most cases, identification will be most difficult.

DRYING PLANT PARTS

Aromatics: These herbs should be dried according to the part that is to be used, but be very careful that they are not piled (a single layer is best here) and that drying is moderate; always in the shade or indoors.

Bark: Most barks are best used fresh, yet they retain their medicinal value well when dry. For easy handling and usage, bark should be cut into moderately small pieces before drying. These may be dried outdoors with moderate sun heat, laying them on sticks, slats, boards, etc. a few inches apart to allow free air circulation, but must be taken indoors at night into a well ventilated room, allowing spaces between pieces for free air circulation. Barks may be tested for dryness by bending slightly, and if no moisture is present, they will snap immediately.

Buds: Dry similar to leaves.

Bulbs: These can be dried in the shade with good air circulation, or better still, they can be hung from rafters in net bags.

Berries: These must be dried in the shade in moderate temperature, and never too quickly. There should only be one layer of berries on the drying rack because they mold very easily.

Excrescents: Appendages of plants (such as burrs, briefs, or galls of oaks) require only a few days' exposure to the air on a table before storing.

Flowers: Flowers are usually used fresh, but can be preserved in the form of syrup (as cloves or poppy), in conserves (cowslip), or dried, although the drying must be done quickly and carefully. Flowers are dried variously—some use only the petals, some are preserved in the whole head, others retain the leaves about them, while still others remove the flower and use only the hip. Flowers should not be exposed to direct sunlight during drying, and the addition of a slight degree of artificial warmth is best to hasten the process. A good test for flowers is that medicinal value is lost when the color and odor are gone.

Fruit: This is dried variously, and in most cases it can be dried in the sun (the fruit should be cut into relatively thin pieces, as chunks that are too large will mold readily), but fan drying and the application of artificial heat is good.

Gum-Resins: These do not have to be dried when they are kept in closed containers, or they may be dried and crystallized (either way is good).

Herbs: Remove dead or decayed matter, spread thinly on a drying rack or tie in very small bunches and hang about one foot apart on lines across a well ventilated room, until completely dry.

Leaves: Pluck from the stem (except those with small leaflets such as thyme and wintry savory). Spread loosely upon a drying rack away from direct sunlight (allowing free air circulation over and under), and stir sufficiently to avoid molding.

Rhizomes: Dry same as roots.

Roots: Most roots may be dried and preserved for a period of time, but certain roots lose their medicinal virtues by drying (such as poke root), and must be used fresh or kept buried in the sand or covered with soil to keep them from deteriorating rapidly. The roots to be dried should be cleaned (a brush is excellent or a little cold water may be used) and the decayed matter, fibers, and little roots removed and, with the exception of certain resinous roots, the worm-eaten roots should be discarded. The thick and strong roots should be split, cut, and sliced immediately into small pieces (while the roots are yet green and fresh), as this will hasten the drying and curing process, and after mold. If the root is covered by a tough bark, peel it off immediately; the longer you wait, the more difficult it will be. Non-aromatic roots (consisting principally of fibers or a small top) may be dried artificially with heat under 100° F. Aromatic roots should be dried in a current of cold air and turned frequently. It is always better to dry roots in a dark room, as sunlight will turn the lighter hue to a darker and more unsightly one. Before storing roots in some appropriate container, always test for dryness, which is—if they snap in two when slightly bent, then they are thoroughly dried.

Seeds: Seeds growing in umbels, naked heads or pods should be left on the plant until ripe, then separated (as heretofore described), spread onto drying screens, on heavy cloth, or on canvas laid on the floor of a well-ventilated, warm room, and left five to six days; then the chaff should be removed (as heretofore described) in a gentle breeze; then the seeds are spread out again on the cloth-covered drying screen another seven to ten days, turning them frequently. The seeds of fleshy fruit, after they are separated from the surrounding membranes and wet matter, should be placed on a table or dry place and rubbed occasionally during the drying process, so that they will be clean when dry. Generally, seeds are gathered when fully ripe. They need little care, and after three to four days on a clean floor or wire mesh (where there is free passage of air, but not exposure to sun), the seeds are ready for storage.

Sprouts: Dry the same as leaves or herbs, indoors, and away from sunlight.
Stems: Dry same as leaves and twigs.
Stalks: Dry same as bark, because they are a tough type of herb.
Tops: Dry carefully, as with leaves and flowers.
Tubers: Dry similar to roots.
Twigs: Dry same as leaves, but slightly longer.
Woods: Dry same as bark, but sunlight will turn the lighter woods dark.

STORING HERBS

Place in a tight appropriate container, not made of formaldehyde or certain damaging plastic types, and seal with sealing wax to keep the air from getting to the herb. Be sure to wrap bottle well for storage, placing sufficient padding between because broken glass from violent jarring, earthquakes, or moving, is dangerous.

The stored herbs should always be labeled, dated, and well organized into an herbal medicine chest, cabinet, or closet.

LONG-RANGE STORAGE

For preserving herbs for long periods of time, the parts and plants should be put into liquid extract, tincture or syrup form. The tincture form will keep indefinitely as long as it is in a dark place, in colored glass bottles (the three-ounce size is good for the average need and easy handling) that should be well-capped and sealed.

YEARLY USE

In most cases, where the herb will be used within the year, just place it into a tight can or other appropriate, closed container. If you desire to keep these herbs a second year, be sure to seal the cans not in current use. Sealing is done by filling the can as full as possible to crowd out oxygen, and then sealing with wax. While the foregoing procedure is generally good for nearly all herbs, there are a few specifics (such as poke root) which lose medicinal potency on the same day they are gathered, so herbs of this type must be put immediately into tincture form.

STORAGE OF OILS

The oils must be stored in brown bottles or in cans, and sealed tightly, kept out of the sun and out of extreme heat.

STORAGE IN POWDER FORM

The length of time that a powdered form will keep depends upon storage conditions; it will last up to a year or more and retain almost full potency when stored in a fairly cool place. Those powders containing oils (such as cayenne) should be put in a container that can be hermetically sealed or waxed (such as a honey can), never placed in paper. A waxed carton, cellophane or plastic container is all right, but the recommended procedure is to store in a can or bottle and then seal. Powdered herbs usually do not need refrigeration, as the covered powder at room temperature should keep well six months to a year, and when hermetically sealed, it should keep two or three years.

PREPARING HERBS

Nicholas Culpeper's *Herbal Improved* quotes Reverend John Wesley in the preface to his "Primitive Physic." Wesley says, "be sure to purchase your drugs from a Druggist who fears God."

This is also stated by the Mormon prophet Joseph Smith in the *Doctrine and Covenants* 42:43:

"And whosoever among you are sick, and have not faith to be healed, but believe, shall be nourished with all tenderness, and with herbs and mild food, and that not by the hand of an enemy."

Be most careful that the medicinal agents you use are genuine and organic. Attempts at curing will be worse than useless, rendering harm to the body if they are not. Whenever possible, collect your own herbs, but if this is not possible, the next best is to be sure to obtain the herbs from a reliable herbalist, botanist, herb shop, or health food store.

GENERAL GUIDELINES

In making your herbal preparations, never use aluminum ware. Aluminum poisons with its gases and acid metallic poison (alum). Use a good grade of stainless steel or Pyrex or a good glassware, providing you handle it with care. Glazed earthenware is adequate. Whenever using enamel pans (which are a basic metal with enamel baked on), always be sure that there are no chips, no cracks, that the pan is fully enamel-covered. Stainless-steel ware is the best because it does not break, although you should watch for over-high temperatures that cause burning. Moist heat is always used, and stainless-steel ware is easiest to control, because you can spin and seal the lid and thereby keep oxygen from going in.

HERBAL PREPARATIONS

The following gives a description of various herbal preparations. General guidelines for dosage are also included, but these are to be adjusted according to need.

Balsam

This is an aromatic, oily, resinous, liquid or semi-solid substance (consisting chiefly of resins and volatile oils containing esters of cinnamic and benzoic acids) that flows by natural exudation from certain trees or is taken by artificial extraction, and is used in expectorants, stomachics, in syrups, etc. The true balsams are such as the balsam of Peru, balsam of Tolu, etc.; but the term is also applied to certain substances that are not true balsams (containing no cinnamic or benzoic acid), but which are resinous and odorous (such as balm of Gilead and copaiba balsam). A balsam is used externally to ease pain, rheumatism (when not inflamed), wounds, etc. and is rubbed on with the warm hand on an affected part or applied by fomentation and renewed every three to four hours. Internally, the balsam is used for asthma, colic, cough, pains in the breast, etc.

Especially in the western mountains of America, there are balsams of pine, spruce, and fir (various resinous gums). Not all resinous gums will work; yet many of the first, pines and spruces, are excellent. "Balsam" is in many instances changeable with the term "balm." Balsams are made variously according to the area where they are to be used. Internally, the balsam resins are often put into capsules and taken directly. Externally, they are mixed in with other types of lubricating oils, such as olive oil or tallow. Often balsams are mixed into liniments, but this must be done carefully.

Bolus

Technically, this is defined as a rounded mass, or a large pill, intended for internal use; but the term "bolus" as it is used by herbalists has connection with the term "poultice"—i.e., it is an internal poultice. The bolus is used internally in the sinus, rectal or vaginal areas and either draws the toxic poisons to it, or is the carrier for healing agents. They are generally composed of powdered herbal agents mixed with a base and may have various therapeutic actions.

The bolus is made in several ways. Powdered herbs added to a base of slippery elm powder is one of the earliest, oldest, and best forms. Water is added to the combination to make a dough-like mass that is easily-formed. The bolus is given the desired shape then left to air-dry till it is rigid enough to be inserted. Just prior to use, submerge the bolus in water to make it slippery to slide easily into the orifice. The slippery elm type will hold its form for quite some time but be sure to adequately rehydrate the bolus if it has been left to completely dry.

You may use cocoa butter (made from coconut in the butter form) as a base for the bolus. Melt the cocoa butter over hot water (never put it directly over the heat, because it burns so quickly and unexpectedly). When the cocoa butter is liquid, stir in the herbs until they reach a heavy gravy consistency. Then let this cool enough to roll into boluses. Set these aside to harden. Another way to shape the bolus is to use an ice cube tray. Stir the mixture till it thickens to the point where the herbs and the cocoa butter will not separate and then pour it into the tray filling each compartment from 1/4 to 1/2 inch up. When cooled and firm you can cut them down to the desired width.

These are easily inserted and will melt at body temperature. Boluses for the vagina are generally made the size of the middle finger of the person using it and about an inch long; and with an adult, the bolus is used in a series of three (which is easier for the patient than one long three-inch bolus in the vaginal area). This, of course, is not used in individuals where the hymen has not been broken. The vaginal boluses are generally prepared in fair quantities at a time, where they will be changed three times a week. If kept in a cool place, they will last for long periods of time—the cocoa butter will not melt except at higher temperatures.

Olive oil can be used as the base for boluses, but it requires hard freezing to make the bolus firm enough for insertion.

Dosage: Series of three, size of user's middle finger and one inch long, inserted fresh every two days, three times a week.

Capsules

Take the herbal powders and other materials that, because of their nauseous taste or smell (oils, tars as with pine gum, bitter powders as with golden seal), would otherwise be difficult to administer, and place them into a soluble gelatin shell or capsule. These capsules are made in different sizes for easy swallowing, with numbers 1 to 4, 0, and 00 being the most common. (For herbal agents that are taken quite regularly in the capsule form, a large quantity of the capsuled preparation may be placed in a labeled container kept tightly covered.) To fill the capsule, simply take the two halves of a capsule apart (one in each hand), and push these halves into the powder and toward each other, pressing the halves together again and at the same time compressing the powder. With a little practice, you can fill several hundred capsules in one single evening.

Small devices that help to encapsulate herbs into 50 capsules at a time are available on the market.

Dosage: This depends on the age, size, vitality, condition being treated, and the strength of the ingredients in the capsule itself, of which the following would be typical:

No. 4: is a small size and usually taken often (golden seal).
No. 0: two to three, two to three times a day (less powerful herbs).
No. 00: two, morning and night (female corrective).
Generally, use the amount specified.

Cataplasm

This is an old term for a form of poultice, made of various herbal agents, usually applied hot. Refer to"poultice."

Dosage: 1/2 to 1 inch thick over inflamed area; add an oil or glycerine to prevent caking and to retain heat (covering with oiled silk is excellent).

Cerate

This is an unctuous (oily, fatty) preparation for external use, consisting of wax (sometimes resin or spermaceti) mixed with oils, fatty substances or resins, and medicinal agents. It is made so that it can be readily spread on linen or muslin, yet firm enough that it will not melt or run when applied to the skin. To keep the oils from running or soaking through, a little slippery elm is often put into the cerate. This preparation is used where one must wear a bandage for long periods of time, and keep the skin from drying out—generally for heavy scaling types of dermatitis or incrustation, and often for a phlebitis condition, a hardening of the surface of the skin and flesh where varicose veins have broken and, over a period of time, become more solidified.

Dosage: Amount needed to cover the specific area, increasing the thickness of the compound according to the severity of the condition.

Collyria

Or eyewash or eye lotion. This is a medicinal application for the eyes. Botanical eye washes include bayberry, eye bright, golden seal, raspberry leaves (all of which may be accentuated with a small quantity of cayenne, which will produce extreme warmth but do no damage to the area). Do not be afraid of the cayenne in the eye, for even if smarting becomes severe cayenne is very beneficial and will never damage the eye—even if accidentally a full handful of cayenne would be thrown into the eye.

Dosage: Eyecupfull, or small amount by eye-dropper, or use a tea bag compress. When first starting, it is best to use for just a very short period of time (maybe two or three seconds and increase as you go along), especially when cayenne or some other powerful healer is combined with the formula.

Combination infusion and decoction

Often the infusion and the decoction processes are combined into one herbal preparation. An example is a medicine for nausea, where you would take cloves, turkey rhubarb, cinnamon and make a decoction of these by simmering them for five to ten minutes; then you take this decoction and pour it over spearmint leaves (making an infusion of the latter), and let this steep. The infusion is required with aromatics, because they have volatile, effervescent oils that escape when heat is applied. Never boil a decoction hard (unless definitely specified in rare cases). Too much heat will destroy the active medicinal properties. If the tea is too strong, then add more water to dilute.

Dosage: Generally one cupful three times a day.

Compound

This is a preparation composed of two or more agents having organic affinity, and in definite proportion to each other; an herbal formula. A given therapeutic action may not be obtained by a single herb, but the use of a number of them together in definite formula proportion are most beneficial and curative. Do not use compounds, however, in "shotgun fashion," (making an herbal preparation with a hodgepodge variety of ingredients. Though they be of the same therapeutic class, nervines for instance, they may be either stimulants or sedatives), for only those combined herbs that have compatible active therapeutic properties will work. You may not do any harm by the shotgun approach, but you may not get the best results, either, due to incompatible or neutralizing action.

Most herbs are ascribed double or multiple medicinal actions. Which particular virtue comes to the fore in actual application depends largely on the other agents with which it is combined. Thus, the alternative properties of an herb may be more pronounced in one combination, while in a different prescription its value as a diuretic might become more operative. As stated by Harold Ward:

"In the effective allocation of his various medicinal agents to meet precise individual requirements lies an important department of the work of the skilled prescribing herbalist."

A good example of compatible functions of different herbs in a compound is in the removal of kidney stones (for which gravel root and uva ursi are excellent); unless you add a demulcent to soothe the mucous membrane (such as marshmallow), there will be excruciating pain. Working on the liver area, one will generally stir up a lot of gas in the cleansing process, so you must include an herb to alleviate the flatulence or gas (such as wild yam)—so in an herbal formula, the second herb is often just as important as the first. Another area where compound compatibility is important is with the kidney. Herbs such as juniper berries or parsley are generally combined with ginger which acts as a carrier to the kidney area and an accentuator (i.e., a stimulant added to a diuretic). You may want to add a third type, golden seal, as a tonic to tone up and heal the area.

Dosage: Generally used in infusions and decoctions, one teaspoon of the herb to a cup of water; give dosage according to type of preparation.

Concentrate

A concentrate is a type of fluid extract with the evaporation of the extractive agent (as with alcohol) from the liquid solution. This preparation refers to the preparations by means of water, distillation, etc. This preparation usually carries one or more, but not all, of the therapeutic virtues in the original herb from which it was made. Concentrates must never be boiled at a high rate. Rather a distilling heat should be used so that the fumes or the steam will evaporate gradually. You must always watch carefully, or you will likely have only burned tar with no medicinal value, because the dry heat destroys the life-giving organic bonds. When you want to make concentrates from a liquid, simmer slowly in a covered vessel so that the volatiles are not lost, but instead evaporate onto the lid and condense back into the concentrate itself.

Watch carefully and stir occasionally, so that the precipitating solids do not stick to the sides of the vessel as you simmer the liquid down to the consistency required. Concentrates are often brought from the original matter of six ounces down to two ounces or ounce concentrate—so again, as a word of caution: be very careful not to burn the preparation, use a temperature of under 160° F. Some of the volatile oils will disperse and evaporate at 120-160° F., while others take more heat to disperse them. If the oils are of an extremely light and volatile nature (spearmint, peppermint and most other mints cannot take much heat), then use a double boiler so that direct heat is not applied.

Dosage: Varies according to the specific herb and its degree of concentration. 1 to 60 drops is usually specified.

Conserve

This is a sweetmeat (candied or crystallized food or fruit), prepared by impregnating sugar into the pulpy mass of the herb or fruit. One method used for example, is to boil sloes (fruit of blackthorn or Prunus spinosa; or any variety of American wild plums—Prunus Americans, Prunus alleghaniensis, etc.), being careful to remove the fruit before the skin bursts in the process, and then to beat this with three times its weight in sugar. This makes an excellent gargle and is a relaxant to the uvula and glands of the throat. Another well-known type of conserve is candied ginger, borrowed from the Chinese. Conserves have some bad side-effects because of the sugar content, but the herbs are in a more pleasant form. Conserves can be made with honey, but this is a little harder to do, as the finished product must be rolled into a powder base to keep it from being sticky. Conserves made with honey are superior to those made with sugar.

Dosage: Varies, use amount specified.

Decoction

This is a process used with roots and barks, chips, etc. Some must be boiled in water while with others, boiling water must be poured over them and then a simmering heat applied over a period of time. Decoctions are intended for immediate use within a twenty-four hour period (with a 72-hour maximum limit when stored in a very cool place.) Some herbs, however, do not sour within seventy-two hours, but if the souring or scum starts, make a fresh preparation. An herbal decoction is the chief basis for preparing enemas, ointments, spirits, fomentation, etc.

A decoction is generally made by pouring cold water upon fresh or dried (cut, bruised, or ground) herbal agents. The usual preparation is one ounce of the botanical herb placed into 1½ pints (24 ounces) of cold water (the ½ pint will be lost in the extractive process). The herb and liquid is then brought slowly to a boil. The decoction differs from the infusion in that heat is applied and continued over a period of time (boiling or simmering), because roots and barks generally need longer heating to extract their active principles.

Water generally extracts the gummy and saline parts of herbal agents but heavy gums must be extracted with alcohol. The oily and resinous properties are also intimately blended with the gummy and saline elements, and many may be extracted by infusion, but a decoction is superior where there is tenacious cell structure. The harder the material, the longer the simmering and extractive period will be. This must be determined by your own careful observation, ingenuity, intuition, and experience, if not specified.

In making a decoction of dry roots and barks, pulverize them first by mechanical means or pounding; next, soak the ingredients for twelve hours; then set this liquid on the fire and gradually heat to a slight boil. After the extractive period, drain off the liquid while hot and press the herb hard to make sure that all of the therapeutic ingredients are removed; then let stand until cool. When cool, pour off the clear liquid on top, separating it from the settlings; and, finally, sweeten to taste. When fresh herbs are used in a decoction, the roots should be cut into very thin slices and the barks and woods should be shaved down, but the leaves and whole herbs need only slight cutting. Again, add more water when decoctions are too strong.

Dosage: Depending on age, size and temperament, 2 fluid ounces to a cupful of liquid three times a day.

Draft or drought

This is a small quantity of medicine, usually in a liquid form, that is taken by the mouthful and swallowed. It is generally not delicious and therefore taken in a hurry. With intense pain or cramps for example, one must take some tincture of lobelia (anywhere from a few drops up to a teaspoonful, as the condition requires), taken in one mouthful and swallowed. There are anodyne drafts for excessive pain and restlessness (25 drops tincture of lobelia, 1 ounce cinnamon water, 2 teaspoons common syrup, mixed); diuretic drafts for obstruction in the urinary tract causing a deficiency of urine (2 drops tincture of juniper berries, 2 teaspoons poppy syrup, 1 ounce water), etc. This is a very quick and efficacious way to administer a remedy.

Dosage: One mouthful generally is enough for a period of time, repeated as necessary.

Electuary

This is an herbal preparation incorporated into honey, or syrup, conserve or mucilage to form a soft or pasty mass which can easily be rolled into a ball. They are generally composed of the lighter powders (chiefly mild unpalatable alterative agents). When a child does not like to take capsules or resists drinking strong teas, you can make up an electuary (such as 1/4 teaspoon of worm seed powder, in case of needing a worm medicine) by just mixing the powder in a little honey, stiffening it with a small quantity of coconut or slippery elm powder, and then having the child chew or wash it down with a liquid. Even cayenne can be made an embedded pasty mass using peanut butter and honey as a base, and the cayenne embedded into it. Electuaries may be made from powders of barks, roots, seeds, conserves of flowers, tops of fresh herbs, etc., but astringent electuaries (having pulps of fruit in them) should be prepared only in small quantities, as the medicinal virtues in these are rapidly lost, and the fruit pulps are apt to ferment. Generally, store this preparation in a cool place.

Dosage: Varies with mixture type, patient, vitality, etc. from pea-size up to marble-size.

Elixir

This is a sweetened, aromatic, spirituous preparation containing soluble medicinal agents in small amounts; it is usually a tincture or mixture of various herbal agents held in solution by alcohol in some form. One of the best examples of an elixir is the hawberry heart tonic (see page 581), a rich syrupy preparation, mixed with enough brandy (of a fine type such as apricot, blackberry, etc.) to serve as a preservative, with glycerine and any other materials needed. You only use one-half teaspoon at a time in this highly concentrated form, which will do just as much good as one-half cup of the juice, because of the concentration.

Dosage: Varies according to age, and size, one-fourth teaspoon up.

Emulsion

This is a preparation of tiny globules of one liquid interspersed within another liquid (the former is called the internal, dispersed or discontinuous phase; and the latter liquid is the external or continuous phase, or dispersion medium). This is a type of homogenization where heavy material is suspended in an oily liquid. It is used for certain substances that would not otherwise be taken in a liquid form—for instance, pure oils, balsams, resins and other similar substances. An example of a common emulsion is:

1 ounce	Sweet almonds.
1 teaspoon	Bitter almonds.
2 pints	Water.

Blanch almonds (remove skin by scalding) and beat up, adding water little by little to form an emulsion; strain and bottle. This particular formula (using a teaspoon a day, six days a week, over the years) is a wonderful cancer preventative.

Dosage: Varies, teaspoonful to tablespoonful.

Enema or Clyster

This is a way to administer copious amounts of liquid into the bowel itself (as much quantity as can be accepted), including such herbal preparations as infusions or decoctions, etc. having a laxative or peristaltic action upon the bowels. It is also used as a means of conveying fluids, nutritive food and herbal medicines into the system. Medicines and nourishment are administered by enema when persons cannot take anything orally. Also, an enema of warm herbal liquid may serve as a fomentation or wash, doing much good for inflammation of the bladder, lower intestines, etc. There are anti-putrefaction enemas, diuretic enemas, emollient enemas, laxative enemas, and enemas for various other problems. If a hot or a warm enema is given, then the anus will relax, causing the rectal area to discharge immediately, so, in most cases, a cold preparation is preferred, as it will soak through the waste concentrations.

Dosage: Prepare in strength of 1½ teaspoons of herb to each cup of water. Use 1½ cups to 1 pint (one quart maximum) solution for children. Administer to a child according to age, vitality, etc. Adults can use 1 to 3 quarts.

Extract

This is an herbal preparation made by boiling the herbal agent in water and evaporating the strained decoction to a desired consistency. By this process, some of the more active principals of the medicinal herb are liberated from the useless insoluble, pulpy matter (which comprises the larger share of the bulk). The solvents used are alcohol, glycerine, water, etc. Make extracts at the lowest temperature possible, because, if care is not taken, many of the light balsam oils and precious ingredients can be lost. The preparation vessel should always be tightly covered until the extract is sufficiently cooled. See also "fluid extract" and "solid extract."

Dosage: A few drops (according to need), generally put into another liquid; the dry extract would be a few grains of powder (as specified).

Fluid extract

Fluid extracts are more concentrated forms of other preparations done variously through evaporation, allowing a suitable solvent (such as spirits or alcohol) to pass through a column of the powdered substance (cold percolation), or high pressure, etc. The extract results so that the medicinal strength of the active properties in one fluid ounce of liquid will be equal to the medicinal value of one ounce of the crude herb. One simple common method is to soak, soften, and separate (macerate) crude herbs in water and alcohol containing a small quantity of glycerine and then to evaporate this solution until the desired strength is reached. In the evaporative procedure, low heat is applied. A fluid extract of an herb tea would be where the liquid has been simmered so that just the water is evaporated.

Wherever it is feasible and compatible, glycerine is a more preferred extraction medium than alcohol (which does not add to the remedial properties of an extract, but simply serves as a vehicle for them and as a preservative). Glycerine has medicinal value. Undiluted glycerine is an irritant and a stimulant, and well-diluted glycerine is demulcent, emollient, soothing and healing. An extract of glycerine solution is superior to alcohol, etheric, or any other extract made for most purposes, but it is incompatible with resinous or oily herb extracts which require alcohol as the solvent. Another valuable characteristic of glycerine is that it unites with and helps to remove many of the insoluble, inorganic drugs, such as those containing mercury, iodine, mineral sulfates, arsenic, strychnine, etc.

A glycerine extract can be made in various ways as follow: Soak four ounces of ground herb in 12 ounces of water and 4 ounces of glycerine (3 parts water to 1 part glycerine), macerate for ten days, strain as with the alcohol tincture (see page 545), and bottle.

Another way is to add enough distilled water to cover one pint of the crude herb and simmer on low heat for 20 minutes. Strain and set aside the solution. Add one gallon distilled water to the same herb and simmer (unless a heavy root or bark, which would be boiled) down to one-half gallon; then strain and mix the two solutions. Slow simmer the combined solutions down to 1/2 gallon and add from 16 to 32 ounces of pure vegetable glycerine; let stand until cool, then bottle. The amount of glycerine you add depends upon the length of time you plan to store the preparation. If it is to be used within a few weeks time, one pint is sufficient (store in refrigerator to extend shelf life). If you wish to store the preparation for months you will need to add a full quart of glycerine and shake the preparation from time to time to be sure the glycerine and solution do not separate.

Still another way to prepare an extract in a glycerine base is to first make a grain alcohol extract from the desired herb(s) and then remove the alcohol from the solution by low heating and add back 30 to 50% vegetable glycerine.

Fluid extracts save storage space, and also provide the practitioner with a compact and concentrated medicinal aid that is readily available and fast-acting. A fluid extract is generally used as a syrup, in liniments, and in fomentation. It is more concentrated than an infusion or a decoction, but less than the concentrate or solid extract.

Dosage: Internally, generally administered in teaspoonful doses; externally apply as needed.

Fomentation

This is generally an external application of herbs to convey heat, moisture, and medicinal aid in order to relieve pain, reduce inflammation, and to relax affected areas. Fomentation are usually made from bitter herbs, sometimes with cayenne added, steeped in vinegar or water, and placed hot in muslin cloth over the affected area. A fomentation of apple cider vinegar alone will often take the pains out of arthritis, rheumatism and similar conditions. Soak a Turkish towel or gauze or similar material in hot tea, lightly wring it out (just enough that the water will not run off the body), and place as hot as possible without causing blistering. Generally keep the fomentation moist and warm by placing plastics, oilcloth, etc. over fomentation.

Dosage: Wet enough that the moisture will not run off the body; keep damp and change periodically.

Gargle

This is a solution of herbal agents used in rinsing the pharynx.

Dosage: One mouthful (not for very young children).

Infusion

An infusion extracts the active principles of herbs in water, or other fluid, without simmering or boiling; and it also refers to the liquid product of such a process. Pour a liquid (hot water, juice, glycerine, vinegar or alcohol) over the crude or powdered herb. The liquid may be hot, cold, or lukewarm (depending upon the type of herb and problem condition) but the flavor of the herb is generally much stronger and the action is much faster when made and administered hot rather than cold.

Generally a standard infusion is used with the lighter herbs (such as the leaves, flowers, etc.), and is made by placing one teaspoonful of finely cut dried herb or two teaspoonfuls of bruised fresh herb into a cup and adding boiling, distilled water; cover and let steep for 15 minutes; strain and drink. For larger amounts of infusion use 1 ounce of the herb to each pint of water. Heavier herbs (such as woody stems, barks, and roots) will need to be coarsely ground or, if tenacious, pulverized; then pour the boiling water over them and allow to stand or steep for fifteen to thirty minutes. Be sure to cover the vessel and stir occasionally, then carefully strain off the clear liquid (though some sedimentation will not hurt in most cases).

Aromatic herbs contain effervescent or volatile oils which will be lost if infused in hot or boiling water, so steep in warm water for 30 minutes or more. With some herbs (such as buds, husks, and dried herbs like thyme), the only way medicinal value can be properly extracted is by infusion; other herbs that yield their medicinal value best by infusion are the pectorals (such as coltsfoot, ground ivy, etc.), aromatics (such as balm, mother of thyme, etc.), and bitters (such as gentian root, orange peel, wormwood, etc.). The bitter herbs do not require so large a quantity of the crude herb to the pint as do other herbs, and with something like cayenne, just a few grains are effective.

Dosage: Don't be afraid of over-concentrating organic herbal medicines or remedies. We do recommend, however, that you follow any instructions that are provided. Dosage varies according to type of herb and problem condition, etc. usually one cupful three times a day. Regulate the quantity to fit the patient's strength. In kidney problems, extreme debilitation, etc. smaller doses should be given.

Injection

Injection is the old English term for a small enema, where medicinal aids are put in the rectum in very limited amounts (one-half to one cupful), the small amounts of liquid are retained in the bowel for a time. Because the modern usage of the term "injection" is always thought of as being an intravenous use of the needle, when you refer to an "injection" be sure to specify that an herbal injection is only an enema.

Julep

This is a stimulating drink-type preparation flavored with aromatic herbs (but this is not the alcoholic drink referred to by the same term), and could be defined as "a large draft." An example of a julep would be: four ounces (eight tablespoonfuls) cinnamon water, two ounces (four tablespoonfuls) Jamaica cayenne, two teaspoons (one-fourth ounce or one dessert spoonful) compound spirit of lavender, one ounce (two tablespoonfuls syrup of orange peel, mixed; (this is for general weakness and depression).

Dosage: 2 fluid ounces to one-half glass at a time.

Juice or express

Fresh herbal juices expressed from leaves or roots are probably the best medicinal aid when available. These are sometimes obtained from an entire herb having a juicy stalk (such as brooklime and watercress); or sometimes, where the stalk is dry and yields almost nothing (such as nettle) from the leaves. Juice may be obtained by using an electrical appliance (such as a blender, juicer, or press), or the old-fashioned, "hand method". The hand method of expressing juice is as follows: thoroughly grind or beat the herb to a pulp with wooden pestle and a marble mortar (which is superior to any metal, unless stainless steel is available), and then wring the juice from the pulp into a vessel through muslin or other appropriate cloth. If the freshly-drawn juice is too thick, too coarse, or too harsh for the patient's stomach, let the liquid stand until the heavier sedimentation goes to the bottom, and then give the clear liquid only off the top.

Sweetening may be added into the juice while beating the herb; and for some roots (such as beets) it is better to add carrot, celery, or some other more bland and light juice in the beating, or a few grains of powdered ginger may be added instead. With some nutritional-type herbs (such as carrot, apple and others which are also highly medicinal), do not add sweetening or anything else. You may wish, however, to include various flavoring and aromatic herbs (such as parsley or peppermint) in some of the more bland herbs (such as types like celery juice). Juices are far superior to plain water in supplying needed liquid to the body, because the appetite diminishes. Juices do not wear out and tire the body in digestion; they are in composition similar to a transfusion. They go almost directly into the blood stream, while furnishing rapid nutrition. Juices are especially valuable because the growing herb filters out all the inorganic poisons (such as the chlorine and fluorine) in the water.

Dosage: Varies with specific cases (but not in large amounts, swished and well-mixed with saliva before swallowing).

Ketone

This is an herbal preparation wherein an organic compound is derived by oxidation from a secondary alcohol.

Dosage: Small amounts, usually a few drops up.

Liniment

This is an herbal preparation of an herbal oil or liquid intended for skin application by gentle friction or massage; it is thinner than the ointment and is usually rubbed on the skin as an anodyne or counter-irritant. Liniments can be mixed with alcohol extracts or with other oils and herbal ingredients.

Dosage: Sufficient so that little is left on the skin surface when massaged thoroughly into the skin.

Lotion

This is a weak aqueous solution of herbs used for external and local application. Lotions are often used to tone up the skin, to bring back a youthful condition and appearance (remove wrinkles and blemishes), and to make hands smoother. In preparing lotions, glycerine or various oils are used to provide the lubricating base, to which the herbal aids are added.

Dosage: According to individual judgment, as often as needed.

Mixture

This is an herbal preparation that is either a complex of two or more active ingredients which are not at fixed formulary proportion to each other; and though they are thoroughly commingled, they retain separate identities, or a suspension of two or more herbal agents in a liquid, which do not readily settle out. Often these are insoluble agents suspended in water by emulsion. It is erroneous, however, to think that the more herbs there are in the preparation, the better. Often only an herb or two appropriately selected is sufficient, and better than too many. Mixtures should be used, generally speaking, in the same proportion as individual formulas, wherein you mix a number together and take as one dose, using one teaspoon of the combined herbs (after they are mixed) to the cup, and then taking just one cup of the tea. At times you will find an herbal mixture in a bag or box on a shelf of health stores and other places, boasting a large number of beneficial herbs for healing the body. This is like trying to shoot an enemy at a distance with a shotgun, it is practically worthless.

Dosage: Varies, but generally one cupful three times a day; smaller doses for weak cases.

Oil

This preparation is made from the plant oils. For instance, the best oils from sassafras come from the root and the bark, but you can also take the oils from the chips and woods. With the mints (peppermint, spearmint, etc.), the oils come from the leaves. The oils from eucalyptus usually come from the leaves and some from the bark; and in many cases, oils are taken from flowers (as in lavender and various others), extracted almost to a gum consistency from red cover blossoms. Many of these oils, when properly made, do not go into rancidity easily (such as when made with olive oil). The amount of herbs used depends on the quantity of oil desired. Often a pound of fresh herbs to a pint of olive oil is used. Simmer the herbs for hours until the oil comes out of the herb. In the case of cloves, grind up fine, and simmer the powder in olive oil at a temperature of 125-150° F. Never use mineral oils.

Dosage: Do not overdo; varies according to type and need, a few drops to one tablespoonful. For olive oil, which is high in nutritional value, massage as much as the skin will absorb; olive oil is generally used in small doses internally, except when used for gallstones or kidney stones (here an adult dosage is four ounces or more at a time after a few days of preliminary herbal liquids).

Ointment or salve

This is a soft, semi-solid fatty herbal preparation used for a protective and emollient effect, liquefying when applied externally. Ointment bases are generally composed of various mixtures of waxes, animal and vegetable oils (olive, wheat germ, almond, coconut, etc.), solid and liquid hydrocarbons, or the so-called water-solubles in which there may be 50-70% water incorporated into an emulsified product. The medicinal substances are mixed with the oils and wax; the oils allow ready absorption of the medicines, and the wax gives firmness to the mass.

With nearly all combinations, start with a melted base, such as olive oil and beeswax, and combine with herb. A good standard is fourteen ounces of olive oil, two ounces of beeswax, and one pound of fresh or one-half pound of dry herbs. Place into a closed container (stainless steel, earthenware, unchipped or unbroken enamel, glassware), put into the oven and leave there at low heat (under 200° F, preferably around 180° F.) for three or four hours. Periodically, if desired, take a fork and lift the fresh herbs to see if they are getting browned and brittle, and whether the oil has drawn the value from the herb.

Vaseline as a base is generally inferior to animal or plant oils, but may be used if you do not want the preparation to be absorbed quickly into the skin (as when used on the internal membranous tissue of the nose). You will soon learn what works best (each ointment formula given in the text suggests the proper base). Ointments in most cases should be massaged in except for counter-irritant ointments that are high in cayenne and require no massaging.

Dosage: Amount needed but do not leave too much on the skin surface unless the area is covered to protect clothing from being soiled.

Oxymel

This is an herbal mixture of honey (five parts) and vinegar (one part), acting as a vehicle or carrier for a water solution (one part) of some herbal aid (which is in infusion, decoction, etc.) used as a gargle or a vehicle for nauseous medicinal aids, such as cayenne, garlic, squills, etc. Common oxymel is made of a pint of vinegar, and two pounds of honey boiled together to the consistency of a syrup.

Oxymel of garlic: put a quarter of an ounce of caraway seeds and a quarter of an ounce of sweet fennel seed into half a pint of vinegar, and bring it to a boil; remove from heat and add 1½ ounces of fresh garlic clove; cover and steep for 10 minutes, then press out the liquid and add ten ounces of honey; and return to a boil till you have a syrup consistency.

Oxymel of squill: put into a pint of vinegar three ounces of dried squills; let it stand two days in a gentle heat, then press out the vinegar, and when it has stood to settle, add a pound-and-half of honey, and boil it to a syrup consistency.

Dosage: As a gargle, usually a mouthful internally, according to the dosage of medicinal aid in the oxymel carrier.

Pessary

This is a suppository, such as a bolus that is placed in the vagina to apply herbal remedies to the internal organs. Pessaries must be made with demulcent or emollient-type herbs; harsh herbs should never be used. Refer to "bolus."

Pill or Lozenge, Pastil

This is an herbal preparation that, for the most part, is composed of concentrated extracts and alkaloids in combination with the active crude herbs. The herbal agent is ground into a very fine powder and mixed with a mucilage of gum Arabic (made by dissolving gum Arabic in water), slippery elm, or a syrup, etc. which is then worked up into a pill mass. A portion is then cut off, sliced into small strips and then into smaller pill sized pieces, which are then rolled into little round balls for easy administration. A small amount of powdered rhubarb or flour on the board in preparation will keep the mass from sticking, but keep the pill mass in a quite firm consistency, else the excess mucilage or syrup will absorb too much rhubarb or flour.

Pills can be coated or uncoated, but the pearl-coated pill is a favorite and is readily soluble in the stomach. Pills are usually made so that one pill equals about 300-400 milligrams of the herbal compound. There are specialty-type pills, such as enteric pills (dissolve in the duodenum or intestines), and concentric pills (formed of different ingredients in concentric layers so as to dissolve at various points in the intestinal tract). A pill differs from a tablet in that a pill needs a mucilage or other substance added to keep the herbal agent in an adhesive mass, whereas the tablet will adhere by its own characteristics upon compression.

Dosage: Varies, and must be administered as specified.

Plaster

This is an herbal preparation for external application that is harder than an ointment, but soft enough to be spread on linen, silk, etc. and adhere to the skin when applied to the body. The consistency of a plaster will vary according to the intended purpose—those applied to the breast or stomach will be soft and yielding, while those applied to the extremities should be firm and adhesive. Plasters must always be watched guardedly, so that they are not left on too long, as types such as the mustard plasters left on the area too long will cause blisters, burns.

Dosage: Usually one-fourth to one-half inch thickness to cover the problem area (varies according to the condition, toughness of the skin, etc.); however, use caution not to make plasters stronger than the patient can stand.

Poultice

This herbal preparation is a soft, semi-liquid mass made of some cohesive substance mixed with water, vinegar or other substances, and used for supplying heat and moisture to an area, or to act as a local stimulant. Have the herbs ground or granulated. When using fine powder, just use enough moisture to make a thick paste; and when using the granulated form, a thick paste may be made with a mixture of water and cornmeal (or flaxseed meal). If fresh green leaves are used, simply heat, bruise, triturate or chop them up finely, and apply to the affected parts. Poultices are excellent for enlarged or inflamed glands (neck, breast, groin, prostate, etc.), and also for eruptions, boils, carbuncles, and abscesses. A simple ripening or suppuration poultice is made as follows: prepare a soft composition with slippery elm powder and warm water, adding a quantity of boiled or raw onion. This can be softened with vegetable oil or fresh butter where necessary.

Dosage: Be generous in making poultices, covering the afflicted area thickly.

Powder

This preparation consists of the fine particles of any dried herbal agent that have been reduced or pulverized by pounding, grinding, etc. The herbal powders may be placed in capsules, electuaries, emulsions, mixtures, etc. and used in hot or cold water. If the stomach is very sensitive to a particular powdered agent, begin with 1/8 teaspoon doses of the preparation every fifteen minutes and increase the amount until the full dosage is reached. Aromatic powders contain volatile oils and should be prepared only in small quantities, and these should be kept in tightly-sealed glass vessels to maintain potency.

Dosage: Varies according to the type of powder used, the condition of the patient, etc. and must be specified for each case.

Preserve

This is a preparation wherein the herb (usually fruit) is cooked with sugar (use dehydrated cane juice) to preserve its shape and value. Steep or boil the fresh herb first in water, then afterwards in a syrup. Take out and dry so that the sugar may candy upon it. Often pectin is used to accentuate the action of the herb and to hold the medicinal aid intact.

Dosage: See "conserve."

Sinapism

This is a counter-irritant poultice made with vinegar and a stimulant-type herb. The common sinapism is made with equal quantities of flaxseed meal (slippery elm powder or bread crumbs) and powdered mustard seed, mixed with sufficient vinegar. It can stimulate blood circulation into areas afflicted with a palsy or atrophy. It is also beneficial for deep-seated pains (such as sciatica), gout attacks of the head or stomach, or low fever (where the poultice is applied to the soles of the feet).

Spirit

This is an alcoholic or hydro-alcoholic preparation containing ordinary alcohol and a watery liquid that has been distilled from an alcoholic tincture or mash. It is a volatile prepared by distillation, whereas a tincture is prepared by infusing the volatile substance in alcohol. These are used as tonics, etc.

Dosage: A few drops on up, as specified.

Soft cast

This is an herbal preparation consisting of layers of medicinal aid coated or painted on body surface and wrapped with a protective covering. As a good example, for a case of phlebitis from varicosity, the soft cast is made in the following manner: paint an alcohol tincture of burdock (the other docks are also good here), on the area. Let the tincture dry and follow with another coat, continuing until a heavy shellac-type thickness has been applied. Next, very carefully and not too tightly, wrap this with white bandages in a spiral motion, covering the entire area with many layers of bandage, tying them with adhesive tape to hold the soft cast in place. The adhesive tape is attached to the skin and the cast itself to act as a tie. Then take an elastic-type bandage and cover the soft cast. This application is left on for a period of weeks, until all the brown tincture or coating is absorbed into the skin, the bandage becoming white and the skin clean.

Solid extract

This is a solid preparation obtained by dissolving the herbs with a suitable solvent, juice of a plant, etc. to a point that the potency in one part of the extract generally equals four to six times the medicinal value of one part of the crude herb. With this preparation, the fresh juice or strong infusion is evaporated to the consistency of honey, or is sometimes reduced to a solid state through distilling the alcoholic agent from a tincture. Ordinarily, however, this would be made by steeping the dry powder of a crude herb for long periods of time in hot water (or in alcohol or in any other suitable menstruum), then evaporating the water or alcohol until only the solid materials remain. This preparation is used for making concentrated and potent aids (such as ointments, pills, plasters, syrups, tablets), as in a cough syrup, whereby the extract of onion and honey is concentrated into a thick consistency, to which some nervine and antispasmodic herbs may be added. This makes a high potency remedy.

Dosage: Varies and must be specified.

Suppository

This is an easily fusible preparation of some convenient and soluble base, in the shape of a cone, cylinder, globular, oviform, or pencil, used to apply an herbal agent into the nostrils, rectum, urethra, or vagina. This may also be a preparation of nutrient ingredients where the patient is unable to take nourishment in the usual manner. Generally, slippery elm is one of the better bases (or cocoa butter or olive oil being hardened by freezing may be substituted). These solid formations (of various weights, sizes, and shapes) are introduced into the different body orifices where they soften or melt at body temperature. The rectal suppositories are tapered and weigh about two grams (this can vary, depending on the size of the individual, from a baby to a large adult); urethral suppositories are pencil-shaped, pointed at one end, seven centimeters in length, and weigh about two grams or fourteen centimeters in length and weigh four grams; and vaginal suppositories are globular or oviform (oval, egg-shaped) and weigh about five grams.

Syrup

A syrup is a thick, sticky liquid preparation made by dissolving sugar into distilled water, decoctions, infusions, juices, or other aqueous solution, and is used to suspend medicinal or flavoring agents for easy administration alone, or to combine with other preparations. For making a syrup with herbs, settle out the heavier matter and pour off the clear liquid; then add to that (for every pint of herbal liquid) one and three-fourths pounds of sugar, place into an appropriate vessel, heat until the sugar is melted (some skimming is needed in the process), cool, and store for future use. For a syrup with flowers (such as cowslip, damask roses, peach blossoms, red poppies, violets, etc.), three pounds of the flowers should be picked from their husks with the heels cut off, five pints of boiling water poured over them, let stand all night, pour off the clear liquid in the morning, and then make the syrup as previously indicated.

Another formula for making a simple syrup is to pour one pint of boiling water over two and one-half pounds of sugar, place on hot stove and stir until the liquid begins to boil, and then instantly remove; this makes one quart of simple syrup, to which medicinal aids, one ounce of fluid extract, to three ounces of the simple syrup may be added, adding two ounces of glycerine which has been mixed into two ounces of thick mucilage (such as gum Arabic) for tender stomachs.

Cordial: A weakened form of medicinal syrup, diluted to 1/4 its original potency.

Dosage: Varies according to size and age, one teaspoonful to one tablespoonful.

Tablet or Pellet

This is an herbal preparation wherein the solid extract of an herb is compressed into a very small compass, where an herb is dehydrated down to a point of very fine powdery consistence so that it naturally adheres upon compression in strong metal dies (compressed tablets); and fine powders are triturated with sugar or lactose moistened with a liquid (alcohol, glycerine, syrup, water, vinegar, etc.), and then pressed lightly into molds and dried (tablet triturates). The tablet differs from the pill in that the latter needs an additive to make the herbal agent adhesive, wherein the former does not necessarily. Tablets are superior to pills as they are more easily administered and because they dissolve in the stomach more rapidly.

Dosage: Administer as specified.

Tinctures

This is an herbal preparation that is technically a fluid extract, but the medicinal virtues are generally extracted into solution with grain alcohol or vinegar. These menstruums are preferred over water as certain medicine principles are not retrieved in water alone. Alcohol (usually vodka) or vinegar (unfiltered apple cider) also makes for a better preservative for long term storage of extracts. Alcohol or vinegar tinctures should be made as follows: take approximately four ounces ground dried herbs or eight ounces of finely chopped fresh herbs and place them in a glass bottle with at least 16 ounces of chosen menstruum (alcohol or vinegar). If the herb is not completely submerged under the menstruum, add more. This is tightly capped and each day for ten days to two weeks the bottle is shaken vigorously at least three times a day or more. Extract all liquids, squeezing the herb residue thoroughly, with a regular juice press, or wring out by hand through cloth, canvas, muslin, etc. Cloth is the least effective because it absorbs much of the liquid. After the liquid is extracted, place the tincture extract in dark or painted bottles, stopper thoroughly and store.

To keep tinctures over a long period of time, wax the stopper. When administering a tincture internally, you may evaporate the alcohol from the solution by putting it into hot water, or it can be taken as is. Alcohol is preferred where there are resinous or oily herb extracts, as glycerine will not dissolve or mix with these.

Dosage: Dilute at least one teaspoonful of tincture to each cup of water.

CONGENIAL COMBINATIONS OF HERBS

While many therapeutic actions of herbs can be combined to provide wonderful synergistic qualities, there are others that when combined, neutralize their benefits and even some that have deleterious effect. Use this list to guide you in combining herbs with differing therapeutic actions. Definitions for the therapeutic action is found in Chapter 17 "HERB ALTERNATIVES" on page 638

Absorbents: Used with *antispasmodics* to relieve pain. *Stimulants* such as cayenne assist in drawing toxins to the surface, and *counter-irritants* can assist to relieve pain.

Alteratives: Use in combination with *accentuators*, such as a *stimulant.* For instance, cayenne will speed the action of an alterative. By using ginger, as another example, the accentuating action occurs, combined with action in the genito-urinary area. Often the undesirable taste of an alterative can be covered with an *aromatic,* such as peppermint, which also acts as an alterative.

Analgesics: Use combined with *nervine* and *antispasmodic* herbs. At times *carminative* and *antibilious* herbs such as wild yam or celery seed are added to cut the accompanying gas that is often the source of pain. Where pain results from engorgement or over-activity, a liniment with wormwood oil (a *tonic),* can be used alone or with other pain-relieving agents. Internally ginger, a *stimulant,* is often used for pain.

Anaphrodisiacs: A straight vegetarian diet is the best cure. You can add *alteratives* to clean up the bloodstream as well.

Anodynes: These are congenial with *antispasmodic* and *nervine* herbs, often using cayenne (a *stimulant)* as an accentuator.

Antacids: stimulants, such as ginger and cayenne, carry and accentuate. Also *demulcent* herbs soothe and relieve pain in specific areas.

Anthelmintics: Laxatives are almost always used with anthelmintics. *Nervines* are often added to relax a certain area made tense by worms.

Antiarthritics: Because of nervous debility in the affected areas, use these and *antilithics* to break up calcification, and *alteratives* to purify the bloodstream. Also use *nervines* and *antispasmodics* to relieve the excruciating pain of this condition. *Stimulants,* specifically cayenne, accentuate or speed the action.

Antiemetics: Here we must relieve the vomiting, but also settle the nerves. *Antispasmodics* will ease the area and *nervines* will settle the nerves, as sometimes vomiting results from a nervous condition alone. A *demulcent* will soothe the stomach area, and *hepatic* herbs such as barberry will ease the liver; it depends on the source of the nausea. A cleansing *laxative* enema is always used to clean out the bowel, which greatly reduces the chance for nausea.

Antihidrotics: These are agents that stop the secretion of sweat (deodorants). Never use the pharmaceutical medications which are high in aluminum and can cause sterility and related malfunctions. You can use a congenial *diaphoretic* such as burdock seed to cleanse the sebaceous and sweat glands. Avoid commercial soaps which clog the glands and pores and force toxic waste into the tissue. Excessive perspiration is usually caused by overeating and by high blood pressure, so a *stimulant* is beneficial in a long-term program to correct the condition. The bowel must be kept clean, which can be done with lower bowel *tonics.*

Antihydropics: These are agents that relieve generalized edema or dropsy. Never use in large amounts. Use a small amount combined with the *diuretic* herbs that are specified for the urinary-genital tract to eliminate excess water from the system. *Nervines* are also used when dropsy results from hyper-contracted nerve endings in the urethral tract that need relaxation.

Antilithics: To avoid the possibility of ever having stones, stay with soft water. Hard water as low as 8 grains is gravel-forming. Also avoid eggs, salt and milk—especially milk, which acts as a stone former. Be sure to use *demulcents* and *emollients* when cutting stone adhesions loose or breaking them up from a stony mass, for passing them through the urethral or gall ducts is very painful. Olive and natural *oils* are excellent to ease the passing, but never use mineral oil. *Nervines* relax tension in the tract itself, wherein the tubes expand and the stones are more easily discharged.

Antiperiodics: stimulants accentuate and speed the therapeutic action, *nervines* relax, and *alteratives* help cleanse the particular area.

Antiphlogistics (counteracts inflammation): Use bayberry, a powerful *astringent,* and cayenne, a *counter-irritant,* to reduce the swelling. A *nervine* and an *antispasmodic* can be added.

Antipyretics: Stimulants are used to increase circulation as rapidly as possible and carry off the poisons. *Diuretic* and *diaphoretic* herbs such as raspberry leaf, peppermint and elder flower) combine well. *tonics* rebuild the entire body.

Antirheumatics: See *anti-arthritics.*

Antiscorbutics: Stimulants are used as carriers and accentuators to speed the absorption of vitamins C and D. Also in such an illness, the nerves are often worn down, which requires a *nervine tonic* to help assimilate the food.

Antiseptics: Stimulants speed the healing. Also *antispasmodic* tincture relieves the intense pain which accompanies conditions requiring antiseptics.

Antispasmodics: A *stimulant* accentuates and speeds this along.

Antisyphilitics: Alteratives work well with these to cleanse the blood and organs, and *stimulants* enhance and speed the therapy. *Diuretics* and herbs which specifically work in the genito-urinary tract are also used.

Antivenomous: Antispasmodics and *stimulants* combine here; the *antispasmodic* serves as an anti-tetanus preventative and the *stimulant* speeds the action.

Antimycotics: Use with *antispasmodics, nervines, antivenomous,* or any type to facilitate a cleansing action. *Alteratives* also work here.

Aperients: Use a mild *stimulant* and a *nervine* to assist.

Aphrodisiacs: Use with *alteratives* and *stimulants* to cleanse the body. When the body is healthy, this takes care of itself.

Aromatics: These work well with almost every other class, not altering their medicinal values, but working to make other herbs taste more pleasant.

Bitters: Most bitters are *alteratives* that cleanse and heal the stomach, lymphatics, etc. *Aromatics* are usually added to improve the taste, with *stimulants* added to facilitate the action.

Blisters: Some blisters are formed from too much friction, and others are formed for healing. Cayenne blisters, formed when not enough oil is used before applying, are painless. Blisters bring out toxins from the body. After using a blister, use an *antispasmodic* to ease pain, and a *cell proliferant* such as comfrey or elecampane to speed healing. *Nervines* and *stimulants* will also work with blisters.

Calefacients: Antispasmodics are compatible if there is pain in the area; *stimulants* assist in the rapid flow of blood to the area, and sometimes an herb such as mullein disperses the poisons from a particular area.

Cardiac stimulants and depressants: Use combined with *cleansing* herbs, but particularly those which would *tone* the heart such as hawthorn berry, cayenne, wheat germ oil, etc. *Nutritional* and *alterative* herbs will help heal the heart. At times a *nervine* will work for pain, but an *antispasmodic* can work more quickly to cut the pain.

Carminatives: You can speed the action with a *stimulant*, and *antispasmodics* combine well to help with the pain.

Cathartics: Always use a guiding factor, such as ginger, to carry into the abdominal area. *Stimulants* are used to accelerate the action, *nervines* condition the peristaltic muscles, and *antispasmodics* will alleviate any pain. *Carminatives* such as wild yam or celery seed will cut the gas and always add a *demulcent* or *emollient* to soothe the area, as cathartics may be sharp in action.

Caustics: When caustic materials get into the system, remove them quickly from the stomach with *emetics.* Then *demulcents, emollients, tonics,* etc. soothe and heal, including such items as honey, wheat germ oil, olive oil, Irish moss, comfrey, etc. On an external surface, honey is the number one healing agent, followed by wheat germ oil, comfrey, Aloe vera, etc. With this, a *neutralizer* is used as quickly as possible.

Cell proliferants: Work well with *stimulants* to accentuate and with other *nutritional* herbs. Nearly all cell-proliferants, such as comfrey, elecampane, etc. are *nutritional* herbs. Add *nutritives* such as Irish moss or slippery elm.

Cholagogues: Being similar to *cathartics,* as both work on the liver. Usually a *carminative* is added to relieve gas, *nervines* for pain, *stimulants,* and because most of them are *bitters,* add *aromatics. Antispasmodics* are also added to relieve pain.

Condiments: Compatible with most *nutritional* herbs, also beneficial itself, such as black pepper in case of hemorrhaging, bleeding, or heart trouble, a substitute for cayenne.

Convulsants: Used in emergencies, and it is a matter of getting them down as fast as possible. Combine with *antispasmodics, nervines, stimulants;* and often it is beneficial to add a *demulcent* or *emollient* to give ease.

Correctives: The *demulcents* or *emollients* combine well here, and mild *stimulants* and *nervines* are often a great help.

Cosmetics: One of the greatest aids that can be added to cosmetics is *colloidal sulphur,* obtained from a live sulphur spring, not from commercial flours of sulphur obtained pharmaceutically. *Stimulants* work well with cosmetics to give new life and texture to the skin. Generally, *tonics* such as burdock seed, sunflower seeds, etc. feed the sebaceous and sudorific glands. When the whole body is clean and regenerated, it glows with radiant health, which shows up in the skin as well. The woman with a beautiful, healthy body needs no cosmetics, because she is already beautiful, with naturally-colored lips, rosy cheeks, and silky skin. It is beauty from the inside, not the outside.

Counter-irritants: In nearly every case, *antispasmodics* and *stimulants* speed up the therapeutic process. *Demulcents* will also give ease to the area. Do not mix these with herbs that work specifically on the lymphatics, because counter-irritants draw to the surface of the skin.

Demulcents: Compatible with nearly all herbs.

Deobstruents: Combine with *nervine* or *antispasmodic* herbs, and often a *demulcent* is added to give ease, because some damage is often done to the bowel. Also a *cell proliferant* such as marshmallow or comfrey rebuilds or restores the area.

Deodorants: Similar to cosmetics, in that a clean body doesn't smell repugnant. Heavy meat eaters smell the worst, so a *vegetarian diet* is most important. When the body is clean, eating onions and garlic will not be objectionable to other people. Until then, parsley is a wonderful herb for deodorizing. Some restaurants ask their waitresses to eat parsley before serving. The sweet, clean smell of a vegetarian is much more pleasant than the stench of a person full of uremic acid and toxins from low-vibrating foods.

Depressomotors: These work best by themselves, although at times they need a *stimulant.* This class consists of *sedative* type *nervines,* not the highly active types.

Detergents: These herbs cleanse wounds, ulcers and so forth. Use with *stimulants* and *antispasmodics.* Afterwards, you may need a soothing or *emollient* herb.

Diaphoretics: *Stimulants* such as ginger, mustard or cayenne, must always be added to accentuate the sweating and water treatment. Always use moist heat, plenty of liquids or moisture in teas, in the cold sheet, and whatever therapeutic process you use. *Nervines* relax the tissues, open the pores, and assist the action. Diaphoretics blend with most herbs.

Digestants: Combine these herbs with *stomachics, stimulants,* and *nervines.* They mix well with other herbs too. Most importantly, see that the digestive juices work properly, beginning by chewing thoroughly to mix the saliva with all liquids and solids. One of the big causes of malnutrition and deficiency is due to poor digestion, causing poor assimilation, resulting in nutritional anemia.

Diluents: The *stimulants, alteratives, diaphoretics,* and *diuretics* are all *diluents.* Do not use too much liquid during a meal, because this dilutes the digestive fluids and the glandular fluids.

Disinfectants: These work well with *stimulants* and *nervines. Antispasmodics* are very important combined here. When disinfectants are used internally, you may need to add *demulcents* and *emollients* when the area is severely decayed.

Diuretics: A directive agents such as ginger carries the herbs into the kidney-urethral area. Use *stimulants* to speed up the action, and *nervine tonics* to relax the tube ends to open up the valves for an easier flow of fluids and to tone up the area.

Drastics: Always follow with a *demulcent* and a *nervine* to ease the harshness of the purging.

Emetics: These are mostly used alone, except with a light *stimulant* such as peppermint tea to allay pain due to muscular wrenching.

Emmenagogues: These combine readily with *stimulants, nervines, demulcents* and *emollients.* Emmenagogues depend on the *stimulant* ginger as a carrier. Sometimes gas is generated in this condition, for which a *carminative* is used.

Emollients: Combine well with almost all herb, very friendly and versatile with most herbs and combinations.

Errhines: With bayberry, an *astringent,* or whatever herb is selected to use in the nose, cayenne, a *stimulant,* may be added if the individual is not too sensitive; *nervine* powder can be added to increase nasal secretion. If the *nervine* is used in ointment form, use it with Vaseline to hold it in suspension so it will not be absorbed into the skin too fast and burn; *demulcents* may be added in certain ointments.

Evacuants: See *cathartics.*

Excitomotors: Herbal *oils* are used in combination, such as wormwood oil, oil of cloves, oil of sassafras. Also *antispasmodics, nervines* and *stimulants* may be used.

Expectorants: Combine with *demulcents, emollients, stimulants, antispasmodics,* and *nutritives.*

Febrifuges: These are compatible with *stimulants,* with *antispasmodics,* and with most *diaphoretics.*

Galactogogues: Work best alone.

Hemostatics: Combine well with *stimulants* and *antispasmodics,* but do not combine with any herb that with expand the pore structure, such as *diaphoretics.*

Hepatics: Work well with *stimulants,* with *antispasmodics,* and with *carminatives.* Often *aromatics* are added to cover some of the bitterness.

Hydrogogues: Must be mixed with *carminatives,* in many cases, to keep flatulence down. Also *antispasmodics* and *nervines* work well here.

Hypnotics: Combine readily with most *nervines*, with *stimulants,* and with *antispasmodics.*

Laxatives: Combine with *emollients, demulcents, stimulants, nervines, antispasmodics, carminatives,* and often *aromatics* are added.

Local Anesthetics: Combine with *stimulants* and *antispasmodics.*

Mucilages: These combine with *nutritional* herbs, *demulcents,* and most herbs, as *mucilages* act as carriers.

Mydriatics: Here *stimulants* are frequently added to accentuate and at times *antispasmodics* and *nervines* assist.

Narcotics: Similar to *mydriatics.*

Nauseants: A *stimulant* controls the contraction of the abdominal muscle and prevents soreness.

Nephritics: There are so many different herbs that have partial diuretic tendencies which are compatible with each other, but in nearly all cases a *stimulant* such as ginger or cayenne is used, the ginger for a carrier and the cayenne as an accentuator.

Nervines: Combine with *antispasmodics, stimulants,* and at times with *natural opiates.*

Nutritives: All herbs are partially nutritive, as they all contain certain ingredients that feed specific areas of the body, although many of them are disagreeable. With specifically nutritive herbs, add *demulcents* and *emollients* to soothe the digestive area and sometimes a *stimulant* is added to speed the absorption.

Ophthalmics: Often require *nervines* because the pain in the eyes is so severe, *antispasmodics,* an accentuator such as a *stimulant,* and in many cases a *demulcent.*

Parturients: Here *nervines* combine well, *antispasmodics, stimulants,* and nearly always such an herb as raspberry leaf to relax the pelvic area.

Pectorals: Use with *antispasmodics, nervines, demulcents, emollients,* and add *aromatics* if the taste is disagreeable.

Peristaltics: Use *stimulants* and *antispasmodics,* and add *carminatives* to cut down the gas. *Emollients* and *demulcents* are added to soothe raw areas where there may be ulcers, abrasions, etc.

Protectives: Work compatibly with most *stimulants, nervines, antispasmodics, demulcents,* and *emollients.*

Pungents: Generally combine with soothing herbs to carry, such as *emollients, demulcents,* in ointments or liniments.

Purgatives: These need *antispasmodics* and *emollients* and *demulcents. Nervines* mix well and *carminatives* will cut the flatulence.

Refrigerants: Among the *nutritives,* celery juice is one of the best to combine with this class.

Revulsants: Combine with *stimulants* and *antispasmodics.*

Rubefacients: Stimulants combine well here.

Sedatives: Combine certain *stimulants* that work on the capillary ends instead of the heart area with the sedative type that soothes.

Sialogogues: Ginger and a few of the other *stimulants* work well with sialogogues to excite the salivary glands, as do many seasoning herbs.

Soporifics: Always combine well with *nervines.*

Specifics: With some of the harsher specifics, *emollients* and *demulcents* are used; with others, *stimulants* serve as accentuators. In some cases, *aromatics* are added, and some combine with *carminatives* to cut gas.

Stimulants: Combine with most herbs.

Stomachics: *Demulcents* and *emollients* are often needed for soothing. Also *nutrients, mucilage,* and in most cases *stimulants* are added. If there is severe pain, *nervines* and *antispasmodics* can be mixed with them.

Styptics: *Stimulants* can be used to speed the action.

Sudorifics: *Stimulants* are nearly always combined to accentuate and speed. Usually copious quantities of liquid are taken.

Teniacides: After killing the tapeworms, a quick purge with a *purgative* cleans them out.

Tonics: Use *demulcents* and *emollients* to soothe, and often *mucilage* herbs combine with *stimulants, antispasmodics,* and *carminatives* to cut gas. These combine well with most herbs, and usually require *aromatics* to make them more pleasant.

Vulneraries: *Stimulants* such as cayenne and black pepper can be used alone as vulneraries. When there is pain, add *antispasmodics* and *nervines* with it. For fresh wounds, *oils* and *mucilage* herbs keep the vulneraries fresh for faster healing. A favorite here is slippery elm.

ABOUT ADMINISTERING HERBS

As a general rule, the warm infusion preparation of a medicinal aid will manifest the quickest and most effective results. The nearer the herbal preparations approach the liquid form, the quicker they will assimilate and take effect and the smaller will be the doses required.

ANAL OR RECTAL

Herbal preparations administered via the anus: bolus, compound, combination, concentrate, decoction, enema, infusion, injection, mixture, oil, suppository or wash. The absorption by this method generally is twice as slow as for the aids administered orally and entering via stomach.

Colonics

A general and accepted method for colonics is the use of a mechanical device to pump the enema material in and out of the body. This is a therapeutic crutch which can eventually weaken the system more than it will give aid; its proper use is only in providing temporary relief as in telescoping of the bowels. Do not depend on this procedure, as it becomes habit-forming. The colonic does not get deep into the pockets or ballooned areas of the intestine. It merely washes out matter obstructing the middle of the intestine channel.

Enemas

Enemas should be used in emergencies, and not as a crutch. Remember that a warm-water enema relaxes the anus and consequently the liquid is retained for only a very short period (with no time to soak through the encrusted fecal matter). With a cold enema, the anus contracts and the rectal area becomes tight, such that the water will stay in the body longer, thereby giving the bowel a chance to soak through and break loose the old toxic fecal matter that must be removed from the system if permanent relief and healing is to take place. The enema is mainly a cleansing procedure and generally is not used medicinally. The low enema is used where there is trouble in the sigmoid and the rectal area itself. Where the problems are higher in the colon, a long catheter is called for to better reach and clean (in every case, a long hose made of rubberized material is best). In using enemas, be very careful not to use caustic or harsh, injurious ingredients in the anus.

Injection

An injection is actually a minimal enema, generally given with a small syringe and the liquid is retained in the bowel for a period of time without immediate evacuation. The reason the injection is used in a small amount instead of having a full bowel of water (or tea, or other liquid) is to avoid having it discharged too quickly. Injections are given both for medicinal and nutritional reasons. For example, the injection given during convulsions (1 cup to 1 pint maximum is what is generally used, according to age, condition, and size) using a tea made from such herbs as catnip, scullcap, lobelia, or hops will give very good and fast results. When the injection is being used for nutritional reasons, such herbs as slippery elm, marshmallow, or sea vegetation (such as Irish moss, Iceland moss, sea-wrack), etc. are used. One can get better effect and results by using the injection or the enema in a knee-chest position (laying on back); and by using cool enema solution.

Ointments

These are very easily used in the anus area where a person has piles or hemorrhoids. To apply ointments into the anal area, administer them by finger, or put them onto a suppository-type piece of cotton and insert (it can also be put onto a Tampax and left in, although this can be uncomfortable).

Sitz baths

There are a number of differing opinions on sitz baths. The common sitz bath is merely sitting in a tub, wherein just the buttocks, the lower back into the sacroiliac and the upper thighs are immersed and the feet are in another tub. In this way, the buttocks would be in cold water and the feet should be in hot water; or vice versa. The most important part of the sitz bath, of course, is soaking the anal area in herbal aids to give relief. This is used for itching, piles, hemorrhoids, acid burning from urine and rectal discharges, or toxic conditions wherein the flesh is raw.

Suppositories

Again, these are crutches which we do not want to depend on, because, with a cathartic-type suppository, one will be forced to use it after a period of time and never get a bowel movement started unaided. When a person is not able to take food orally (from being unconscious or otherwise afflicted), food may be put into the rectum. People can be kept alive with this type of assistance for considerable periods of time. Suppositories are used when one has hemorrhoids, painful ulceration, itching, etc.

Tinctures

These are often used in the anus to save lives, because after a person has gone into spasms or convulsions, nothing can be put into the body through the mouth. Never use a tincture at full strength, always dilute. Be very careful, for, although the tincture injection will not do any critical damage, it may cause the inconvenience of a loose stool. To administer an average strength tincture in the rectum, the dilution should be 1 teaspoonful to each cup of water or tea combination.

NASAL

Herbal preparations administered via the nasal passage: bolus (small), decoction, infusion, oil, ointment, powder, tincture.

Camel hair brush

A small camel hair brush is often used to paint the inside of the nose with an ointment (the nose ointment of essential oils of peppermint and spearmint mixed in Vaseline found on page 263 is used this way) or a tincture.

Inhalants or Vapors

Often when one has lung congestion, along with the vapor or steam bath, a good inhalant will be very beneficial in cutting loose the mucus from the bronchial-lung areas. The inhalant can be steam from apple cider vinegar or vapors from oils (such as eucalyptus, peppermint, spearmint, etc.). These will help heal and clear congested areas. There are electric vapor dispensers, but inhalants may also be administered simply with a pan of water (with the oil poured on the surface of the water) and a towel placed over the head, wherein the oils are carried with the water vapors, and the patient breaths over the vessel to inhale the effervescent fumes of the various essence used. Volatile herbal aids can be rapidly absorbed into the system through this procedure.

Insufflations or powder snuffing

This procedure uses the fine powders of various herbs (with bland or non-irritating bases such as bayberry and white oak) by snuffing directly into the nose or allowing another person to gently blow the powder into the nostril with a straw or, by means of a flexible straw, blowing it in one's own nostrils. This procedure can be combined with a nasal spray of herbal infusions.

Liquid snuffing

Often bayberry and other herbal teas are used as astringents and antiseptics to clear and purify the nasal passage, or to reduce the pulse rate in cases of adenoidal problems.

Massage

If only a small amount of nose ointment (see page 263) is to be applied, then the easiest way is to take a small quantity on the end of the little finger and massage it gently into the nose area, next closing off one nostril and inhaling and then repeating the process for the opposite side.

Sprays

Sprays are very easy to administer in an atomizer or nebulizer with the right type of ingredients; light, fixed (non-volatile) oil, a decoction, or an infusion will work very well. Powders are also used in nasal sprays (such as bayberry, golden seal, etc.).

ORAL

The most convenient way of administering herbs and herbal correctives is through the mouth and down the throat (the gastrointestinal route). Preparations used is this manner are in the form of balsam, concentrate, conserve, decoction, capsule, draft, electuary, elixir, emulsion, essence, fluid extract, gargle, infusion, julep, juice, mixture, oil, pill, powder, preserve, spirit, solid extract, syrup, tablet or tincture.

In oral administration, the herbal aids are absorbed through the walls of the blood vessels (that copiously permeate the mucous membrane of the intestinal tract), portal veins (carrying blood from the digestive organs and spleen to the liver), and lacteals (lymphatic vessels of the small intestines conveying chyle to the thoracic duct). Herbal aids that are gelatinous (Irish moss, slippery elm), gum resinous (asafetida, myrrh, pine, scammony), oleo resinous (copaiba), starchy, or fatty substances are passed into the duodenum, where they are acted upon by bile, intestinal and pancreatic juices. As a rule, herbal aids enter circulation much quicker when taken on an empty stomach, and the systemic receptivity is better at night than in the morning.

Electuaries

Electuaries are generally made up in individual pieces, small enough so that they can be swallowed with ease. They are not always chewed. However, some of these "sweets" (such as a children's laxative), are made with ground fruits and herbs in them and are quite tasty when chewed. The manner of administration would depend on the taste of the herbal compounds placed or concealed in them.

Gargle

One mouthful is generally sufficient for gargling, and the best effect may be obtained by injecting the solution into the throat area by syringe, gargling in the throat until a cleaner or more relaxed feeling is sensed in the area, then spitting out the solution. Thereafter, it is beneficial to take a tablespoonful or more of a demulcent-type aid after the gargle (such as bayberry or raspberry leaf tea). Small children who are not old enough to comprehend the procedure should never gargle, because they generally choke and the liquid invariably gets into the bronchi.

Juices

All juices should be sipped slowly, chewed almost like solid food, and swished through the mouth (long enough to insure that saliva is well-mixed with the juices in order to get the value, and to avoid discomfort or regurgitation) before swallowing. This procedure is most important to the digestive process since many juices are very rich and are not compatible with gastric juices unless sufficient saliva is present. Juices should not be gulped or drunk in large amounts, as this may result in irritation to the system. Some people who throw up after rapidly drinking rich juices are not properly mixing the juice with their saliva before swallowing.

Liquids

Liquids (extracts, decoctions, infusions, etc.) should not be so hot that they damage or scald the mucous membrane, yet should be taken as hot as possible. A warm liquid via the oral cavity is the fastest procedure of getting herbal medicinal aids into the body itself. As the tea or liquid enters the oral cavity (from the mouth into the intestinal tract), the blood stream immediately starts absorbing the medicinal value from the solution going into the area. In emergencies, it is always best to use a hot tea (with heart attack, put a teaspoon of cayenne in a cup of boiling water, and when it is cool enough to drink without burning the interior surfaces, administer promptly for immediate results). Teas or liquids that are cool are somewhat slow in absorption, but are excellent for a long-range corrective program.

Oils

Oils must not be overdone. There are certain types of oils that should never be used internally or externally (mineral oil will rob the body of its nutritive values by draining them off before they are assimilated). Vegetable oils of other types taken internally, however, are acceptable to the human body when taken from a few drops up to a tablespoonful at a time (depending on the condition being treated, patient vitality, etc.), and a tablespoon every hour of olive oil with lemon juice can be used to pass gall stones.

Ointments

This procedure is used less often internally, yet the black ointment (see page 354) or the cayenne ointment (see page 539) placed on the base of the tongue or on the teeth is very effective in healing a sore throat; or placed on the tongue or lip-cheek area, it is good for canker sores, cuts in the mouth and various types of mouth diseases (such as thrush or mycotic stomatitis); and alleviating throat irritations, the power in the herbal salve will travel a long way, even into the bronchial and lungs.

Never use any type of "external only" ointment in the mouth that has been mixed with rubbing alcohol or with caustics (irritating, destructive, and poisonous drugs). It is best for the herbalist to supervise and prepare his own ointments, and then he will eliminate the difficulties and risks with commercial practices and procedures of additive poisons, preservatives, etc. (even some under "organic" labels), in multitudinous, attractively-named concoctions and made so often of highly questionable and destructive ingredients. Many of these have not been tried and tested, and later (after usage by the public) have proven to be very damaging to the body. The deadly, inorganic preparations used commercially should never be used orally at any time, for any reason.

SKIN

Herbal aids may be applied externally by rubbing or massaging them directly on the skin (epidermic or epidermatic). Passage of the medicine (liniment, oil, ointment, etc.) is facilitated through and between the epidermal cells with the best results achieved when an herbal application is applying with friction where the skin is the thinnest (abdomen, axillae or armpits, groins, and insides of thighs). Aqueous solutions pass slowly into the tissue (this can be accelerated with mullein on the lymphatic and cayenne elsewhere), and alcohol causes an outward osmotic flow.

The subcutaneous injection (hypodermic or hypodermatic) and blistering (endermic or endermatic) procedures are not used by herbalists, as these are unnatural to normal body functions. Herbal correctives are administered in the form of: balsam, cataplasm, cerate, collyria, compound, combination, concentrate, decoction, emulsion, fluid extract, fomentation, infusion, juice, ketone, liniment, mixture, oil, ointment, plaster, poultice, powder, sinapism, solid extract, soft casts, syrup, tincture, or wash.

If two-thirds of the skin is clogged, a person will die because there is not enough oxygen entering through the nose and lungs to meet the full body requirement, so the skin must be kept clean and clear at all times. The use of many commercial soaps, dusting powders, skin lotions, etc. will obstruct and close the pores, and the skin vitality is too important to allow careless deterioration. Rather than using caustic types of commercial soaps and cleansing agents, just plain water or a biodegradable agent should be used to keep the skin fresh. With occupational problems of dust, dirt, grime, oil, etc. that get on the skin, a covering or glove will partially protect the skin from inorganic poisons and filth. One of the most important responsibilities in life is to maintain a clean body, for "cleanliness is next to godliness!"

There are many therapeutic procedures for treating the human body through the skin. In applying herbal aids to the skin, always be careful that the delicate tissue is not damaged with improper herbs and combinations. Often if a liniment, ointment, plaster, etc. that is too strong is used (for instance, with a mustard plaster), then blistering will occur. Also be very careful with the types of applications that are used after a hot sweating bath, so that the exposed pores are not damaged or burned.

Bathing

The best procedure in either retaining or restoring skin vitality is to take a good hot bath, then a cold one to close the pores. "What's one man's meat is another man's poison," as far as how much bathing a person should do. There are some who feel that to wash their hair once a week, or to take a bath on Saturday night, is adequate. There are many like me, however, who do not feel the day has started off right without the early morning bath and meditation. As far as the hair is concerned, a woman with long tresses will have a more difficult time washing hair every day as a man with short hair does, but I personally wash my hair every day, and it always feels good and clean, and lends to clear thinking. The water acts as a good tonic to the skin, because it goes in, flushes and cleanses the skin, and in the process, much of this water will go right on into the blood stream.

It is relaxing to have the right temperature of water, which would be tepid to slightly warmer, but water that is too hot is not relaxing. The heat expands the body tissue and brings toxic poisons to the surface, and after that is discharged and eliminated, then the cold water will contract the tissue, close the pores and cause the skin to be sealed again where it will not allow a cold, exposure, flu or pneumonia to set in. Our advice (where one is just starting to take cold baths) is to sponge the body with a cold wash cloth for a few days after bathing, then go into a quick, cold shower, and eventually a longer one; then, if you want to really enjoy the bath properly, try lying in a cold tub of water after the hot bath. This will be very beneficial to the body if done gradually, but if done too soon, it may cause a shock to the heart.

Clothing

The skin being so very important and sensitive, it pays to stop a moment to think seriously of how to cover the skin when we do not desire to leave it over-exposed to the sun. True, the more we can let the sun rays bathe on the skin, the better off we are, but the clothing materials should be of the highest vibration possible. Silk is one of the greatest and best materials that can be used, as it is a live substance, spun from the body of the silk worm using organic vegetation. The next in preference would be materials from animals (sheep wool, camel hair, etc.), as these are still of a higher vibrating nature and can be used without killing the animal, and yet give mankind the advantage of its use. Next, and lower in vibrancy, come the higher vegetable types (including linen such as Christ was wrapped in), cotton, hemp, nettles, etc.

Then we get to man-made or chemical synthetics, which have a very sluggish and low vibration and are very damaging to the body. The lower vibrational materials should be avoided as much as possible—as the nylon and many other man-made synthetics will not allow the skin to breathe properly and in addition are highly combustible and a definite fire hazard to the skin. Much unaccounted for sickness can be attributed to the use of nylon (undergarments, hose, etc.) and other synthetic clothing. These do damage to the physical system, and this results in a waning and deterioration of the health. The Law of Moses advises against mixing or blending different fibers together; pure, organic clothing is best. It is absolutely imperative for air to circulate between the skin and clothing, so a free and loose-fitting, organic-type clothing is superior. Many people even become covered with itches and rashes and are poisoned from wearing "economical" and "long-wearing" man-made cloth.

Collyria

The method of administering the eye wash or eye lotion is generally with an eye cup, filled and placed up to the eye, then holding the head back so that the eye is immersed, open the eye and exercise in the liquid. If the eye cup is unavailable, use an eyedropper to administer the dosage, or use an eyelid compress (a regular tea bag works great). When using a powerful healer such as cayenne, the administration should last only a few seconds at first and gradually increase the time of each successive treatment.

Fomentation

Soak a natural fiber cloth or Turkish towel in an herbal compound (fresh or dried herbs, emulsions, essences, fluid extracts, spirits, tinctures) that has been prepared in a decoction or infusion. Apply the cloth to the skin and allow the solution to be taken in by the body. Heat will facilitate this process and generally we prepare a fomentation as warm as can be comfortably tolerated by the individual. Fomentations are also prepared using juices such as carrot, onion, garlic, etc. Castor, olive and other oils may also be used in a fomentation. Here many types of oils are used hot: oil of wormwood, sassafras and peppermint make a very good combination for rheumatism, arthritis, sore joints, muscular spasms, and muscular soreness from exercise you are not accustomed to, and a fomentation with ointment is used occasionally in specific cases.

The effectiveness of the fomentation can be speeded by using a hot water bottle during the warm application. Alternating this with a cold application in many cases is very beneficial, following again with a hot one. The method to be used will depend on the type of problem, but specifically in sprains and sore muscles, the alternate hot-and-cold applications are very excellent. Generally, fomentations are covered with oiled silk, plastic, or wax paper, and a hot water bottle placed over this to keep the application warm, changing periodically when the potency and value of the tea itself has been absorbed out of the toweling. For a glandular swelling, the preferred procedure is a hot fomentation—always with moist heat.

In case a hot water bottle is unavailable, then wrap a hot, wet Turkish towel around heated bricks or rocks, or as a last resort, use an electric heating pad (be sure here that there is no danger of an electrical short). Be sure there is moisture between the body and the dry heat and the electric pad is rated for moist applications. Along with the fomentation, an internal tea used in combination with the external aid will greatly facilitate the healing process.

Foot baths

Put the feet into hot apple cider vinegar and let them soak; if faster action is desired, then place the sole of one foot on garlic or in a strong decoction of garlic and place the other foot in hot apple cider vinegar. This will start a circulating movement within the body system that will afford quick relief. The use of apple cider vinegar and honey internally (a teaspoonful, three times a day) will help facilitate and speed the process of toxic elimination.

Herbal baths

In the bath water (hydrotherapy) we oft times use decoctions, infusions, tinctures, dry powders, etc., using herbs such as ginger, cayenne, mustard, and others. We also use foot baths and/or hand baths in heated apple cider vinegar for arthritis and rheumatism.

Liniments

Massaging oils, tinctures, and teas on the skin are very beneficial. This may be done anywhere on the external tissue, but where rapid absorption is critical, an accentuating aid must be added. Massage the preparation in thoroughly and see that very little medicinal agent is left on the skin surface but rubbed well into the skin and flesh itself. Liniments are excellent for sore muscles and sprains, and often lobelia is used here in combination with other herbal preparations, to ease the pain (see "Fomentation").

Lotions

With the skin it is so important to keep those pores clean (as we stated before), for the body can be choked to death when the skin becomes unclean. The body must not be painted with nonporous substances that will smother the skin. Many of the sun lotions on the market today do just that; they do great damage by shutting off that source of oxygen supply to the system.

Oils

Medicinal oils can be used for healing the body externally, and for many internal problems as well. Only high grade vegetable oils (generally olive oil) are used as these are most readily absorbed through the skin and into the blood stream. These are very beneficial when used with knowledge and skill.

Ointments

There are many ointment combinations, and generally the healing ointments are used externally. We have had many cases of cancer, skin rashes, eruptions, etc. that have been healed using ointments. The ointments can be used for acid urine, all types of dermatitis, blood-poisoning, boils and carbuncles (bring the toxins to a head), diaper rash, felons, infections, in-grown hair, etc. Ointments are applied either by rubbing the preparation directly onto the skin, or the aid is smeared onto gauze and placed over the area.

Plasters

Never make plasters stronger than the individual can endure. For example, when making a mustard plaster, softening agents should be used (such as mixing the mustard with slippery elm, flax seed meal, whole wheat flour, or even egg whites) and olive oil should be thoroughly massaged into the skin prior to the plaster application to prevent blistering or burning the skin.

Poultices

The poultice action is similar to the fomentation, but where the fomentation ingredients are in the liquid form, the poultice uses herbal solids or often the entire herb itself is placed on the inflicted area. Before applying a poultice, one should first bathe the affected part thoroughly with herbal teas (such as mugwort, apple cider vinegar, or an antiseptic or astringent herb). The poultice is usually heated prior to application whereby, besides providing medicinal aid, it yields secondary value in maintaining warmth and moisture on the afflicted area over a period of time. Oft times in using poultices, we have to watch that only the proper and congenial herbs are used, because in cases where the pus should continue to flow, an astringent (or an aid that would stop the flow) should not be used. A hot poultice can be prepared with apple cider vinegar (which is good with nearly all herbs), and if no vinegar is available, then use hot water.

In an emergency (such as a bee sting or poisonous bite), simply chew up some plantain or comfrey leaves in the mouth (without swallowing the saliva), make into a soft mass, and apply pulp and juice immediately on the wound. Cover the injury with a plastic-type material when possible to retain the moisture, and repeat the application as often as necessary for a number of hours, until the herbal action has had time to draw the poison out. Be careful not to suck the value out of the plantain, of course, as the value is in both the pulp and the juice itself. The fastest method of bruising for stings, snake bites, rabid dogs, etc. (where the herb must be applied quickly), is to simply chew it and place it. There are several ways to bruise an herb without losing any medicinal value in the mouth such as crushing it with a rock, a hammer, a pestle, or even rubbing between the hands. Where only dried herbs are available, moisten them, and apply as quickly as possible.

The poultice can be changed quite frequently, if needed, or it can be left on longer and changed only once or twice a day until healing is assured. It is always best to cover any poultice application with a plastic material or some type of covering which will not allow the moisture to escape.

Soaps

Inorganic soaps are very damaging to the skin and obstruct the pores. A little dandruff scraped off the scalp, for example, and placed into distilled water (which is zero grain hardness) will often shake into a heavy foamy lather or suds, showing that the major part of dandruff is composed of soap that has not been washed out. There are very few rinses that can thoroughly cleanse the inorganic, commercial-type soaps out and these will often cause rashes and do considerable damage to the skin tissue and the body itself (through epidermal absorption). It is better to use a cleansing agent of a biodegradable type, such as yucca root soap, pine tar soap, castile soap, Dr. Shaklee's Basic-H, etc. all of which are made of soluble vegetable bases. If biodegradable soaps are unavailable, then lemon juice, vinegar, and wild sage are very effective. The commercial soaps give the appearance of beauty by cleaning and perfuming the surface, while the pores remain dirty still from toxic matter.

Steam baths

One of the most important procedures of water therapy (hydrotherapy) are the steam or sweat baths. These will bring the poisons out of the body wonderfully. There are various types of steam baths, and these are all very valuable, very invigorating and health giving. This therapeutic procedure is recommended for arthritis, asthma, bursitis, colds, flu, hay fever, neuritis, pneumonia, rheumatism, sinusitis, stiff joints, etc. Someday, I hope to see a steam cabinet in every home (not a chicken on every plate and a car in every garage). In sweat therapy, we also have the cold sheet treatment—a positive remedy for colds, flu, and pneumonia—which can be effectively used even in advanced and chronic cases.

Sun

Helio-therapy on the skin is very important, as the sun is the Great Doctor of all times. But this therapy must always be done with caution because the sun (though a healer) is like any fire, which can either provide gentle warmth or it can burn a city down. The sun will heal where medicinal aids, herbs and other procedures are slower. In many instances, it will bring skin cancer to the surface; and various other skin problems (such as acne, eczema, etc.) are beneficially aided by bathing in the sun. The internal use of tea or other herbal aids and often an herbal wash before the sunbathing are congenial and excellent. When there is moisture in the body, sunbathing is much more beneficial—for instance, burdock seed and burdock root may be used internally (which work on the lymphatic and oil glands of the body), while at the same time using sun therapy for the outside.

Indiscreet exposure can cause third-degree burns, shock, and death. The light-skinned individual must be most careful, but even a person with dark skin can get a very heavy burn. Helio-therapy is used on bright days, but we do advise against sunbathing at midday, between the period 11:00 to 1:00, when sun might be quite toxic to the user. A blonde person who has never done sunbathing before should never be out over one minute on the first day, adding a minute each day. This should be measured by stop watch or clock, and accuracy is important, because the feel of the sun is so luxurious that one will desire to stay in it just a little bit longer, and that can cause serious trouble. This may not sound like very much, but within thirty days a person can be sunning up to an hour total time! Brunettes can often start with two minutes front and two minutes back without any injury at all, and add four minutes a day. A person who has been sunbathing years before and has sunbathed regularly each season may start with a little more, five minutes front and five minutes back for the brunette, and two minutes front and two minutes back for the blonde. If done gradually and judiciously, this can give power to the body.

The propaganda in daily newspapers and national publications each year (although promoted often by people with doctoral degrees) stating that "the sun causes cancer" is as ridiculous as saying "the tonsil is poisoning the whole body." It is the putrid condition of the body that is poisoning the tonsil, or the skin! All the sun does is to ripen and bring the cancer that is already there to the surface, wherein the waste matter can slough off, so that the body may heal. This is why we must work inside the body with herbs, as well as outside the body with the sun, which will harmoniously speed the curative process and eliminate the problem so there is no recurrence.

Wash

When medicinal aid needs to be applied to an area (exterior surface) where bandages, a cast or a soft case (poultice) cannot be applied, a liquid herbal preparation (decoction, infusion, or tincture, etc.) can be applied as a wash for the area. In some cases, only one application is used, but sometimes the area is washed repeatedly. The liquid herbal preparation is applied over the afflicted area and left to dry between coats.

Phlebitis (which is a varicose condition in an advanced stage, wherein the pressure is intense and the pain is excruciating) is often corrected with just a wash of white oak bark decoction (or some other appropriate herb). Washes give immediate relief within minutes. A wash is similar to a "paint job" since a tincture of myrrh, pine, kino, etc. could be applied in layered coatings (twelve to fifteen or more) and each layer (like a coating of paint) would be allowed to dry before adding the next one. Often a juice extract (in the Old English called an "express") made by squeezing the medicinal liquids from mullein, plantain, or black walnut (excellent), etc. is washed on. Herbal washes are generally hot or very warm. Herbal aids are administered here in the forms of: compound, combination, concentrate, decoction, douche, infusion, mixture, ointment (thinned with olive oil), or tincture.

VAGINAL

Bolus

One of the valuable procedures in a healing program for women is the vaginal bolus. The bolus is a mass of herbs suspended in viscus oils (coconut oil or even olive oil hardened by freezing), cocoa butter, or just plain slippery elm powder (moistened, shaped and partially dried to give firmness) and shaped for insertion into the vagina. There are two types of bolus: one that dissolves at body temperature spreading nutritional herbs to feed the reproductive organs and the other type which acts more as a poultice. The poultice-type is made with healing herbs to draw out poisons and toxins and bring out cysts, tumors, and cancerous conditions even as far up as the abdominal area. The bolus has a widespread influence, affecting not only the vagina, but also other organs, such as the bowel and the urinary tract. This drawing-type bolus generally consists of a group of expectorant and drawing herbs.

Douche

This well known method is an internal cleansing and healing bath used in the vaginal area. Yellow dock tea is one of the most potent of all douches for strengthening, cleansing and purifying the female genital area; and it is a well-established fact that lemon juice or vinegar alone has far more strength than most commercial products, with none of the harmful effects of these inorganic compounds.

CHAPTER 15

THE CLEANSING PROGRAM

This cleansing program purifies the body so it can heal more easily. If you are overweight, this program will take you down to your normal weight; if you are underweight, it will bring you up to normal. The entire purpose of the program is to eliminate mucus from the body, which will simplify healing.

Dr. Christopher always said that there are no incurable diseases, but only people who think they are incurable. He offered this cleansing program as an essential part of healing virtually any infirmity.

The cleansing program will:

- Clean the mucus out of the body; mucus is the source of polyps, tumors, cysts, etc. and also the cause of allergies, disease, pain, and death.

- Give you foods that are alive, nutritious and healthful, foods which can rebuild your body.

- Provide you with herbal formulas and corrective aids to facilitate healing and regeneration of the body.

- Release static electricity from the body to eliminate frustrations and confusions.

THE THREE DAY JUICE CLEANSE

Detoxication:
To begin, you will have three days detoxication (body purification) therapy, and then proceed with the diet outlined hereafter. This three-day cleanse is taken in part from Dr. N. W. Walker's book, *Raw Vegetable Juices,* "To Detoxicate," Phoenix, AZ: Norwalk Press, Publishers, P.O. Box 13206.

Supreme cleanliness is the first step towards a healthy body. Any toxins within us will retard our progress towards recovery. The natural eliminative channels are the lungs, the pores of the skin, the kidneys, and the bowels. When we perspire, our sweat glands throw off toxins which would be toxic to us if retained. The kidneys excrete the end products of food and body metabolism from the liver. The bowels eliminate not only the food waste but also matter known as body waste, in the form of used-up cells and tissues, the result of our physical and mental activities, which if retained can cause protein putrefaction, resulting in toxemia or acidosis.

Retaining such body waste is much more damaging to our health than is generally suspected, and when we begin to cleanse it, we experience perceptible progress. One efficient method to eliminate it quickly, particularly for adults, is the following procedure:

First thing in the morning upon arising, drink 16 ounces or more of prune juice. The purpose of this is not primarily to empty the bowels, which it will do anyway, but rather to draw into the intestines from every part of the body such toxic matter as may be there, and eliminate it through the bowels.

Take one or two tablespoons of olive oil three times a day, to aid in lubricating bile and liver ducts.

To prevent dehydration, and to alkalinize the body as it cleanses, drink at least two quarts of fruit juices, preferably freshly made. You might choose apple, carrot, grape, citrus, tomato, etc. but for the one chosen, use it exclusively for the three days, and *chew* each mouthful thoroughly.

CARROT JUICE
Use this without diluting as directed below.

CITRUS JUICE
If you live where citrus is grown, make a combination. Use four to six grapefruit, two to three lemons, and enough oranges to make two quarts. Dilute with two quarts of water, making one gallon. Proceed as below.

GRAPE JUICE
Use unsweetened juice without additives or preservatives. Bottled juice is better

than frozen, which often contains sugar and usually contains additives not listed on the label. The best juice would be homemade, unsweetened, but you can buy organic grape juice at the health food store which is excellent. People have had good results using grape juice from the grocery, such as Welch's, Church, Tea Garden, Queen Isabell—just check the label to be sure it has no additives. Dilute half and half with water.

APPLE JUICE
Use freshly pressed apple juice if available, from unsprayed, organic apples if possible. Making your own apple juice is ideal. You can also use bottled apple juice, if it contains no preservatives or chemicals of any kind. Do not use frozen juice, which can contain preservatives without being labelled.

Drink one 8-ounce glassful, beginning half an hour after having taken the prune juice, being sure to swish or "chew" each mouthful thoroughly. This is very important, so that the juices can mix with the saliva for easy digestion. If you are hypoglycemic, "chewing" the juice will prevent an unpleasant sugar reaction. You can drink a glass of plain water, preferably distilled, a half hour after that. Follow this with a glass of juice every thirty minutes or so, alternating with water every half hour, throughout the day. You can follow this outline, but take more or less as your case requires; it is a rule of thumb and not a specific rule. However, many people have followed it this way, with excellent results.

Do not eat anything all day, although if very hungry towards evening, take an apple if you are using apple juice, an orange with citrus, grapes with grape, carrot or celery with carrot juice, etc. Chew it thoroughly.

As you detoxify, you may likely experience constipation. If you do, use more prune juice, or take some of our lower bowel formula, two or more capsules three times a day.

Continue this program for three consecutive days. Approximately three gallons of toxic lymph will have been eliminated from the body and will have been replaced by three gallons of alkaline juices. As your system becomes more alkaline, you will experience healing of your particular complaints.

On the fourth and subsequent days, begin taking vegetable juices and vegetables and fruit, preferably all raw. For breakfast, for example, eat three or four fruits in season, sliced, chopped or grated, with some honey for sweetening and one or two tablespoonfuls of finely grated unsalted almonds sprinkled over them. Also drink one or two glasses of fresh fruit or vegetable juices. For lunch, eat more fruit and one pint of fresh raw vegetable juices, thirty minutes before or after eating the fruit. For dinner add any of the salads given hereafter, or as in *The Mild Food Cookbook* by Michael Tracy, Springville, UT: Christopher Publications.

You will probably feel somewhat weak during or after this detoxication. Don't let this alarm you. Nature uses our energies for a housecleaning within us, and we soon regain greater energy and vitality as a result of a cleaner and heal their body. You can do the three-day cleanse monthly or several times a year.

If there is the slightest tendency toward appendicitis, take high enemas, using catnip tea or a tea of three parts red raspberry leaf and one part lobelia. Do this two, three or more times a day as needed. Only use enemas in the case of possible appendicitis. If you are experiencing trouble with constipation, use more prune juice or the lower bowel tonic (see page 578).

Continued Fast:
Once you have completed several three day juice cleanses, you can, if you want to try, and feel up to it, fast one to three more days using only distilled water, then a day of juice, before returning to salads and other regular foods. Do not eat any heavy foods immediately after a cleansing period or a fast, but add these to your diet gradually. This is the best and smoothest way to get back onto solid foods. Such a continued fast will greatly accelerate the cleansing and healing process.

Cleansing Symptoms:
As your body begins to cleanse, you will probably experience periodic aches and pains in the areas where the cleaning action is most acute and the wastage is loading the elimination system; there are times when you will feel very, very rough! Do not panic on the days after cleansing or during your periods of healing.

In fact, the cleaning action may produce all symptoms and effects of severe illness, but don't blame the temporary problem onto the cleansing. Be comforted that the healing process is well underway, and the sooner such discomforts come, the better, for this means that the toxins and poisons are being eliminated—and the faster the cleansing, the quicker the healing.

But this cleansing will not be instantaneous; do not expect the toxic accumulations of a lifetime to be miraculously flushed out of the tissues and organs in some colonic fashion. This will all take time working with the body's normal cyclic functions. You will have high days and low days, usually in cycles. These "cleansing sicknesses" come in cycles of seven days, seven weeks, seven months, and seven years in most cases. As the toxic poisons break loose and are dumped into the bloodstream so they can be eliminated, you will feel pretty rough; and quite frequently during a crisis, you may feel worse than you did before you ever started the program. But do not panic! The bad days will become fewer and fewer and the good days greater and greater, if you are faithful to the program. Professor Arnold Ehret's book, *Mucusless Diet Healing System* (which can be purchased from any health food store) may help you to understand some of the reactions you might experience while ridding the body of toxins, waste and mucus.

THE MUCUSLESS DIET

Now you can eliminate the mucus-forming foods from your diet, so as not to put mucus into the body faster than it can be eliminated. This mucusless diet removes constipating mucus (catarrh) from the tissues of the body from the heart to the bottom of the feet. Use this guide as an ideal diet. Some people can undertake this diet completely from the first with great results; others require a "transition period," using the mucusless diet as a guide as they move more and more to the ideal. Don't let yourself become filled with guilt as you make this transition, but do the very best you can as you work to rebuild your health.

ITEMS TO ELIMINATE:

Processed salt:
Use only unrefined salt with no additives or chemicals of any kind. This may be sun-evaporated sea salt, or one of the natural, unrefined earth salts that are mined without additional chemicals. Do not add salt during cooking, but salt to taste at the table. You will find your craving for excessive salt immediately begins to disappear. For those accustomed to large amounts of salt, this may sound difficult, but you can add coarsely ground pepper and savory herbs, and perhaps some powdered kelp or dulse. Black pepper is a good nutritional herb and helps rebuild the body when used in its natural state. But when pepper is cooked in food, the molecular structure changes, so that it becomes an inorganic irritant; high heat changes cayenne, black pepper, and spices from organic to inorganic. You can also use seasonings from a vegetable or potassium base, such as Dr. Jensen's, Dr. Bronner's, and other various ones, which in some cases contain some sea salt.

Eggs:
No eggs should be eaten in any form.

Sugar and all sugar products:
You may use honey, sorghum molasses, blackstrap molasses, or unrefined, dehydrated cane juice, but even these should be used sparingly. Never use refined sugar of any type.

Meat:
Eliminate all meats from the diet. Some people include a little white fish once a week, or a bit of young chicken that has not been fed commercial food or inoculated with formaldehyde and other antispoilage serums, but recent research has shown that most meats are contaminated with organisms of various kinds, and the fish with heavy metals. If you wish to add meat-like products to the diet, you can look into the variety of soy-based products available in health food stores. These can give the texture and taste of meat without the threat to your health.

Milk:
Eliminate all dairy products: butter, cheese, cottage cheese, milk, yogurt, etc.

These are all mucus-forming substances and in most cases, can be high in cholesterol, especially butter. As a substitute for butter or margarine—which is one of the worst junk foods known, as the hardened oils cannot be digested— you can train your taste buds to enjoy a good, fresh, bland olive oil on vegetables and salads. Soymilk and tofu can add taste, texture and protein to the diet in a variety of ways; you can learn to use them creatively to be good substitutes for dairy foods.

Flour and Flour Products:
Flour and flour products such as pasta are eliminated because, when heated and baked at high temperatures, it changes to a mucus-forming substance. It has no more life. All wholesome food is organic, where unwholesome food is dead and inorganic.

These are our "don'ts"; now for the "do's":

SUPPLEMENTS AND HEALING AIDS

Cayenne:
Take 1 teaspoonful of cayenne 3 times a day. Start gradually with 1/4 teaspoonful in a little cold water; drink this and follow with a glass of cold water. Add 1/4 teaspoonful to this dosage every 3 days, until you are taking 1 teaspoonful 3 times a day. The graduated dosages will accustom your system to the pungency of the herb.

Honey and Apple-Cider Vinegar:
Place 1 teaspoonful of honey and 1 tablespoonful of undiluted, apple cider vinegar in warm water, so that the honey will liquefy. Sip this amount 3 times a day so that at the end of the day a total quantity of 3 tablespoonfuls of vinegar are consumed. This must be apple cider vinegar; do not use distilled or other types of vinegars, as these are damaging to the body. The apple cider vinegar is medicinal and very beneficial.

Kelp:
Take two or more kelp tablets a day, and sprinkle kelp on food if desired. Dulse is similar in nature and very delicious; some people eat the dried leaves out of hand as a snack, and it is excellent added to soup. Kelp helps to build and strengthen the thyroid. If you have a hypothyroid problem, take five to ten kelp tablets a day.

Molasses:
Take 1 tablespoonful 3 times a day of either sorghum or blackstrap molasses. If you are trying to cut down on sugars, use the molasses instead of honey in the vinegar beverage above.

Wheat Germ Oil:
Take 1 tablespoonful of a good, fresh wheat germ oil three times a day.

DIETARY SUGGESTIONS: REGENERATIVE FOODS

If you follow this diet as outlined, we guarantee that after a short period of time you will have much more satisfaction from your food than you ever had from the food of your former diet. Remember, you do not have to count calories or fat grams in this type of diet; just eat as instructed and you will come to your normal weight, with plenty of physical strength.

Do not be overly concerned because this diet omits meat and dairy food, and don't worry about adding protein, as you will get all that you need in these foods. The gorilla is built on the same order as the human being, and he gets all the protein he needs from just fruit and nuts—and for the human, the greens will round out the body requirement. Don't panic; just prove this program to yourself!

Morning:
It is best not to "break-the-fast" (breakfast) until at least noon, except in cases of young or very active people. You will find that this will not be hard to do when you take your wheat germ oil, cayenne, etc. These will lower the appetite while providing the needed nutrition, so you will feel satisfied. You may take these items even the second time during the morning before it is time to eat the regular noon meal. But if after taking the lower bowel tonics, wheat germ oil, cayenne, apple cider vinegar, honey, molasses, herbal teas, etc. you are hungry, you can eat fresh fruits.

Dr. Christopher taught that the best food to start the day is a good low-heated whole-grain cereal. This should be cereal in its wholesome state, with life in it. Soak the whole grain in water 8-20 hours, then heat in a stainless steel double boiler at a very low heat, 130° F. or under, 12 to 14 hours, or longer if needed. It can also be prepared in a thermos bottle, which is done as follows: take a thermos bottle for an individual or couple. Fill it in the early afternoon or evening one-third full of high-protein turkey red wheat or other grains or combinations; then finish filling the thermos bottle with water that has been brought to a boil, and turn the container on its top and back once or twice, so that during the evening the water circulates completely into the bottom, or else some wheat in the bottom will not be treated. When you uncover the wheat in the morning, after low heating the grain all night long, it should be ready: the wheat popped open, soft and very tasty. Add a little oil and honey, and it is a very delectable food. Some people like to add cinnamon, allspice, or other flavorings.

Wheat contains all of the potential nutrients needed in the human body. The wheat herb of wheat grass is a complete food, as it provides you with protein, calcium, and all the needed enzymes, vitamins, minerals, etc. to regenerate the cell structure of your body. The grain is alive until it is killed in some chemical storage procedure or at high heat.

You can tell if wheat is alive by planting it to see if it will grow. This test is also valid for testing cooked wheat; when it is low-heated in stainless steel, it will retain the life power and will grow! Wheat and other foods prepared in this manner, are organic; consequently, this is the manner that grains must be prepared for use. We are told in holy writ that "all wholesome grains and herbs are for man," and "grain is the staff of life," but it does not say that it is permissible to grind wheat to a face powder fineness or to heat it above 212° F., and change the molecular structure from organic to inorganic, and thereby make it very mucus-forming. You can also sprout the grains if you prefer.

Noon:

If you prefer only a light lunch, then have a tossed salad of mixed vegetables and leafy greens as large as you want, using a homemade olive oil dressing:

1 cup	olive oil
2 tablespoonfuls	apple cider vinegar or lemon juice
Pinch	herbs, black pepper, etc.

Make this dressing to your own taste, for there are so many varieties you can make; avocado, onion, garlic, etc. but do not use the processed dressings of the commercial market. You will be surprised how delicious this will come to taste.

You can take juices during the afternoon: carrot, grape, apple, etc. Together, dried fruits and nuts make a very nourishing and beneficial snack, but for a whole protein, nuts are better when used in combination with garden greens.

If you have cancer or if you are inclined towards cancer, do not overdo eating any protein, such as nuts. Excess protein does damage to the pancreas, so in these cases, eat nuts only in the morning. Stay away from peanuts and instead use almonds, cashews, or other mild nuts. A person with a cancerous condition should use from 8 to 10 almonds in the morning and the same at noon. But do not take any protein from evening time until the next morning, allowing 16 to 18 hours for the pancreas to clear and start to work on enzymes again. All protein should be taken early in the morning. In cancer cases *never* use any secondary protein such as meats.

Regular meals can start off with a cup or bowl of potassium broth. Dehydrated vegetables in the form of potassium powder or broth can be purchased from most health stores or you can prepare your own. You do this by simmering onions, celery, carrots, and potatoes (particularly the skin) in pure water until soft and soupy. You can add tomatoes and seasoning herbs for flavor. For minerals and potassium, include some dulse with the vegetables. You can also add the left-over, low-heated vegetables from the day before to the broth. This delicious soup can become a favorite food of the family.

The broth starts the meal off, and is followed with a salad. There are thousands of salad combinations, and with some experimentation, you will never run short of interesting ones.

After that, serve low-heated vegetables. Eat at least five or six vegetables each day, of which two should be green, leafy ones. Add a small amount of olive oil to a baked potato, baked squash, etc. and use herbs, Spike, or other seasonings. Make casseroles with vegetables and whole grains. Use tofu, vegetables, and whole grains. Low heat legumes, such as lentils and beans, preferably sprouted or semi-sprouted before you cook them. You can put together very interesting, intriguing meals with a little daring and imagination. And you will never need to worry if you eat until you are satisfied; you will have all the nutrition you need for ample physical strength.

Evening:
This is generally the heavy meal of the day, but you can reverse this if you like, eating the heavy meal maybe at noon, then the light meal with a salad at night. Start off with a cup of potassium broth. Follow with a salad, then with the main course of steamed vegetables that have been prepared at low-heat. Be sure to always cook in stainless steel, Pyrex, or some other safe pan, but *never* in aluminum. You may also have vegetable juices, or a baked potato or baked squash with some olive oil in place of butter.

Juice or nuts, dried fruits or fresh fruits are all excellent. Whenever you use a fresh fruit, use it alone. When you want to eat some other type of fruit, or other food, wait for one-half hour or more at least before eating it; this will prove much easier on your digestive system.

CORRECTIVE AIDS

Castor Oil Fomentation:
In order to get rid of hardened mucus in the body, which may appear as cysts, tumors or polyps, use the following fomentation:

Soak a piece of outing flannel or baby's diaper in castor oil, squeeze slightly so it won't drip much, then place over entire frontal torso (neck to groin and side to side). Place a hot water bottle—over the castor oil application—over the liver area (the liver is on the right side just above the waist). If you use a heating pad, place a wet towel between it and the skin—but even then, a wet heat, such as the hot water bottle, is best. Leave all this on for 90 minutes; the hot water bottle may have to be refilled with hot water several times, because it cools rapidly. The next three days, over the same area covered by the outing flannel and castor oil, massage in circular motion toward the heart with olive oil for 5 to 10 minutes. This castor oil fomentation is excellent for any ailment where the liver is congested—and that can be with most of our illnesses. More than one family has used this fomentation, in connection with other therapies, to treat a child's appendicitis!

The seventh day is a day of rest, not only from the fomentation, but every part of the program, drinking only water the entire day—and every seventh day thereafter will be done the same way. On the eighth day then, begin again with the castor oil for three days and so forth, along with the mucusless diet, the herbs, etc. until healing is accomplished. In the use of the fomentation, the castor oil goes through the skin into the liver area and lymph glands and starts drawing out the poisons and flushing them out, while the olive oil goes in and heals and rebuilds new tissue. This procedure may have to be continued between six weeks to six months to properly clean up the system, depending on the case.

Exercise:
Everyone should do some jogging, which is a bouncing motion. This helps to improve circulation, tone the organs, and slough off the dead cell accumulations faster. Each person should work up to a mile of jogging a day, but start out with one-fourth mile or less. Never jog to the point of exhaustion because all the good that is done each day will be undone as a result of overexertion. If for some reason you cannot jog outside, do it inside the house in front of an open window. This will especially vibrate the peristaltic colon muscle and give it tone, will revive the uterus from a prolapsed state in the female, and help heal the prostate in the male. Some people use the mini-tramp to jog in the same way.

Deep Breathing:
We are not going to give you scientific Yoga breathing exercises or anything difficult. The main thing is deep breathing fresh air in through the nose and out through the mouth. Breathe deeply enough that it actually hurts when you breathe. Do this morning and night, no less than 5 or 10 minutes, and this will start the day with pep and energy and finish the day off with complete relaxation. Try this just before retiring at night for the best sleep you have ever had. Deep breathing gives the "breath of life," taking this breath to every cell in the entire body. Each cell will die unless it gets the breath of life, and the only way you can get this life-giving element is through inhaling oxygen and air through the nose. This principle is absolutely vital, and yet so overlooked. A person can live up to 110 days without food and 16 days without water, but only a few minutes without breathing.

The Vital Circuitry:
All of us accumulate static electricity in the body, which can be released by removing the shoes and socks and shuffling the feet through the lawn or grass ten or fifteen minutes a day. What happens is this: the hair acts as antennae and pulls the electrical energy from the atmosphere. As this electrical force comes in through the top of the head, it distributes so many amps and/or ohms to each organ, cell, gland, etc.; then the rest of the electricity is supposed to pass out of the body again into the earth through the feet. But when we wear rubber-soled shoes and wear nylon stockings or socks, that electricity cannot be grounded properly, so it collects as static electricity in the body, and we become mentally confused and frustrated from it. Ideally, we can go barefoot throughout our work

day, including some outside work. Some of our associates might laugh, but it is an excellent way to release tension and maintain a quiet equilibrium. Try it; you can get used to it easily, and you might be surprised what a difference it makes to your mental state.

POSITIVE ATTITUDE

Some people follow a very clean diet, take herbs, and are still uncomfortable or even sick. Why? Because they toxify themselves with unhappy, negative thoughts or behaviors. You already possess a degree of health right now. Thank God for that, and then go forward to build even better health. Train yourself to live with an "attitude of gratitude," live positively and generously, and be sure to nurture your spirituality, including prayer and meditation. We consider this to be so important that it is equal to your dietary and herbal programs.

EXTENDED HERBAL CLEANSE

When we are dealing with long-standing health problems we cannot expect to totally cleanse or cure the body with one or so three-day cleansing routines. Therefore to rid the body of chronic conditions or to prevent their occurrence, an extended herbal cleanse is an excellent path to follow. This should be used in conjunction with the aforementioned mucusless diet.

Upon arising we take one or two (more if needed!) of the lower bowel formula. This would then be repeated one hour before lunch, and prior to retiring for the night.

Then, twenty minutes before eating we would take two of the liver-gall bladder formula, which would then be repeated prior to each meal.

Next on the program, take two of the kidney-bladder formula mid-morning and also mid-afternoon. This routine would be followed six days, resting on the seventh.

We resume taking the herbs on the second week, adding two capsules of the blood purifying formula one hour after each meal. We would again do this for six days, resting on the seventh day. This procedure would then continue every week for six weeks, after which we would rest one week. We would repeat these intervals for six months and then rest for one entire month. At the end of this seven month program we will assess our progress and determine if another seven month program would be beneficial.

The one week delay in adding the blood purifying formula is absolutely essential because of the extreme effectiveness of the formula. What we are doing is opening the eliminative channels of the body, allowing a pathway of elimination for the ensuing toxins eliminated by the blood cleansing formula.

HERBAL COMBINATIONS ON THE MARKET

Herbs are food. Just as carrots, potatoes, cabbage, and onions are herbs, so are comfrey, yellow dock root, and lobelia. There are thousands of these precious herbs growing around us and some even in our doorways waiting patiently for us to use them for our better health.

The following are a few of Dr. Christopher's cleansing and rebuilding herbal formulas that may aid you in creating better health and happiness. The formulas have been released in print for personal home use only. They are not released for commercial enterprise. These combinations are not intended to be used as a replacement for competent medical attention but within a full health program. Consult a competent health practitioner for any uncommon health problems not found within the scope of these formulas. At the end of each formula is listed the names used by various vendors who supply Dr. Christopher's formulas commercially. If you can not find these formulas in you local health food store, they may all be obtained from The Herb Shop by calling 1-800-453-1406.

1. Lower bowel formula.

1 part	Barberry bark (Berberis vulgaris)
2 parts	Cascara sagrada bark (Rhamnus purshiana)
1 part	Cayenne (Capsicum frutescens; C. minimum)
1 part	Ginger (Zingiber officinalis)
1 part	Lobelia herb and/or seeds (Lobelia inflata)
1 part	Red raspberry leaves (Rubus idaeus)
1 part	Turkey rhubarb root (Rheum palmatum)
1 part	Fennel (Foeniculum vulgaris)
1 part	Golden seal root (Hydrastis Canadensis)

Take according to how many you need. As there are no two people alike in age, size, or physical construction (and the bowel itself will differ in persons as much as the finger prints), most cases will START with two number 0 capsules or 30 drops of the glycerine based extract three times a day, and then regulate the dosage from there. If the stool seems too loose then cut down, but if it is difficult to get a bowel movement and the stool is hard and takes a long time, then increase the amount until the movements become soft and well-formed (and here, in very difficult cases, you could take even up to 40 of these capsules a day, for these herbs are FOOD and can do no damage to you).

After the hard material has broken loose and is eliminated (these are hard incrustations of fecal matter that have been stored in the bowel for many years that are breaking loose and soaking up intestinal liquids), you can gradually decrease but do not taper off the lower bowel formula dosage so much at this point that you lose this advantageous momentum and continuity of elimination. In most cases, the improper diet has caused the peristaltic muscles of most people to quit working, and it will take six to nine months with the aid of the lower bowel formula for the average individual to clean out the fecal matter and to rebuild the bowel structure sufficiently to have the peristaltic muscles work entirely on their own.

Most people have pounds of old dried fecal matter that is stored in the colon which is toxifying the system and keeping the food from being assimilated. Because of this putrefied condition, most people engorge themselves with many times more food than the actual body requirements. In the process they wear out their bodies in trying to get sufficient nutrition and are still always hungry and eating; whereas, after the bowel is cleaned, the food is readily assimilated and a person can sustain himself on about one-third the quantity of his current food consumption at some four or five times more power, vitality and life. Herein, the clean body is able to normally assimilate the simple food values through the cell structures in the colon instead of it being trapped in a maze of waste and inhibited by the hard fecal casing on the intestinal wall, which causes the large part of nutrition to be pushed on and eliminated before it can do any good. When the body is completely clean, these aids will no longer be necessary and then your food will be your medicine and your medicine will be your food. After following this program properly and the bowel is cleansed, this formula should only be used when needed. Sources: Herbal L.B., FEN LB, Naturalax 2.

2. Blood purifying formula.

2 parts	Red clover blossoms (Trifolium pratense)
1 part	Chaparral (Larrea tridentata)
1 part	Licorice root (Glycyrrhiza glabra)
1 part	Poke root (Phytolacca americana)
1 part	Peach bark (Prunus Persica vulgaris)
1 part	Oregon grape root (Mahonia aquifolium; M. repens)
1 part	Stillingia (Stillingia sylvatica)
1 part	Cascara sagrada (Rhamnus purshiana)
1 part	Sarsaparilla (Smilax officinalis)
1 part	Prickly ash bark (Zanthoxylum americanum)
1 part	Burdock root (Arctium lappa)
1 part	Buckthorn bark (Rhamnus Frangula).

The blood stream is life itself and it is our job to keep it clean and pure so that we can have a good circulatory system for delivering food to the body properly and to carry off the waste materials. After years of using this blood cleansing formula, we discovered it to be the same type of formula used by Hoxey.

This herbal blood rebuilder is made up of herbs that are cleansers, herbs that give astringency, others aid in removing cholesterol, kill infection, and build elasticity in the veins and strengthen the vein and artery walls. Use a cup of this tea or two #0 capsules or 5 to 15 drops of the glycerine based extract three time a day, six days a week, week after week, until the blood stream is flowing as it should to bring health and give one more pep and energy.

This blood purifier in teamwork with the bowel cleansing and rebuilding formula, the liver-gall bladder formula and the kidney formula, makes a wonderful combination. These four, with a good mucusless diet, can renew the body and add years to a healthy life (see “EXTENDED HERBAL CLEANSE” page 577). Sources: Red Clover Combination, R.C.C.

3. Formula for liver-gall bladder.

3 parts	Barberry (Berberis vulgaris or Mahonia aquifolium)
1 part	Wild yam (Dioscorea villosa)
1 part	Cramp bark (Viburnum trilobum; V. opulus)
1 part	Fennel seed (Foeniculum vulgare)
1 part	Ginger (Zingiber officinalis)
1 part	Catnip (Nepeta cataria)
1 part	Peppermint (Mentha piperita).

To speed up the blood purifying process, it is good to have a clean liver and gall bladder area. When the liver does not function properly, the bile does not excrete freely into the intestinal tract, and so it passes off into the blood stream and throughout the rest of the system, causing a toxic condition called cholemia, causing indigestion, sluggishness, fatigue, constipation, upset stomach, chills, vomiting and fever. Why wait until it gets to this condition? This combination will help relieve this condition.

Suggested dose: 1 cup of the tea or one or two capsules or 15 to 30 drops of the glycerine based extract, 15 or 20 minutes before a meal. Sources: Barberry LG, Hepatean, LG.

4. Formula for the kidneys.

1 part	Juniper berries (Juniperus communis)
1 part	Parsley (Petroselinum crispum)
1 part	Uva ursi (Arctostaphylos uva-ursi)
1 part	Marshmallow root (Althaea officinalis
1 part	Lobelia (Lobelia inflata)
1 part	Ginger (Zingiber officinalis)
1 part	Golden seal (Hydrastis Canadensis).

Approximately 80% of the body is liquid, and much of this fluid must be pumped, filtered, etc. through the urinary system of the individual. We generally do not take the best care of this delicate tract. Through it circulates irritating and clogging-type materials, i.e., tea, coffee, soft drinks, hard water, alcohol, etc.

Over the years we have used a formula of herbs with people who have been afraid to be out in public because of lack of control over the urinary tract and unknowingly voiding urine. After using this formula, many people have found relief from this condition and are living normal lives again.

Suggested use is a cup of tea morning and evening, or two capsules or 30 to 60 drops of the glycerine based extract morning and evening taken with a cup of parsley tea. Sources: Juni-Pars, Renatean, KB.

5. For more severe cases of incontinence, neurosis (bed wetting, etc.).

1 part	Parsley root (Petroselinum crispum)
1 part	Juniper berries (Juniperus communis)
1 part	Marshmallow root (Althaea officinalis)
1 part	White pond lily (Nymphaea odorata)
1 part	Gravel root (Eupatorium purpureum)
1 part	Uva ursi (Arctostaphylos uva-ursi)
1 part	Lobelia (Lobelia inflata)
1 part	Ginger root (Zingiber officinalis)
1 part	Black cohosh root (Cimicifuga racemosa).

This formula is a specific for controlling or overcoming bed wetting and to strengthen the entire urethral canal, kidneys, bladder, etc.

Recommended dosage: Two No. 0 capsules three times a day with a cup of parsley tea. Upon retiring at night fasten about a six or eight inch ball of yarn or string or cloth onto night clothes in the middle of the back. This is for the purpose of preventing the individual from lying on the back, as this is generally the time the valves release to void urine. Sources: DRI.

6. Formula for the heart.

The heart is our life pump, and when it is not properly fed (with wholesome foods) it suffers malfunction (weakness and heart attacks) causing the heart failure condition that is one of the worlds greatest killers. The mucusless diet used over a period of time can rebuild a heart to a good strong condition, but if the heart, its valves, and other working parts are in a weakened condition and need quick help, we use a great heart food or tonic to assist it back to health. This food is the hawthorn berry (Crataegus laevigata). We refer back to Potters Cyclopaedia of Botanical Drugs and Preparations, one of the old herbals out of England (published by Potter and Clarke, Ltd., 60 Artillery Lane, London), which lists hawthorn as a “cardiac” tonic. This herb is claimed to be a curative remedy for organic and functional heart disorders such as dyspnoea, rapid and feeble heart action, hypertrophy (valvular insufficiency), and heart oppression.

Hawthorn berry syrup is made by putting fresh hawthorn berries into a stainless steel, Pyrex glass, or porcelain pan and filling the pan with distilled water 2 inches above the original level of the berries. If you have dried berries, reconstitute the berries in distilled water then strain off the excess water and treat the reconstituted berries as fresh (use the water that was strained off adding more distilled water if needed to reach the level of 2 inches above the berries). Heat the mixture on low to about 120° F. and low simmer (under 130° F.) for about 15 to 30 minutes. Stir while simmering. Remove the mixture from the heat and let it steep (covered) for 15 to 30 minutes. Strain the liquid off and set it aside in a clean container.

Mash the remainder of the berries and cover them with distilled water, adding an additional inch of water to the solution. Heat again and simmer this mixture for 20 minutes, stirring while you are simmering. Remove pan from heat and let steep (covered) for 20 minutes. Strain off the liquid and press the excess liquid from the solids.

Combine the second batch of liquid with the first batch of liquid in a clean pan and heat on low with the lid off. While stirring regularly, simmer into a syrup by reducing it to 1/4 its original volume (if you started with one gallon, you should reduce it to one quart). Take off the heat and add 1/4 amount of vegetable glycerine and stir well (if you have one quart of syrup you should add 1 cup of glycerine). Let cool and add 1/4 amount of grape brandy (again 1 cup of brandy if you ended up with 1 quart of syrup). Mix well and store in amber bottles in a cool place (for long term storage, keep in the refrigerator). Recommended dosage is one half teaspoon three times a day.

In an emergency heart attack, a teaspoon of cayenne in a cup of hot water taken quickly has saved many peoples lives. To save time, the extract should be kept on hand. Sources: Hawthorn Berry Syrup.

7. Aid for pancreas.

1 part	Golden seal (Hydrastis Canadensis)
6 parts	Uva ursi (Arctostaphylos uva-ursi)
2 parts	Cayenne (Capsicum frutescens; C. minimum)
16 parts	Cedar berries (Juniperus monosperma)
3 parts	Licorice root (Glycyrrhiza glabra)
3 parts	Mullein (Verbascum thapsus)

Malfunction of the pancreas and other affiliated glands causes high or low blood sugar (namely diabetes or hypoglycemia). This combination has assisted many that have had hypoglycemia. Use two or three capsules or 15 to 30 drops of the glycerine based extract three times a day, six days a week. (All herbal aids give faster results in six days a week instead of seven, using the same days of each week.) Many have had a glucose tolerance test with a clean bill of health on the pancreas area. Many reports have come in about heavy insulin users who continue using the insulin but by watching litmus paper or other types of diabetic checking have gradually tapered down on the insulin; and many within a year, have found complete relief using two to three or more capsules, or 30 to 60 drops of the glycerine based extract of the pancreas formula three times a day, six days a week. Of course, the closer a person stays on the mucusless diet and eliminates from the diet the unnatural sugars, soft drinks, candies, pastries, bread, etc. the quicker the results. Sources: Panc Tea, Pancratean, PC.

8. Calcium formula.

6 parts	Horsetail grass (Equisetum hyemale)
3 parts	Oat straw (Avena sativa)
4 parts	Comfrey root (Symphytum officinale)
1 part	Lobelia (Lobelia inflata)

A wonderful natural calcium formula which can be made up in capsule, tea or glycerine based extract form. As explained in the book *Biological Transmutations*, the silica in horsetail grass converts to calcium, and the other herbs work in close conjunction with this master calcium herb. We need calcium for nerve sheath, vein and artery walls, bone, teeth, etc. This combination is all pure herbs. It is also used for cramps, charlie horses, and for all calcium needs in the body.

Children with crowded, crooked teeth who later must have the wisdom teeth pulled because their jaw is too narrow are lacking calcium in the body. The pregnant woman should increase her natural calcium intake now for two people, so as to build for the child a good wide jaw and tooth material. Sugars, pastries, soft and alcoholic beverages, breads, candies, etc. leach the calcium out of the body, causing varicose veins, cramps, charlie horses, loss of teeth, nervous upsets, etc. Sources: Calc Tea, Calctean, Kid-E-Calc, CA-T.

9. Formula for allergies, sinus, hayfever.

1 part	Brigham tea (Ephedra species)
1 part	Marshmallow root (Althaea officinalis)
1 part	Golden seal root (Hydrastis Canadensis)
1 part	Chaparral (Larrea tridentata)
1 part	Burdock root (Arctium lappa)
1 part	Parsley root (Petroselinum crispum)
1 part	Lobelia (Lobelia inflata)
1 part	Cayenne (Capsicum frutescens; C. minimum)

This is an aid for clearing up the malfunctions of the sinuses. This is a natural aid that works as a decongestant and natural antihistamine to dry up the sinuses and expel from the head and bronchial-pulmonary tubes and passages the offending stoppage and mucus. Take two capsules or 20 to 40 drops of the glycerine based extract three times a day or as often as needed.

To speed up this cleansing procedure, use the following combination in addition to the above: blend fresh, chopped-up horseradish roots mixed with apple cider vinegar into a thick pulp and chew thoroughly before swallowing. Take 1/3 teaspoon three times in a day. Increase this amount 1/3 teaspoon each three days, up to one teaspoon three times a day. (For a sinus preparation that contains horseradish, see formula #58 on page 597). Sources: SHA Tea, Sinutean, HAS.

10. Blood circulation combination.

2 parts	Ginger (Zingiber officinalis)
3 parts	Cayenne (Capsicum frutescens; C. minimum)
1 part	Golden seal (Hydrastis Canadensis)
1 part	Ginseng (Panax quinquefolius)
3 parts	Parsley (Petroselinum crispum)
1 part	Garlic (Allium sativum)

This group of herbs feeds cayenne (a stimulant) and ginger (stimulant) into the circulatory system where the cayenne works from the bloodstream to the heart and arteries and out into the veins. The other herbs in the formula assist these two herbs and work together to equalize the blood pressure (whether high or low) bringing it to a good systolic over the diastolic reading. Blood flow is life itself. This formula is given to assist blood purifying teas to work more efficiently and to also aid the clearing up of allergies, etc. (available in capsules and glycerine based extract). Sources: BPE, Circutean, B/P.

11. Anti-obese herbal food combination.

6 parts	Chickweed (Stellaria media)
4 parts	Saffron (Crocus sativus)
3 parts	Burdock (Arctium lappa)
3 parts	Parsley root (Petroselinum crispum)
3 parts	Kelp (Laminaria saccharina or Fucus vesiculosis)
2 parts	Echinacea (Echinacea angustifolia; E. purpurea)
2 parts	Black walnut (Juglans nigra)
2 parts	Licorice (Glycyrrhiza glabra)
2 parts	Fennel (Foeniculum vulgare)
2 parts	Papaya (Carica papaya)
1 part	Hawthorn berries (Crataegus laevigata)

Combine this anti-obese aid with the mucusless diet and you have a winner. This is not a crash program for fast loss of weight, but graduated and accurate loss without robbing the body of the needed nutrients like so many fad diets do. This acts as a blood purifier, aids kidneys in relieving excess fluids, feeds the body for relief from nervous tension generally caused by diets, appeases the appetite, feeds the thyroid and other malfunctioning glands and thus gains a healthier state for holding weight control. Take two or three capsules morning and night with a cup of chickweed tea. Sources: CSK Plus, SLM.

12. Formula for malfunctioning glands. Through the accumulation of toxic waste in the body from improper diet, poor blood stream and sluggish circulation, the glands become congested and infected and swell up to cause much pain and misery. (There are glands that swell on the neck, breast, groin, under arm, etc.) Make a tea of three parts mullein (Verbascum thapsus) and one part lobelia (Lobelia inflata) herb and use as a fomentation over swollen or malfunctioning glands. Leave on all night (covering fomentation with plastic), six nights a week until relief is obtained. Use a fresh fomentation as warm as possible each night.

This can be used as an aid to relieve mastitis, thyroid malfunction, etc. In addition to the external fomentation, also drink a cup of this tea two or three times a day or take two of the capsules with a cup of steam-distilled water. Source: Mullein & Lobelia.

13. Nerve herbal food combination.

1 part	Black cohosh (Cimicifuga racemosa)
1 part	Cayenne (Capsicum frutescens; C. minimum)
1 part	Hops flowers (Humulus lupulus)
1 part	Lady's slipper root (Cypripedium calceolus var. pubescens)
1 part	Lobelia (Lobelia inflata)
1 part	Skullcap (Scutellaria lateriflora)
1 part	Valerian (Valeriana officinalis)
1 part	Wood betony (Stachys officinalis)
1 part	Mistletoe (Viscum album)

Here is a formula we have used with great success for well over thirty years and is used for relieving nervous tension and insomnia. It is mildly stimulating and yet lessens the irritability and excitement of the nervous system, and also lessens or reduces pain. This formula contains herbs that feed and revitalize the motor nerve at the base of the skull (medulla area and upper cervicals), and also herbs that help rebuild or feed the spinal cord. This group of herbs will also rebuild the frayed nerve sheath, the nerve itself, and its capillaries. The suggested amount for an adult's use would be one to three cups of the tea, or two or three capsules, or 15 to 30 drops of the glycerine based extract, three times a day, taken with a cup of celery juice or steam-distilled water. Sources: Relax-Eze, Nervean, Ex-Stress.

14. Hearing loss and earache formula.

1 part	Blue cohosh (Caulophyllum thalictroides)
1 part	Black cohosh (Cimicifuga racemosa)
1 part	Blue vervain (Verbena hastata)
1 part	Skullcap (Scutellaria lateriflora)
1 part	Lobelia (Lobelia inflata)

When this procedure is used as explained here, it can be an aid in assisting an improvement of poor equilibrium, failure of hearing, aiding the motor nerve, etc. With an eye dropper put into each ear at night four to six drops of oil of garlic (it is important that the oil of garlic be used first) and four to six drops of the herb tincture listed below, plugging ears overnight with cotton, six days a week, four to six months, or as needed. On the seventh day, flush ears with a small ear syringe using warm apple cider vinegar and distilled water half and half. Source: B & B.

15. Formula for lungs and respiratory tract.

1 part	Comfrey root (Symphytum officinale)
1 part	Mullein (Verbascum thapsus)
1 part	Chickweed (Stellaria media)
1 part	Marshmallow root (Althaea officinalis)
1 part	Lobelia (Lobelia inflata)

This combination of herbs is an aid to relieve irritation in the respiratory tract, lungs and bronchials. This is an aid in emphysema as well as other bronchial and lung congestions such as bronchitis, asthma, tuberculosis, etc. This formula is extremely valuable in strengthening and healing the entire respiratory tract. It promotes the discharge of mucus secretions from the bronchopulmonary passages. Suggested amount for an adult is a cup of tea two or three times a day, or two or three capsules or 10 to 20 drops of the glycerine based extract two or three times a day with a cup of comfrey tea. For additional help in the program, it is good to add three to six drops of tincture of lobelia to each cup of tea. Sources: Resp-Free, Respratean, Breathe-Aid.

16. Formula for colds and infections.

6 parts	Garlic (Allium sativum)
1 part	Parsley (Petroselinum crispum)
1 part	Watercress (Nasturtium officinale)
1 part	Rosemary (Rosmarinus officinalis)
6 parts	Rosehips (Rosa species)

This formula acts as an aid to assist in relieving colds, etc. or wherever garlic is needed to help stop infection! The adult amount can vary from one to six or more cups in a day or two or more capsules six or more times per day taken with a cup of steam-distilled water. Sources: Garlic, Rosehips & Parsley; Winter Formula C&F.

17. Herbal aid for eliminating intestinal parasites (worms, etc.).

1 part	Wormwood (Artemisia absinthium)
1 part	American wormseed (Chenopodium anthelminticum)
1 part	Tame sage (Salvia officinalis)
1 part	Fennel (Foeniculum vulgare)
1 part	Malefern (Dryopteris filix-mas)
1 part	Papaya (Carica papaya)

This combination acts as a vermifuge (herbal agent that will cause expulsion of worms from the body) and/or vermicide (herbal agent that destroys worms in the body). It is generally made into a syrup. The recommended dosage is to take one fluid teaspoon each morning and night for three days. On the fourth day drink one cup of senna and peppermint tea (combine the herbs using 2 parts senna powder and 1 part peppermint powder) using a teaspoon of the herbs in a cup of hot, distilled water. Rest two days and repeat two more times. Source: VF Syrup.

18. Herbal tooth powder.

3 parts	Oak bark (Quercus alba)
6 parts	Comfrey root (Symphytum officinale)
3 parts	Horsetail grass (Equisetum hyemale)
1 part	Lobelia (Lobelia inflata)
1 part	Cloves (Syzygium aromaticum)
3 parts	Peppermint (Mentha piperita)

This herbal food combination is used to help strengthen the gums (bleeding and pyorrhea-type infections of the gums), and assist in tightening loose teeth. This type of tooth powder will brighten tooth luster and make for a healthier mouth. For severe cases place this powder combination between the lips and gums (upper and lower) around entire tooth area and leave on all night, six nights a week (as well as brushing regularly) until improvement is evident. Then continue on with regular brushing with this herbal food combination. Source: Herbal Tooth Powder.

19. Herbal composition powder (also see page 147-148) .

4 parts	Bayberry bark (Myrica cerifera)
2 parts	Ginger root (Zingiber officinale)
1 part	White pine bark (Pinus strobus)
1 teaspoon	Cloves (Syzygium aromaticum)
1 teaspoon	Cayenne (Capsicum frutescens; C. minimum)

As quoted by Dr. Nowell, instructor at the Dominion Herbal College, Ltd. of Vancouver, British Columbia in this textbook:

> We have made and used composition powder for over forty years. When we state we regularly mixed it in batches of sixty pounds the student will readily see that we have had at least some experience with it. As a remedy in colds, beginning of fevers, flu, hoarseness, sluggish circulation, colic, cramps, etc. We believe it has done more good than any other single preparation ever known to man.
>
> If this compound were kept in every home, and used as the occasion arose, there would be far less sickness. Give it freely in your practice and your patient will bless you. Look over the ingredients, and consider how it will clear canker, ease cramps and pains in the stomach and bowels, raise the heat of the body equalizing the circulation, and removing congestions. It is safe. It is effective. We have on numberless occasions given a cup of composition tea every hour as warm as the patient could drink it, until the patient has perspired freely, and after four or five doses have seen our patients in a free perspiration, thereby removing colds and febrile trouble.

20. Herbal eyewash combination.

    1 part Bayberry bark (Myrica cerifera)
    1 part Eyebright herb (Euphrasia officinalis)
    1 part Golden seal root (Hydrastis Canadensis)
    1 part Red raspberry leaves (Rubus idaeus)
    1/8 part Cayenne (Capsicum frutescens; C. minimum)

This formula is excellent for brightening and healing the eyes, and it is known to remove the cataracts and heavy film from the eyes. Using the powder or the extract, make into tea form and put into an eye cup made of glass. There will be a burning sensation when using the eyewash at first. This is due to the stimulating effect of the cayenne pepper and will do nothing but good to the eyes. Tip head back and apply the eye cup to eye. Exercise eye while doing this as though you were swimming under water. Do this three to six times a day and take two capsules or a cup of the tea, morning and evening. Source: Herbal Eyebright.

21. Herbal aid for female reproductive organs (female corrective).

    3 parts Golden seal root (Hydrastis Canadensis)
    1 part Blessed thistle (Cnicus benedictus)
    1 part Cayenne (Capsicum frutescens; C. minimum)
    1 part Cramp bark (Viburnum trilobum; V. opulus)
    1 part False unicorn root (Chamaelirium luteum)
    1 part Ginger (Zingiber officinalis)

1 part Red raspberry leaves (Rubus idaeus)
1 part Squaw vine (Mitchella repens)
1 part Uva ursi (Arctostaphylos uva-ursi)

This is an amazing combination of herbs to aid in rebuilding a malfunctioning reproductive system (uterus, ovaries, fallopian tubes, etc.). Over the years herbalists and patients have seen painful menstruations, heavy flowing, cramps, irregularity, etc. change to a painless menstrual period, good menstrual timing, and a new outlook on life by using these aids to readjust the malfunctioning areas.

Recommended dosage is one cup of tea or two capsules or 30 to 60 drops of glycerine based extract three times a day or more if desired, six days a week for as long as required to get the desired results. We have seen many severe cases who have had many years of suffering cleared up in ninety to 120 days. Some get relief sooner, some take longer—no two cases are alike. This is a food to rebuild the malfunctioning organs. Sources: Nu Fem, FEM.

22. An aid for the prostate area.

1 part Cayenne (Capsicum frutescens; C. minimum)
1 part Ginger (Zingiber officinalis)
1 part Golden seal root (Hydrastis Canadensis)
1 part Gravel root or queen of the meadow root (Eupatorium purpureum)
1 part Juniper berries (Juniperus communis)
1 part Marshmallow root (Althaea officinalis)
1 part Parsley root or herb (Petroselinum crispum)
1 part Uva ursi leaves (Arctostaphylos uva-ursi)
1 part Ginseng (Panax quinquefolius)

In case of malfunction we suggest this combination to assist the male. This will dissolve the stones that are in the kidneys, as well as clean out other sedimentation and infection in the prostate. Mix the powders and place in No. 0 capsules and take two or more morning and night, with parsley tea when possible. Sources: Prospallate, PR.

23. Hormone herbal combination.

1 part Black cohosh (Cimicifuga racemosa)
1 part Sarsaparilla (Smilax officinalis)
1 part Ginseng (Panax quinquefolius)
1 part Licorice (Glycyrrhiza glabra)
1 part False unicorn (Chamaelirium luteum)
1 part Holy thistle (Cnicus benedictus)
1 part Squaw vine (Mitchella repens)

These are natural herbal foods that are needed by both men and women at all ages. Being natural herbs, the human body can accept, assimilate and use these needed materials to produce estrogens and other hormones naturally. This formula will assist in rebuilding the weak malfunctioning areas and help keep the organs healthy so they can supply the proper amounts of hormones and estrogens themselves. The critical times when this formula is necessary are when entering puberty, during pregnancy, during the weeks and sometimes months following the birth of a child, and during menopause. Herbs are a natural food, so they do not have the negative side effects and after effects as are so evident in man-made synthetic drugs.

Whenever malfunction shows in the female reproductive areas, it is good to use formulas No. 21 and No. 23 together. For male reproductive problems use formulas No. 22 and No. 23 together. Sources: Changease, Fematean, Change-O-Life.

24. Herbal bolus.

1 part Squaw vine herb (Mitchella repens)
1 part Slippery elm bark (Ulmus rubra)
1 part Yellow dock root (Rumex crispus)
1 part Comfrey root (Symphytum officinale)
1 part Marshmallow root (Althaea officinalis)
1 part Chickweed herb (Stellaria media)
1 part Golden seal root (Hydrastis Canadensis)
1 part Mullein leaves (Verbascum thapsus)

Here is another excellent aid for both men and women who have problems in the reproductive areas. Boluses are made with healing herbs that feed malnourished organs and draw out the toxins and poisons making the malfunctioning area clean and healthy, so that scavengers like cysts, tumors, and cancerous conditions will not have waste material to survive on or live in. Herbalists who use this formula have found that these scavengers will release and be eliminated. The bolus spreads its herbal influence widely from the vagina or bowel through the entire urinary, genital and reproductive organs.

The herbs are to be used in powder form. Coconut butter should be melted down so that it will mix well with the herb powder. Mix a small quantity of this powder, and wet to pie dough consistency with coconut butter (which can be purchased from the drug store, health food store, or herb shop). Next, roll this mass between hands until you have a pencil-like bolus approximately the size of the middle finger in about inch-long pieces. Harden in a refrigerator. These are to be inserted into the vagina or rectum much the same as suppositories would be. It may be necessary to wear a sanitary napkin.

Insert upon retiring and leave in all night, six nights a week. The coconut butter melts at body temperature, leaving only the herbs, and these are easy to douche out. The following morning use the routine in formula #25. Sources: V.B., Herbal Bolus.

25. Prolapse formula.

6 parts	Oak bark (Quercus alba)
3 parts	Mullein herb (Verbascum thapsus)
4 parts	Yellow dock root (Rumex crispus)
3 parts	Walnut bark or leaves (Juglans nigra)
6 parts	Comfrey root (Symphytum officinale)
1 part	Lobelia (Lobelia inflata)
3 parts	Marshmallow root (Althaea officinalis)

To build and relieve prolapsed uterus, bowel, or other organs or for hemorrhoid problems, make this formula into a concentrated tea (simmer down to half its amount) and inject a cup or more with a syringe (while head down on a slant board) into vagina or rectum. Leave in as long as possible before voiding. When the tea is injected into the abdominal area and while on the slant board, knead and massage the pelvic and abdominal area to exercise muscles, so the herbal tea (food) will be assimilated into the organs. It is helpful to drink one fourth cup of tea concentrate in three fourths cup of distilled water three times a day or take 2 capsules three times a day. Sources: Yellow Dock Combination.

26. Anti-miscarriage formula. The anti-miscarriage formula consists of two herbs: 3 parts False unicorn root (Chamaelirium luteum) and 1 part Lobelia (Lobelia inflata). Unless otherwise specified, teas are always made with one teaspoon of herbs to a cup of distilled water if obtainable. If hemorrhaging starts during pregnancy, stay in bed, use a bed pan when needed, and use cup of the tea each hour until bleeding stops, then each waking hour for one day, while in bed as much as possible, and then three times in a day for three weeks. If bleeding continues instead of decreasing, see a doctor. Source: False Unicorn & Lobelia.

27. Prenatal formula.

1 part	Squaw vine (Mitchella repens)
1 part	Holy thistle (Cnicus benedictus)
1 part	Black cohosh (Cimicifuga racemosa)
1 part	Pennyroyal (Mentha pulegium)
1 part	False unicorn (Chamaelirium luteum)
1 part	Raspberry leaves (Rubus idaeus)
1 part	Lobelia (Lobelia inflata)

Using this tea (or two or three capsules) morning and evening is an aid in giving elasticity to the pelvic and vaginal area and strengthening the reproductive organs for easier delivery. The formula should be used only in the last six weeks before time of birth as follows: 1 capsule per day of the first week, 2 capsules per day the second week and 2 capsules three times a day from the third week on. Six capsules a day is the maximum dosage suggested. Source: Pre-Natal Tea, PN-6.

28. Bone, flesh, and cartilage (comfrey combination fomentation).

6 parts	Oak bark (Quercus species)
3 parts	Marshmallow root (Althaea officinalis)
3 parts	Mullein herb (Verbascum thapsus)
2 parts	Wormwood (Artemisia absinthium)
1 part	Lobelia (Lobelia inflata)
1 part	Skullcap (Scutellaria lateriflora)
6 parts	Comfrey root (Symphytum officinale)
3 parts	Walnut bark or leaves (Juglans nigra)
3 parts	Gravel root (Eupatorium purpureum)

This is an aid for malfunction in bone, flesh, cartilage, and is excellent for varicose veins, sprains, curvature of the spine, tremors, skin eruptions, pulled muscles, blood clots, calcium spurs, etc. Soak this herb combination in distilled water (at the rate of one ounce of combined herbs to a pint of distilled water), four to six hours, then simmer for thirty minutes, strain and reduce the liquid down to its volume by simmering over low heat. To retard spoilage of large batches, add vegetable glycerine. Example: one gallon of tea simmered (not boiled) down to two quarts and add one pint of glycerine.

Soak flannel, cotton or any natural material cloth in the solution—never use synthetics. Wrap the fomentation (soaked cloth) around the malfunctioning area and cover with plastic to keep it from drying out. Leave on all night six nights a week, week after week, until relief appears.

Severe cases: Drink cup of finished concentrated tea with 3/4 cup of distilled water three times a day (Also see formula No. 51). Source: BF&C.

29. Hair conditioner formula and procedure. To help restimulate hair growth, for two evenings massage scalp deeply with warm castor oil, apply hot, wet towel over head thirty minutes or more. Leave oil on all night. Next morning wash hair with pine tar soap or a good biodegradable soap and rinse. Wash again and rinse with tea made from this combination which contains equal parts of sagebrush, chaparral and yarrow. Massage well and leave tea in hair. The next two evenings do same procedure but use olive oil instead of castor oil and the next two evenings use wheat germ oil. Rest one night and repeat six days a week as needed. Use shoulder stands. Drink one or two tablespoons of wheat germ oil morning and night, and also drink cup of this tea made with distilled water, two times a day. Source: Desert Herb Combination.

30. Formula for arthritis-rheumatism.

4 parts	Brigham herb (Ephedra species)
6 parts	Hydrangea root (Hydrangea arborescens)
4 parts	Yucca (Yucca species)
4 parts	Chaparral (Larrea tridentata)
1 part	Lobelia (Lobelia inflata)
1 part	Burdock root (Arctium lappa)
1 part	Sarsaparilla (Smilax officinalis)
1 part	Wild lettuce (Lactuca scariola)
1 part	Valerian root (Valeriana officinalis)
1 part	Wormwood (Artemisia absinthium)
1 part	Cayenne (Capsicum frutescens; C. minimum)
1 part	Black cohosh (Cimicifuga racemosa)
3 parts	Black walnut (Juglans nigra)

This is a combination of herbs that detoxify, act as a solvent for the accepted but not assimilated calcium deposits, relieve pain, provide a rich supply of organic calcium that can be assimilated and useful, kill fungus and infection and give wonderful relief. This relief is not immediate because this type of condition requires rebuilding of the tissue, yet gradual relief can come, and full healing, if the program is followed faithfully. Take two capsules three times a day with a cup of Brigham tea or steam-distilled water. Use hot fomentations of this formula in tea form and formula No. 28 called bone, flesh, and cartilage over extremely painful or crippled areas. Also drink one or two quarts of kidney bean pod tea daily. In addition for relief, an external application of formula No. 44 is recommended. If one uses these aids yet continues with an improper diet, one may get some help but not as much. Remember the teachings for years have been—"No healing in this condition." We are giving you hope if you will follow through with these formulas and the mucusless diet. Sources: AR-1, Yucca AR.

31. Infection formula.

4 parts	Plantain (Plantago major)
4 parts	Black walnut (Juglans nigra)
4 parts	Golden seal root (Hydrastis Canadensis)
2 parts	Bugle weed (Lycopus americanus; L. virginicus)
1 part	Marshmallow root (Althaea officinalis)
1 part	Lobelia (Lobelia inflata)

This wonderful formula kills infection, clears toxins from the lymph system, and is a natural infection fighter. Dose 2 capsules three times a day or make a tea (empty 2 capsules into a cup and pour in boiling hot water). Sources: INF Combination, IF.

32. Kelp combination.

1 part	Parsley (Petroselinum crispum)
4 parts	Watercress (Nasturtium officinale)
5 parts	Kelp (Laminaria saccharina)
1 part	Irishmoss (Chondrus crispus)
1 part	Romaine lettuce (Lactuca sativa)
1 part	Turnip tops (Brassica rapa)
1 part	Iceland moss (Cetraria islandica)

This is an aid for the thyroid and assisting glands. These herbs assist in controlling metabolism and give herbal feeding to the thyroid glands to help them do their job more efficiently. This is a very fine glandular aid. For additional help, use with formula No. 12. Source: T Caps.

33. Antispasmodic tincture (also see page 399).

1 part	Skullcap herb (Scutellaria lateriflora)
1 part	Lobelia (Lobelia inflata)
1 part	Cayenne (Capsicum frutescens; C. minimum)
1 part	Valerian root (Valeriana officinalis)
1 part	Skunk cabbage (Symplocarpus foetidus)
1 part	Myrrh gum (Commiphora myrrha)
1 part	Black cohosh (Cimicifuga racemosa)

To be used in cases of convulsions, fainting, cramps, delirium, tremors, hysteria, etc. also good for pyorrhea, mouth sores, coughs, throat infections, tonsillitis, etc. Dose to one teaspoon to glass of steam distilled water as a gargle and use until throat clears, also take one teaspoon in steam distilled water morning and evening. Source: ANTSP.

34. B and B tincture.

1 part	Black cohosh (Cimicifuga racemosa)
1 part	Blue cohosh (Calophyllum thalictroides)
1 part	Blue vervain (Verbena hastata)
1 part	Skullcap (Scutellaria lateriflora)
1 part	Lobelia (Lobelia inflata)

Used to aid in nervous conditions, sore throat, hiccups, restore malfunctioning motor nerves, assist in adjusting poor equilibrium and hearing, and a great blessing to epileptics. Massage into the medulla (base of skull), and upper cervicals, follow instructions in formula No. 14, and take six to ten drops in a little water or juice two or three times a day. Source: B & B.

35. Formula for relief of minor pain. This is a tincture or tea consisting of equal

parts of wild lettuce (Lactuca scariola) and valerian (Valeriana officinalis). It is to be taken orally or massaged externally as relief of minor pain. It is a natural sedative, quiet and soothing to the nerves. Source: Wild Lettuce & Valerian.

36. Asthma formula. An excellent asthma syrup—very helpful to expel mucus from the respiratory system. Can be used for sore throats and mucus. Excellent for fighting toxins. This is made of extracts of comfrey, mullein and garlic, and vegetable glycerine. Recommended use—a teaspoon or more, as required, as often as needed. Source: Comfrey-Mullein-Garlic syrup.

37. A fine, old fashioned combination for coughs. Made up with fresh onion juice, licorice, honey and vegetable glycerine. Recommended use—a teaspoon or more, as required, as often as needed. Source: Herbal Cough.

38. Drawing ointment. For use externally on old ulcers, tumors, boils, warts, skin cancers, hemorrhoids, excellent for burns and as a healing agent. This is made with chaparral, comfrey, red clover blossoms, pine tar, mullein, beeswax, plantain, olive oil, mutton tallow, chickweed and poke root (see page 354). Source: Black Ointment.

39. Healing ointment. Made of comfrey, marshmallow, marigold, beeswax and oils, this is an antiseptic to be used on lesions, eczema, dry skin, poison ivy, abrasions, burns, hemorrhoids, bruises and swellings. Very soothing to inflamed surfaces. Good to have on hand at all times. Source: CMM.

40. Chickweed ointment. This is made of chickweed herb and beeswax and oils. Excellent for eczema and/or other skin infections, sores, burning, itchy skin or genitals, swollen testes, acne, hives, also for ulceration of mouth and throat. This is a wonderful healing ointment. Source: Chickweed ointment.

41. Nose ointment.

1 part Oil of spearmint (Mentha spicata)
1 part Oil of peppermint (Mentha piperita)
4 parts Vaseline (petroleum jelly)

This is a natural anti-histamine. Apply to the inside of nose when it is congested, dry, sensitive or chapped. Source: Nose ointment.

42. Catnip and fennel tincture. A blessing for infants. A fine combination for colic, teething pain, flatulence, spasms, etc. Use a few drops, or as much as needed when desired (available in alcohol and glycerine based extract). Source: Catnip & Fennel Tincture, Kid-E-Kol, Kol-X.

43. Black walnut tincture. This is one of the best known remedies for fungus. Use externally and apply frequently. Source: Black Walnut tincture.

44. Cayenne salve. This penetrating salve contains olive oil, cayenne, oil of wintergreen, pure distilled mint crystals and other herb oils, in a beeswax base. It is excellent for stiff necks, sore muscles, headaches, pain, stiff joints, arthritis, etc. Source: Deep Heat Balm.

45. Antiseptic tincture. This is our first-aid tincture. Good for infection, both external or internal. The formula is: oak bark, golden seal root, myrrh, comfrey, garlic and capsicum, in a grain alcohol base. Source: X-Ceptic.

46. Heavy mineral formula: Contains bugleweed, yellow dock, and lobelia. This is the herbal combination for combating pollution, both external and internal. It helps draw out minerals, drugs, and other pollutants trapped in our system. The dosage is two #0 capsules daily in conjunction with 6 #0 chaparral capsules taken three times a day. (This formula including the chaparral, is available in extract form.) Every other day bathe in 1 to 3 pounds of Epsom salts in a tub of hot water. The bathing routine should continue for three weeks then rest a week but continue taking the herbs. Source: Bugleweed combination.

47. Adrenals formula. Contains mullein, lobelia, Siberian ginseng, gotu kola, hawthorn berries, cayenne and ginger. As this formula corrects any imbalance in the adrenal glands it also compensates for any stress placed on the heart. Source: Adrenetone, Adr-NL.

48. Colitis formula. Contains marshmallow, slippery elm, comfrey root, lobelia, ginger and wild yam. This formula is for relief of colitis, and should be used in conjunction with the lower bowel formula and the mucusless diet. Source: CC.

49. Ulcer formula. Contains bayberry, chickweed, slippery elm and mullein. This formula is designed to soothe the discomforts caused from stomach ulcers. It should be taken with hops or chamomile tea. Please note; to cure an ulcer, take three teaspoons of cayenne pepper per day. This cayenne may be mixed in water or tomato juice. It is recommended that you start with only 1/8 teaspoon three times a day, then gradually work up to one teaspoon three time a day. Source: ULC.

50. Anti-gas formula. Contains fennel, wild yam, catnip, ginger, peppermint, spearmint, papaya and lobelia. This formula was designed to relieve flatulence. Source: AT-GS.

51. Bone, flesh and cartilage ointment. Convenient form of formula No. 28. It is made into an ointment using an olive oil and beeswax base. Apply formula No. 41 after this for better penetration and quicker healing. Source: BF&C ointment.

52. Anti-plague. The best remedy for colds, flu, or any communicable disease. This formula strengthens and stimulates your immune system and should be used as a tonic and preventative at the dosage of 1 tablespoon of syrup per day. If

infected, the dosage changes to one tablespoon every hour. Anti plague syrup contains fresh garlic juice, apple cider vinegar, glycerine, honey, fresh comfrey root, wormwood, lobelia, marshmallow root, oak bark, black walnut bark, mullein leaf, skullcap and uva ursi. Source: ANT-PLG.

53. Cold Sore Relief. This formula, in extract form, is taken orally two droppers full 3 times a day and applied topically. Contents: fresh golden seal root, garlic and skullcap. Source: CSR.

54. Immune stimulating formula. Designed to enhance the body's ability to prevent the spread of bacteria and viruses. It consists of echinacea, calendula and red clover blossoms (available in alcohol extract or glycerine based extract for children). Sources: Imunacea, Kid-E-Mune, Immunaid.

55. Immune calming formula. Designed to calm yet strengthen the body's immune responses. Many times we believe that we are allergic to certain foods, plants or animals, but in reality our immune system may be just overreacting. This simple combination of marshmallow root and astragalus has made life easier for those who suffer from allergies, hayfever, asthma, rheumatoid arthritis or any hyperactive immune response. Sources: Imucalm, Kid-E-Soothe.

56. Memory formula.

3 parts Blue vervain (Verbena hastata)
3 parts Gotu kola (Centella asiatica)
3 parts Blessed thistle (Cnicus benedictus)
1 part Brigham tea (Ephedra species)
1 part Ginkgo (Ginkgo biloba)
1 part Cayenne (Capsicum frutescens)
1 part Ginger root (Zingiber officinalis)
1 part Lobelia (Lobelia inflata)

A great combination of old fashioned herbs used to cleanse, build and increase circulation to the brain. Source: MEM.

57. Vitamin and Mineral formula. Nature balanced, whole food vitamin and mineral supplement. This combination of alfalfa, barley, and wheat grass (flash dried extract powder), dandelion, kelp, purple dulse, spirulina, Irish moss, rose hips, beet, nutritional yeast, cayenne, blue violet, oatstraw, carrot juice powder, and ginger is an organic source of vitamins and minerals that are easy to assimilate because they are whole foods. Source: Vitalerbs.

58. Formula for sinus congestion. This very powerful formula consists of Brigham tea, horseradish, and cayenne. For immediate relief of sinus pressure due to cold or allergies, use 20 drops (1/4 teaspoon) in 2 ounces of hot water. May be taken every 30 minutes. Source: Ephedratean.

59. Rubefacient ointment. As the name indicates, this balm brings blood circulation to the surface of the skin causing it to turn red. Used to relieve tension and pressure. Great for tension headache or sinus pressure. Use sparingly as this formula is strong. Contains: olive oil and natural oils of cassia, eucalyptus, cajeput, pure menthol and camphor crystals and other fragrant natural oils. Source: Sen Sei balm.

60. Greens combination. A blend of alfalfa, barley grass, and wheat grass herbs grown organically in virgin soil and separated from urban agricultural pollutants by the same mountains that provide its pure source of water. These herbs reduce acidity, provide needed chlorophyll and wholesome nutrients to the body. Source: Jurassic Green.

61. Energy combination. Rather than being an energy jolt that shocks the body, this formulation of Siberian ginseng, bee pollen, licorice root, gotu kola, Brigham tea, yerba mate, and ginger root provides energy and vitality through wholesome nutrition. Source: Bee Power.

CHAPTER 16

THE REGENERATIVE DIET

The ideal diet consists of natural food, eaten in moderation and simplicity. The fruits are especially good for cleansing the system after your night's fast during sleep. They will satisfy the need and craving for sweetness. The green herbs of the garden, used fresh and tender in salads and chewed well, will build strength and vitality in the body tissues. The bulbs, roots, and starches in grains will provide fire and heat for the body, but these should be eaten only as needed for those who work hard physically. The sprouted seeds are nourishing tonics to restore the body constitution and in resisting ill health. The nuts of the trees will provide the nutrient "meat" (protein) for man and will season other foods. The culinary herbs will provide variety, flavor, and seasoning. And in the whole of your daily activities, you can achieve a varied and harmoniously-blended whole: fresh air, sunshine, exercise, work, play, song, prayer, reading, meditation, recreation, etc.

More people have died of malnutrition and constipation than from all the wars, automobile accidents, earthquakes and fires to date. Yet you seldom hear of it, and the poor, suffocating and victimized organ that gives out is generally given the official blame. When we speak of constipation, we usually think of only the lower bowel area, but this is only a small part of it. The entire body is composed of flexible systems of tubing, much like the intestines. This tubing varies in size, some of which is even smaller than a hair. The Great Planner equipped the body structure with these rubber-like pipes of all kinds and sizes, from the largest intestine, which can expand to a terrific size, down to the arteries, veins, and minute capillaries. Though the capillaries are smaller than hairs, they are perfectly constructed and pliable; but when they are not properly cared for, they age like an old rubber hose and eventually break at the weak spots. Varicosity is a good example of this, as the life-line gets clogged up like lime inside household plumbing.

Toxic matter can form a hard lining in the bowel so that the peristaltic action ceases, and this solid shield inhibits peristaltic action upon the fecal materials. We have seen this mucus lining taken from patients that appeared like hard, black plastic, shaped to the curvature of the colon walls.

As you progress in this program, do not be surprised to see some of these linings coming from your body also. Usually a person takes little notice of constipation and, instead of getting at the real cause, just starts using laxatives, enemas, bulk and volume remedies to break a passage through for temporary relief. When constipation goes throughout the entire body, it may build up congestion in one area. The discomfort will increase until a peak of pain is reached, and this is really the nature of what we term "disease." Do not allow yourself to become confused with thousands of seemingly-sophisticated medicinal terms; just remember that there is only one disease, and that is systemic constipation. This mucus constipation will back up not only in the arterial structure, but also into the cells and tissues; and it can become so severe that it will eventually bring the entire system to a standstill.

Where does all of this mucus and waste come from? It comes from those things that we eat with our eyes and taste-buds, from what we put into the body and incorrectly call food.

Some people's taste buds cause problems when they are changing to a health-building diet. Other people hesitate because of fear. We have heard persons say, "Why, I enjoy the type of food I am used to, and I would rather risk ill health than change." Well, at that moment, they have made the choice of living to eat, instead of eating to live. The average individual has grown up on the "great American diet" of meat, potatoes, and gravy, and may panic at the very thought of missing a meal—let alone fasting a few days—he is deathly afraid that he will starve to death! The truth is that very few persons ever starve to death, but die first from fear and panic. Some people have gone over a hundred days without food and over two weeks without water and lived, so missing a few meals cannot hurt you. Instead, fasting wisely can truly benefit you. Some sacrifice usually accompanies getting something really worthwhile, and though abstinence from food or from indulgence in over-eating may seem like a sacrifice and a burden, the supposed "sacrifice" will be realized as a blessing instead after the goal has been reached.

Proper low heating of some fruits and vegetables will bring out the natural sweetness. Notice how cabbage or cauliflower tastes sweeter after low-heating or steaming a short while. If overcooked, it becomes yellow and strong-tasting. There is a savory sweetness in squash, pumpkin, and apples when baked just right and not too much. And even the sour lemon can be "ripened" with dry heat to be as sweet as an orange, yet when it is heated a bit more, it will turn bitter. The reason for heating foods is to get the benefit and value of the natural grape sugar.

Softened foods are easier on delicate digestive systems. And it will be much easier for those who are culturally-accustomed to eating cooked foods for so many years.

FASTING

The "no breakfast" procedure:
So many times people say, "But breakfast is my main meal; start the day with a big breakfast and you start the day off right." This "big breakfast" idea is pushed hard by the breakfast-food, egg, milk, and coffee merchants, and some of their advertising plays on emotional fears.

But this is not always true, as better health is found in countries where people have the custom of not eating breakfast, except maybe a warm cup of liquid, and the first meal of the day is eaten at noon. There are even places where the evening meal is the first and only one, as the partaking of food is considered a privilege only after the work has been done and the right to eat is earned. So as you try the "no breakfast" experiment, the first few days may be a little rough, with headaches, light-headiness, grumpiness, etc. This will only last a few days and you will see great improvement in health. People who gain experience in fasting realize that occasionally feeling hungry is really only a *feeling;* you can become accustomed to that feeling, knowing that it doesn't signal starvation.

Some health teachers champion the fast as a cure for anything and everything, or that fruit alone will answer your health problems, or juice therapy alone, or all raw fruits and vegetables. But in your properly-balanced program, some of the food will be raw, while some of it will be steamed, baked or low-heated.

A bodily famine is not required:
Periodic fasting is good to cleanse the body, but a bodily famine is not required for cleansing. A cross-country runner would be committing suicide to make a grueling competitive twenty or thirty mile run without preparation and so it is with the fast; a person must work up gradually to the longer fasts.

UNWHOLESOME SUBSTANCES

Vegetation is the source of nourishment for all animal life. Some of the birds, animals—and men—live on the carcasses of other higher animal life, but these carcasses received their health and vitality from vegetation. This is second-hand or secondary food has lost a lot of its value, but its nutrient value can be traced back to the original or primary food source, vegetation. The bird that eats the insect gets its real food value from the tree, plant or shrub that the insect has fed on, and not from the insect itself.

MEAT AND ANIMAL PROTEIN

The great dietitian Moses warned against eating the carnivorous animal types, for these have strong odoriferous meat from concentrated uremic acids and other poisons that result from their secondary diet of flesh, and this carries the essence of death. High amounts of uremic acid lead to gout, rheumatism, and bursitis.

You may believe that meat and milk are absolute dietary necessities; most people react immediately, "Yes, but what about protein?" And where do most people go to get their main source of protein? From the lower animal kingdom, steaks from the carcasses of slaughtered animals. And where does the meat-providing cow obtain its protein? From eating grass. These animals, when left to select their food in the wilds or on the open range, are mono-eaters of herbs, and green vegetation. The cow gets from grass, the herbs, all of the necessary materials for hard hooves, hair, horns, teeth, hide, muscle (which people eat), blood and life itself.

When the cow suckles her baby calf, she does not drink milk to make milk; it all comes directly from the green vegetation. So when this cow is killed to get the meat for protein, you are getting what the animal ate, only second-handed, and you also eat the uremic acid poisons and the fear vibrations which penetrate the animal when it is killed. Then your system must work many times harder to wrest the value from the meat than you would by going to the original food source in nature's vegetation. It is like wearing out your expensive ore-processing machinery on low grade ore, when you could get the more precious metals from readily-accessible higher grade deposits, with less work, and with less wear and tear on the equipment.

Recent research shows that meat contains bacteria and viruses which can undermine your health, eventually making you very sick. In 1993, you might have heard of the deaths caused by E. coli. organisms in improperly cooked hamburger in fast-food establishments and from private sources. These are only the publicized stories; there are many, many more illnesses caused by meat that no one ever hears about. Meat herds and dairy herds are commonly given "by-pass" protein, which contains ground-up beef products, chicken feathers, offal, and waste products, and other materials. This feed directly assaults the naturally-vegetarian cow, and produces various diseases, including "mad-cow" syndrome, which occurs throughout the world in meat and dairy herds, and is now beginning to occur in man. Much of the meat in the United States is imported, and if it is inspected at all, it is only given a brief "look-and-smell" inspection. So much of our meat is imported that only a small percentage is even inspected. For those who think chicken is a better meat than beef, tests now show that at least 50% of all slaughtered poultry contains significant contamination with salmonella.

Dr. Christopher was a member of the Church of Jesus Christ of Latter-day Saints (Mormons), and he frequently quoted references from its scriptures. He wrote that the Lord has given us the key concerning meat in verse thirteen of the Word of Wisdom (Doctrine and Covenants, section 89): "And it is pleasing unto me that they [meat] should not be used, only in times of winter, or of cold, or famine." During the cold and winter, the flesh from animal cadavers does not rot quite as quickly in the long herbivorous intestines of man as it will in hot weather—but still, it is only to be used as an emergency measure, as a secondary resort, for even in cold or winter, we are admonished in verse twelve that such should be used "sparingly." If you would at least begin to follow this portion of the inspired counsel, you will be on the way to eliminating the chief cause of disease in your body. Your intake of uremic acid and other toxic poisons will be reduced, giving the body less work to do. And that will make energy available that can be put to work in healing and regenerating the body, instead of spent struggling, on a heavy diet, for survival alone.

Avoid the use of blood:
Throughout the Holy Scriptures, prophets have taught and warned against the use of blood, that it is the soul or life of the animal, and it should be spilled upon the ground. If all the blood were out of the meat, it would be a different color; the tissue, muscle, and the flesh without blood is colorless, with a grayish tinge. Many people will say, "But who would even think of using blood as a food?" The old European blood puddings are still very popular, even in some locations in the Americas. Certain sausages and liver rolls contain blood. Not too long ago in the news we heard that a number of meat packing plants were using fat and other generally discarded parts of the animal carcass to make hamburger, and that large amounts of blood were being added for coloring. A few of these concerns were caught, but how many others have not been caught and are still selling this over the counter?

A death-carrying food:
All animals can sense death, and when an animal is driven into the stock yards for slaughter, it senses that death is close by. When the butcher's mallet hits the death blow, fear is carried by the nerves to every tissue in the system. Thoughts are real substantive things for man or animal, and these fears remain as poisons in the cadaver of the beast. So when you buy the meat, you not only take on the vibrations of death and constantly decomposing tissue, but you also take on fear.

It is generally accepted that the higher the uremic acid in beef, the richer the flavor, yet these toxins and poisons in meat are a main contributor to gout, rheumatism, bursitis, and many other mucoid ailments. The fat of the animal is the hardest part for the body to eliminate, and Moses in particular condemns the use of fat. Notice that very few animals will eat fat at all. Again, the only value in meat is what the particular animal has received from eating green herbs, and this is why the range animal is so much better than the stockyard-fattened beef.

MILK AND DAIRY PRODUCTS

Milk, the infant's life-line:
Milk is a very jealous food, to be used only at the correct time. It is intended to feed the infant mammal. A newborn babe is equipped with red corpuscle-making facilities in the bone marrow which is ready to go to work immediately, but there are at first no gastric juices present to digest solid foods such as protein or starch. Consequently, a baby must have predigested food. Nature amply provides for each stage and condition of life, so the mother eats and digests the food, which is transferred via the blood stream into the mammary glands or breasts where only the red corpuscles are filtered out; the infant is actually given an oral blood transfusion by the mother.

This is a perfect arrangement, since the child and mother are of similar flesh and blood, the vibration of the milk is compatible with the baby. The first feedings from the breast, colostrum, were provided by the Lord as a mild laxative that cleans out the baby's bowels and eliminates the tar-like black substance—meconium—that previously could not be evacuated. Man never will synthetically match this perfect prescription that God has provided for the newborn suckling baby. Many doctors have confidently said: "Oh, we will feed the baby the first day or two while you rest up and your milk is coming in, for all you have to offer is this watery substance." But God provides colostrum to cleanse the body, and then the mammary gland automatically switches to a light milk formula, as this is all the baby needs at first, and then the milk becomes richer feeding by feeding as the baby grows older.

Many doctors have placed their puny knowledge above God's and have advised: "Oh, don't bother nursing your baby; we have far better formulas than what comes from the breast." "Your milk is too thin and blue; you cannot feed this baby." The poor little fellow is then put onto an inorganic, man-made concoction that is really not fit for man nor beast—or the mother is told to give the babe plenty of cow's milk (which suits the dairy interests just fine).

Cow's milk was made for baby calves and not for humans; it has over 20 times more casein in it than can be utilized properly by humans. So right off, the newborn begins life in a struggle, with a mucus and acid-forming diet, which produces those big, fat, roly-poly babies about which people say, "Oh, how nice and healthy!"

The natural milk from the mother is the best food for the young infant, alkaline and nonmucus-forming; and if the mother is eating properly and leaving harmful substances such as coffee, liquor, drugs and tobacco alone it will build good teeth, healthy tissue, and strong bones. The baby's body will accept this perfect alkaline diet, needing nothing else, until it cuts its eye teeth and its stomach teeth, usually at 18 to 20 months of age. When these teeth come through, it is nature's signal that the gastric juices have started to flow, and as these begin to mix with the milk, it now becomes acid to the baby. From that time on, the milk will have the opposite and unhealthy effect. It forms into mucus, causing sinus problems, allergies, colds, tooth deterioration, etc. So at this time, the child must be taken off milk and put onto an alkaline diet; the mucusless fruits, vegetables, and juices. Many babies have been suffocated as a result of adults forcing mucus-forming foods and improper formulas down them before they were equipped with the digestive juices to handle them. These harmful substances include bread, meats, and baby cereal foods that are so commonly recommended by medicinal practitioners long before the baby has even a fighting chance.

No milk after weaning time:
The human is the only mammal on the face of the earth that tolerates milk after weaning, that is, with the exception of our domestic animals that we have led astray. The cow on the range will kick the calf away when it is time for weaning; and man is so disgusted to see a mature cow getting milk from another one that he shoots her, but he goes home for lunch and sits down to a big pitcher of milk. All wildlife, like the range cow, have the natural instinct that tells them that milk is not a proper food after weaning time.

Pasteurization renders milk inassimilable:
About 1850 Louis Pasteur discovered a process called "pasteurization," by heating a substance such as milk around 140-145° F. for one-half hour so that the so-called "pathogen" bacteria were destroyed. Of course new discoveries have varied the temperature and time elements, but the general principle remains the same. Thus, while these "pathogenic" organisms are well taken care of, so are the beneficial bacteria that are so necessary for proper digestion and assimilation.

Here is what you can do yourself to compare the processed milk with unprocessed milk as a test for vitality. Take a glass bottle of fresh "raw" milk (non-pasteurized) and a glass bottle of pasteurized milk, and set these both in the sun for a day or two and carefully observe the results. The raw milk will clabber or go sour. This is still a healthy condition and is not so mucus-forming in this state, and though it is not our recommended first-class type of food, it is still a product with life in it. The other bottle containing the pasteurized milk, however, will not sour or clabber—it will only do one thing, rot. The stench is horrible, and the rotted milk goes from green to black.

When you drink pasteurized milk, you are taking a dead product into the body. Raw milk is at least a live food. As for other dairy products, cottage cheese is almost free from mucous and can be used, but not in excessive amounts, while butter is a mucus-former and is hard to digest. Yogurt is also mucus-forming and should be avoided for better health.

Swam in his problems:
A young man came as a patient to Dr. Christopher when his office was in Salt Lake. He was not feeling well, but the medical doctors had not been able to help

him, so he finally came to Christopher's for help. He was only 18 years of age and had suffered 17 broken bones, one at a time, and at this early age had false teeth. This young man had grown up on a dairy farm in Smithfield, Utah (a dairy center), and as he said, he "practically swam in milk," for it was his main food during most of his life. And if lots of milk was supposed to make good teeth and strong bones, with the amount of milk he had consumed, he should have been "king for the year," but here he was, a really sick young man.

Her own beautiful teeth:
One day a lady brought three of her married daughters into Dr. Christopher's office to teach them concerning milk. She told how two of these ladies were very good little girls and had drunk their milk faithfully and would at times ask for more, but she had one that was not so cooperative and would not drink her milk, and in fact would almost vomit when the milk was forced upon her, until the family finally gave up with the threat that she would be the family weakling and lose all her teeth! Well, these three little girls grew up, and here they sat in our office as young women, the two good little milk drinkers with false teeth and the one that could not tolerate milk had all her own very beautiful teeth. One of the ladies was a bit perplexed and said, "But we must drink milk when nursing a baby!" And our answer was: "Do you give a cow milk so she can nurse her calf? No she gets the milk from the grass alone—and you have a good choice of green foods to pick from."

Easier than amputation:
A young man came to Dr. Christopher's office in Olympia, Washington to ask for help. He had played professional soccer for years, and his shin bone areas were so roughed up that they had been raw for several years. All types of treatments had been tried, and failed. Dr. Christopher told him that it was evident from the sinus inflations on the nose and brows that he was a milk fiend, and that he would take no patients unless they discontinued using milk completely.

This young man was so badly addicted (and you can become a milk addict) that they did not care to work with him. He immediately became angry and stated that he did drink large quantities of milk and that he would not quit for any reason, as it was good food as far as he was concerned. Dr. Christopher told him that he would welcome him back when this problem got so bad that it would mean amputation and he was frightened enough to follow our prescribed instructions. And with that he stormed off.

But he was back in a few weeks, scared to death, because he had been told by his surgeon that one of the legs would have to come off, and maybe the other one also. He was now ready to do anything we said in order to save his legs. And within six weeks those sores were completely healed and he was a happier, healthier man by far, without the milk. Weaning from milk and using herbs were much easier than amputation!

EGGS

A sickly-looking type of people:
Dr. Christopher often commented that vegetarians often were sickly-looking, extra thin and gaunt, overly-heavy and sallow, accompanied by a forced gaiety that has not been very good advertising for the vegetarian program in general. Watch the type of people in a health store. A large majority of them appear as though they should look elsewhere if it is health they are looking for. And why?

There are many good products in a health store, but there are also a lot of over-advertised man-made money makers. Many people who want to be vegetarian wrongly think that all there is to being a vegetarian is not using meat. Without the health store, they would probably be in even worse condition. When you change your diet, you need to find out what your particular body requires.

Trying to replace meat, many vegetarians buy protein that is mostly man-made and too highly concentrated. All the protein that a clean body needs can be derived from fresh fruits, vegetables, grains, nuts, and seeds in the natural and organic state. Otherwise, the extra protein becomes burdensome work and waste in the body. A weight-lifter who uses great amounts of protein may temporarily build large muscles, but if he quits exercising, this type of protein will not hold its firmness in the body, whereas the muscles that are built from protein of herbs and fruit will hold their own and remain firm and in good tone.

Many "vegetarians" still feel that they should eat eggs and milk products when they stop eating meat. This can make for a sickly condition. The average novice vegetarian turns to eggs, because they are easy to prepare and considered "the perfect protein." Eggs are far too concentrated in protein and are highly constipating; the mucus that is formed is far more gluey and sticky than meat. To test the excellence of egg whites as glue, drop a carton and when dry, try to get the egg shells loose from the carton. Eggs are one of the main contributors to arthritis, kidney stones and gall stones. Dr. Christopher commented that many of his patients, when told to give up eggs, replied, "Oh, that won't be hard because each time I eat eggs the pain flares up and gets worse in my joints and muscles." Dr. Christopher taught that the hard boiled egg is the least harmful of any of the forms in which it is used, but that is still quite harmful when used too often.

Often times true vegans (those that eat no animal products of any kind) do not have access to a wholesome range of organic fruits, vegetables, grains, nuts, and seeds or do not take the time to enjoy them and can suffer thereby. Things are changing, however, and in most cities, you can find wonderful organic produce and vegetarian restaurants that will serve vegan meals, as well as those rich in vegetables and grains and containing a minimum of dairy products. Even government dietary recommendations are emphasizing whole grains, fruits and vegetables, and minimizing animal foods.

SPICY CONDIMENTS, SALT

The fine art of culinary camouflage:
Much food in the average person's diet would not be very palatable in its raw state, and most people would probably prefer to go hungry rather than be forced to eat it. For this reason, the fine art of seasoning with spicy condiments was developed. This art was especially useful prior to refrigeration, to hide the putrefaction of meats. The average heavy meat-eater does not like the taste of good ripe fruits or salads. The taste bud is such a demanding little organ, and gourmets tell us that by tasting the soup in a restaurant they can tell the age of the chef, because the older he gets the more salt he must add to get the flavor through while sampling. So with improper diet and salt, the taste buds become more and more dulled, eventually becoming paralyzed as the years progress.

Rebuild the taste buds:
Each morning as our children (ages 2 and 3) were growing up, we would give them orange juice made from organically grown, tree-ripened oranges that we generally had shipped to us from the Garlets Citrus Groves in Florida. One particular morning when we had run out of these oranges, we went down to a fruit market not far from our lodging and bought some beautiful "orange" oranges (the tree-ripened oranges do not look the same as those with the color added). As usual, we had breakfast when the children awakened, and started the meal with the fresh orange juice. Nothing had been said of running out of oranges and substituting the other type, but as the children eagerly grasped their glasses for a drink of their favorite beverage, they both made faces of disgust and pushed away the juice. An adult that has used a lot of salt would not have discerned much difference in the juice, whereas the bright new taste buds of children and youth (or the clean rebuilt ones of the vegetarian) can notice the difference immediately.

STARCHY FOODS

Rice—temperamental and capricious:
If you have had much experience in preparing rice dishes, you will know what a temperamental grain this is. If it is not cooked just right, you will have a sticky glue which will be one of the worst mucus-forming foods there is. Brown rice is better than the white or polished rice, but we still will not recommend it very highly; it adheres to the venous structure and capillaries as do all other mucus-type foods.

The cold cereals or "Pied Piper" foods:
The cold cereals are dead, and they are mucus- and toxin-forming. Besides, they are loaded with inorganic "enrichments," many of which are derived from cancer-forming coal tar, plus many poisonous additives to insure longer shelf life for the commercial interests. These are rightfully labeled as "Pied Piper" foods, as they are leading children (and adults) cheerfully down the road to ill health and physical ruin.

FOODS FOR THE HEALTHY

Dried beans, peas, lentils, etc.
For people who are seriously ill, dried beans, peas, and other lentils are far too rich in protein. When mixed with other foods they can almost be as detrimental as meat and eggs. Of this group, the soybean is the best, but the proper use of any of these would be to consume only the sprouts and throw the harmful seed itself away. To best use the legumes, soak with several changes of water until the beans are semi-sprouted, then low heat for ten to twelve hours. The peanut, though a tuber, is also mucus-forming.

However, for the generally healthy person, the legumes are a great addition to the mucusless diet. Soak them overnight in cool water, drain the water, and then low-heat for 12-15 hours. You can also soak them, drain, and allow them to just begin to sprout, then low-heat. You can puree or mash pinto beans cooked this way to make delicious refried beans; just heat in a pan coated with a little oil. Salt to taste; you can season with chili powder, garlic powder, cayenne, etc. Serve with cooked grains, fresh salad things, and hot salsa. *The Farm Vegetarian Cookbook* suggests a brewer's yeast-based "cheese" which is nice on top of the beans. Use any kinds of cooked beans to create casseroles with grains, vegetables, and seasonings. Soymilk is a wonderful substitute for milk to make sauces. You can also puree tofu and season it to make sauces for your casseroles. Try tomato sauces too. Look at your regular casserole recipes and substitute whole food ingredients to make familiar comfort foods.

Potatoes—the pigs are better fed:
Most of the nutrients of potatoes are in the peeling and approximately 1/4 inch under it, so if you peel potatoes, be sure to use the peeling for vegetable broth. One lecturer told of a small village in Nova Scotia where all of the adults were found dead from scurvy and beriberi, but the little children were found alive. The main food was potatoes, and the parents peeled and boiled them and threw the skins or peelings away. The small children who hungrily picked up and ate the peelings survived, while the adults received no food value and died.

The peeled potato serves as a basis for the great American diet, and with the peelings thrown to the pigs, they are better fed than ourselves. The best way to prepare potatoes is to bake them till soft, serving with some pure olive oil, salt and pepper, etc. This can be the basis for many a vegetarian meal; it is healthy, satisfying, and easy to do. Sweet potatoes, however, are far better than Irish potatoes—they are less starchy and less mucus-forming.

Nuts, a highly energizing food:
Nuts are rich in protein and high in fats. They are most beneficial as a winter food or where you must work hard physically. They should be used sparingly with some type of dried sweet fruits or honey, and thoroughly chewed together to aid in digesting them. Do not use nuts with juicy fruits, because the water of the

fruit and the fat in the nuts do not mix. When eating nuts, chew them so finely that no small pieces are left and only a smooth, slick liquid enters the throat.

WHEATGRASS
(Triticum species; GRAMINEAE)

Common name:
Wheat grass.

Identifying characteristics:
This is the grass of the common, hard or soft, cereal-type wheat that has been a staple food of man for many, many centuries.

Part used:
The tender blade (the first 5-7 inches before the first joint appears) of soil-grown wheat.

Therapeutic action:
Nutritive, tonic.

Dr. Ann Wigmore quotes the late Dr. G. H. Earp Thomas, a great soil scientist of New Jersey, in her book, *Why Suffer?:*

> Wheatgrass grown in good soil up to about six inches in height absorbs well-balanced nourishment from the sunlight, air, and earth and its LIVE minerals, LIVE vitamins and LIVE trace elements have a total acid content that comes very close to the pH 7.4 which symbolizes healthy human blood. This indicates an extraordinary connection between the green blood of the wheat grass and the red blood of the healthy human bloodstream and shows that the distribution and the amounts of nutrients come very close to being identical.

Medicinal uses:
Arthritis, bruises, burns, cancer, constipation, emphysema, gangrene, leukemia, poison oak, skin abrasions, rheumatism, wounds, etc.

The wheat grass chlorophyll, when taken in conjunction with the Cleansing Program will do much as a tonic aid toward relieving the pain and suffering of all so-called “incurable” diseases, and will promote general healing to the body.

Preparations:
Dr. Wigmore found that the best device for extracting wheat grass chlorophyll is a meat grinder or a rather inexpensive grain mill, but she advised that electrical blenders and juicers require the use of too much water, and neutralize a great por-

tion of the vital potency; the fast moving blades or paddles mix in too much air and oxidize the liquid. We have found an excellent device in the fruit press for expelling the most juice with the least effort. The preparation of the wheat grass chlorophyll is made in the following manner:

First wash the newly-gathered wheat grass to remove any dust and soil.

Second place a reasonable amount of grass, say 3 ounces, into the grinder or mill and pulverize it; this could also be done with a pestle and mortar. Be sure to save any drippings around the handle, as every drop is precious. For the addition of flavoring agents during the pulverizing process, see "Congenial combinations."

Third squeeze the juice from the pulp with a spoon and place into an appropriate vessel, then wash the remaining pulp in another vessel with a minimum of water, so that as much of the residual chlorophyll as possible may be extracted into solution.

Fourth mix these two liquids together, strain, and place into the appropriate drinking vessel. **Note:** This procedure is not necessary with the expeller press.

Dosage:
1-2 glasses a day before the morning and/or evening meals.

ADMINISTRATION

Whatever the problem condition, the wheat grass chlorophyll will serve as an excellent restorative aid and nutritive tonic.

Place the juice in a glass and drink it straight or add some distilled water (and flavoring agents if you like). Wheat grass chlorophyll drink should be sipped slowly, swishing each mouthful so that the liquid and the saliva juices are thoroughly mixed together. This is especially important when taking the juice straight. The more you swish, the less feedback (burping) you will get from this powerful elixir.

Morning:
Upon arising, drink 1 quart of warm water, mixed with 2 tablespoonfuls of unsulphured molasses and 1/2 lemon to clear any left-over digestive liquids from the stomach. One-half hour later, drink the first glass of wheat grass chlorophyll, then wait another one-half hour before a cleansing raw fruit breakfast.

Evening:
Drink the second glass of wheat grass chlorophyll before the evening meal, which will be a low-heat vegetable preparation. Drinking this prior to the meal will aid in digestion and cut down the appetite.

Skin

Burns, skin abrasions, bruises, wounds: The wheat grass chlorophyll is both healing and antiseptic. The juice is applied either directly onto the afflicted surface, or it is soaked in a cloth and bandaged to the area. At the same time, the chlorophyll should be taken internally.

Poison oak, running ulcers: Place a poultice of freshly crushed wheat grass pulp on the afflicted area and cover with thin gauze.

FORMULAS

Wheatgrass paste

1 part Wheatgrass (Triticum species) chlorophyll (juice)
Mixed with equal parts wheat germ oil and honey.

Administration: For external and internal use.

Congenial combinations:
The chlorophyll flavor may be altered several ways without interfering with the natural value and healing potency:

a. Add a small shoot of scallion (any onion without a bulb) not over an inch long to the wheat grass during the pulverizing process. This will lend an onion flavor, but not the onion odor, as the chlorophyll nullifies this.

b. Add a tiny sprig of parsley or some mint leaves while pulverizing the wheat grass.

c. Add a spoonful of sassafras tea to the extracted chlorophyll itself for flavoring.

d. Use honey as flavoring in equal parts with the pure wheat grass chlorophyll.

e. Add 2-3 celery leaves to the wheat grass while pulverizing.

f. Flavor the wheat grass chlorophyll with 1/2 teaspoonful of brewer's yeast.

g. Cut the wheat grass fine with scissors, and mix this with vegetable food, salads, or casseroles.

Note: Do not mix the wheat grass chlorophyll with fruit or fruit juices, as these are known to effectively kill the potency of any vegetable juices.

Growing characteristics:
The wheat herb itself is an annual plant that will grow almost anywhere with

moderate warmth, indoors or outdoors. The thick rootlet, which appears first, has the characteristic of quickly building a very durable sod, while picking up the widest variety and balance of human nutrients possible, live minerals, vitamins, and trace elements. Next, the wheat berry itself sprouts, and quickly pushes its blade through the thin earth into the light within 2-3 days after planting. Some 6-7 days after planting, this round shaft, now full of vital strength, attains the height of 5-7 inches before the first joint comes into view.

Indoor soil: Procure several wooden boxes (best at 8 inches deep, 20 inches wide, and 30 inches long), and for convenience of handling, line each box with oilcloth, or plastic sheets, or tar paper. Obtain some good loamy soil, and finely crumble about 6 inches of this into each box, then mix some "plant food" such as Azomite (a natural composition of colloidal silicate minerals and trace element catalysts which are highly synergistic), and, if possible, add earthworms to tend the soil, though this is not absolutely essential for growing satisfactory wheat grass if the green wheat grass stubble and roots are carefully tucked under after each harvesting.

Indoor planting: Soak 2 cupfuls of wheat in plain water; the hard wheat should be soaked overnight and soft wheat only 3-4 hours. Spread these soaked seeds in the box in all directions, so that they are in a single layer and almost touching each other. Cover them with 1/2 inch of earth, and place several thicknesses of newspaper on top of the earth to hold in the moisture until the first blade appears; then remove the newspaper. Irrigate the planted seeds amply once a day with plain water morning or evening until the first blade appears. Then reduce the watering to a moderate moisture until the blades are ready to harvest at 5-7 inches tall. Be careful not to completely "drown" the seeds and plants in watering, as this may cause mildew and spoilage. Dr. Wigmore found that the chlorophyll extracted from sturdy, round-stemmed, shade-grown (indirect light) wheat grass was softer, sweeter, and had a more pleasant aroma than the chlorophyll from wheat grass blades that were exposed to direct sunlight and had fallen limply upon the ground. Use only the first blade growth, as the second blades produce a more bitter chlorophyll, which in the opinion of Dr. Thomas contains only about 40% of the nutrients present in the first growth.

Replanting:

Replant immediately after harvesting. Soak the wheat as indicated above before placing them into the ground. Obtain two containers to hold the soil while you "rework" it. Break up the sod that is in your box and place these larger pieces into one of the containers, then pour out the loose soil remaining in the box into the other container. Arrange the larger pieces of sod in the bottom of your indoor box, spreading the loose soil over the top of the larger pieces, but save back some 2 quarts of the loose soil to cover the seeds. Smooth the top surface flat, then spread the wet wheat as indicated above. Cover the wheat with the loose earth which was set aside. Dr. Wigmore suggests that an old ash sifter with a screen of about 3/4 inch squares is ideal to distribute the cover soil over the seeds. Your fingers alone will do a fine job. Then continue the procedure as described above. Harvest the sixth day and let the soil rest on the seventh.

Fertilizing: We have already indicated the excellence of using a colloidal silicate such as Azomite, yet the stubble of the wheat grass alone is a superior agent for soil enrichment. Dr. Wigmore indicates that through the months, as you turn under this green stubble of the wheat grass and break the roots into small chunks, this will make each crop of wheat grass grow better, and the soil, even rather poor soil, will gradually take on a texture of rich, sweet-smelling loam. She has used the same soil in her boxes as many as 140 successive times, with all indication that the effects were constantly regenerative!

Collection: Just 6 days from planting, the wheat grass should be ready for harvest. When the wheat grass is about 5-7 inches tall, before the first joint of the blade has appeared above the surface of the soil, you can cut the grass with ordinary scissors. For convenience of handling, have some rubber bands handy and bind the freshly-cut wheat grass into small, 3-ounce bundles (the amount needed to make each drink). The greatest potency is obtained from the growing wheat grass that is harvested immediately before converting it into the wheat grass chlorophyll drink. The vital potency may be stored and preserved in the cut grass form for nearly a week in a bag in the regrigerator. Once extracted, however, the precious chlorophyll is only live and electrically positive for about three hours.

MENU PLAN AFTER CLEANSING

THE FIRST TWO WEEKS

Here is a sample diet program which you can use as a guide. As no two people are alike, it is impossible for everybody to follow the same diet. As another old saying goes, "What's one man's meat is another man's poison." A person with a "touchy" stomach, who is bothered with indigestion and stomach discomfort, should use far more vegetables, and more steamed or baked vegetables and fruit, than raw; whereas the person with a compatible stomach condition can use more fruits and less vegetables.

After finishing a three-day fast, your first two weeks dietary program will be as follows: Make a practice of retiring to bed before 11 and arising each day before 7, as this cycle gives better rest for most people than any other. After rising, drink a glass or two of distilled water but do not break your fast from food until noon, when you proceed with lunch as given below.

Lunch

Cayenne pepper and apple cider vinegar: Start your day by taking the supplements of cayenne pepper and apple cider vinegar as explained in the "SUPPLEMENTS AND HEALING AIDS" section (see page 572).

Prune or fig juice: In about 10 minutes, follow the cayenne and apple cider vinegar with a small glass of prune or fig juice. About 15 minutes thereafter comes your first meal of the day. If you do not need the prune or fig juice as a bowel regulator, leave out the juice and have your meal about 15 minutes after the cayenne and vinegar drink.

Combination salad: Make up either a cabbage coleslaw or grated carrots salad, adding 2 or 3 tablespoonfuls of a stewed or canned vegetable such as string beans, red beets, peas or spinach, any type that is acid-binding. Add to this one of the following for flavoring and as a touch of variety: green onions, tomatoes, cucumbers, chives, celery, or any other green-leaf vegetables.

For a dressing, use pure fresh olive oil, flavoring it with a touch of apple cider vinegar or lemon juice, black pepper (a very good herb unless cooked), plus a little sweet basil, thyme, or any of your favorite salad herbs as described. If you like garlic, you may squeeze or grate a few garlic cloves finely to taste. As no two people are alike, the tastes will vary, so you may use more or less of this or that, or leave any or all out and use the salad just plain and tossed.

Vegetable: The rest of the meal can be one only of either baked or stewed vegetables, such as cauliflower, parsnips, squash, turnips, beets, or any other of the vegetables that are "plus" or acid-binding.

If you have been a big eater and still feel hungry, have in addition a small baked potato, but no bread. For flavor, put on the potato a little olive oil and coarse black or regular pepper, and natural salt, and eat skin and all, or else do not have the potato.

Kitchen notes: When greens are not in season, use canned or frozen. When thirsty, along with your distilled water you can enjoy the fresh juice of vegetables. Whatever type of vegetable you choose for this meal, mix in the solid part with the salad stock (root and leaf/stalk and florescence). This combination of raw and stewed or baked vegetables supplies the necessary "cleaning tool or broom" to aid in mechanically cleansing the digestive tract. The low-heating of the vegetables aids in bringing out the grape sugars which may not be available when eaten raw.

Dinner

Fruit: Use a stewed fruit such as stewed prunes, applesauce, stewed dried apricots or peaches or, if you have no stomach trouble, very ripe bananas. Sweeten to taste with honey or unrefined sugar. This helps to satisfy the craving for the wrong kinds of food, and yet is in no way mucus-forming.

This is the menu plan for the first two weeks. Remember to step up the dosage of cayenne 1/4 teaspoonful every three days, until you are using at least 1 teaspoon (minimum) before each meal. This may feel warm going in and going out for a few days, but after a period of time with regular usage, it will not be objectionable or discomforting at all.

THE SECOND TWO WEEKS

Lunch

Cayenne and apple cider vinegar: Have your cayenne and apple cider vinegar just before your lunch and dinner as before, except you should be up to a teaspoon of cayenne by now. The cayenne and vinegar do not have to be taken together, so if preferred, drink the cayenne before the meal in water and the vinegar between meals. Never drink during a meal; always wait at least 1/2 hour after the meal is finished to drink.

Fruit: Stewed fruit, applesauce or a baked apple to start. Sweeten this with honey or with unrefined sugar.

Combination salad: Wait for 10 or 15 minutes; then have a combination salad like the ones used during the first two weeks' period. But use variety, and change your salad each day with a little different combination. This procedure not only proves challenging, but it will transform your mealtime into a more pleasant, exciting, and anticipated experience. Use the liquid from your steamed vegetables as a drink between meals as your thirst requires. Your cooked vegetables can be used on your salad and will serve as a good dressing substitute.

Dinner

Serve a baked or stewed vegetable as in the first two weeks menu, followed by a vegetable salad made of lettuce with celery, green peppers or cucumber. Or, if preferred, you may have a small serving of coleslaw or carrot and raisin salad.

THE THIRD TWO WEEKS

Lunch

Mono-diet (summer): Now is the time to start on a mono-diet. If this is during the summer, you can choose the fruit you want to use for lunch today. Be sure it is ripe and stay with that one kind. As an example, if it is peaches, eat all you want, cantaloupes the same, or apricots, apples, berries, etc. The type of fruit you choose doesn't matter; just be sure it is good and ripe, and it is better still when these foods are selected and eaten only "in the season thereof," and that you use only one kind for your meal. If you are still not satisfied, have a stalk of celery, some lettuce leaves, some other leafy vegetable (raw or cooked), but just a small quantity. Be sure to wait 10 or 15 minutes after the fruit before you eat the vegetable.

Mono-diet (winter): During winter a sweet dried fruit can be chewed together with a few nuts (very few) and then followed by some fresh fruit. Figs, prunes, raisins, or dates may be eaten with oranges or apples. You have a wide variety in dried fruits to choose from.

Dinner

As before, serve a combination salad, followed preferably by a baked or steamed vegetable. Again, there is a wide variety to choose from, so just rotate them to make each meal different.

THE FOURTH TWO WEEKS

Lunch

Fruit: Use fruit in mono-diet as in the previous menu.

Dinner

For a starter, use fresh, baked or stewed fruit. Then after 10 or 15 minutes, have either a cold cooked vegetable, or, better still, a vegetable salad.

Curbing the craving for meat: A person who has been a heavy meat-eater may get the craving for meats during this program, just as an alcoholic will want the bottle, because the cleansing is stirring up stored poisons and uremic acids. When these are broken loose, the craving is intensified. If at dinnertime the craving is hard to handle, use vegetables only—no fruits—and these will help to satisfy. If you feel that your weight is going down faster than desired, use a baked potato more often, eating skin and all, but do not use butter or margarine. The best flavoring is olive oil, but be sure that it is new and fresh stock.

CLEANSING

Cleansing crisis: At this cleansing time, don't let the taste buds rule again, because at this period of the physical cycle, you will have intensely strong cravings for the wrong kinds of food—the very ones which have been your favorites in the past and have led to a degenerative downfall. When your body is trying to eliminate toxins, "like calls for like."

This is the most important of all times to see that these wastes causing the cravings are eliminated quickly and not allowed to remain in the body.

Keep the bowels clean: Use any positive, live, and non-mucus forming food which acts as a laxative for you. This same food might not have the same effect on someone else. With many people, a few dried prunes just before other fruit does a very effective job, but with others, it does not. We suggest prune or fig juice as a starter for your meals, drinking it a few minutes before eating any other food. We have found this is best for most of the patients we have worked with, but if raspberries do the job better, or something else, then use these other nutritive aids. And don't forget the lower bowel tonic. In Dr. Christopher's early years of lecturing, people wrote from foreign countries to have this herbal aid sent to them at great expense when their supply had run out, and they needed it especially while traveling. This one formula alone will be worth more to you, many times over, than the price you have paid for this text.

Do not let other people's opinions sway you in your new program. If you are earnest and seek God's counsel, you will have the strength to carry on no matter what people say.

FASTING

Fast once a week: This procedure of eight weeks that we have just outlined is the "No breakfast, mucusless diet plan." After a time, if you want to speed up your healing and you have a good, solid footing in what you are doing, so that you feel you can take a bit heavier load dumping waste without panic, you may slip in a one-day fast each week to hurry your health-building process along.

Always remember, for the best results when you are using a special addition to your diet routine, such as the one-day juice therapy, one-day fast, or two, three, or more days of fast, be positive to have these days fall on the same starting day of the week, so that you can keep up a smooth rhythm. A good rhythm is just as important in this program as it is in good music. If you have your 24-hour fast on Monday, keep it on Mondays; or if on Saturday, always keep it on that day each week. Before starting, figure out which day is your least rushed and frustrating day, and then choose that one for your fast, as some people will need to rest or at least not work so hard during the fast period.

After your evening (or late afternoon) dinner, eat nothing until the same time the next day. If this is a 24-hour fast once a week, try not only to have it on the same day of the week, but also the same hour of the day, when possible. During this day of fasting 24 hours (or longer), all that you will have will be your water, as much as desired. Cayenne and lemonade, apple cider vinegar, or other liquids that will be further specified hereafter, are for children, the febrile, and rare cases.

When breaking your fast at mealtime, start your dinner with fruit; then, after 15 or 20 minutes, eat the salad or vegetables. Remember not to overeat or to side-step from the recommended course.

Fasting is like fire: Throughout the scriptures the Lord advises to fast and pray.

All of the great prophets from the beginning of time have fasted. And, through prayer and being close to the Maker, they were guided in how to fast. Most of them lived the simple life in the first place, and they were not contaminated with the toxins, wastes, and man-made concoctions that we today call food and medicine. In our present condition we are mostly incapable of walking and talking with God and being led directly by Him as were the leaders of old. This is where we are given the blessed way of compassion, shown in the patience of the Lord, such as: "For those who cannot be healed by faith, heal them with herbs and mild food." Also, He tells us to use fasting and prayer. But first things first, of course, as fasting improperly can be a killer as well as a savior. It is like fire, it can either gently warm you, or, if not understood and kept under control, it can kill you.

Long fasting—use with prudence and skill: If a person should undertake a long fast without first cleaning out a lot of the waste matter that has been stored and deposited in the body for years, the fast will break this loose so fast that the avenues of elimination will completely clog up, and the well-meaning person will strangle and suffocate in his own toxins. Bowel movements are usually hard to come by while fasting. Fasting will break loose mucus, poisons, and drugs from years ago, but because of the glue-like stickiness of this unleashed slime, the natural bowel movements will not be able to bring it out, so you must pave the way for such drastic cleansing with a modulated or transition diet. After much of this waste is removed in a gradual process, then is the time to have a fast, short ones at first, then gradually working up to longer ones.

Liquid intake during a fast: The dictionary defines "fast" as: "To abstain from all or certain foods." Many theologians believe that in a spiritual fast you can use only water, and this is very good. But for a healing procedure, it is permissible to use some various forms of liquid, but no solid food. This is not a strict fast but a liquid diet. You may use any cleansing herbal tea, such as alfalfa, mint, yarrow, desert or Brigham tea, sassafras, etc. sweetened with honey. You may use over 2-3 quarts a day. One more type of drink is permissible, vegetable broth. Drink it warm and do not exceed the 2-3 quart limit. When using any of these drinks, do not gulp them down, but sip them slowly, rolling the liquid around the mouth, swishing it and chewing it like you would solid food. With drinking, even with water alone, learn to be at ease; take your time and enjoy your beverage.

JUICE

Quenching the thirst: The roots of the plant go down into the earth and take in food and minerals in solution via osmosis into the plant. Here these ingredients changed from inorganic to organic, and if properly selected, this natural "blood" or life-line in the plant is a perfect food and liquid for man, both for the required nourishment and liquid used by the system. During summertime, for instance, drinking celery juice not only quenches the thirst, but also supplies the natural organic salts in proper quantities so that the heat is not noticed (this should be used instead of the inorganic salt tablets). While others are in misery and sweltering with the heat, you are enjoying life. This simple procedure properly thins down a sluggish and heavy bloodstream so that it flows rapidly through the body to carry off the poisons and wastes. And this is the reason why a heavy meat and starch eater will suffer apoplexy and strokes long before the heat even bothers the vegetarian or fruitarian.

Energy without stress: Juices supply energy without overworking the body. This is because nearly all fresh juice from fruits and vegetables is partly assimilated immediately upon entering the mouth, going directly into the bloodstream through the mouth. The juice will not wear out the digestive organs with a lot of excess materials that are difficult to digest and burdensome to eliminate.

Juice therapy: Though Dr. Christopher had years of experience in juice therapy and saw miraculous healings with it, nevertheless problems often arose with patients that juice therapy could not handle. We found the reason for the distress, was our mistake with using a straight juice therapy. With fruit juice especially—but with almost any type vegetable juice also—the sticky mucus and waste materials would break loose from the tissues and be carried out to be eliminated, but there it stayed, in large, gluey deposits. Liquids only cannot clean out all the accumulated filth from the body. So with all of your cleansing aids, these should be used in moderation and with prudence and skill! We highly recommend the use of fruit and vegetable juices—and for them to be used copiously—but they were intended to nourish the tissue and break loose the waste, so they should always be coupled with raw and cooked (low heated) fruits and vegetables as aids in elimination. After a person's body is completely cleaned of all waste—up to 7 years on the program—and during the long cleansing process, more and more juice can be used, but the roughage will always be needed. In addition, herbal aids can help move out the toxins.

A transition program: After eating the way most of us do, we cannot change to a mono-diet overnight. This is why we recommend a modulation process or transition program. In the following menus that you will see that some of the combinations are slightly more complex than the mono-diet. These may serve you for a start, or can be used for entertaining, but after you are firmly on the path, your own intuitive desires will lead you naturally to simplicity in diet.

One cooked food: As a general rule, build your meals around one cooked food. This gives a wonderful variety with something different each day. The principle of one cooked vegetable will make digestion simple and easy, and will eliminate the kitchen burden of planning, preparing, and cleaning. This vegetable may be eaten warm or cold, mixed with raw vegetables and green salads, or eaten as a separate dish by itself. Carrots, cabbage, beets, cauliflower, onions, or turnips, for example, become sweet when low-heated, steamed or carefully baked; the carbohydrates are developed into sugars and the mineral salts are not extracted.

Your immediate goal at this time is to enjoy your change of diet during the transition period, until your condition and tastes have improved. In this way, it will be a pleasurable experience and not a dreaded hardship.

RECIPES

Make your own salad dressing: Your salads will be brightened in flavor with a dressing. The following are some of the ingredients to use in your dressing; vary them and make different combinations according to your taste:

1. The best of all oils is olive oil, but always be sure it is fresh, first-pressed, and of a good name brand. Safflower oil and some of the other vegetable oils are good, though not in the same class as olive oil. But do not use animal fats or oils from mineral products, such as mineral oil.

2. The next ingredient for the base is either fresh lemon juice or apple cider vinegar to taste. Do not use malt or other types of vinegar.

3. Almost all herbal condiments—those that are not man-made—are good to use. A touch of cayenne, paprika (also good for color), freshly ground black pepper, parsley, celery seed, thyme, sweet basil (our favorite—grow your own and enjoy it fresh in salads, too): you can go on and on with wonderful tasty herbs. For those who like the sweet touch, honey, raw sugar, maple sugar, or a little sorghum may be used.

And for us, no salad dressing is complete without garlic. Either use a garlic press or grate the garlic finely from the fresh clove. Use a little or as much as you like, to taste. Some people just like a rub of a garlic clove on the dish before tossing the salad, but to us this is like washing your hands with gloves on; we like it either in the dressing or in the salad itself. Finely-grated onion or onion juice, a good tomato paste, a touch of good sea salt (without iodine or other additives), or vegetable broth powder may be used for variety. From these ingredients you can do wonders in making numerous dressing combinations.

To make mayonnaise: This is one time a raw egg can be used without creating mucus, as the lemon juice or vinegar will offset its bad traits to some extent. Put the egg in a blender; add two tablespoons lemon juice or apple cider vinegar; add about one cup of salad oil to this, in a thin stream, continuing to beat while the oil is being added. Then mix in salt and pepper to taste. This is the basic formula for mayonnaise, but by adding substitutes, you can create a wide variety of dressings to your own liking.

If you wish to avoid eggs entirely, try this tofu mayonnaise: 6 oz. tofu, 2 tablespoons lemon juice, 2 tablespoons oil, 1/2 teaspoon sea salt, 1 tablespoon dill weed, 1 tablespoon mustard, 1 clove garlic. Blend in blender 20 seconds or till smooth. This is a delicious salad dressing.

You can also buy mayonnaise and salad dressings without any animal products.

Fresh Salsa:
4 tomatoes, 1 chopped onion, 1/2 chili pepper, 1 teaspoon herb seasoning, 1 red bell pepper, 1 garlic clove. Chop ingredients and mix. Store in fridge. Good as a condiment.

Create your own salads: The standard transition salad is based on coleslaw or carrot, or in combination. Here are a few combinations you may like and wish to use, but enjoy the challenge of creating your own, remembering that simplicity is always best. You will notice that proportions are in parts, not cups or pounds. This is so you can make the amount you desire, for 1 or 20, simply by enlarging the parts in the same proportion. A part would be the equivalent of a cup.

SALADS

Standard or Natural Combination Salad:

Large bowlful	Lettuce
4 parts	Radishes (3 parts if strong)
4 parts	Tomatoes, chopped
2 parts	Parsley, cut extra fine

Cut or shred lettuce very fine and add the other three ingredients; add desired dressing.

Cabbage Salad:

2 parts	Cabbage
1 part	Peppers (green sweet), finely chopped
2 tablespoons	Lemon juice or apple cider vinegar
2 tablespoons	Mayonnaise dressing (our recipe only)
Sufficient	Paprika or chopped pimento
Sufficient	Lettuce

Toss first 3 ingredients well and serve on fresh crisp lettuce leaves. The paprika or chopped pimento may be sprinkled on for decoration (a pretty salad is a pleasant one to eat).

Spring Salad:

Large bowlful	Cabbage, chopped
1 part	Radishes, cut fine
1/2 part	Peppers (sweet green), finely chopped
1 part	Green onions, chopped fine
1/2 parts	Tomatoes, chopped
1/2 part	Cucumbers, chopped with skins
Garnish	Olives
Garnish	Radishes

Toss well with your favorite dressing. Garnish with olives and/or radishes.

Apple and Celery Salad:

2 parts	Apples, cubed (Sprinkle immediately with fresh lemon juice to preserve coloring)
1 part	Celery, chopped
1/4 part	Parsley, chopped
1 part	Seedless raisins
2 tablespoonfuls	Mayonnaise dressing (our recipe)
Sufficient	Lettuce

Mix well all ingredients and serve on bed of crisp lettuce.

Cooked Combination Salad:

1 part	Carrots, cooked and diced
1 part	Peas, cooked
1 part	String beans, cooked and chopped
1/2 part	Celery, raw and finely chopped
	Mayonnaise (our recipe only)
	Lettuce

Mix all ingredients, add mayonnaise to taste, and serve on crisp leaves of lettuce. *Please note:* Whenever the word "cooked" is used, it means low heated.

Carrot and Raisin Salad (an old favorite):

2 parts	Carrots, coarsely shredded
1/2 part	Seedless raisins (soak for 2 hours)
1/2 part	Celery, finely chopped
	Mayonnaise (our recipe)

Mix thoroughly and add mayonnaise to taste.

Stuffed Prune Salad:

Prunes
Almonds
Paprika
Mashed tofu or soy yogurt
Lettuce
Mayonnaise (our recipe)

Cook prunes, cool thoroughly, and fill the center with tofu or soy yogurt. Place one blanched almond in center of cottage cheese. Serve on lettuce leaves with mayonnaise and a touch of paprika.

Pea and Cauliflower Salad:

2 parts	Cauliflower
1 part	Peas, cooked
1 part	Parsley, finely chopped
	Mayonnaise (our recipe only)
	Lettuce

Low heat cauliflower until sweet and break into small pieces; add peas and parsley. Place on bed of lettuce leaves and add mayonnaise to taste.

Coleslaw, Mexican Style:

2 parts	Red cabbage, finely sliced
1/2 part	Celery, chopped
1 part	Red kidney beans, cooked
1/4 part	Onions, chopped
1/4 part	Chives, chopped
1/4 part	Peppers (sweet green), chopped
	Lemon juice and Olive oil to taste
	Paprika

Toss together first 8 ingredients and sprinkle with paprika.

Asparagus Salad:

Asparagus, low heated and cut into 2 or 3 inch lengths
Mayonnaise or your choice of dressing
Pimento, chopped or in shreds
Lettuce
Arrange asparagus on a bed of lettuce leaves, add dressing and decorate with pimento.

Coleslaw, Serbian Style:

1 part	Cabbage, finely sliced
1 part	Celery, coarsely chopped
1/4 part	Onions, finely chopped
1/4 part	Olives, minced
1 tablespoon	Pimento, chopped
	Olive oil
	Lemon juice or apple cider vinegar

Toss all ingredients together and serve.

Russian Salad:

2 parts	Carrots (raw), diced
1/2 part	Onion, finely chopped
1/4 part	Watercress chopped (use more or less as desired)
2 parts	Celery, diced
2	Tomatoes, sliced (ripe)
	Mayonnaise (our recipe)
	Lettuce

Mix first four ingredients add mayonnaise and garnish with tomato slices. Arrange on a bed of lettuce leaves.

Apple and Carrot Salad :

1 part	Apples, cubed (soaked in lemon juice)
1 part	Carrots, chopped
1/2 part	Celery, chopped
1/4 part	Onions, finely chopped (more or less to taste)
1/2 part	Dates, finely sliced

Olive oil
Lemon Juice

Mix all ingredients and soak for 15 minutes for flavor accentuation.

Fruit Salad a la Apple Shell:
Apples, of your choice
Grapefruit
Pineapple equal parts
Cherries
Lemon juice
Honey

Cut off tops of apples and scoop out meat. Chop the apple hearts with grapefruit, pineapple and cherries; add lemon juice and sweeten with honey. Place into the apple shells and sprinkle with grated coconut.

Summer Salad:
1 part Watercress, chopped
1/2 part Cucumbers, diced with skins on
1/2 part Tomatoes, chopped
1/2 part Celery, diced
Olive oil
Lemon juice or apple cider vinegar
Pimento strips
Lettuce

Toss well and serve on crisp lettuce leaves; garnish with pimento strips.

Waldorf Salad:
1/2 part Lemon juice
1 1/2 parts Apples, diced (tart and crisp)
1 1/2 parts Celery, diced
Mayonnaise (our recipe)
English or Black Walnuts
Lettuce

Mix first three ingredients well and drain off lemon juice. Add mayonnaise and serve on lettuce leaves. Garnish with walnuts.

Asparagus and Cauliflower Salad:
Asparagus, cut into 2 or 3 inch lengths
Cauliflower, break into small pieces
Pimento
Lettuce
Mayonnaise (our recipe)

Low heat asparagus and cauliflower separately. Serve on lettuce leaves with mayonnaise; garnish with pimento.

Spinach and Carrot Salad:

1 part Carrots, raw grated
1 part Spinach, raw chopped
1 part Coleslaw
Lemon juice
Mayonnaise (our recipe)
Ripe olives
Lettuce

To spinach and coleslaw add lemon juice and let soak for 10 minutes. On leaves of fresh, crisp lettuce arrange a layer of coleslaw first, then a layer of chopped spinach, and last a layer of grated carrots. Place a spoonful of mayonnaise in the center for decoration.

Brazilian Style Salad:

1 1/2 parts Strawberries, ripe
1 1/2 parts Pineapple, cubed (fresh, if possible)
12 Brazil nuts (blanched and thinly sliced)
4 tablespoonfuls Lemon juice
Lettuce leaves
Mayonnaise (our recipe)

Marinate first three ingredients in lemon juice. Arrange lettuce on plates in rose shape; fill crown with above mixture. Cover with spoonful of mayonnaise. Decorate with strawberries.

Date Celery Salad:

Celery Equal parts
Dates
Lettuce leaves

Chop celery and dates and serve on lettuce with mayonnaise.

Elimination Salad:

2 parts Coleslaw
2 parts Spinach, chopped
1 part Peas, fresh green
1 part Celery, chopped
Olive oil
Apple cider vinegar or lemon juice

Toss well and serve.

Onion Salad:

2 parts Cabbage, finely sliced
1 part Red onions, sliced
1 part Tomatoes chopped
1/2 part Parsley, coarsely chopped
2 tablespoonfuls Mayonnaise (if desired, add more to taste)
Radishes

Paprika

Toss well first five ingredients and add paprika and radishes for garnish.

Watercress Salad:
Watercress, chopped
Tomatoes, chopped
Lettuce
Toss watercress with tomatoes and place on bed of lettuce.

Mock Chicken Salad:

2 parts	Cabbage, sliced finely
1 part	Celery chopped
2 tablespoons	Onion, finely chopped (or more to taste)
1/2 part	Peppers (sweet green), finely chopped
1 part	Nut loaf (cold), cubed (See Nut Loaf recipe), or cubed tofu
2 tablespoonfuls	Mayonnaise (our recipe)
	Olives
	Lettuce leaves

Mix first six ingredients thoroughly. Arrange on fresh, crisp lettuce leaves and decorate with olives.

Tossed Salad:

Large bowlful	Lettuce leaves
2 parts	Tomatoes, chopped
1 part	Onions, finely chopped
1 part	Celery, chopped
1/2 part	Chives, chopped
1/2 part	Spinach, raw chopped
1/2 part	Parsley, chopped
	Oil and vinegar dressing

Toss vegetables well and add dressing.

COOKED RECIPES

Serbian Vegetable Goulash (a favorite from the Balkans):
Onion, sliced and lightly browned in olive oil
Cabbage (red or white), coarsely sliced
Sweet peppers, sliced
Tomatoes, sliced or chopped
Touch of salt or pepper (if desired)
Low heat browned onions, cabbage, and sweet peppers using a little olive oil or a very little water. Add tomatoes and salt and pepper, and finish stewing.

GUEST RECIPES

Sometimes you need to prepare a meal when company is coming. These recipes suggest dinners that your guests will enjoy whether they are vegetarians or not. Some of them contain ingredients which are not strictly on the mucusless diet; when this is the case, we include suggestions to make them mucusless, especially important if you are working with serious illness.

Using Combinations: Use cauliflower, red or white cabbage, carrots, Brussels sprouts, zucchini squash, or beets (use tops and all). Each can be baked or broiled with onions in a little olive oil and tomato paste or sauce as the gravy. You may use just one vegetable or any combination, with or without onions. Onions are the standard seasoning base and also the world's greatest known antihistamine. Bake as dry as possible and you will find it will satisfy as a meat substitute.

Other meat substitutes: Loma Linda and a number of other companies have made meat substitutes from soybeans, and have done a remarkable job of it. These soybean substitutes may be used in combination if not used to excess. Dr. Christopher had two naturopathic doctor friends to dinner in Evanston, Wyoming and his wife served soybean broiled cutlets for dinner. One of the doctors commented that these were the best cutlets he had ever eaten and wanted to know if they were veal, or what type of meat it was. We had not mentioned that it was a meat substitute we were using, and they thought it was real meat. Were these men surprised when told it was a soybean substitute!

In recent years, more meatless meats have become available. On occasion, you can enjoy slices which resemble deli cuts, soy bacon, soy hot dogs (with no objectionable chemicals) and other substitutes to use in stir-fry and casserole dishes. Further, you can easily buy tofu—and it is not that difficult to make yourself—for a protein base in your foods.

The main reason for giving the following recipes is to offer variety in your eating program, and to satisfy any cravings you might have for unhealthy foods. These are mostly for the cravings of the beginner or if you have a special family dinner or when guests drop in, etc. but we still advise you to stay with the simple monodiet the major part of the time, or you will slow down the progress.

Note:
In the cooked recipes, it is the same as in the salad—a part is the same as a cup.

Carrot Nut Loaf:
2 parts Carrots, coarsely chopped
1 part Celery, chopped
1/2 part Crumbs, toasted bran or whole wheat
3/4 part Walnuts, chopped
1 part Tomatoes, mashed
1/2 part Onions, sliced and braised
soy butter or a good margarine
Mix together all ingredients and bake 1/2 hour in a loaf pan.

To make mucusless, replace the crumbs with low-heated grains, chopped in your food processor after cooking.

Bell Peppers, Stuffed:

4	Green sweet peppers, large
1/2 tablespoon	Soy butter or good margarine
1/2 tablespoon	Flour, whole wheat or graham
1 part	Soymilk or vegetable broth
1/2 part	Nut meats, chopped
1 part	Bread crumbs, whole wheat
1/2 part	Celery, diced
2 tablespoons	Onion, grated
	Tomatoes (chopped) or tomato paste

Remove seeds from peppers and parboil 10 minutes, drain well. Mix together celery, nutmeats, bread crumbs, onion, milk, flour, salt and pepper to taste, if desired. Add tomatoes or tomato paste. Fill peppers and add additional crumbs on top. Bake in margarine or olive oil.

To make mucusless, use low-heated grains, chopped in food processor after cooking. Top with chopped nuts or lightly-toasted sesame seeds instead of crumbs.

Tomatoes, Baked:

Tomatoes
Garlic, if desired
Pepper, coarse ground
Lettuce or Watercress
Beets, cooked and sliced
Onions (grated)
Parsley
Salt, touch
Choice of dressing

Cut tops off tomatoes and scoop out pulp. Season pulp with grated onion and a little garlic (if desired), parsley, pepper and salt. Put stuffing into tomato shells, place on lids, cover, and bake for 25 minutes, basting with olive oil or good vegetable oil. Place tomatoes on bed of lettuce and/or watercress for decoration surround with ample sliced cooked red table beets. Add your choice of dressing.

Italian Mock Meat Balls:

2 parts	Spaghetti, whole wheat
2 parts	Nutmeat loaf
1/2 part	Chives, finely chopped
1/2 part	Celery, chopped
1/8 part	Peppers, hot Spanish (or to flavor of preference)
1/4 part	Tomato sauce or paste
	Onion to taste

Braise onions and add ingredients (except nut meat loaf) to make a sauce. Form nut meat loaf into balls, using some of the Spanish sauce. Bake balls, spaghetti,

and some of the Spanish sauce in a baking dish and serve with the remaining Spanish sauce.
To make mucusless, replace the whole grain spaghetti with cooked spaghetti squash.

String Beans and New Potatoes:
New potatoes with skins
String beans
Parsley, chopped
Salt, small amount
Pepper, coarse ground (black), to taste
Paprika
Olive oil, Italian
Low heat new potatoes and string beans (with very little water) in separate pans. Place both in baking dish and add parsley, salt and pepper. Sprinkle a showing of paprika on top. Pour olive oil over the top and warm in oven for 15 minutes, then serve.

Sauerkraut and Vegetable Sausage:

2 parts	Rice, natural brown
1/4 part	Peanuts, finely chopped
1/2 part	Bread crumbs, toasted whole wheat
1 part	Onion, sliced and braised in olive oil
	Flour, whole wheat, soy or unbleached
	Olive oil
	Sauerkraut

Soak rice overnight or at least six to eight hours, pour water off add fresh water and boil until soft. Mix together rice, peanuts, crumbs, and onions. Mold into shape of sausages, dip in egg and roll in flour. Have oil hot, then dip sausages in until golden brown. Serve with warm sauerkraut.

Strictly speaking, the mucusless diet would not include even brown rice. If you are being very careful, replace this cooked grain with low-heated wheat or barley, lightly-chopped after cooking. You can replace the bread crumbs with lightly-toasted wheat germ. Instead of rolling in flour, roll in sesame seeds or ground sunflower seeds. These alterations change the taste considerably, but produce a comparable product.

Note: As you can see, these recipes are to be used only occasionally when one feels strong cravings for meat, or on special occasions. But it is far better to use these recipes than to lose ground by returning to meat in desperation.

Mock Halibut Cutlets with Tartar Sauce:

2 parts	Lima beans, soaked and low heated
Amount desired	Onions
Amount desired	Peppers, green bell

Salt and pepper
Breadcrumbs, whole wheat
Tartar sauce, made with apple cider
Parsley

Braise onions and peppers, add beans, mold to the form you desire, dip in bread crumbs and bake. Use olive oil in the baking. Serve with tartar sauce, garnished with sprigs of parsley.

To make mucusless, replace breadcrumbs with low-heated grains, chopped after cooking.

Zucchini, Italian Style:

2 Zucchini squash (large) sliced in about 1/2 inch thickness
1 Tomato (large)
1/2 Onion (red), sliced
1 or 2 Garlic, small clove (if desired)

Low heat zucchini, garlic and onion until soft (about 30 minutes). Add tomatoes and low heat another 10 minutes; serve.

Corn Beef, Vegetarian Style:

1 part Cabbage, coarsely chopped
1 part Carrots, cubed
1/2 part Potatoes
1/2 part Celery, chopped

Steam (low heat) vegetables until sweet and soft. Fill baking dish one-half full of vegetarian brown gravy (purchase at health food store), add vegetables, brush lightly with olive oil or margarine, and bake for 10 minutes at 400° F.

Sweet Potatoes and Carrots Sauteed:

2 parts Carrots, diced fresh
2 parts Potatoes, diced (sweet)
Olive oil or vegetable oil
Parsley

Low heat carrots and sweet potatoes separately until tender. Combine and saute in frying pan, using olive or vegetable oil. Season with flavoring to taste, then before serving, sprinkle with finely chopped parsley.

Boiled New England Dinner:

4 1/2 parts Potatoes
1 part Turnips
2 parts Onions
1 3/4 parts Carrots
2 1/2 parts Cabbage

Cube carrots, turnips and potatoes to 1/2 or 3/4 inches. Low heat onions and potatoes together. When practically done, add cabbage, carrots, and turnips and finish cooking until tender. When all are done, mix together and serve.

Hash a la Vegetarian:

1/2 part	Lima beans, cooked
1/2 part	Peas, cooked
1/2 part	Celery, chopped
1/2 part	Bread crumbs, toasted whole wheat
2 parts	Potatoes, boiled or baked and diced
1/2 part	Beets, cooked and diced
4 tablespoons	Oil, olive or vegetable
2	Onions (large) boiled, (low heated) and chopped
2 tablespoonfuls	Flour, whole wheat or graham
	Vegetable broth, stock or hot water

Brown onions and flour in onion, add vegetable broth or hot water, and cook until done. Add rest of ingredients and bake until brown.
To make mucusless, replace bread crumbs with low-heated grains, chopped after cooking. You can omit the bread crumbs without harming the recipe, or replace with chopped walnuts.

Egg Plant Hash:
Egg plant
Onions, fried
Salt and pepper
Cut egg plant in half lengthwise; place in oven until baked to a mushy pulp; remove and peel. Mash and add fried onions, salt and pepper.

Chicken a la King, Vegetarian Style:

1 part	Celery, sliced (or more to liking)
2 parts	Bell peppers, chopped
1/2 part	Pimento, chopped
1/2 part	Green peas
1/2 part	Carrots, cubed
	Onion, sliced
	Whole wheat flour cream gravy

Low heat vegetables, add gravy, and serve on whole wheat toast.
To make mucusless, make a sauce with soymilk, thickened with arrowroot and seasoned with tamari sauce and/or vegetarian bouillon.

Vegetable Chop Suey:
Use the following ingredients in equal parts or to your liking:
Onions, coarsely chopped and braised
Bean sprouts
Celery, chopped
Bell peppers, chopped
Water chestnuts
Mushrooms, dried (soak mushrooms for 3 or 4 hours before using)
Tomatoes, enough to flavor
Mix all ingredients, place in ovenware pot, and bake in olive oil until golden

brown.

Cabbage and Lima Beans en Casserole:
2-8 ounce cans, or 1 package Lima beans, fresh-frozen
2 parts Cabbage, shredded
Margarine or olive oil
Bread crumbs, toasted whole wheat
Low heat cabbage until tender, using very little water. Prepare Lima beans same way if frozen; if canned, drain liquid to drink later. Alternate the layers of vegetables in an oiled baking dish. Dot with margarine or olive oil, add toasted bread crumbs and bake in moderate oven for fifteen to twenty minutes. Serves 6.
To make mucusless, top with chopped nuts or seeds instead of crumbs.

Spinach Loaf:
Spinach, very thoroughly washed
Onion, finely chopped
Celery, finely chopped
French dressing
Low heat spinach in its own juice and the water drops left on from washing until tender. Drain and chop. When chilled, add onion and celery. Moisten with French dressing. Mold and bake in pan. Serve hot or cold.

French Dressing:

1 teaspoonful	Lemon juice
1/4 teaspoonful	Honey
4 teaspoonfuls	Olive oil, fresh
1/4 teaspoonful	Salt
1/4 teaspoonful	Paprika
	Garlic, pressed (if desired)

Mix 1-1/4 tablespoonfuls of oil with other ingredients (except lemon juice); stir well and add lemon juice. Continue stirring until dressing thickens and add rest of oil slowly.

Baked Beet Tops:
Beet tops, washed thoroughly equal parts
Spinach, washed thoroughly equal parts
Onions, braised
Celery, chopped
Low heat beet tops and spinach separately until tender. Drain and chop, add onions and celery, mix together and put into an oiled baking dish. Cover with whole wheat bread crumbs and bake.
To make mucusless, top with chopped nuts or seeds.

Baked Artichokes:
Artichokes
Garlic cloves

Olive oil
Low heat artichokes until tender, remove from water, spread open a few of the leaves on outside and add garlic cloves. Place in baking dish, pour olive oil over the tops and bake in oven about 25 minutes.

Mock Chicken Croquettes:
Onions, braised
Celery
Carrots
Bell pepper
Potatoes, baked and mashed
Peas
Bread crumbs, toasted whole wheat
Make a base of onions, pepper and celery; add potatoes, carrots, peas, or other cooked vegetables if preferred, and the bread crumbs. Mold into croquettes and bake in oil until a nice golden brown.
To make mucusless, replace bread crumbs with low-heated grains, chopped after cooking, or chopped nuts or seeds.

Mock Country Sausage:
Brown rice, soaked overnight
Bread crumbs, whole wheat (toasted)
Celery, chopped
English walnuts, chopped
Peanut butter
Onions, sliced and braised
Salt and black pepper
Garlic
Sage
Mix all ingredients and mold into round balls. Bread and dip in hot oil until a golden brown. (Vary the proportions to your liking.)
To make mucusless, replace the rice and the bread crumbs with low-heated grains, chopped fine after cooking.

Spinach Cutlets:

Equal parts	Spinach, washed thoroughly
	Beet tops, washed thoroughly
1 part	Beets, fresh (diced after low heating)
1 part	Celery, chopped and braised
1 part	Onion
1 part	Bell peppers, chopped
1 part	Bread crumbs, toasted whole wheat or wheat cracker crumbs
1 part	Walnuts, chopped (or peanuts—walnuts preferred)
	Olive oil
	Pimento strips

Low heat spinach and beet tops separately in their own juice until tender. Drain

off water (save for a beverage later) and chop. Use canned or frozen spinach if not in season. Braise beets, celery, onion in olive oil until golden brown. Combine spinach, beet tops, braised vegetables, bread crumbs, walnuts; place in chopping bowl, chop and mix thoroughly. Mold into round patties or cutlets. Dip in whole wheat cracker crumbs or whole wheat flour and fry in hot olive oil. Serve either cold or hot. Garnish with pimento strips.
To make mucusless, replace crumbs with low-heated grains, chopped after cooking. Roll in sesame seeds instead of bread crumbs.

Vegetable Hamburger:
Onions
Garlic
Bell peppers
Celery, chopped fine
Walnuts, chopped
Hominy, chopped
Bread crumbs, toasted whole wheat
Salt and pepper to taste
Braise onions with bell peppers and add remaining ingredients. Mold and bake in oiled baking dish. Serve with onion.
To make mucusless, replace crumbs with low-heated grains, chopped after cooking.

Stuffed Onions:
6 Onions (large and firm)
Breadcrumbs, whole wheat
Bell peppers, chopped
Tomato pulp
Seasoning, to suit taste
1/2 cup soymilk
Slice off the top of each onion and parboil until almost tender. Strain and remove centers, making 6 onion cups. Chop scooped part of cut onion, add soft bread crumbs, peppers, tomato pulp, and seasoning. Refill onion cups with mixture. Place in baking dish and cover with onion tops and toasted crumbs. Add milk and bake until tender.
To make mucusless, replace crumbs with low-heated grains, chopped after cooking. As a variation, replace soymilk with tomato juice.

Nut and Vegetable Loaf:
1 part Pistachio or cashews, coarsely ground
1 part Almonds, coarsely ground
1 part Coconut, ground (if desired)
1 part Celery, finely chopped or grated
1 part Carrots, finely chopped
1/4 part Minced parsley
6-8 Spinach leaves

1 part Tomato, put through food chopper
1 Avocado
1/2 part Raisins (if desired)
Salt and pepper to taste
After all ingredients except avocado have been through food grinder, mix well together. Mash avocado and mix with other ingredients and form into a loaf and garnish with parsley and green onions. For flavor variations, substitute thyme, dill, sage, oregano, etc. for parsley, adjusting the portion to suit personal taste requirement.

SAMPLE MENUS

Please note: In all menus, allow 10 or 15 minutes between finished fruit and the remainder of the meal, and during this time discuss pleasant happenings of the day, items read, people talked to, or pleasant plans for outings or programs for the afternoon or evening. Remember that a crust of bread in a cottage is better than a large feast in a castle of unhappiness. "A merry heart doeth good like a medicine, but a broken spirit drieth up the bones."

Menu #l
Dried fruit (apricots, dates, raisins, figs, etc.) and pecans or walnuts (use nuts sparingly) chewed together with the fruit.
Russian salad (page 624)
Baked Irish potato, with olive oil and black pepper

Menu #2
Cottage cheese and applesauce mixed
Elimination salad (page 626)
Baked banana squash

Menu #3
Fresh fruit in season (apricots, grapes, cherries, peaches, etc.)
Serbian Goulash (page 627)

Menu #4
Baked apple with honey
Natural vegetable combination salad (page 622)
Baked sweet potato

Menu #5
Carrot and raisin salad (page 623)
Vegetable Chop Suey (page 632)

Menu #6
Stuffed prune salad (page 623)
Baked beet tops

Menu #7
Fresh strawberries with ripe mashed banana and honey
Cooked combination salad on bed of lettuce (page 623)

Menu #8
Cottage cheese and apricot jam
Ripe olives, sliced tomatoes and cucumbers
Baked artichoke

Menu #9
Baked apple with raw sugar or honey
Lettuce and tomato salad
Baked Irish potato

Menu #10
Applesauce with raisins
Mexican coleslaw (page 624)
Baked acorn squash

CHAPTER 17

HERB ALTERNATIVES

At times you may not be able to procure a specific herb for one reason or another but, since many herbs have multiple effects, you can always find a good substitute. This chapter provides a listing of therapeutic properties and the different herbs which may be used to achieve the desired effect. We recommend that you become familiar with the cause of the malfunction and become knowledgeable of which therapeutic action is needed so that you may be selective in the particular herb or combination you choose rather than simple choosing from the herb lists at random. Your ability to transcend from simple use of various herbs to knowledgeable use of them with reference to their therapeutic characteristics and action will determine how skilled and useful you may become as an herbalist.

ABSORBENTS:
Herbs used to produce absorption of exudates or diseased tissues. Black elm, Mullein, Slippery elm.

ALTERATIVES:
Herbs used to alter the existing nutritive and excretory processes and gradually restore normal body functions. Abscess root, American bittersweet, balm of Gilead (bark), Barberry, Bayberry, Beth root, Bistort, Bittersweet, Black alder, Black cohosh, Black haw, Black hellebore (small), Black horehound, Black spruce, Black walnut, Bladderwrack, Blue cohosh, Blue flag, Blue violet, Borage, Brigham tea, Brooklime, Buckbean, Bugleweed, Bullnettle root, Butternut, Carob, Carrot, Cascara amarga, Cascara sagrada, Cayenne, Celechium, Condurango root, Chaparral, Chickweed, Chicory, China root, Cleavers, Comfrey, Common speedwell, Cramp bark, Culver's root, Cup-plant, Dodder, Dogbane, Dwarf elder, Echinacea, Elder bark (cured), flowers and berries, Elecampane, False Unicorn, Figwort, Fireweed, Fleawort, Fringetree, Frostwort, Fumitory, Garlic, German sarsaparillas, Gea, Golden Seal, Great water dock, Greater celandine, Ground ivy, Guaiac, Hemp agrimony, Herb patience, Hickory, Honeysuckle, Hops, Horsenettle, Hyssop, Indian sarsaparillas, Ipecacuanha, Iron wood, Jerubeba, Lady's bedstraw, Larch, Lippia, Manaca, Mandrake, Meadow anemone, Meadow fern, Mezereon, Milkweed root, Mountain laurel, Oregon grape, Ox-eye daisy, Pansy, Peruvian bark, Pipsissewa, Plantain (cooling), Pokeroot (relaxant), Polypody root, Pomegranate, Prickly ash (dried bark), Pulsatilla, Purple loosestrife, Queen's delight, Red alder, Red clover, Red raspberry, Red-veined dock, Rock rose, Rosinweed, Sanicle, Sassafras, Soapwort, Sorrel, Spikenard, Squaw vine, St. John's wort, Stillingia, Sumach, Swamp milkweed, Tag alder, Tamarack, Turkey corn, Twin leaf, Wahoo, Water dock, Water fennel, Wild indigo, Wild sarsaparillas, Wood betony, Wood sage (wild sage), Yarrow, Yellow dock, Yellow parilla.

ANALGESICS:
Herbs used to allay pain when administered orally. See also "anodynes." Black willow (ovarian), Camomile, Catnip, Dill, Fit root, Flaxseed, Foxglove, Giant Solomon's seal, Indian hemp, Jamaica dogwood (root bark), Lobelia, Mullein, Sassy bark, Scopola, Scullcap, Skunk cabbage, Solomon's seal, Stinging nettle, Twin Leaf, Wild yam, Wood betony.

ANAPHRODISIACS:
Herbs used to lessen sexual functions and desires. American black willow, Black willow, camphor, Celery, Coca, Garden sage, Hops, Life everlasting, Oregon grape, Scullcap, White pond lily.

ANODYNES:
Herbs used to relieve pain when applied externally. Aconite (external only), American hellebore, Bittersweet, Bugle weed, Camomile, Camphore, Catnip, Coca, Corn silk, Elecampane, Figwort, Fireweed, Gladwin, Hemlock spruce, Hops, Horsenettle, Houndstongue, Hydrangea, Indian hemp, Jamaica dogwood, Jamaica ginger, Juniper berry and oil, Life everlasting, Marigold, Mullein (especially flower and oil), Mustard, Passion flower, Peppermint (methyl), Pleurisy root, Poke root, Pulsatilla, Red cedar tops, Red poppy, Saffron, Sanicle, Sassafras oil, Silk weed, Stinging nettle, Stramonium, Sweet-scented goldenrod, Texas snake root, Tobacco juice, Tomato tops, Vervain (with flax seed), Virginia snake root, Water plantain, White lily, White pond lily, White lettuce.

ANTACIDS:
Herbs used to neutralize acid in the stomach and intestinal tract. American angelica, Apple, Barberry, Black horehounds, Bladderwrack, Caraway, Catnip, Cloves, Coolwort, Elder flowers, Fennel, Galangal, Garden carrot, Irish moss, Pereira, Parsley, Peppermint, Slippery elm, Sweet marjoram, White poplar.

ANTHELMINTICS:
Herbs used to expel or destroy intestinal worms. Alkanet, Aloe, Alstonia bark, American centaury, American senna, Apricot seed, Arbor vitae, Areca nut, Asafetida, Azedarach bark, Balm of Gilead (bark), Balmony, Balsam fir, Banana root, Beach wormwood, Bearsfoot, Beech, Bistort, Bitter root, Black alder berries (with red cedar gum for children), Black hellebore, Black mulberry bark, Black walnut, Blue cohosh, Buckbean, Blue flag, Buckthorn, Butterbur, Butternut, Cabbage tree, Cajuput oil, Calumba, Camomile, Camphor, Carolina pink, Carrot, Cascara sagrada, Castor oil, Catnip, Cedar gum, Cloves (especially Eugenol), Colombo wood, Common melon seeds, Costmary, Corsican moss, Cowhage, Culver's root, Devil's bit, Demarara pink root, Double tansy, Dulse, Elecampane, Embelia, European pennyroyal, False unicorn, Feather geranium, Fennel and oil, Feverfew, Gamboge (small dose), Garlic, Gentian, Garden sage, Glycerine (non-herb), Goat's rue, Groundsel, Hedge hyssop, Hops, Horehound, Horseradish, Hyssop, Jalap, Jamaica quassia, Jerusalem oak (American wormseed), Kamala, Knotgrass root, Krousso, Leek, Life everlasting, Lilac leaves &

fruit, Male fern, Mandrake, Marigold flowers, Margosa bark, March woundwart, Mexican tea, Mullein, Onion, Peach, Phlox glaberrima, Phlox ovate, Pink root, Plantain, Polypody root, Pomegranate, Primrose, Pumpkin seeds, Purslane seeds (alcohol tincture), Purslane seeds, Quassia (small dose), Red cedar oil and bark, Red lobelia, Red mulberry bark, Rock broke, Rue, Santonica, Savine, Sea wormwood, Self-heal, Senna, Sorrel, Southern wood, Stavesacre (small dose), Stinging nettle, Swamp milkweed, Tamarind, Tanacetum balsamita, Tansy, Thyme, Thymol, Turkey rhubarb, Turpentine (small dose), Valerian, Vervain, Water ash leaves and young shoots, Watermelon seeds, White birch, White oak, White poplar, Wild carrot, Wood betony (decoction with wine), Wood sage, Wormwood.

ANTIABORTIVES:
Herbs used to counteract abortive tendencies. Cramp bark, False unicorn, Lobelia, Red raspberry, Witch hazel.

ANTIARTHRITICS:
Herbs used to relieve and heal arthritic conditions. Bears foot, Bitterroot, Blackberry, Black cohosh, Buckthorn, Burdock, Cayenne, Chaparral, Dandelion, Hydrangea, Irish moss, Sarsaparilla, Saw palmetto, Scullcap, Wintergreen, Yellow dock, Yucca root.

ANTIASTHMATICS:
Herbs used to relieve asthma. Agrimony, Ammoniac, Angelica, Aniseed, Apple blossoms, Asafetida, Asarabacca, Balm of Gilead, Balsam of Peru, Balsam of Tolu, Beetroot juice, Bethroot, Black cohosh, Blue cohosh, Blood root, Boneset, Brigham tea, Butterbur, Cajuput oil, Cayenne, Chaparral, Cleavers, Coca, Coltsfoot, Comfrey root, Cramp bark, Cubebs, Daisy, Elder bark (cured) and berries, Elecampane, Eucalyptus, Evening primrose, Flaxseed, Garden sage, Garlic, Gelsemin, Grindelia (small dose), Ground ivy, Heartsease, Hickory bark, Holly leaves, Honeysuckle, Horehound, Hyssop, Indian hemp, Indian turnip, Irish moss, Jaborandi (small dose), Jamaica dogwood, Jamaica ginger, Licorice, Lobelia (specific), Lungwort, Maidenhair, Malabar nut, Masterwort, Milkweed, Mullein, Myrrh, Ox-eye daisy, Plantain, Pleurisy root, Poke root, Polypody root, Prickly ash, Pulsatilla, Quebracho, Red clover, Red root, Red sage, Rosinweed, Saw palmetto, Senega, Senna, Silk weed, Skunk cabbage, Slippery elm, Spikenard, Stinging nettle (roots and leaves), Storax, Sundew, Sunflower seeds, Thyme, Tree-of-heaven, Vervain, Water ash, Wake robin, Wall germander, Walnut leaves, Water fennel, Wild cherry, Wild plum bark, Wild yam, Yerba santa leaves.

ANTIBILIOUS:
Herbs used to eliminate a biliary or jaundice condition in the body. Agrimony, Alkanet, American centaury, Angastura, Apple bark, Ash leaves (with wine decoction), Balmony, Barberry, Bayberry, Bistort, Bitter root, Bittersweet, Black alder, Blackstrap molasses, Blessed thistle, Blood root, Boneset, Borage, Broom, Buckbean, Butcher's broom, Button snake root, Calamint, Camomile, Cascara sagrada, Cayenne, Celandine, Chicory, Cleavers, Columbine seeds, Couchgrass,

Dandelion, Dodder, Dyer's madder, Elecampane, European centaury, European ground pine, Fennel, Fringetree, Fumitory, Garden sage, Gentian, Golden seal, Gravel root, Grindelia, Ground ivy, Groundsel, Hedge-hyssop, Hemp agrimony, Henna, Herb Robert, Herb patience, Hollyhock, Hops, Horehound, Horseradish, Hyssop, Ipecacuanha, Jaborandi (small dose), Jamaica ginger, Jewel weed, Lungwort, Mandrake, Marigold flowers, Mountain laurel, Mouse ear, Oregon grape, Origanum, Pareira, Parsley, Peach, Pennyroyal, Peruvian bark, Pichi, Plantain, Poke root, Pomegranate, Prickly ash, Red root, Red sage, Rest harrow, Rue, Salsify, Self-heal, Senna, Sheep laurel, Silverweed, Sorrel, Spearmint oil, St. John's wort, Stinging nettles, Sweet marjoram, Tamarack, Tansy, Texas snake root, Turkey rhubarb, Tumeric, Vervain, Wahoo, Water plantain, White poplar, Wild cherry, Wild yam, Wood betony, Wormwood, Yarrow, Yellow toad flax.

ANTICATARRHAL:
Herbs which heal catarrhal conditions in the body. Acadia, Ammoniac, Angelica, Anise (infantile), Asafetida, Asthma weed, Avens, Balm, Balsam of Tolu, Barberry, Barley, Bayberry, Bistort, Bittersweet, Black catechu, Black Haw, Black mallow flowers, Black walnut, Bladderwrack, Blood root, Boldo, Boneset, Borage, Buchu, Burdock root, Cajuput, Cascara sagrada, Cascarilla, Cayenne, Cheken, Cherry, Cloves, Coltsfoot, Comfrey, Common speed well, Copaiba, Coriander seed, Cough grass, Cramp bark, Cranesbill, Cubebs, Echinacea, Elder flowers and berries, Elecampane, Eyebright, Feather geranium, Fennel seed, Flaxseed, Fringetree, Galla, Garden sage (nasal), Garlic, Golden seal (non-astringing), Greater celandine, Grindelia (small dose, bladder and uterus), Heartsease, Horseradish, Houndstongue, Hyssop, Iceland moss, Indian hemp, Indian turnip, Irish moss, Jaborandi, Juniper berries, Lemon, Lemon balm, licorice, Lily-of-the-valley, Lime flowers, Lobelia, Lungwort, Marshmallow, Matico, Milk thistle, Mother of thyme, Mountain flax, Mullein, Oregon grape, Ox-eye daisy flowers, Parsley, Peppermint, Peruvian balsam, Peruvian bark, Peruvian rhatany, Pichi, Pipsissewa, Polypody root, Pulsatilla, Raisin seed, Safflower, Sanicle, Sarsaparilla, Saw palmetto berries, Senega, Sesame, Skunk cabbage, Sneezewort, Squill, Storax (genito-urinary), Sumach, Sundew, Swamp milkweed, Thyme and thymol, Tolu balsam, Tormentil, Turpentine (small dose), Uva-ursi, Vervain, Vinegar and honey, Virginia stone crop, Wake robin, Watercress, Water fennel, Water plantain, White oak, White pine, White pond, Wild cherry, Wild yam, Wintergreen, Witch hazel, Wood sorrel, Yarrow, Yerba rheumy, Yerba santa.

ANTIEMETICS:
Herbs used to lesson nausea and prevent or relieve vomiting. Adder's tongue, Adrue (pregnancy), Anise, Avens, Balm, Bilberry, Bitter orange, Black hore-hounds, Calumba, Camphore, Cascarilla, Cassia, Catnip, Cayenne, Cinnamon bark, Cloves, Coffee, Colombo, Cramp bark (pregnancy), Fennel, Galangal, Gentian, Giant Solomon's seal, Golden seal, Horsemint, Horseradish, Iceland moss, Ipecacuanha (pregnancy), Irish moss, Jamaica ginger, Knotgrass, Lavender, Lobelia, Marigold, Mountain balm, Nutmeg, Origanum, Peach leaves,

Pennyroyal, Peppermint (pregnancy), Pimento, Red clover, Red osiers (pregnancy), Red raspberry, Sassafras oil, Spearmint (pregnancy), Sweet balm, Sweet basil (fresh), Water plantain, White clover, White oak, White poplar, Wild marjoram, Wild yam.

ANTIHYDROPICS:
Herbs used to eliminate excess body fluids or dropsy. Adder's tongue, Agrimony, American pennyroyal, Angelica, Angostura, Anise, Arborvitae, Asarabacca, Ash leaves, Asparagus, Balm leaves, Balmony, Barberry, Bitter candytuft, Bitter root (cardiac), Black alder, Black bryony, Black cohosh, Black hellebore, Black horehounds, Black mustard, Bladderwrack, Blessed thistle, Blood root, Blue cohosh, Blue flag, Broom, Buchu, Buckbean juice, Buckthorn, Burdock seeds and root, Bur marigold, Butternut, Button snake root, Camomile, Canada flea bane, Canadian hemp (cardiac), Carrot, Celandine, Celery, Chaparral, Cleavers, Copaiba, Coriander, Corn silk, Couchgrass, Cucumber seeds, Culver's root, Daisy, Dandelion, Dwarf elder, Dyer's green weed, Dyer's madder, Elder bark (cured and berries), Elecampane, European ground pine, False hellebore (cardiac), False unicorn, Fennel, Flaxseed, Foxglove, Gentian, Glycerine, Golden seal, Gravel root, Haircap moss, Hawthorn, Hedge agrimony, Hedge-hyssop, Hemlock spruce, Horseradish (steeped in apple cider), Hydrangea, Hyssop, Indian hemp, Indian physic, Irish moss, Ivy, Jaborandi (small dose), Jalap, Jamaica ginger, Jewel weed, Juniper berry and oil, Knotgrass, Larkspur, Leek, Licorice (with thirst), Lily-of-the-valley, Lobelia, Mandrake, Masterwort, Meadowsweet, Milkweed, Mugwort, Mullein, Mustard, Night-blooming cereus, Onion, Origanum, Orris, Pareira, Parsley, Pellitory-of-the-wall, Pennyroyal, Peruvian bark, Pipsissewa, Plantain, Prickly ash berries, Quassia, Quince seed and fruit, Red osiers, Rest harrow, Rosemary, Saffron, Sandalwood, Sassafras, Scarlet pimpernel juice, Senega, Shavegrass, Shepherd's purse, Skunk cabbage, Spearmint, Squill, Stinging nettle, Sundew, Tamarack, Tansy, Twin leaf, Uva Ursa, Wahoo, Walnut leaves, White ash, White birch leaves and bark, White pond lily, White poplar buds, Wild carrot, Wild lettuce, Wintergreen, Wood betony, Yellow dock.

ANTILITHICS:
Herbs used to prevent the formation of calculi in excretory passages. Apples, Buchu, Couchgrass, Elecampane, Golden rod, Gravel root, Horseradish, Hydrangea (powerful), Lily-of-the-valley, Pareira, Pichi, Pleurisy root, Sarsaparilla, Stinging nettle, Sumach, Uva Ursa, Wild violet.

ANTIPERIODICS:
Herbs used to relieve malarial-type fevers and chills. Agaricus, Alstonia bark (powerful), Angostura bark, Apple bark, Ash bark, Avens, Barberry, Beth root, Black alder, Black cohosh, Black mustard, Black pepper, Black walnut, Black willow, Bladderwrack, Blessed thistle, Blue cohosh, Blood root, Boneset (large), Buckbean, Burning bush, Cascarilla, Cassia, Cedron, Calumba, Camomile, Celandine, Ciratta, Cinquefoil, Cramp bark, Dodder, Dogbane, Eucalyptus, European angelica, European centaury, Feverbush, Figwort, Florida dogwood,

Fringetree, Fumitory, Gesemium, Gentian, Germander, Glycerine, Golden seal, Horehound, Horse chestnut, Horseradish, Irish moss, Iron wood, Lady's slipper, Lemon, Life root, Lilac leaves and fruit, Mandrake, Motherwort, Mountain ash, Oregon grape, Parsley juice, Pennyroyal, Peruvian bark (powerful), Persimmon, Pomegranate, Prickly ash, Quebracho, Red raspberry, Rosemary, Rosinweed, Rue, Scullcap, Shepherd's purse, Senna, Silk weed, Squaw vine, Tansy, Vervain, Virginia snake root, Wafer ash (root bark), Wahoo, Water fennel, White ash bark, White birch (inner bark), White poplar (powerful), White willow, Winter cherry, Wintergreen and oil (small dose).

ANTIPHLOGISTICS:
Herbs used to reduce inflammation or swelling. Abscess root, Acacia, Adders tongue, Alder, Alkanet, Arnica (external), Ammoniac, Asphodel root, Balm of Gilead, Balmony (breasts), Bayberry, Bearsfoot, Black cohosh (nerves), Bladderwrack, Blue cohosh (uterus), Boldo, Borage, Buckbean leaves, Burdock root (external), Bugloss, Camomile, Cayenne, Chaparral, Chickweed, Cinquefoil, Comfrey, Couchgrass, Cranesbill, Cubeb oil, Devil's bit, Elder flowers and leaves, Elecampane, European angelica, Fennel and berries, Fenugreek, Figwort, Fireweed, Flaxseed, Fringetree, Galbanum, Garden sage, Garlic juice, Gentian (with sweet flag), Ginseng (urinary), Golden seal, Great white field lily, Grindelia, Heartsease, Hops, Hydrangea, Hyssop, Ipecacuanha, Ivy (glandular), Juniper berry and oil, Kava kava, Kidney wort, Lady's mantle, Lily-of-the-valley, Lobelia, Lemon, Licorice, Marigold flowers (with Myrrh), Marshmallow, Mountain laurel, Mugwort, Mullein leaves & oil, Ox-eye daisy root, Pareira (kidney, bladder), Peppermint and menthol, Peruvian bark, Pleurisy root, Purslane, Sandalwood, Sarsaparilla, Saw palmetto berries, Scopola, Self-heal, Slippery elm, Smartweed, Solomon's seal, Sorrel, Stinging nettle (kidney), Tansy, Tormentil, Uva Ursa, Vervain (with flax seed), Water figwort, White lily, White pond lily, White poplar, Wild marjoram and oil, Wintergreen and oil, Witch hazel, Wood sage, Wormwood, Yellow flag flowers, Yellow loose strife, Yellow parilla.

ANTIPYRETICS:
Herbs used to reduce temperature in fevers. Benzoin, Camphor, Eucalyptol, Soap tree, Thymol, Wild indigo.

ANTIRHEUMATICS:
Herbs used to prevent, relieve and cure rheumatism. Acadia, Alder, Alstonia bark, American bittersweet, American centaury, American pulsatilla, Angelica, Ash bark and leaves, Azedarach, Balm, Balm of Gilead (buds), Balsam of Tolu, Birch, Birthwort, Bitter candytuft, Bitter root, Bittersweet, Black alder, Black berry, Black bryony, Black cohosh, Black pepper, Black willow, Bladderwrack, Blue cohosh, Blue flag, Blood root, Boneset, Boxwood, Brigham tea, Broom, Buchu, Buckbean, Buckthorn, Bugleweed, Burdock, Cajuput, Camphor, Canada flea bane, Candy tuft, Cayenne, Cedar berries, Celery seed, Chaparral, Chickweed, Cloves, Colchicum, Comfrey, Colombo, Coriander, Couchgrass, Culver's root, Dandelion, Dyer's green weed, Elder bark (cured) and flowers and berries,

Embelia, European angelica, European ground pine, Fennel, Fireweed, Galbanum, Garden carrot, Gelsemin, Germander, Gladwin, Glycerine, Gravel root, Guaiac wood and gum, Guarana, Hemlock spruce, Horehound, Horse chestnut, Horsemint, Horseradish, Hydrangea, Hyssop, Indian hemp, Indian physic, Indian sarsaparillas, Indian turnip, Irish moss, Jaborandi (small dose), Jamaica ginger, Juniper berry, Kava kava, Lemon juice, Lobelia, Manaca, Mandrake, Mezereon, Mother of thyme, Mountain flax, Mountain laurel, Mugwort, Mullein, Mustard, Myrrh, Oregon grape, Origanum, Pareira, Peppermint, Pipsissewa, Pleurisy root, Poison oak, Poke root and berries, Prickly ash, Primrose, Quassia, Ragwort, Rest harrow, Rosemary, Rue, Safflower, Sarsaparilla, Sassafras, Scarlet Pimpernel, Scullcap, Senega, Silverweed, Skunk cabbage, Soapwort, Spikenard, Stavesacre, Stinging nettle, Stramonium, Sumach berries, Sweet-scented goldenrod, Tamarack, Thyme and oil, Tormentil, True unicorn, Turkey rhubarb, Turpentine (external), Twin leaf, Uva Ursa, Wafer ash root bark, Wahoo, Wake robin, Watercress, Wheat germ oil, White ash bark, White birch leaves, White pine, White poplar, White willow, Wild cherry, Wild indigo, Wild marjoram, Wild sarsaparillas, Wild yam, Wintergreen (small dose), Wood betony, Wood sage, Wormwood, Yarrow, Yellow dock, Yellow parilla, Yellow poplar bark.

ANTISCORBUTICS:
Herbs used to prevent and cure scurvy. Arrowhead, Balm of Gilead buds, Barberry berries, Bilberry, Black berries, Black currant, Bladderwrack, Blueberries, Brooklime, Buckbean, Burdock root, Burning bush, Chickweed, Citron, Cleavers, Common melon (in large amounts), Common speed well, Cranberries, Crawley root, Daisy roots, Dandelion, Dodder, Elecampane, European mountain ash (berries), Flaxseed, Fleawort, Fumitory, Great water dock, Groundsel, Hemp agrimony, Horseradish, Hydrangea, Juniper berry, Lemon juice, Lily-of-the-valley, Lime, Mandarin orange, Marjoram, Mountain ash, Oregon grape, Origanum, Paraguay tea (large), Pineapples, Poke root, Radishes, Red currants, Sanicle, Sarsaparilla, Scurvygrass, Sheep sorrel, Shepherd's purse, Sorrel, Spinach, Spruce, Strawberry, Stinging nettle, Stonecrop, Tomatoes, Water dock, White pine, Whortleberries, Wild apple, Wood betony, Wood sanicle, Yellow dock, Yellow parilla.

ANTISCROFULOUS:
Herbs used to heal scrofula (Tubercular condition of the lymph nodes). Abscess root, Adder's tongue, Agrimony, Asphodel root, Barberry, Bayberry, Bearsfoot, Bittersweet, Black cohosh, Black walnut, Bladderwrack, Bloodroot, Blue flag, Buckbean, Burdock root, Burning bush, Button snake root, Camomile, Celandine, Chaparral, Cleavers, Coltsfoot, Comfrey root, Culver's root, Dandelion, Dodder, Echinacea, Elder flowers, Figwort, Frostwort, Fumitory, Gentian, Germander, Greater celandine, Guaiac, Horseradish, Hyssop, Irish moss, Iron weed, Ivy, Juniper berries, Lavender, Manaca, Mandrake, Marigold leaves (fresh), Mayweed, Mezereon, Oregon grape, Pansy, Peruvian bark, Pipsissewa, Plantain, Pleurisy root, poke root, Prickly ash, Quince seed and fruit, Red clover, Rock rose, Rosemary, Sarsaparilla, Sassafras, Silk weed, Soapwort,

Sorrel, Stillingia, Stinging nettle, Sumach berries, Tag alder, Turkey corn, Turkey rhubarb, Valerian, Vervain, Water figwort, White pond lily, Wild carrot, Wild sage, Wintergreen, Wood betony, Wormwood, Yellow dock, Yellow parilla, Yellow toad flax.

ANTISEPTICS:

Herbs used to prevent, resist and counteract putrefaction (decay of cells and formations of pus). Amaranth, Anise oil, Arrowroot (mashed rhizome), Avens, Balsam of Peru, Beech, Benzoin, Betel, Beth root, Black alder, Blackberry, Black cohosh, Black walnut hulls and leaves (powerful), Black willow, Bladderwrack, Blood root, Blue violet, Boldo, Buchu, Bugleweed, Burdock leaves, Cajaput oil, Calumba, Camomile, Camphor, Canada flea bane, Caraway oil (powerful), Carline thistle, Cassia, Cayenne, Cinnamon oil, Cloves and oil, Coffee, Colombo, Comfrey, Condurango root (powerful), Coriander oil, Coto bark, Cranesbill, Culver's root, Echinacea (powerful), Elecampane, Elder bark, Eucalyptus & Eucalyptol, European centaury, Fennel oil, Figwort, Fleawort, Florida dogwood root bark, Galla, Garden sage, Garlic in olive oil or steeped in apple cider (powerful), Gentian, Glycerine, Golden seal, Great white field lily, Guaiac, Heartsease, Herb patience, Holly, Horseradish, Hydrangea, Ipecacuanha, Juniper berry and oil, Irish moss, Ivy berries, Lemon, Lily-of-the-valley (powerful), Logwood, Malva, Marigold, Marshmallow, Mullein, Myrrh (powerful), Nux vomica, Olive leaves & young bark, Peppermint (menthol), Peruvian bark, Plantain, Pleurisy root, Prickly ash, Purslane, Quassia (small dose), Quince, Red oak, Rhatany root, Rue, Sandalwood, Sanicle, Saw Palmetto, Smartweed, Southernwood, Stinging nettle, Stockholm tar, Storax, Sumach, Thyme & thymol, Tobacco leaves, Tormentil, Turpentine (external), Uva Ursa, Vervain, Walnut leaves, Water avens root, Water pepper, White birch bark, White oak (slow), White pond lily, White poplar, Wild indigo, Wild marjoram and oil, Wintergreen and oil, Witch hazel, Wood sage, Wormwood.

ANTISPASMODICS:

Herbs used to relieve nervous irritability and reduce or prevent excessive involuntary muscular contractions (spasms). American pennyroyal, Ammoniac, Aniseed (infantile), Apricot seed, Arbor vitae leaves, Arracacha, Asafetida, Asthma weed, Balm, Beth root, Black cohosh (alcohol extract), Black Haw, Black horehounds, Blue cohosh, Boneset, Brigham tea, Bugbane, Bugleweed, Burra gokeroo, Cajuput, Camomile, Camphor, Cascara amarga, Cassia, Catnip, Cayenne, Cedron, Chaparral, Chirata, Cinnamon, Clary, Cloves, Coltsfoot, Cramp bark, Cumin, Dragon turnip, Elder bark, Elecampane, Eucalyptus, European pennyroyal, Evening primrose, Fennel, Firewood, Fit root, Galbanum, Garden sage, Garlic, Gelsemin, Gentian, German camomile, Gladwin, Grindelia (small dose), Heartsease, Horsenettle berries, Indian hemp, Indian turnip, Indian valerian, Ipecacuanha, Jamaica ginger, Jerusalem oak, Lady's slipper, Life root, Linden, Lippia, Lobelia, Malabar-nut, Marigold, Masterwort, Matico, Meadow anemone, Mayweed, Mexican tea, Mistletoe, Mother of thyme, Motherwort, Mugwort, Mullein, Oats, Ox-eye daisy, Parnassia, Parsley, Passion flower,

Pennyroyal, Peony, Peppermint, Pleurisy root, Pomegranate, Prickly ash berries, Primrose, Pulsatilla, Quassia (small dose), Quebracho, Red clover, Red lobelia, Red root, Rosemary, Rosinweed, Rue, Sassafras, Scullcap, Self-heal, Senega, Silverweed, Skunk cabbage, Small cleaver, Small yellow lady's slipper, Spearmint, Squaw mint, Stone root, Stramonium, Sumbul, Sundew, Tansy, Texas snake root, Thyme and oil, Tree-of-heaven, Twin leaf, Valerian, Vervain, Virginia snake root, Water mint, White poplar, Wild ginger, Wild yam, Yellow lady's slipper.

ANTISYPHILITICS:
Herbs used to relieve and cure syphilis or other ventral diseases. American senna, Barberry, Bayberry, Bitter root, Bittersweet, Black catechu, Black walnut, Black willow, Bladderwrack, Bloodroot, Blue flag, Blue violet, Boldo, Boxwood, Burdock, Burra gokeroo, Button snake root, Caroba, Chaparral, Cleavers, Condurango, Copaiba, Corn silk, Cranesbill, Cubebs, Culver's root, Devil's bit, Echinacea, Elder bark, leaves and berries (external), European birch, Fringetree bark, Frostwort, Galla, Golden seal, Guaiac, Hardhack, Hydrangea, Hyssop, Indian sarsaparillas, Ivy, Juniper berry, Kava kava, Krameria root, Lily-of-the-valley, Life everlasting, Manaca, Mandrake, Manzanita, Marshmallow, Marsh rosemary, Matico, Mezereon, Mountain laurel, Mullein oil, Oregon grape, Pansy, Pareira, Parsley, Peruvian balsam, Peruvian rhatany, Pipsissewa, Plantain, Poke root, Prickly ash, Quince, Red clover, Red raspberry, Red root, Rock rose, Sandalwood, Sanicle, Sarsaparilla, Sassafras root bark, Shavegrass, Soapwort, Spikenard, Spruce, Stillingia, Storax, Sumach berries and leaves, Tag alder, Thyme oil, Tormentil, Tragacanth, Turkey corn, Turpentine (small dose), Twin leaf, Uva Ursa, White pine bark, White pond lily, White poplar, Wild sarsaparillas, Yellow dock, Yellow parilla.

ANTIVENOMOUS:
Herbs used as antidotes to animal, vegetable, and mineral poisons. Abscess root, Agrimony, Alkanet, American pennyroyal, Arrow root (mashed rhizomes), Balm, Beth root, Bistort, Black cohosh, Black mustard (narcotic poisoning), Blood root, Blue juice, Borage, Box leaves, Bugbane, Cedron, Chaparral, Coca (narcotic poisoning), Coffee, Condurango (narcotic poisoning), Contrayerva. Cornflower, Echinacea, Elecampane, European angelica, European pennyroyal, Fennel, Fleawort, Garden carrot, Garlic, Gentian, Houseleek, Hyssop, Indian hemp, Jalap, Juniper berry, Life everlasting, Lobelia, Marigold, Marjoram, Mustard (narcotic poisoning), Olive oil, Pareira, Parsley, Plantain (powerful), Rue, Sassafras bark & oil, Scullcap, Slippery elm, Solomon's seal, Sundew, Sweet basil seeds, Tormentil, Virginia snake root, White ash bark (wine decoction), White oak, Wood betony (decoction with wine), Wormwood, Yellow flag.

ANTIZYMOTICS:
Herbs used to destroy or arrest the action of bacterial organisms. Blackberry, Black walnut leaves and hulls, Cinnamon bark, Cloves (Eugenol—powerful), Elecampane, Garlic, Gentian, Glycerine, Horseradish, Lobelia, Mullein,

Peppermint (menthol), Quassia (small dose), Thyme & thymol, White bryony,

APERIENTS OR LAXATIVES:
Herbs used as mild evacuants or laxatives to the bowels. Agar, Almonds, American senna, Apples (stewed), Apricot, Asafetida, Ash, Asparagus, Balm of Gilead, Balmony, Barberry, Bearsfoot, Bittersweet, Black alder, Bladderwrack, Bloodroot, Blue cohosh, Blue violet, Boneset (large), Borage, Buckthorn bark, Burdock root, Butcher's broom, Calumba (small dose), Carob, Cascara sagrada (small dose), Cocillana bark, Coconut milk, Chicory, Chirata, Cleavers, Cocillana, Copaiba, Couchgrass, Culver's root, Damiana, Dandelion, Dodder, Dwarf elder, Elder flowers and berries, Endive, European rhubarb, Fennel, Feverfew, Figs, Flaxseed, Fringetree, Fumitory, Garden sage, Glycerine, Golden seal, Hartstongue, Heartsease, Herb patience, Hickory, Honeysuckle, Hops, Horehound, Horseradish, Hydrangea (small dose), Hyssop, Ivy, Jewel weed, Jujube berries, Larch, Licorice, Lily-of-the-valley, Malva, Manna, Marshmallow, Motherwort, Mountain flax, Mustard, Oats, Olive oil, Oregon grape, Pansy, Pareria (small dose), Parsley, Peach, Pellitory-of-the-wall, Peruvian bark, Pitcher plant, Prickly ash berries, Prunes, Quince, Raspberries, Rest harrow, Rhubarb, Safflower, Salsify, Sassy bark, Senna pods, Sesame, Spinach, Strawberry, Tamarack, Tamarind, Turkey rhubarb, Turtle bloom leaves, Virginia stone crop, Wahoo, Water dock, White birch shoots and leaves, Watermelon, Wood betony, Yellow parilla, Yellow water lily.

AROMATICS:
Herbs that are odoriferous, having a fragrant, pungent and spicy taste, and which stimulate the gastrointestinal mucous membrane. Adrue, American pennyroyal, Angelica, Angostura, Anise, Areca nut, Avens, Balm, Balm of Gilead, Basil, Bayberry leaves, Bdellium, Benzoin, Birthwort, Black pepper, Buchu, Burdock leaves, Cajuput, Calamint, Camomile, Canada snake root, Canella, Caraway, Cardamon, Cascarilla, Catnip, Celery, Cinnamon, Cloves, Condurango, Contrayerva, Coriander, Cubebs, Culver's root, Dill European angelica, European centaury, European pennyroyal, Fennel, Fleabane, Frostwort, Galangal, Garden sage, Goat's rue, Goldenrod, Ground pine, Horehound, Horsemint, Hyssop, Jamaica ginger, Jerusalem oak, Juniper berry, Knotgrass, Lavender cotton, Lemon peel, Lemon thyme, Lovage, Masterwort, Matico, Meadowsweet, Melilot, Mexican tea, Mountain balm, Myrrh, Nutmeg, Olibanum, Orange peel, Orris, Parsley, Peach, Peppermint, Peruvian balsam, Pimento, Pimpernel, Red clover, Rosemary, Rue, Sassafras, Sea wormwood, Southernwood, Spearmint, Sweet nicely, Sweet fennel, Sweet flag, Sweet marjoram, Tansy, Tolu balsam, Tumeric, Valerian, Vanilla, Wafer ash, Wild cherry, Wild marjoram, Wintergreen, Wood betony, Wood sage, Wormwood, Zedoary.

ASTRINGENTS:
Herbs that influence the vital contractility of cell walls, condense the tissues, make them denser and firmer, and arrest improper discharges. Abscess root, Acacia, African ginger, Agaricus, Agrimony, Alder, Alstonia, Amaranth,

American boxwood, American liverwort, American sea lavender, Apple bark and root bark (powerful), Areca nut, Ash bark, Avens, Azalea, Balm, Barberry (root, berries), Bayberry (powerful), Beech bark & leaves, Betel nut, Beth root, Betony, Bilberry, Bistort (powerful), Black alder, Blackberry (powerful), Black catechu, Black cohosh, Black Haw, Black walnut leaves, Black willow, Boldo, Buchu, Bugle, Bugleweed, Burr marigold, Butternut, Button snake root, Cabbage tree, Canada flea bane, Cassia, Catechu, Cayenne, Chaparral, Cherry, Chestnut leaves, Chocolate root, Cinnamon bark, Cinquefoil, Cloves, Comfrey root, Copaiba balsam, Coto bark, Cramp bark, Cranesbill, Cudweed, Culver's root, Cypress tree, Dodder, Dragon's blood, Drameria root, Echinacea, Elecampane, English elm, Eucalyptus kino, European birch, Evening primrose, Eyebright, Farkleberry (root, bark or berries), Figwort, Fireweed, Fleabane, Florida dogwood, Fluellin, Frostwort, Fumitory, Galla, Gambir, Garden sage, Goldenrod, Gold thread, Grape leaves, Gravel root, Great burnett, Great water dock, Great white field lily, Ground ivy, Guarana, Hardhack bark, Hawthorne, Hemlock spruce, Henna, Herb Robert, Hickory bark, Holly, Honeysuckle, Hops, Horse tail, Houndstongue, Houseleek, Hydrangea, Ivy, Jacob's ladder, Jambul, Kino, Knapweed, Knotgrass, Kola, Kousso, Lady's mantle, Larch, Lesser burnet, Lesser celandine, Life everlasting, Life root, Lobelia, Logwood, Lungwort, Magnolia, Maidenhair, Male fern, Mandrake, Manzanita, Marsh rosemary, Matico, Meadow cranesbill, Meadow fern, Meadow lily, Meadowsweet, Mimosa, Mouse ear, Mountain ash, Mountain laurel, Mullein, Myrrh, Nutgall, Nux vomica, Olive leaves & young bark, Paraguay tea, Peony, Periwinkle, Persimmon, Peruvian bark (moderate), Peruvian rhatany, Pilewort, Pipsissewa, Pitcher plant, Plantain (mild), Pleurisy root (slight), Polypody root, Pomegranate, Primrose, Purging cassia (bark —powerful), Purple loose strife, Quassia, Quince, Ragwort, Red maple, Red oak, Red osiers, Red raspberry, Red root, Red rose, Red sage, Red sanders wood, Rhatany root, Rhubarb, Rock rose, Rosemary, Rupturewort, Russian knot grass, Salsify, Sandalwood, Sanicle, Sassy bark, Scrub oak, Scullcap, Self-heal, Shavegrass, Shepherd's purse, Silverweed, Slippery elm (slight), Smartweed, Solomon's seal, Sorrel, Southernwood, Squaw vine, St. John's wort, Stinging nettle, Stone root, Strawberry, Sumach, Sumbul, Sweet gale, Sweet sumac, Sycamore, Tag alder, Tea, Tormentil, Trailing arbutus, Tree-of-heaven, Turkey rhubarb, Uva Ursa (powerful), Virginia stone crop, Wafer ash bark, Wahoo, Walnut leaves & bark, Water avens (powerful), Water dock, Water pepper, Water plantain, White ash bark, White birch inner bark, White oak (strong), White pond lily, White poplar, White willow, White apple, Wild cherry, Wild indigo, Wild mint, Wild rose, Wintergreen (small dose), Witch hazel, Wood betony, Wood sage, Yarrow, Yellow dock, yellow flag, Yellow loose strife, Yellow pond lily, Yellow toad flax, Yerba rheuma.

APHRODISIACS:

Herbs used to correct conditions of impotence and strengthen sexual power. Arracacha, Betel, Black cohosh, Burra gokeroo, Camphor, Carline thistle, Damiana, Echinacea, Coca, False unicorn, Garden sage, Ginseng, Guarana, Jamaica ginger, Matico, Murira-puama, Night blooming cereus, Nux vomica, Quaker button, Saw palmetto berries, Summer savory, Sundew, True unicorn (impotence), Vanilla pods, Virginia snake root, Yohimbe.

BALSAMIC:
Herbs that mitigate, soothe and heal inflamed parts. Avocado leaves, Balm of Gilead buds, Clary, Larch, Ox-eye daisy flowers, Poplar buds, Spikenard.

BITTERS:
Herbs having a bitter taste and serving as stimulant tonics to the gastrointestinal mucous membranes. Angostura, Barberry, Boneset, Bugle, Cachalagua, Camomile, Cascara amarga, Cedron, Chaparral, European birch, European centaury, Feverbush, Feverfew, Gentian, Gold thread, Horehound, Peach, Quassia, Rue, Wild cherry, Wood sage, Wormwood.

BLISTERS:
Herbs that cause inflammatory exudation (blistering) of serum from the skin when applied locally. Black mustard, Blue violet root, Meadow anemone (bruised leaves), Mezereon, White bryony.

CALEFACIENTS:
Herbal agents used as diffusive stimulants and which cause increased capillary circulation, giving an external sense of warmth. Cayenne.

CARDIAC DEPRESSANTS:
Herbs that lessen and are sedative to the heart's action. American hellebore (small dose), Asparagus, Bitter candytuft, Bitter root, Blood root, Bugleweed, Grindelia (small dose), Jaborandi (small dose), Lobelia (large dose), Mountain laurel, Peruvian bark (large), Pleurisy root, Poke root, Saw palmetto, Tree-of-heaven, Wintergreen oil (small dose).

CARDIAC STIMULANTS:
Herbs used to increase and give greater power to the heart's action. Apples, Balsam of Peru, Bitter root, Blackberry, Black cohosh, Black hellebore (small dose), Black mustard, Blessed thistle, Blood root (small dose), Borage, Broom tops, Buchu, Bugleweed (powerful), Butterbur, Cayenne, Cherry, Cinnamon, Cloves, Coca, Coffee, Comfrey, Condurango, Coriander, Cubebs, Dogbane, Elecampane (tonic), Euphorbia (small dose), European centaury, False hellebore, Flaxseed (tonic), Foxglove, Galangal, Garden sage, Garlic, Gentian, Golden seal, Guaiac, Hawthorn berry, Horehound, Horseradish, Jamaica ginger, Jerusalem oak, Knotgrass, Kola, Licorice, Lily-of-the-valley (tonic), Lobelia (small dose), Mescal buttons, Mistletoe, Motherwort, Mustard, Myrrh, Nux vomica, Night-blooming cereus, Nutmeg, Peppermint, Peruvian bark (small dose), Pipsissewa, Prickly ash, Quassia (small dose), Quebracho, Quince seed, Raisins, Rue, Sassy bark, Scullcap, Smartweed, Sorrel, Squill (small dose), Tansy, Turpentine (small dose), Valerian, Vervain, Virginia snake root, Wild cherry, Wild lettuce, Wintergreen, Wood betony.

CARMINATIVES:

Herbs containing a volatile oil that excites intestinal peristalsis, and relieves and promotes the expulsion of flatus or gas from the gastrointestinal tract. Azure, American angelica, American pennyroyal, Anise seed, Asafetida, Balm, Bitter orange, Black mustard, Black pepper, Buchu, Cabbage, Cajuput, Calamus, Calumba, Camphor, Canada snake root, Caraway, Cardamon, Coriander, Canada snake root, Carrot, Cascara sagrada, Cascarilla, Cassia, Catnip, Cayenne, Cedron, Celery, Cinnamon, Cloves, Coriander, Cramp bark, Cubebs, Cumin, Dill, Elecampane, Embelia, European angelica, European pennyroyal, Fennel, Feverfew, Fleawort, Galangal, Garden sage, Garlic, German chamomile, Goldenrod (cold), Golden seal, Herb patience, Horsemint, Horseradish, Hyssop, Indian turnip, Jamaica ginger, Juniper berry, Lemon thyme, Lovage, Masterwort, Melilot, Melissa, Mexican tea, Mother of thyme, Mountain balm, Mustard, Myrrh, Nutmeg, Parsley, Peppermint, Peruvian bark, Pimento, Pleurisy root (mild), Prickly ash (berries), Red rose, Rosemary, Rue, Safflower, Saffron, Sarsaparilla, Spearmint, Star anise, Sumbul, Summer savory, Sweet basil, Sweet nicely, Sweet fennel, Sweet flag, Tansy, Thyme, true unicorn, Turpentine (small dose), Valerian, Virginia snake root, Watermint, Wild carrot, Wild ginger, Wild marjoram, Wild yam, Wintergreen (infantile), Wood betony, Wormwood, Yarrow, Yellow goldenrod, Yerba buena, Zedoary.

CATHARTICS:

Herbs that are active purgatives to the intestinal tract, exciting peristalsis and stimulating glandular secretions, producing semi-fluid bowel movements with some irritation and griping. Agaricus (large), Aloe, American senna (mild), Angostura (large), Asarabacca, Ash leaves, Azedarach (large), Balm of Gilead, Balmony, Barberry (large), Bitter root, Black alder, Black hellebore (drastic, hydragogue), Black walnut, Blood root, Blue flag, Broom seed, Buchu (large), Buckbean (large), Buckthorn, Butternut, Cabbage tree, Calumba (large), Camomile, Canada snake root, Carline thistle, Cascara amarga, Castor oil plant (drastic), Cascara sagrada (large), Celandine, Cocillana bark, Colchicum, Colocynth (drastic, hydragogue), Common buck thorn, Copaiba, Croton oil, Cubebs, Culver's root, Daffodil, Dogbane, Dyer's green weed, Elder root and bark (hydragogue), Euphorbia (small dose), Fever root, Fireweed, Gamboge (drastic, hydragogue), Garlic, Gentian, Gladwin, Goat's rue, Gourd root, Greater celandine, Groundsel (large), Heartsease root & seeds, Hedge-hyssop, Hemp agrimony, Herb patience, Hickory, Holly, Horehound (large dose), Hydrangea, Indian hemp, Indian physic, Indian podophyllium (hydragogue), Ivy berries, Jalap (hydragogue), Jerubeba, Kamala, Kousso, Licorice, Lobelia, Mandrake (large, hydragogue;, Mezereon, Morning glory, Mountain flax, Mulberry, Myrrh (large), Orris (fresh, large), Pansy, Paraguay tea (large), Pareira (large), Pleurisy root (mild, large), Poke root, Polypody root, Prickly ash (fresh bark or berries), Purging cassia (mild and pleasant), Red raspberry, Sarsaparilla, Scammony (drastic and hydragogue), Senega (large), Senna leaves, Squill (small dose), Stavesacre, Stillingia (large), Swamp milkweed, True unicorn, Turkey rhubarb, Turpentine (small dose), Uva Ursa (large), Valerian, White ash bark, White bryony (hydragogue), Wild indigo, Wild senna, Wild violet, Yarrow (large), Yellow dock, Yellow flag, Yellow parilla, Yellow toad flax.

CAUSTICS:
Herbs that burn or destroy living tissues. Cashew juice, Celandine juice, Lesser celandine leaves, Yellow anemone herb.

CELL PROLIFERANTS:
Herbs that promote rapid healing and restoration. Aloe vera, Comfrey, Elecampane, Saw palmetto.

CEPHALICS:
Herbs that are particularly healing to cerebral conditions and diseases. Almonds, Apple (unpeeled), Bee balm, Black mustard, Bladderwrack, Blessed thistle, Broom, Canada snake root, Catnip, Cowslip, Flaxseed, Garden sage, Garlic, Gelsemin, Irish moss, Jacob's ladder, Jalap, Juniper berry, Kola, Lemon balm, Lily-of-the-valley (powerful), Onion, Parsley, Peruvian bark, Red sage, Rosemary, Rue, Scarlet pimpernel, Scullcap, Stinging nettle, Sumach leaves, Sweet marjoram, Wood betony.

CHOLAGOGUES:
Herbs used to promote a flow and discharge of bile into the duodenum by contracting the bile ducts, and to produce purgation of the bowels. Aloe, Ash bark, Balmony, Barberry, Beets, Blue flag, Boldo leaves, Boneset, Butternut, Colocynth, Culver's root, Dandelion, Fennel, Fringetree, Fumitory, Gamboge, Gentian, Golden seal, Hedge hyssop, Herb patience, Hops, Horseradish, Ipecacuanha, Jalap, Mandrake, Manna, Parsley, Pichi, Purging cassia, Scammony, Self-heal, Stillingia, Tamarack, Turkey rhubarb, Wahoo, Wild yam, Wood betony.

CONDIMENTS:
Herbs used to season or flavor foods. Angelica, Asafetida, Basil, Bay leaves, Bitter almonds, Black mustard, Black pepper, Borage, Boteka, Calamus, Canella, Caraway, Cardamon, Cassia buds, Cayenne, Celery seed, Chervil, Cinnamon, Clary, Cloves, Coriander, Costmary, Cumin seed, Curry, Dill seed, European pennyroyal, Fenugreek seed, Galangal, Garden sage, Garlic, Horehound, Horseradish, Jamaica ginger, Juniper berries, Lavender, Lemon grass, Lemon peel, Lemon verbena, Mace, Marigold flowers, Mugwort, Mustard seed, Nasturtium flowers, Nigella, Nutmeg, Olive, Onion, Orange mint, Oregano, Paprika, Paradise seed grains, Parsley, Peppercorns, Peppermint, Perilla, Pimento (allspice), Pineapple sage, Poppy seed, Rose geranium, Rose hips, Roselle, Rosemary, Rue, Safflower, Saffron, Salad burnet, Salad mint, Sesame seed, Smartweed, Southern wood, Spanish thyme, Spearmint, Star anise, Summer savory, Sweet basil, Sweet marjoram, Tansy, Tarragon, Thyme, Tonka beans, Tumeric, Vanilla.

COLORING AGENTS:
Herbs used for coloring or dyeing purposes. Agrimony leaves—yellow,

Alder—reddish-brown, Alder bark—brown, Alkanet root—red, Annatto—bright yellow, Apple tree bark—brown, Bilberry—dark blue or purple, Black catechu—brown, Black malva flowers—red, Black oak bark—yellow, Black walnut hulls or root—brown, Blood root—deep red or bronze, Bugbane berries—black, Butternut leaves and bark—brown, Cardoon artichoke—yellow, Cedar bark—red, Cedar roots—green, Cochineal—red, Crab apple bark—yellow, Dyer's broom—yellow, Gamboge—yellow, Garden sage leaves—brown, Golden seal—yellow, Golden seal and indigo—green, Hazel nut hulls—mordant, Hemlock bark—reddish-brown, Henna—orange-red, Henna leaves—reddish-brown, Indigo leaves—blue, Juniper berries—brown, Logwood chips—purplish-red, Madder root—scarlet-red, Marigold flowers—yellow, Mesquite gum—mordant, Mountain mahogany—reddish-brown, Oregon grape bark—yellow, Pecan hulls—brown, Poinsettia flowers—scarlet-red, Pokeberries (unripe)—reddish-purple, Pokeberries (ripe)—purplish-black, Rabbit brush bark—green, Rabbit bush flowers—yellow, Red hibiscus—red, Red hibiscus flowers—black, Red maple bark—brown, Red sunders wood—blood red, Safflower (water)—yellow, Safflower (alkalines carbonates)—red , Saffron flowers—red, Smooth sumac inner bark and pith—orange-yellow, Smooth sumac roots—yellow, Sumach—brown, Tumeric—golden yellow, White angelica—yellow, Wild cherry—purple, Yellow dock—yellow, Zedoary—yellow.

CORDIALS:
Herbs that combine the properties of a warm stomach and a cardiac stimulant. Angostura, Avens, Basil, Bdellium, Blackberries, Boldo, Borage, Calamint, Calamus, Camomile, Canella, Cardamon, Carline thistle, Cinnamon, Clary, Clove bark, Coriander, Costmary, Cubebs, Damiana, Dill, Flaxseed, Flowering dogwood, Gentian, Galangal, Ginseng, Great burnet, Hops, Hyssop, Jamaica ginger, Juniper berries, Kava kava, Lemon grass, Lemon thyme, Masterwort, Orange peel, Rosemary, Saffron, Spikenard berries, Tarragon, Virginia snake root, Wood betony, Woodruff, Wormwood, Wild cherries, Yarrow, Zedoary.

CORRECTIVES:
Herbs used to alter and lessen the severity of action of other herbs, especially cathartics or purgatives. American pennyroyal, Aniseed, Bay leaves, Bee balm, Caraway, Cascara sagrada, Catnip, Cinnamon bark, Cloves, Coriander, Fennel, Flaxseed, Jamaica ginger, Licorice, Manna, Nutmeg, Olive bark, Peppermint, Sweet fennel, Thyme, Tormentil.

COSMETICS:
Herbs which are skin tonics and are used to improve the complexion and beautify the skin. See also "emollients". Agar agar, Balm of Gilead, Black walnut, Bladderwrack, Comfrey, Cowslip flowers, Cranesbill (with non-irritating oils, resins, gums), Cucumbers, Elder leaves and flowers with linseed oil & oil of lavender, Elecampane, Horseradish (with butter-milk and glycerine), Irish moss, Lily-of-the-valley, Potato starch, Saffron, Tragacanth, Watercress juice, Witch hazel, Yellow flag.

COUNTER-IRRITANTS:
Herbs that cause irritation by local application in one part and therapeutically relieve pain in another more deep-seated part. American hellebore, Balm of Gilead (buds), Cajuput oil, Ipecacuanha, Lobelia, Night-blooming cereus, Pine tar, Prickly ash, Rue, Tamarack gum, Turpentine.

DEMULCENTS:
Herbs having mucilaginous properties that are soothing and protective internally to irritated and inflamed surfaces and tissues. Acadia, Agar, Almond, American liverwort, Apricot seed, Arrowroot, Balm of Gilead (buds), Barley, Bitter almond, Black elm, Bladderwrack, Blue cohosh, Borage, Broom corn, Bugloss, Burdock root, Burra gokeroo, Calumba (slight), Canna, Cayenne, Chickweed, Coconut oil, Coltsfoot, Comfrey root, Corn silk, Couchgrass, Deer's tongue, Devil's bit, Elm, English elm, Fenugreek, Figs, Flaxseed, Fleawort, Ginseng, Glycerine, Golden seal, Great white field lily, Grindelia, Heartsease, High mallow, Hollyhock, Hops, Houndstongue, Irish moss, Iceland moss, Jujube, Karaya gum, Licorice, Lippia, Litmus, Lobelia, Malva, Manna, Marshmallow, Meadow lily, Mimosa gum (gum acacia), Mountain flax, Mugwort, Mullein, Oats or oatmeal, Okra, Pareira, Parsley pier, Peach, Pellitory-of-the-wall (slight), Plantain, Polypody root, Pomegranate seeds, Prunes, Psyllium, Purple loosestrife, Pumpkin, Quince seed, Ragwort, Red poppy, Rice water, Salep, Sage, Sarsaparilla, Sassafras pith, Scabious, Sesame leaves, Slippery elm, Solomon's seal, Sorrel, Sundew, Sweet cicely, Tansy, Tapioca, Tragacanth, Virginia stone crop, White pine, White pond lily, Yellow pond lily.

DENTAL ANODYNES:
Herbs used locally to relieve pain from an exposed nerve filament in the tooth (toothache). Bee balm, Black mustard, Boxwood oil, Broom, Bull nettle root (chew), Cajuput, Camomile, Camphor, Canada snake root, Galangal, Hops, Jamaica ginger, Mullein, Mustard, Oil of cajuput, Oil of capsicum, Oil of caraway, Oil of cloves, Oil of origanum, Oil of peppermint, Oil of Rosemary, Oil of sassafras, Pennyroyal, Pellitory root, Prickly ash bark (chew), Prickly ash berries (tincture), Silverweed, Stavesacre seeds (local), Summer savory, Sweet marjoram, Tansy, Thymol, Tormentil, Wild marjoram (oleum origanum), Yarrow (fresh leaf), Yellow flag.

DEOBSTRUENTS:
Herbs that remove alimentary and other body obstructions. American liverwort, Asparagus, Barberry, Bayberry, Bittersweet, Buckbean, Butcher's broom, Culver's root, Dyer's madder, English liverwort, Eternal flower, Golden seal (glandular), Great water dock, Horsemint, Lobelia, Mandrake, Plantain, Poke root, Prickly ash, Red clover, Red dock, Salsify, Sarsaparilla, Southernwood, Succory, Turkey rhubarb, Vervain, White pond lily, Wild carrot, Winter green.

DEODORANTS:
Herbs that eliminate foul odors. Blackberry, Charcoal (activated), Chlorophyll

(wheat grass), Echinacea, Lovage, Mandrake, Thymol.

DEPRESSO-MOTORS:
Herbs that diminish muscular movement by action on the spinal centers. See also "nerve sedatives" and "antispasmodic". Gum wood, Lobelia, Poke root.

DEPURANTS:
Herbs that clean or purify the blood by promoting eliminative functions. Agrimony, American sarsaparillas, Apple (unpeeled), Bitter root, Bittersweet, Black alder, Blackberry, Blessed thistle, Blue cohosh, Blue flag, Borage, Brooklime, Buckbean, Buckthorn, Burdock root, Chaparral, Chickweed, Cleavers, Coconut milk, Couchgrass (large), Culver's root, Dandelion, Dulse, Echinacea, Elder flowers, European centaury, European pennyroyal, Fennel, Figwort, Fireweed, Fringetree, Gentian, Guaiac, Heartsease, Hemp agrimony, Herb patience, Hickory, Hyssop, Kava kava, Linden, Marsh rosemary, Meadow fern, Meadowsweet, Oregon grape, Pansy, Plantain, Poke root, Prickly ash, Queen's root, Red clover, Red dock, Sanicle, Sarsaparilla, Sassafras root bark, Senna pods, Sorrel, Spikenard, St. John's wort, Stillingia, Stinging nettle, Turkey corn, Water cress, White clover, Wild violet, Wood betony, Yellow dock, Yellow parilla.

DESICCANTS:
Herbs which are able to dry surfaces by absorbing moisture. Agar, Bladderwrack powder, Corn starch, Great white field lily, Marshmallow powder, Slippery elm powder.

DETERGENTS:
Herbs that are cleansing to wounds, ulcers, etc. or the skin itself. Amaranth plant, Balm of Gilead, Balmony, Balsam fir, Birth wort, Bistort, Bitter root, Black horehounds, Black walnut, Black willow, Blood root, Butternut flower, Cranesbill, European pennyroyal, Goa, Golden seal, Great water dock, Hyssop, Plantain, Poke root, Prickly ash, Red clover, Red dock, Rest harrow, Shepherd's purse, Soap tree, soapwort, Southernwood, Water dock, Water figwort, White clover, White oak, White pond lily, Wormwood, Yellow dock, Yellow loose strife, Yellow toad flax.

DIAPHORETICS:
Herbs that produce insensible perspiration and increased elimination through the skin. Abscess root, American bittersweet, American centaury, American hellebore, American pennyroyal, American spikenard, Angelica, Anise, Arbor vitae (thuja), Ash leaves, Asparagus, Bayberry, Bee balm, Betal, Beth root, Bittersweet, Black birch, Black cohosh, Black currant, Black pepper, Blessed thistle, Boneset, Brigham tea, Buchu, Bugloss, Burdock root, and seeds, Burr marigold, Butcher's broom, Button snake root, Cajuput, Calamint, Camomile, Camphor, Canada snake root, Canadian hemp, Carline thistle, Carob, Catnip, Cayenne, Celandine, Centaury, Coca, Colchicum, Coltsfoot, Common speedwell, Contrayerva,

Crawley root (powerful), Cuckoopint, Culver's root, Cup plant, Deer's tongue, Devil's bit, Dill, Dogbane, Dwarf elder, Echinacea, Elder (flowers, cured bark, berries), Elecampane, English chamomile, Eryngo, European angelica, European ground pine, European pennyroyal, False boneset, Fennel, Fleawort, Gelsemin, Garlic, German chamomile, German sarsaparillas, Germander, Ginseng, Goat's rue, Goldenrod, Groundsel, Guaiac, Heartsease, Hemlock spruce, Hops (somewhat), Horehound, Horsemint, Horseradish, Hydrangea, Indian physic, Indian turnip, Ipecacuanha, Ivy, Jaborandi (small dose), Jacob's ladder, Jamaica ginger (hot), Jerusalem oak, Juniper berry, Kava kava, Kino, Knapweed, Lady's slipper, Lemon balm, Life everlasting, Life root, Linden flowers, Lobelia, Magnolia, Mandrake, Marigold, Masterwort, Meadow anemone, Melissa, Mezereon, Motherwort, Mountain balm, Mungwort, Peppermint, Pleurisy root, Prickly ash, Pulsatilla, Purple loosestrife, Ragwort, Rosin-weed, Safflowers, Saffron, Sarsaparilla, Sassafras, Sassy bark, Savin, Scabious, Scarlet pimpernel, Sheep sorrel, Skunk cabbage, Small cleaver, Smartweed, Soapwort, spearmint, Spikenard, Squaw mint, Stillingia, Stone-root, Sumach berries, Sweet goldenrod, Tansy, Texas snake root, Thyme, Turpentine (small dose), Valerian, Vervain, Virginia snake root, Wake robin, Water germander, Watermint, Water plantain, White ash bark, Wild ginger, Wild lettuce, Wild marjoram, Wild sarsaparillas, Wild yam, Wood sage, Yarrow (powerful), Yellow lady's slipper, Wormwood.

DIGESTANTS:
Herbs containing ferments and acids, that aid in the solution and digestion of food. Apples, Balm of Gilead bark, Barberry, Cachalagua, Calumba, Caraway, Cinnamon bark, Cloves, Coriander, Dandelion, Fennel, Galangal, Garden sage, Garlic, Gentian (with dried orange peel), Golden seal, Horseradish (powerful), Nutmeg, Onion, Orange peel, Quassia (small dose), Star anise, Wild cherry.

DILUENTS:
Herbs that dilute secretions and excretions. Flax seed.

DISCUTIENTS:
Herbs that dispel or resolve (dissolve) tumors and abnormal growths. Adder's tongue, Ammoniac, Arnica, Asarabacca root, Balm of Gilead (bark), Bayberry, Betel leaves, Bethroot leaves, Birthwort, Black willow, Bladderwrack, Blood root, Blue violet, Burdock root, Calamint, Celandine, Chickweed, Columbine, Coltsfoot, Condurango root, Crawley root, Cudweed, Elder (leaves, flowers), Flaxseed, Galbanum, Garden sage, Garlic, Golden seal, Greater celandine, Heartsease, Hops, Ivy, Life everlasting, Lily-of-the-valley, Marigold flowers, Masterwort, Mountain balm, Mugwort, Mullein, Pansy, Periwinkle, Plantain, Pipsissewa, Red clover, Red root, Rock rose, Sanicle, Sarsaparilla, Skunk cabbage, Slippery elm, Snapdragon leaves, Solomon's seal, Sorrel, St. John's wort, Tansy, Tobacco leaves, Tormentil, Walnut leaves & hulls, White clover, White lily, White melilot, White oak, White pond lily, Wild sage, Wintergreen, Witch hazel, Wormwood, Yellow dock, Yellow pond lily.

DISINFECTANTS:

Herbs that eliminate or destroy the noxious properties of decaying organic matter and thereby prevent the spreading or transfer of toxic matter or infection. Apples, Balsam of Tolu, Benzoin, Black walnut (hulls, leaves), Calumba, Cajuput, Cloves (Eugenol—powerful), Copaiba and oil, Cubebs, Eucalyptus, Garlic, Horseradish, Myrrh, Rue, Sandalwood, Storax, Thymol, Turpentine, Uva ursi.

DIURETICS:

Herbs that increase the secretion and flow of urine. Agrimony, Alder buck thorn, American bittersweet, American centaury, American senna, Ammoniccum (mild), Anise root, Arbor vitae, Arenaria rubra, Arnica, Arrowhead, Artichoke, Ash leaves, Asarabacca, Asparagus, Balm of Gilead, Balsam fir, Barberry, Bayberry, Betel, Bilberry, Bistort, Bitter root, Bittersweet, Blackberries, Black bryony, Black cohosh, Black currant, Black Haw, Black hellebore, Black horehounds, Blood root, Blue cohosh, Blue flag, Boldo, Boneset, Borage, Brooklime, Broom, Broom-corn, Buchu, Buckbean, Buckthorn, Bugloss, Bugleweed, Burdock, Burdock seeds, Burra gokeroo, Burr marigold, Butcher, Butterbur, Button snake root, Cajuput, Calamint, Camomile, Canada snake root, Canadian hemp, Caraway, Carline thistle, Carob, Carrot, Catnip, Cayenne, Cedar berries, Celery, Chaparral, Cheken, Chicory, Cleavers, Coca, Colchicum, Cococynth, Columbine, Common melon (seeds, fruit), Common speedwell, Condurango, Colewort, Copaiba, Corn silk, Couchgrass, Cramp bark (relaxant), Cranberry (fruit, leaves), Cranesbill, Cubebs, Cucumber seed, Cudweed, Culver's root, Cup plant, Currant leaves, Damiana, Dandelion, Deer's tongue, Dogbane, Double tansy, Dwarf elder, Dyer's green weed, Dyer's madder, Dwarf elder, Elecampane, Elder (cured bark, flowers, berries), Elm, Embelia, English elm, Eryngo, European angelica, European ground pine, False hellebore, False unicorn, Fennel, Fever root, Flaxseed, Fleabane, Fleawort, Foxglove, Fringetree, Fumitory, Garlic, Germander, Goat's rue, Goldenrod, Golden seal, Gravel plant, Gravel root, Greater celandine, Great water dock, Great white field lily, Grindelia (small dose), Ground ivy, Groundsel, Guaiacum, Guarana, Haircap moss, Hartstongue, Hawthorn berry, Heartsease, Hedge hyssop, Hemlock spruce, Hemp agrimony, Herb patience, Herb Robert, Hollyhock, Honeysuckle, Hops, Horehound (slight), Horsemint, Horseradish, Huckleberries, Hyacinth bulb, Hydrangea, Hyssop, Indian hemp, Indian sarsaparillas, Ipecacuanha, Jaborandi (small dose), Jacob's ladder, Jalap, Jambul, Jerusalem artichoke, Jerusalem oak, Jewel weed, Juniper berry, Kava kava, Knapweed, Knotgrass, Kola, Lady's bed straw, Lady's slipper, Larch, Leed, Life root, Lily-of-the-valley (powerful), Linden, Lobelia, Lovage, Malva, Manaca, Manzanita, Marshmallow, Masterwort, Matico, Meadow cranesbill, Meadow lily, Meadowsweet, Mezereon, Mistletoe, Mugwort, Mullein, Mustard, Night-blooming cereus, Onion (lithotriptic), Oregon grape, Orris, Ox-eye daisy, Paraguay tea, Pareira, Parsley, Parsley pier (lithotriptic), Peach, Pellitory-of-the-wall (lithotriptic), Peruvian bark, Pichi, Pipsissewa, Pitcher plant, Plantain, Pleurisy root, Polypody root, Prickly ash, Pulsatilla, Pumpkin seeds, Purple loosestrife, Purslane, Radishes, Ragwort, Red cedar berries, Rest harrow, Rosinwood, Rue, Rupturewort, Russian knot grass, Safflower, Saffron, Samphire,

Sandalwood, Sarsaparilla, Sassafras, Savin, Saw palmetto, Scammony, Scarlet pimpernel, Scullcap, Scurvygrass, Self-heal, Senega, Shave grass, Sheep sorrel, Shepherd's purse, Skunk cabbage, Slippery elm, Smartweed, Soap tree, Sorrel, Spearmint, Spruce, Squaw vine, Squill (small dose), Star anise, Stillingia, Stinging nettle, St. John's wort, Stone root, Storax, Stramonium, Strawberry, Sumach, Sumach berries, Sunflower, Swamp milkweed, Sweet fennel, Sweet marjoram, Sweet sumac, Tamarack, Tansy, Trailing arbutus, True unicorn, Turkey corn, Turpentine (small dose), Twin leaf, Uva Ursa, Valerian, Vervain, Virginia snake root, Wahoo, Water fennel, Watermelon (seeds, fruit), Water plantain, White ash bark, White birch leaves, White Melilot, White oak (lithotriptic), White pine, White poplar, Whortleberry, Wild carrot, Wild lettuce Wild yam, Winter cherry, Wintergreen (small dose), Woodruff, Wood sage, Wood sorrel, Yarrow, Yellow daisy, Yellow goldenrod, Yellow parilla, Yellow toad flax, Yellow water lily.

DRASTICS:
Herbs that are hyperactive cathartics producing violent peristalsis, watery stools, and much griping pain. Black hellebore, Castor oil, Colocynth, Croton oil, Gamboge, Hedge hyssop, Jalap, Red bryony, White bryony.

EMETICS:
Herbs that induce vomiting and cause an evacuation of stomach contents. American hellebore, Asarabacca, Azedarach, Bayberry (large dose), Birthwort, Bitter root, Bittersweet, Black bryony, Black cohosh (overdose), Black mustard, Blessed thistle (large dose), Blood root, Blue flag, Blue violet, Boneset (large dose given warm), Broom, Buchu (large dose), Buckthorn, Bugleweed (large dose), Button snake root, Cabbage tree (overdose), Calumba (large dose), Camomile (large dose), Canada snake root, Canadian hemp, Cayenne (large dose), Celandine, Centaurea, Chaparral, Cocillana bark, Colchicum, Contrayerva, Culver's root, Dogbane, Dwarf elder root, Dyer's green weed, Elder (cured bark, flowers, berries), Elecampane (large dose), Euphorbia, European angelica, False unicorn (large dose), Fever root, Fireweed, Foxglove, Gentian (large dose), German camomile (large dose), Groundsel, Heartsease root & seeds, Hedge hyssop, Hyacinth bulb, Indian hemp, Indian physic, Ipecacuanha, Ivy berries, Jaborandi, Jalap, Larch, Lily-of-the-valley (large dose), Lobelia, Mandrake (large dose), Marqosa bark, Mayweed (small dose), Meadow lily, Mescal buttons (small dose), Milkweed root, Mistletoe, Mustard seeds, Orris (fresh, large), Pansy (large dose), Pleurisy root (large dose), Prickly ash (fresh bark), Primrose, Poke root, Pulsatilla, Quassia (overdose), Rock rose (large dose), Rosinweed, Rue, Saffron, Senega, Skunk cabbage, Solomon seal, Squill, Stavesacre, Stillingia, Swamp milkweed, Tag alder, Tragacanth, Tree-of-heaven, True unicorn, Twin leaf (large dose), Uva Ursa (large dose), Vervain, White bryony, Wild indigo, Wild mint, Wild yam (large dose), Wintergreen (large dose), Wood betony, Yarrow (large dose), Yellow adder's tongue.

EMMENAGOGUES:
Herbs that are female correctives to the reproductive organs, which stimulate and

promote a normal menstrual function, flow and discharge. Acadia, Aloe, American angelica, American centaury, American pennyroyal, Ammeniacum, Arbor vitae, Arrach, Asafetida, Bamboo juice, Bayberry, Bee balm, Beet, Bethroot, Birthwort, Bistort, Bitter root, Bittersweet, Black cohosh, Black Haw (anti-abortive), Black hellebore, Black horehounds, Black mustard, Blessed thistle, Blood root herb (fresh), Blue cohosh, Boneset, Brooklime, Buchu, Buckbean, Button snake root, Burnet, Cajuput oil, Calamint, Camomile, Canella, Carline thistle, Carrot, Catnip, Cedar berries, Celandine, Columbine, Comfrey, Cornflower, Contrayerva, Cotton root, Cramp bark, Crawley root, Cubebs, Culver's root, Dandelion, Devil's bit, Double tansy, Dyer's madder, Elecampane, European angelica, European ground pine, European pennyroyal, Evening primrose, False unicorn, Fennel, Fenugreek, Fever root, Feverfew, Figwort, Fringetree, Galbanum, Garden sage, Garlic, Gelsemin, Gentian, German camomile, Ginger, Goldenrod, Golden seal, Gravel root, Ground pine, Guaiac, Guarana, Hemlock spruce, Horehound, Horsemint, Jacob's ladder, Jamaica dogwood, Jamaica ginger, Jerubeba, Jerusalem oak, Juniper berry, Lavender cotton, Lemon, Lemon thyme, Life root, Linden, Lobelia, Lovage, Lungwort, Magnolia, Mandrake, Manzanita, Marigold, Masterwort, Mayweed, Meadow lily, Mistletoe, Motherwort, Mugwort, Myrrh, Oregon grape, Parsley seeds, Peach, Peppermint, Peruvian bark, Peruvian rhatany, Pilewort, Pitcher plant, Plantain, Pleurisy root, Prickly ash, Pulsatilla, Ragwort, Red cedar berries, Red raspberry, Red sage, Rosemary, Rue, Saffron, Safflower, Sanicle, Santonica, Sassafras root bark, Savin, Scabious, Senega, Shepherd's purse, Slippery elm, Smartweed, Sneezewort, Solomon's seal, Sorrel, Southern wood, Spruce, Squaw vine, St. John's wort, Stinging nettle, Storax, Stramonium, Sumach berries, Sumbul, Summer savory, Sweet cicely, Sweet gale, Sweet marjoram, Sweet-scented goldenrod, Tamarack, Tanacentum balsamita, Tansy, Thyme, True unicorn, Turkey corn, Uva Ursa, Valerian, Vervain, Virginia snake root, Wake robin, Watercress, White ash, White bryony, White pond lily, White poplar, Wild carrot, Wild columbine, Wild indigo, Wild marjoram, Wild mint, Wild yam (anti-abortive), Wintergreen (small dose), Witch hazel, Wood betony, Wood sage, Wormwood, Yarrow, Yellow flag.

EMOLLIENTS:
Herbs that are softening, soothing and protective to external surfaces. Adder's tongue leaves, Almond oil, Apricot oil, Balm of Gilead (buds), Bean leaves, Black elm, Blue violet, Borage, Bugloss, Chickweed, Coltsfoot, Dates, Elecampane, English elm, Fenugreek, Fig, Flaxseed, Garlic, Glycerine, High mallow, Hollyhock, Leek, Licorice, Linseed oil, Litmus, Malva, Marshmallow, Melilot, Mullein, Oats or Oatmeal, Olive oil, Onion, Pareira, Plantain, Poppy capsules, Potato starch, Quince seed, Rose petals, Sassafras pith, Sesame, Slippery elm, White lily, White melilot, White pond lily, Yellow pond lily.

ERRHINES:
Herbs that increase nasal secretions from the sinuses. American hellebore, Asarabacca, Bayberry, Blood root, Canada snake root, Cayenne, Cubebs, Ginger, Horseradish, Ipecacuanha, Oil of lavender, Pellitory, Sassy bark.

EXANTHEMATOUS:
Herbs that are healing to skin eruptions or to skin diseases of an eruptive nature. Alkanet, Asafetida, Beech, Bistort (hot), Black elm, Bloodroot, Burdock (root, seeds), Brooklime, Camomile, Catnip, Cayenne, Cleavers, Contrayerva, Elecampane, European birch, Eucalyptus, Evening primrose, Figwort, Fumitory, Garden sage, Garlic, Golden seal, Ground ivy, Heartsease, Henna, Hyssop, Jaborandi (small dose), Jamaica ginger, Labrador tea, Lady's slipper, Licorice, Linden flowers, Lobelia, Lovage, Marigold flowers, Mullein oil, Peppermint, Peruvian bark, Pipsissewa, Pleurisy root, Red sage, Safflower, Saffron, Sesame, Slippery elm, Soapwort, Stockholm tar, Storax, Strawberry, Sweet marjoram, Thymol, Tormentil, Turkey corn, Valerian, Vervain, Virginia snake root, Wild indigo, Wild marjoram & oil, Yarrow, Yellow toad flax.

EXCITO-MOTORS:
Herbs that increase motor reflex and spinal activity. Nux vomica.

EXPECTORANTS:
Herbs that promote and facilitate discharge of mucus secretions from broncho-pulmonary passages. Anise seed, Asafetida, Balm of Gilead, Balsam of Peru, Balsam of Tolu, Benzoin, Beth root, Bitter root, Black cohosh, Black elm, Black horehounds, Blood root, Blue violet, Boneset, Bugleweed, Bugloss, Button snake root, Calamint, Canada snake root, Canadian hemp, Celandine, Cheken, Cherry, Chestnut leaves, Cloves, Cocillana bark, Coltsfoot, Colchicum, Comfrey, Common speedwell, Copaiba, Cramp bark, Cubebs, Cuckoopint, Dogbane, Dwarf elder, Elder flowers, Elecampane, English elm, Eryngo, Eternal flower, European angelica, Feather geranium, Fennel, Flaxseed, Fleawort, Galbanum, Garden sage, Garlic, Ginger, Ginseng, Golden seal, Greater celandine, Grindelia (small dose), Guaiac, Hawthorn, Heartsease, Honeysuckle, Hops, Horehound, Horseradish, Hyssop, Iceland moss, Indian hemp, Indian physic, Indian turnip, Ipecacuanha, Irish moss, Ivy, Jaborandi, Jerusalem oak, Labrador tea, Licorice, Lippia, Life root, Lobelia, Lungwort, Maidenhair, Malabar nut, Manna, Marshmallow, Mouse ear, Mountain balm, Murillo bark, Mullein, Myrrh, Olibanum, Onion, Orris, Pansy, Parsley, Peach, Pearl moss, Peruvian balsam, Pimpinella, Pleurisy root, Polypody root, Pomegranate, Pulsatilla, Purple loosestrife, Ragwort, Red poppy, Red root, Red sage, Rock brake, Rosinweed, Sandalwood, Sanicle, Sassafras, Saw palmetto, Scarlet pimpernel, Senega, Shepherd's purse, Silk weed, Skunk cabbage, Slippery elm, Small cleaver, Soap tree, Solomon's seal, Spikenard, Squill (small dose), Stillingia, St. John's wort, Stockholm tar, Storax, Summer savory, Sundew, Sunflower, Sweet cicely, Sweet fennel, Sweetwood, Thorja, Tragacanth, Turpentine (small dose), Twin leaf, Virginia snake root, Vervain, Wahoo, Wake robin, Water fennel, White melilot, White pine, White pond lily, Wild cherry, Wild chestnut, Wild ginger, Wild indigo, Wild lettuce, Wild sage, Wild thyme, Wild yam, Yellow loosestrife, Yarrow, Yerba santa.

FEBRIFUGES:
Herbs that reduce fever. Acadia, Alstonia bark, American angelica, American boxwood, American centaury, American hellebore, Angostura bark, Anise root, Apple bark, Arbor vitae, Avens, Balm, Barberries, Barley, Beech wormwood, Birthwort, Bitter orange, Bitterroot, Black alder, Black currant, Black pepper, Black walnut, Blessed thistle, Blue cohosh, Blood root, Boldo, Boneset, Borage, Brigham tea, Brooklime, Buckbean, Buckthorn, Bugloss, Burr marigold, Butternut, Cabbage tree, Cajuput, Calamint, Calumba, Camomile, Cascara sagrada, Catnip, Cascarilla, Cayenne, Cherry bark, Chestnut bark, Chirata, Cinquefoil, Cleavers, Colombo, Coltsfoot, Common melon, Coriander, Couchgrass, Crawley root, Culver's root, Cypress, Dandelion, Deer's tongue, Devil's bit, Echinacea, Elder flowers, European centaury, Eucalyptol, Fenugreek, Fever root, Feverwort, Fir root, Fireweed, Florida dogwood, Fringetree, Gelsemin, Gentian, Hemp agrimony, Herb Robert, Holly, Hops, Hyssop, Indian hemp, Ivy berries, Jamaica ginger, Jerusalem oak, Life everlasting, Life root, Lilac leaves and fruit, Lily-of-the-valley, Lobelia (powerful), Magnolia, Mahogany, Malabar nut, Mandrake, Marigold flowers, Masterwort, Mugwort, Olive (bark, leaves), Pareira, Parsley seeds, Pennyroyal, Peppermint, Peruvian bark, Plantain, Pleurisy root, Prickly ash, Purple loosestrife, Quassia (small dose), Red osiers, Red raspberry, Red sage, Sarsaparilla, Scabious, Sea wormwood, Shepherd's purse, Stinging nettle, Sumach berries, Sweet balm, Tansy, Thyme, Turpentine (small dose), Valerian, Vervain, Virginia, Wahoo, Water avens, Watermelon, White oak, White poplar, Wild cherry, Wild ginger, Wild sage, Willow, Winter cherry, Wormwood, Winter green.

GALACTAGOGUES:
Herbs that increase the secretion of milk. Anise seed, Blessed thistle, Buckwheat poultice (flowers with buttermilk), Centaurea, Fennel, Garden carrot, Goat's rue, Jaborandi (small dose), Mild thistle, Red raspberry (enrich), Vervain.

GALACTOPHYGA:
Herbs that diminish or arrest the secretion of milk. Agaricus, Betel, Bilberry (huckleberries), Cassia bark, Cranesbill, Garden sage, Parsley (poultice).

HEMETICS:
Herbs rich in iron and manganese and which augment and enrich the red corpuscles of the blood (blood-builder). Agrimony, Apple (unpeeled, sour), Barberry, Blackberries, Black walnut leaves, Comfrey, Dandelion, European centaury, Fenugreek, Gentian, Hydrangea, Lily-of-the valley, Quassia (small dose), Red raspberry, Watercress, Wild apples, Yellow dock.

HEMOSTATICS:
Herbs that are generally astringent and arrest hemorrhaging or internal bleeding. Amaranth, American liverwort (lungs), Avens, Bayberry (uterus), Beth root (general), Bistort (powerful), Black berry (uterus), Black catechu, Black cohosh (lungs), Black pepper, Black walnut, Blood root (lungs), Bugleweed (lungs), Burr

marigold (lungs, uterus), Canada flea bane (uterus, bowels), Cayenne (powerful), Cinnamon bark (uterus), Cranesbill (general), Dandelion (general), Elecampane, False unicorn (uterus), Fireweed, Fleabane (uterus, bowels), Galla, Gambir, Gentian (uterus), Golden rod, Golden seal (uterus, rectum), Ground ivy (urinary), Groundsel (nose, bowel, urinary), Grape leaves, Hardhack, Herb Robert, Ipecacuanha, Jamaica ginger, Kino, Krameria root (stomach, intestines, uterus), Lady's mantle (uterus), Lemon juice (cold—uterus), Life everlasting, Lily-of-the-valley, Logwood (uterus, lungs, bowels), Lungwort, Marshmallow (lungs, urinary), Marsh wonderwort, Matico (lungs), Meadow cranesbill, Mountain laurel, Mullein (bowels, general), Onion juice, Peruvian rhatany, Pomegranate, Red raspberry, Red rose (uterus, etc.), Rock brake, Sanicle (lungs, bowels), Sassy bark (passive), Self heal (lungs), Senega (uterus), Shavegrass (general), Shepherd's purse (lungs, uterus, stomach, bowels), Solomon's seal (lungs), Sorrel, St. John's wort, Stinging nettle root (general), Tag alder cones, Tormentil (bowel), Turkey rhubarb, Turpentine (small dose), Uva Ursa (uterus), Vervain, Walnut leaves, Water avens, Watercress, White oak (general), Witch hazel, Yarrow, Yellow dock (lungs), Yellow loosestrife.

HEPATICS:
Herbs used to strengthen, tone and stimulate the secretive functions of the liver, causing an increased flow of bile. Agrimony, Aloe, American angelica, American liverwort, Apple (tonic), Balmony, Barberry, Bayberry, Bee balm, Beech, Bitter root (stimulant), Bittersweet, Blessed thistle, Black alder, Black cohosh, Black root, Blue cohosh, Blue flag (powerful), Boldo (stimulant), Boneset, Broom, Buckbean, Butternut, Calumba, Carrot, Cascara sagrada, Celandine, Celery, Chicory, Chirata, Cleavers, Coolwort, Cramp bark, Crawley root, Culver's root (relaxant, tonic), Cup plant, Daisy roots, Dandelion, Dodder, Dyer's madder, Elder, Elecampane (stimulant), European centaury, Evening primrose, Fennel, Fringetree, Fumitory, Garden sage, Gentian (tonic), Golden seal, Gravel root, Greater celandine (stimulant), Hedge-hyssop, Honeysuckle, Hops, Horehounds, Horseradish, Hyssop, Ipecacuanha, Jerubeba, Lemon, Liverwort, Lobelia, Magnolia, Mandrake root (specific), Marsh watercress, Milk thistle, Motherwort, Olive oil, Oregon grape, Pareira, Parsley, Peony, Pichi, Pitcher plant, Plantain, Poke root, Prickly ash, Purple loosestrife, Quaker button (small dose), Quassia (small dose), Red maple, Red root, Red sage, Rosin-weed, Scarlet pimpernel, Sea wormwood, Self-heal, Stillingia, Tamarack, Turkey rhubarb, Uva Ursa, Wahoo (stimulant), White poplar, Wild indigo, Wild yam (powerful), Wood betony, Wood sage, Wormwood, Yarrow (stimulant), Yellow dock, Yellow parilla, Yellow toad flax.

HERPATICS:
Herbs that are healing to skin eruption and scaling diseases (such as ringworm, etc.). Agrimony, Azedarach, Balm of Gilead buds, Barberry, Beech, Betel leaves, Bittersweet, Black alder, Black bryony, Black catechu, Black hellebore, Black walnut (hulls, leaves, and bark), Blood root, Blue flag, Boneset, Borage, Buckbean, Buckthorn bark, Burdock, Cashew oil, Celandine, Chickweed,

Cleavers, Comfrey, Couchgrass, Culver's root, Dandelion, Devil's bit, Elder (leaves, berries), Elecampane, Fringetree, Fumitory, Garlic, Glycerine, Goa, Golden seal, Greater celandine, Heartsease, Henna, Hydrangea, Indian sarsaparillas, Indian turnip, Irish moss, Jalap, Jewel weed, Kamala, Kino, Labrador tea, Lily-of-the-valley, Lobelia, Magnolia, Mezereon, Mountain laurel, Mullein, Myrrh, Oleander leaves (external only), Oregon grape, Pansy, Pennyroyal, Peppermint & menthol, Peruvian balsam, Peruvian bark, Pine tar, Pipsissewa, Plantain, Poison ivy (obstinate conditions—alcohol tincture), Poison oak (obstinate conditions), Poke root, Prickly ash, Red clover, Red root, Rock rose, Saffron, Sarsaparilla, Sassafras root bark, Soap tree, Sorrel, Spikenard, Stillingia, Stinging nettle, Soap tree, Storax, Sweet marjoram, Tag alder, Tamarack, Thymol, Turkey corn, Turpentine (external), Vervain, Wake robin, White birch bark, White clover, White lily, White pond lily, Wild sarsaparillas, Wintergreen, Wood sage, Yellow dock, Yellow parilla.

HYPNOTICS:
Herbs that are powerful nervine relaxants and sedatives that induce sleep. Bittersweet, Boldo leaves, Bugleweed, Hops (slight), Indian hemp Lachnanthes, Mistletoe, Passion flower, Scopols, Stramonium, Valerian, Wild lettuce.

INSECTICIDES:
Herbs that are used to destroy insects. Anise oil (with sassafras oil), Black cohosh, Black walnut hulls and leaves, European centaury, Field larkspur Jamaica quassia, Pine tar, Rue, Tobacco, Tonka bean, White hellebore.

IRRITANTS:
Herbs that produce a greater or lesser degree of vascular excitement when applied to the epidermis or skin surface. See also "rubefacients," "blister," "counter-irritants". American hellebore, Arbor vitae, Black mustard, Cascara sagrada bark (fresh), Colocynth, Coto bark, Cubeb oil (local), Culver's root (fresh), Elder bark (fresh), Goa, Henbane, Kava kava resin, Mandrake resin, Mustard, Orris root (fresh), Poison ivy, Poison oak, Quassia (overdose), Senega, Soap tree, Squill, Stavesacre, Stinging nettle, Stone root, Vanilla pods, Turpentine (strong vapors), White bryony.

LITHOTRIPTICS:
Herbs that dissolve or discharge urinary and biliary concretions (gravel or stones) when formed in excretory passages. Alkanet, Apple bark, Arenaria rubra, Ash leaves (white wine decoction), Bilberry (berry or root steeped in gin), Bitter root, Blackberries, Black currant, Broom tops, Buchu, Burr marigold, Butcher's broom, Butterbur, Button snake root, Canada flea bane, Capsella leaves, Carrot, Cascara sagrada (gall), Chaparral, Cherry bark (gall), Cleavers, Common speedwell, Coolwort, Corn silk, Couchgrass, Damiana leaves, Dandelion, Elecampane, Flaxseed, Fleabane, Fringetree, Goldenrod, Grave root, Heartstongue, Hops, Horseradish, Hydrangea (powerful), Hyssop, Irish moss, Jalap, Knotgrass, Lady's bed straw, Maidenhair, Marshmallow, Milkthistle, Mugwort, Onion, Pareira,

Parsley, Parsley pier, Pellitory-of-the-wall, Pichi, Pipsissewa, Radishes, Ragwort, Sarsaparilla, Scullcap, Shavegrass, Slippery elm, Smartweed, Sorrel, Spearmint, Spruce, Squaw vine, Stinging nettle, Stone root, Tormentil, Trailing arbutus, Uva Ursa, Valerian, Vervain, Water plantain, White birch leaves, White oak, Wood betony (gall).

LOCAL ANAESTHETICS:
Herbs that produce anesthesia (loss of sensation) where applied locally to a surface. Caraway oil, Coca (powerful), Eugenol (feeble), Eucalyptol, Honey locust (twigs and leaves), Kava kava, Soap tree, Thymol.

MATURATING:
Herbs that promote the maturation or ripening of tumors, boils, ulcers, etc. Bayberry bark, Bee balm, Birch bark, Black alder, Burdock root, Camomile, Chickweed, Comfrey, Cubebs, Echinacea, Fenugreek, Figs, Figwort, Flaxseed, Galbanum, Garlic, German camomile, Leek, Linden, Lobelia, Meadow lily, Onion, Oregano, Pine gum, Pine tar, Plantain, Sarsaparilla, Turkey corn, Vervain (with flax seed), White lily (fresh bulb), White pond lily (leaves & roots with eucalyptol), Wild carrot, Wild cherry bark, Wild sage, Wintergreen, Yellow dock.

MUCILAGES:
Herbs having mucilaginous properties. Acadia, Agar, Amaranth, American liverwort, Black elm, Bladderwrack, Blue violet, Borage, Bugloss, Chickweed, Clary (seeds), Comfrey, Common (musk) melon, Contrayerva, Couchgrass, Cucumbers, Cudweed, English elm, Evening primrose, Fenugreek seed, Flaxseed, Fleawort, Great white field lily (bulb), Heartsease, High mallow, Hollyhock, Houndstongue, Iceland moss, Irish moss, Lily-of-the-valley, Lungwort, Maidenhair, Male fern, Malva, Marshmallow, Meadow lily, Okra, Pansy, Purple loosestrife, Quassia, Quince seeds, Ragwort, Salep, Sesame, Slippery elm, Solomon's seal, Tragacanth (generally not recommended), Uva Ursa, White lily, White pond lily.

MYDRIATICS:
Herbs that cause dilation of the pupil (eye). Belladonna, Coca, Grindelia (large dose), Gelsemin, Scopola, Stramonium.

MYOTICS:
Herbs that cause contraction of the ciliary muscles of the pupil (eye). Arena nut, Jaborandi.

NARCOTICS:
Herbs that are powerful anodyne-hypnotics. Bayberry wax (slight), Birthwort root, Bittersweet, Black cohosh (slight), Black hellebore (powerful), Bugleweed (mild), Cabbage tree, Camphor gum, Coca, Culver's root, Grindelia (large dose), Hedge-hyssop, Horse chestnut, Hound's tongue herb, Indian hemp, Ipecacuanha root, Jamaica dogwood root bark, Mayweed, Mescal buttons, Mistletoe (slight),

Mountain laurel leaves, Mullein, Passion flower, Oleander leaves, Poison oak, Potato plant tops, Quassia (slight), Rue (overdose), Sassy bark, Skunk cabbage, Spotted wintergreen, Squill, Stinking glad wine root, Stramonium, Tobacco leaves, Yellow lady's slipper, Tonka bean.

NAUSEANTS:
Herbs that produce nausea or an inclination to vomit. Chirata (large dose), Copaiba, Ipecacuanha, Lobelia, Orris, Quassia (overdose), Ragwort, Tomato tops, Vervain, Wintergreen (large dose).

NEPHRITICS:
Herbs that influence the kidneys and are healing in kidney complaints. Almond, Aloes, Balm of Gilead (buds), Bee balm, Beech, Bethroot, Bilberry, Birch, Bitter root, Bittersweet, Black birch, Black cohosh, Bladderwrack, Blessed thistle, Blood root, Broom, Buckbean, Buchu, Burr marigold, Button snake root, Camomile, Carrot, Cayenne, Celandine, Chicory, Comfrey, Corn silk, Couchgrass, Cranesbill (powerful), Dandelion, Elder, Elecampane, European centaury, False hellebore, False unicorn, Fennel, Fleabane, Fringetree, German camomile, Golden rod, Golden seal, Gravel plant, Greater celandine, Grindelia (small dose), Hart's tongue, Hawthorne, Hemlock spruce, Hollyhock, Hydrangea, Hyssop, Indian hemp, Irish moss, Jaborandi (small dose), Juniper berry, Lady's bed straw, Linden, Lobelia, Maidenhair, Marshmallow, Masterwort, Milkweed root, Oregon grape, Pansy, Pareira, Parsley root, Parsley pier, Partridge berry herb, Peach, Peppermint, Pichi, Pipsissewa, Pitcher plant, Pleurisy root, Poke root, Samphire, Sanicle, Sassafras, Saw palmetto berries, Scarlet pimpernel, Sesame, Shavegrass, Smartweed, Sorrel, Spearmint, Stinging nettle, Sweet balm, Tansy, Trailing arbutus, Turpentine, Uva Ursa, Virginia snake root, Watermelon seeds, Water plantain, White oak, White pine, White pond lily, White poplar, Whortleberry, Wild carrot, Wild sage, Yarrow.

NERVINES:
Herbs that are tonic and healing to the nerves. American hellebore (small dose-sedative), Apples, Arrach, Asafetida, Bee balm, Bitter orange (mild stimulant), Black cohosh (sedative), Black Haw, Black hellebore, Black horehounds, Bladderwrack, Blue cohosh, Blue violet, Boneset, Buchu, Bugleweed (sedative), Burdock seeds, Burning Bush, Camomile (sedative), Camphor (sedative), Catnip (sedative), Cedron (sedative), Celery, Coca (stimulant & tonic), Condurango, Cramp bark (sedative), Crawley root (sedative), Damiana, Dill, Dittany, False hellebore, Fennel, Fit root (sedative), Foxglove (sedative), Garden sage (sedative), Garlic, Gelsemin (sedative), German camomile (sedative), Ginseng, Golden seal, Gravel root, Guarana (stimulant), Hops, Horsemint, Ignatius beans, Indian hemp, Indian valerian (sedative), Jerusalem oak, Kola, Lady's slipper (relaxant), Lavender oil, Lemon balm, Lily-of-the-valley, Lime flowers, Lobelia (sedative), Marshmallow, Meadow anemone, Mistletoe, Motherwort, Mullein, Mugwort, Muira-puama, Nux vomica, Oats, Onion, Oregon grape (tonic), Parsley, Passion flower (sedative), Peach, Pennyroyal, Peony, Peppermint (sedative), Peruvian

bark, Pleurisy root (slightly sedative), Prickly ash, Pulsatilla (sedative), Pumpkin, Quassia, Quince, Radix valerianae majoris, Red Clover, Rosemary, Rue (stimulant), Sage, Sanicle, Scullcap (sedative), Skunk cabbage, Small cleavers, Small yellow lady's slipper, Southernwood, Spearmint (sedative), Stavesacre (depressant), Sumbul (sedative), Sweet basil (mild), Tansy (relaxant), Texas snake root, Thyme (sedative), Tormentil (sedative), Turpentine (depressant), Twin leaf, Valerian (sedative), Vervain, Virginia snake root, Wild celery seed, Wild cherry (sedative), Wild indigo (stimulant), Wild lettuce (sedative), Wild marjoram, Wild sage, Wood betony, Wormwood, Yarrow, Yellow lady's slipper, Yellow parilla, Yerba mate (stimulant).

NUTRITIVES:
Herbs that are nourishing and building to body tissues. Agar, Almond, Amaranth, Acacia, Apple, Apricot, Arrach, Arrowroot, Artichokes, Balm of Gilead (buds), Bladderwrack, Barley, Beet, Bistort shoot, Bitter almond, Burdock (root, and stalks-stripped of rind), Canna, Carob, Carrot, Cayenne, Chickweed, Cloves, Comfrey, Common melon, Dandelion leaves, Dates, Fennel (peeled stalks), Fig, Garden sage, Glycerine, Herb patience, Holberd leaves, Horseradish, Iceland moss, Irish moss, Jerusalem artichoke, Jujube berries, Lamb's quarter, Lentils, Licorice, Mangos, Manna, Mimosa gum, Marshmallow, Mullein, Oats, Olive oil, Pleurisy root (shoots, flowers, and seed pods-boiled), Poke root (tender leaves), Prune, Pumpkin seeds, Purslane, Red clover, Rest harrow shoots, Rice, Rye, Sage, Salep, Salsify, Saw palmetto, Sesame, Sheep sorrel, Slippery elm, Sorrel, Sweet basil, Sweet potato, Tamarind, Tapioca, Wafer ash fruit (seed), Watercress, Wood betony (leaves, flowers), Yellow dock (leaves).

OPHTHALMICS:
Herbs that are healing to disorders and diseases of the eyes. American angelica, Angelica, Borage, Camomile, Canada snake root, Cayenne, Chickweed, Cornflower, Cranesbill, Dandelion, Elder, Eyebright, Farkleberry root bark & berries, Fennel, Golden seal, Greater celandine (for deposits & opacities), Grapevine leaves, Hyssop, Lily-of-the-valley, Marigold flowers, Marshmallow, Morning glory flowers, Mullein (flower, oil), Peruvian rhatany, Plantain, Purple loosestrife, Quince seed, Red maple, Rosemary, Rose petals, Rue, Sarsaparilla, Sassafras, Slippery elm, Squaw vine, Summer savory juice, Sycamore, Tormentil, Vervain, Violet, White poplar, White willow, Wild clary, Wild rose, Wintergreen, Witch hazel, Yellow dock, Yellow loosestrife.

PARASITICIDES:
Herbs that kill or destroy animal and vegetable parasites within the body. Balsam of Peru, Blackberry, Black cohosh leaves, Cajuput oil, Cassia oil, Cinnamon oil, Cloves (Eugenol-powerful), Gentian, Ipecacuanha, Larkspur seed, Mullein, Quassia (small dose), Red cedar oil, Rue, Storax, Thymol.

PARTURIENTS:
Herbs that stimulate uterine contractions, which induce and assist labor, and pro-

mote and hasten childbirth. American angelica (afterbirth), Bethroot, Birthwort (afterbirth), Black cohosh, Blue cohosh, Cedar berries, Cinnamon bark, Cinnamon oil, Cotton root, Cramp bark (after pains), Crawley root (fever, after pains), Honeysuckle, Horehound (after birth), Lobelia, Red raspberry, Rue, Shepherd's purse, Spikenard, Squaw vine, St. John's wort (after pains), Sweet gale, Uva Ursa (large dose).

PECTORALS:
Herbs that are healing to complaints or affections of the broncho-pulmonary area. Abscess root, Acacia, Alfalfa, Almond, Ammoniac, American angelica, American liverwort, Anise, Apple blossoms, Apricot seed, Asafetida, Asthma weed, Avocado leaves, Balm of Gilead buds, Balsam of Peru, Balsam of Tolu, Barley, Benzoin, Betel, Beth root, Bitter almonds, Bitter candytuft, Bitter orange, Black elm, Black horehounds, Black mustard, Blood root, Boneset, Borage, Bugleweed, Bugloss, Burdock root, Cauliflower leaves, Cherry, Chickweed, Chirata, Clary, Cocillana bark, Coconut oil, Coltsfoot, Comfrey, Copaiba, Cubebs, Cup plant, Elder flowers & berries, Elecampane, Eucalyptus, European angelica, Fennel, Flaxseed, Galbanum, Gambir, Garden sage, Garlic, Gentian, Ginseng, Golden seal, Ground ivy, Groundsel, Hartstongue, Hollyhock, Hops, Horehound, Horseradish, Hyssop, Iceland moss, Irish moss, Ivy, Jamaica ginger, Jerusalem oak, Kava kava, Labrador tea, Lachnanthes, Lady's slipper, Lavender oil, Licorice, Life everlasting, Life root, Lily-of-the-valley, Lungwort, Maidenhair, Malva, Marshmallow, Meadow anemone, Mouse ear, Mullein, Mustard, Myrrh, Onion, Orris, Pansy, Paraguay tea, Peppermint, Peruvian bark, Pimpernel, Pleurisy root, Polypody root, Pomegranate, Ragwort, Red root, Red sage, Rock brake, Rosin-weed, Sanicle, Saw palmetto, Senega, Shepherd's purse, Skunk cabbage, Slippery elm, Solomon's seal, Spikenard, Spruce, Squill, Stinging nettle, Storax, Sumbul, Sunflower, Sweet cicely, Thymol, Turpentine (external), Vervain (with flax seed), Wake robin, Water fennel, White melilot, White pine, White pond lily, Wild sarsaparillas, Yarrow, Yerba santa.

PERISTALTICS:
Herbs that stimulate and increase peristalsis, or muscular contraction (as in the bowels). Aloe (powerful), Balm of Gilead buds, Camphor, Cascara sagrada, Cloves (Eugenol), Horseradish, Jalap, Nux vomica, Olive oil, Peruvian bark, Prickly ash, Quaker button (small dose), Sassy bark, Turkey rhubarb (powder), Turpentine (powerful).

PROTECTIVES:
Herbs that serve as protective coverings to abraded, inflamed, or injured parts when applied locally to a surface. Acadia, Benzoin, Castor oil, Corn starch, Flaxseed, Marshmallow, Myrrh (alcohol extract), Olive oil, Tragacanth.

PUNGENTS:
Herbs that cause a sharply pricking, acrid, and penetrating sensation to the sensory organs. Black pepper, Cardamon, Cayenne, Contrayerva, Coriander,

Horseradish, Jamaica ginger, Mustard, Prickly ash, Rue, Self-heal, Sneezewort, Wake robin, Water mint.

REFRIGERANTS:
Herbs that have cooling properties, lower the body temperature, and relieve thirst. Barberry, Bee balm (Melissa), Bilberry, Black currant, Borage, Burnet, Catnip, Cherries, Chickweed, Cleavers, Couchgrass, Cranberries, Elder flowers, Groundsel, Houseleek, Licorice, Lemon juice, Limes, Maidenhair, Mandarin oranges, Oranges, Pellitory-of-the-wall, Pimpernel, Plantain, Pomegranate seeds, Prickly pear cactus, Prune, purslane, Red currants, Red mulberries, Red raspberries, Rice water, Salsify, Sheep sorrel, Sorrel, Strawberries, Sumach berries, Tamarind, Watermelons, Wild strawberries, Wood sorrel, Yellow flag, Yellow water lily.

RESOLVENTS:
Herbs that promote the dispersion of inflammatory deposits, and their absorption into excretory channels. Ammoniac, Balm of Gilead (bark), Barberry, Bittersweet, Black horehounds, Blue flag, Blood root, Camphor, Chickweed, Daffodil roots, Elder (leaves, and berries), Field scabious, Galbanum, Greater celandine, Great white field lily, Horehound, Lily-of-the-valley, Mandrake, Marigold flowers, Milk thistle, Pareira, Poke root, St. John's wort, Tormentil.

RUBEFACIENTS:
Herbs that, upon local application, stimulate capillary dilation and action, and cause skin redness (drawing blood from deeper tissues and organs and thereby relieving congestion and inflammation). Ammoniac, Black bryony, Black mustard, Black pepper, Cajuput oil, Camphor, Cayenne, Cloves, Cowhage, Croton oil, Garlic, Horsemint, Horseradish, Jamaica ginger, Mustard, Pellitory, Peppermint (oil), Pine gum, Pipsissewa, Rue, Rosemary (oil), Sassafras (oil), Squill, Stinging nettle, Sweet scented golden rod, Turpentine, Wild marjoram.

SEDATIVES:
Herbs that lower the functional activity of an organ or part of the body, thereby tending to calm, moderate or tranquilize. Adrue, American hellebore, American pennyroyal, Aniseed, Apricot seed, Belladonna, Bitter almonds, Black cohosh (arterial & nervine), Black Haw, Black hellebore, Bladderwrack, Blue cohosh, Blood root, Boldo leaves, Boxwood, Bugleweed (arterial, nervine), Camomile, Caroba, Cedron, Colchicum, Cowslip, Cramp bark, Crawley root, Evening primrose, European pennyroyal, Fit root, Fox glove, Garden sage, Gelsemin (arterial, nervine), Hemlock spruce, Hops, Horsemint, Horsenettle, Houndstongue, Ice plant, Jamaica dogwood, Lady's bed straw, Lobelia, Meadow lily, Meadow saffron seed, Motherwort, Muira puma, Mountain laurel, Night-blooming cereus, Passion flower, Peach, Peppermint, Pleurisy root (slight), Primrose, Pulsatilla, Red clover, Red maple, Red poppy, Red root, Saw palmetto berries, Scullcap, Spearmint, St. John's wort, Stone root, Stramonium, Sumbul, Thyme, Tormentil, Turpentine, Valerian, Wafer ash fruit, Water avens, Wild cherry, Wild lettuce, Wild yam

(relaxant), Witch hazel, Yarrow, Yellow pond lily.

SIALAGOGUES:
Herbs that promote the secretion and flow of saliva and buccal mucous. Balmony, Bayberry, Betel leaves, Blood root, Blue flag, Button snake root, Cayenne, Echinacea, Elder bark, False sweet flag, False unicorn (fresh), Gentian Horseradish, Hydrangea, Indian hemp, Jaborandi (small dose), Jamaica ginger, Licorice, Mandrake, Mezereon, Pellitory root, Peruvian bark, Prickly ash, Senega snake root, True unicorn, Turkey rhubarb.

SOPORIFICS:
Herbs that induce a relaxing sleep. Black cohosh, Catnip, Elder flowers, Hops, Indian hemp, Jamaica dogwood root bark, Lady's slipper, Motherwort, Mullein, Passion flower, Peppermint, Primrose, Scullcap, Valerian, Vervain, Wafer ash fruit.

STERNUTATORIES:
Herbs that are irritating to the mucous membranes in nasal passages, which cause sneezing. American hellebore, Asarabacca, Bayberry, Cayenne, Jamaica ginger, Lily-of-the-valley, Marigold juice, Pellitory, Sassy bark, Senega, Sneezewort, Soap tree, Soap wort, Wood betony, Yellow flag juice.

STIMULANTS:
Herbs that increase functional activity and energy in the body. American pennyroyal, Ammoniac, Angostura bark, Aniseed, Arbor vitae, Asafetida, Asarabacca, Asthma weed (respiratory), Balm of Gilead, Balmony (gastric), Balsam fir, Balsam of Tolu, Bayberry, Bdelliulm, Bee balm, Benzoin, Birthwort, Bitter root, Black alder (digestive), Black horehounds, Black pepper, Bladderwrack (glandular, thyroid), Blessed thistle, Blood root, Blue cohosh (diffusive, relaxant), Blue flag, Boldo, Boneset (powerful), Brigham tea, Buchu (slightly diffusive), Button snake root, Cajuput (diffusive), Calumba (gastric), Camomile, Camphor, Canada flea bane, Canada snake root, Canella, Caraway, Carrot, Cassia, Cascarilla, Catnip (diffusive, relaxant), Cayenne, Celandine, Celery, Chirata, Cloves (relaxant), Coca, Cocash root, Colombo (mild), Contrayerva, Copaiba, Cornflower, Cubebs, Cup plant, Damelena, Dandelion, Dill, Dwarf nettle, Echinacea, Elder flowers, Elecampane (gentle), European angelica, European ground pine, European pennyroyal, False unicorn, Feverfew, Galangal, Galbanum, Garden sage, Garlic, Gentian, German camomile, Ginseng, Goldenrod, Gold thread, Gravel root (relaxant), Ground ivy, Guaiac, Guarana, Hops (relaxant), Horehound, Horsemint, Horseradish (powerful), Hyssop (diffusive), Indian turnip, Jaborandi, Jamaica ginger (diffusive), Jerusalem oak (diffusive), Juniper berries, Kava kava, Labrador tea, Lady's slipper, Leek, Lemon, Lemon thyme, Licorice (slight), Life root, Linden, Lobelia (diffusive, relaxant), Lovage, Mace, Marigold, Masterwort, Mayweed, Meadow fern, Mezereon, Mountain laurel, Mugwort, Muira puma, Myrrh (diffusive), Mustard, Nutmeg, Nux vomica, Oats, Onion, Oregon grape (slight), Orris, Paraguay tea (Yerba mate), Peppermint, Peruvian balsam, Pimento,

Pine tar, Pleurisy root, Prickly ash, Quebrado (cardiac, respiratory), Queen's root, Ragwort, Raspberries, Red clover (mild), Red raspberry, Red root, Rosemary, Rue (gastric), Saffron, Sandalwood, Santonica, Sarsaparilla, Sassafras (relaxant), Senega, Senna (slight), Smartweed, Snapdragon leaves, Southernwood, Spearmint, Spikenard, Star anise, Stinging nettle, Stone root, Storax, Strawberry, Sumbul, Summer savory, Sundew, Sweet cicely, Sweet fennel, Tansy, Thymol, Tonka bean (small dose), True unicorn, Tumeric, Turkey rhubarb powder, Turpentine (small dose), Valerian, Virginia snake root (diffusive), Wafer ash, Wake robin, White oak (slight), Wild carrot, Wild cherry (digestive), Wild ginger, Wild marjoram, Wild sarsaparillas, Wild yam (relaxant), Wintergreen (small dose), Wood sage, Wormwood, Yarrow, Yellow dock, Yohimbe bark, Zedoary.

STOMACHICS:
Herbs that are stimulative tonics to the stomach. Agrimony, Allspice, Aloes, Angelica, Aniseed, Avens, Azedarach, Balm of Gilead (bark), Balsam of Peru, Balsam of Tolu, Barberry, Bay leaves, Betel leaves, Bitter orange, Bitter root, Black cohosh, Blessed thistle, Boneset, Burdock root, Calamint, Calumba, Camomile, Canella, Caraway, Cardamon, Cascarilla, Cassia, Cayenne, Centaurea, Cherry, Chirata, Cinnamon, Clary, Cloves, Colombo, Condurango, Contrayerva, Coriander, Costmary, Cubebs, Dandelion, Dill, Elecampane, European angelica, European centaury, European rhubarb, Fennel, Florida dogwood berries, Gentian, German camomile, Ginseng, Gladwyn, Gold thread, Grindelia (small dose), Hops, Horehound, Horsemint, Ipecacuanha, Juniper berry, Linden, Lovage, Mouse ear, Nutmeg, Nux vomica, Peppermint, Peruvian bark, Pimento, Pitcher plant, Quassia (small dose), Red raspberry, Rue, Sea wormwood, Swamp milk-weed, Sweet fennel, Sweet flag, Tansy, True unicorn, Turkey rhubarb, Virginia snake root, Wafer ash root bark, White cedar leaves, Wild carrot, Wild yam, Wood betony, Wormwood, Yellow parilla, Zedoary.

STYPTICS:
Herbs that astringe the blood vessels when applied to an external surface, and thereby arrest local bleeding or hemorrhaging. Avens, Bayberry, Bistort (power-ful), Blackberry (powerful), Black walnut, Bluebell bulb, Bullace, Canada flea bane, Cinquefoil, Comfrey, Cranesbill, False sweet flag, Fleabane, Grapevine leaves, Knotgrass, Lady's mantle, Lesser Burnett, Marsh woundwort, Matico, Plantain, Self-heal, Stinging nettle, Tormentil, Witch hazel, Wood sage.

SUDORIFICS:
Herbs that stimulate the sudoriferous glands and produce visible and profuse per-spiration when taken hot and act as tonics when taken cold. Avens, Birthwort, Bitter root, Black walnut, Blue cohosh, Blue violet, Boneset, Boxwood, Carline thistle, Cayenne, Columbine, Crawley root, Cudweed, Dogbane root, Dwarf elder leaves, Elder flowers, False boneset, Garden sage, Garlic, Goat's rue, Great bur-net, Horsemint, Hyssop, Indian hemp, Indian physic, Ivy, Jacob's ladder, Mayweed, Mouse ear, Pennyroyal, Peppermint, Pleurisy root (powerful, relaxant), Rough boneset, Safflower, Saffron, Scarlet pimpernel, Skunk cabbage, Vervain,

Wild sarsaparillas.

TAENIAFUGES and TAENIACIDES:
Herbs that expel (taeniafuges) or kill (taeniacides) tapeworms in the intestinal tract. Areca nut, Bearsfoot leaves, Boneset, Castor oil, Cucumber seeds, Demerara pink root, Embelia, False unicorn, Gamboge (small dose), Goa, Kamala, Kousso, Male fern, Pink root, Polypody root, Pomegranate, Primrose, Pumpkin seeds, Santonica, Self-heal, Watermelon seeds.

TONICS:
Herbs that stimulate nutrition and permanently increase systemal tone, energy, vigor, and strength. Agrimony, Alder, Almond, Astonia, American angelica, American boxwood, American centaury, American liverwort, Anise, Apricot (flowers, seed), Asarabacca, Ash bark, Avens, Balm of Gilead bark, Balmony, Balsam of Tolu, Bayberry, Bee balm, Beech, Bethroot, Bistort, Bitter orange, Black alder, Black catechu, Black cohosh, Black currant, Black elm, Black haw (uterine), Black horehounds, Black pepper, Black swamp ash, Black walnut, Black willow, Bladderwrack, Blue ash (bark, and leaves), Blue cohosh, Blood root, Boldo, Boneset, Brigham tea, Buchu, Buckbean, Buckthorn, Bugleweed, Burdock, Butterbur, Butternut, Button snake root, Cachalagua, Calumba, Camomile, Canada snake root, Canella, Carrot, Cascara amarya, Cascara sagrada, Cassia, Carline thistle, Cayenne, Centaurea, Chaparral, Cherry, Chestnut, Chicory, Chirata, Cinquefoil, Cleavers, Colombo, Coltsfoot, Columbine, Comfrey, Condurango, Contrayerva, Coolwort, Cornflower, Couchgrass, Cramp bark, Cranesbill, Culver's root, Cup plant, Damiana, Dandelion, Deer's tongue, Dodder, Dogbane, Echinacea, Elecampane, Endive, European angelica, European pennyroyal, Eyebright, False boneset, False unicorn, Feverfew, Fleabane, Fireweed, Fit root, Florida dogwood, Fringetree, Fumitory, Garden sage, Garlic, Gentian, German camomile, Ginseng, Golden seal, Gravel root, Great water dock, Grindelia (small dose), Ground ivy, Hardhack, Hawthorn, Hemp agrimony leaves, Herb patience, Hickory, Hops, Horehound, Horse chestnut, Horseradish, Hydrangea, Hyssop, Iceland moss, Ignatius beans, Indian physic, Ipecacuanha, Ivy, Jamaica quassia, Jerusalem oak, Kino, Krameria root, Labrador tea, Lady's slipper, Larch, Licorice, Life root, Lime flowers, Logwood, Mace, Magnolia, Maiden hair, Male fern, Manna (gentle), Mandrake (liver, intestines, uterus), Marigold, Matico, Meadow cranesbill, Milkweed root, Mistletoe, Mother of thyme, Motherwort, Mountain flax, Mugwort, Mustard, Myrrh, Oats, Oregon grape, Pareira, Parsley, Passion flower, Periwinkle, Pichi, Pipsissewa, Pleurisy root, Poke root, Pomegranate, Prickly ash, Purple loosestrife, Quassia (small dose), Quebracho, Quince, Ragwort, Red clover, Red maple, Red osiers, Red raspberry, Red rose, Rhubarb, Rock rose, Rue, Safflower, Sanicle, Sarsaparilla, Scabious, Scullcap (nervine), Sea wormwood, Self-heal, Senna, Shrub yellow root, Slippery elm, Smartweed, Solomon's seal, Southernwood, Squaw vine, Stinging nettle, Stone root, Strawberry, Sumach, Sumbul, Sweet marjoram, Tag alder, Tamarack, Tamarind, Tansy, Texas snake root, Thyme, Tormentil, True unicorn, Tumeric, Turkey rhubarb, Twin leaf, Uva ursi (soothing), Valerian, Vanilla,

Vervain, Virginia snake root, Wafer ash root bark, Wahoo, Walnut leaves & bark, Water avens, Water dock, White oak, White pond lily, White poplar, Wild cherry, Wild marjoram, Wild yam, Witch hazel, Wood betony, Woodruff, Wood sage, wormwood, Yarrow, Yellow dock, Yellow lady's slipper, Yellow parilla, Zedoary.

VULNERARIES:
Herbs that promote healing of fresh cuts, wounds, etc. Adder's tongue, Agar, Agrimony, Alkanet, Aloes, American pennyroyal, Apricot seed, Apple honey, Arnica flowers, Avocado leaves, Balm of Gilead (buds), Balsam of Tolu, Bayberry, Bee balm, Beech, Benzoin, Bilberry, Bistort, Bittersweet, Black elm, Black walnut, Black willow, Bladderwrack, Blessed thistle, Bloodroot herb (fresh), Buchu, Burdock plant, Cajuput, Camomile flowers, Carrot, Cayenne, Celandine, Chickweed, Cleavers, Comfrey, Copaiba, Couchgrass, Cranesbill, Cudweed, Daisy leaves, Echinacea, Elder (leaves, and flowers), Elecampane, English elm, European pennyroyal, Fenugreek, Figwort, Flaxseed, Fleabane, Fringetree, Garden sage, Garlic, Gentian Glycerine, Golden seal, Great burnet, Great white field lily, Greater celandine, Groundsel, Heartsease, High mallow, Horsetail grass, Houseleek, Hyssop, Irish moss, Ivy, Kidneywort, Knapweed, Knotgrass root, Lady's mantle, Lesser burnet, Life everlasting, Life root, Lily-of-the-valley, Male fern, Malva, Marigold flowers, Marshmallow root, Marsh woundwort, Matico, Meadow cranesbill, Meadow fern, Milkweed root, Mullein, Myrrh, Olive oil, Ox-eye daisy root, Pansy, Parsley, Peach, Peruvian balsam, Plantain, Pleurisy root, Poke root, Prickly ash, Quince, Ragwort, Red oak, Red rose, Rhubarb root, Rice, Rosemary, Rue, Russian knot grass, Sanicle, Self-heal, Shepherd's purse, Slippery elm, Solomon's seal, Sorrel, Southernwood, Spruce, St. John's wort, Stone root, Sumach, Sweet clover, Sycamore, Tansy, Thyme, Tormentil, Turkey rhubarb, Turpentine (external), Vervain, Water figwort, White lily, White oak, White pond lily, White poplar, Wild carrot, Wild indigo, Witch hazel leaves, Wood betony, Woodruff, Yarrow, Yellow loosestrife, Yellow parilla.

GENERAL TERMINOLOGY

Therapeutic properties describe the active principles in herbs that effect healing, restorative, and curative changes within the tissue and organs.

Health is a dynamic, positive, regenerative, and elevating attribute of a functioning system. A healthy condition in the human body is one wherein there is no mucus in the body.

An herbalist is a botanic physician who uses medicinal agents in their organic and unprocessed state—herbs, roots, barks, seeds, flowers, and berries. The medicines are alive and organic, and therefore are endowed with life-giving properties harmonious with and assimilable in man's body chemistry. The herbalist is opposed to unnatural and inorganic procedures of administering serums, vaccines and drugs that have serious side effects and after effects on cell functions and which eventually result in the induction of systemal malfunction and the smothering of life. Herbalists can become adept in this natural science in a relatively short period of time because they work only with nonpoisonous, beneficial agents and can therefore concentrate on cleansing out the few causes of disease without having to learn individual therapies for the thousands of clinical terms of disease.

Herbology is that branch of natural science that deals with the therapeutic properties of herbs. *In the practice of herbology, we do not use poisonous herbs or caustic medicinal aids of any kind.*

A medicinal herb is any plant or vegetation used beneficially in therapeutic treatment. Herbs are classified under two categories, medicinal and nutritional. The nutritional herb is the common herb normally eaten for food such as the turnip, beet, carrot, potato, etc. But in each of these nutritional herbs are medicinal qualities or active therapeutic principles which may be quite valuable. These mild, pleasant herbs are eaten for their palatability. The medicinal herb is generally more pungent and distasteful due to its selectivity and concentrations. Although one herb may be classed as more nutritional and the other as more medicinal, the classification is relative because the medicinal herb is also nutritional, rebuilding the cell structure of the body with great speed because its highly concentrated materials are specific for particular conditions.

Organic matter is used as food for animal life. Inorganic matter is that which the plant life consumes. Man is equipped to handle the organic, the elements which have been processed by plants from the raw chemicals in rocks, earth, and air into the living tissues of plants. These elements become natural foods for man, and can be readily taken into the blood stream. The inorganic are in the raw state, or they are those plant tissues which have been subjected to man's inventive designs wherein a chemical or molecular change has taken place such as through heat or by unnatural and caustic catalyzing agents such as inorganic acids or alkalies. These processes alter the plant substance into inorganic, dead, and inassimilable material. Herbs are organic materials with the life in them as in their chlorophyll-processed state. Inorganic may seem to give quick healing but generally only give relief from symptoms instead of health.

REFERENCES

Bailey, L.H., & E.Z. Bailey. *Hortus Third, A Concise Dictionary of Plants Cultivated in the United States and Canada*. Rev. ed. New York: Macmillan, 1976.

Brooks, Richard. *A New Family Herbal*. N.d.

Brown, O. Phelps. *Complete Herbalist*. London., 1871.

Christopher, John R. *Just What is the Word of Wisdom?* Springville, UT: Christopher Publications, 1974.

Deschauer, Thomas. *Complete Course in Herbalism*. Self-published, 1940.

Doctrine and Covenants. Salt Lake City, UT: Church of Jesus Christ of Latter-day Saints, 1989.

"1833 Guide for Preventing Heart Disease." *Improvement Era*. Aug. 1969: 60-3.

Kloss, Jethro. *Back to Eden*. 1939. Rev. ed. Loma, CA: Back to Eden Books, 1994.

Meyer, Joseph E. *The Herbalist*. 11th ed. Glenwood, IL: Meryerbooks, 1976.

Nowell, H. *Post Graduate Course*. Vancouver: Domican Herbal College, 1926.

Shook, Edward. *Advanced Treatise in Herbology*. Springville, UT: Christopher Publications, 1994.

——. *Elementary Treatise in Herbology*. Springville, UT: Christopher Publications, 1994.

Walker, N.W. *Raw Vegetable and Fruit Juices*. Rev. ed. Prescott, AZ: Norwalk, 1978.

——. *The Vegetarian Guide to Diet and Salads*. Rev. ed. Prescott, AZ: Norwalk, 1986.

Wigmore, Ann. *Why Suffer?* Wayne, NJ: Avery, N.d.

Wren, R.W. *Potter's New Cyclopedia of Medicinal Herbs and Preparations*. New York: Harper Colophon, 1972.

INDEX

Entries in capital letters indicate the name of a commercial formulation or that an entire section is devoted to the entry (where more than one page number is listed, the section reference will be underlined). Case histories can be located under the heading, "Case History," beginning on page 681. Formulas are listed under the heading, "Formula," beginning on page 690. Botanical names are listed under the heading "Herb" beginning on page 696. When looking for an herb, the most comprehensive page reference will be found under its botanical name. To cross reference the common name of an herb with its botanical name, turn to page 722.

CROSS REFERENCE
COMMON TO BOTANICAL NAME OF HERBS

This list includes only the common names of herbs used within formulas. The index is the main source for common name entries. However, the index places more emphasis on listing herbs by their botanical name. For this reason we've included this cross reference. Botanical names can be found under "herb" on pages 696-701 of the index.

acacia	Acacia senegal
agrimony	Agrimonia eupatoria
almond, sweet	Prunus dulcis, var. dulcis; Amygdalus dulcis
aloe	Aloe vera
allspice	Pimento officinalis
amaranth	Amaranthus hybridus
Amer. boxwood	Cornus florida
Amer. hellebore	Veratrum viride
American ivy	Ampolopsis quinquefolia; Vitis hederacea
Amer. pennyroyal	Hedeoma pulegioides
angelica	Angelica atropurpurea; A. archangelica
aniseed	Pimpinella anisum
Arabic gum	Acacia senegal
asafetida	Ferula assa-foetida
asparagus	Asparagus officinalis
asthma weed	Euphorbia pilulifera; E. hirta
avens	Geum urbanum
balm	Melissa officinalis
barley	Hordeum vulgare
bay	Laurus nobilis
bethroot	Trillium erectum; T. pendulum
bitter root	Apocynum androsaemifolium
bittersweet	Solanum dulcamara
black alder	Prinos verticillatus
blackberry	Rubus villosus
black catechu	Acadia catechu
black current	Ribes nigrum
black haw	Viburnum trilobum; V. opulus
black walnut	Juglans nigra
bladderwrack	Fucus vesiculosus
blood root	Sanguinaria canadensis
blue vervain	Verbena hastata
bogbean	Menyanthes trifoliata
bramble	Rubus villosus
Brigham tea	Ephedra species
broom pine	Pinus palustris
broom tops	Cytisus scoparius
buckbean	Menyanthes trifoliata
buckthorn	Rhamnus frangula
bugle weed	Lycopus virginicus; L. americanus
bull nettle	Solanum carolinense
bur marigold	Bidens tripartita
cactus grandiflorus	Selenicereus grandiflorus
camphor	Cinnamomum camphora
Canada snake root	Asarum canadense
caraway	Carum carvi
cardamon	Elettaria cardamomum
cascarilla	Croton eleuteria
cassia	Cinnamomum cassia
castor	Ricinus communis
catechu	Acadia catechu
celandine	Chelidonium majus
celery	Apium graveolens
chamomile	Chamaemelum nobile
chestnut	Castanea sativa; C. dentata; Fagus castanea
chiretta	Swertia chirata
cicely	Osmorhiza longistylis
cinnamon	Cinnamomum zeylanicum
clover, white	Trifolium repens
club moss	Lycopodium clavatum
colt's foot	Tussilago farfara
coriander	Coriandrum sativum
cornus	Cornus florida
couchgrass	Agrogyron repens
cranesbill	Geranium maculatum
cubeb	Piper cubeba
cucumber	Cucumis sativus
cudweed	Gnaphalium obtusifolium
Culver's root	Veronicastrum virginicum
current, black	Ribes nigrum
dandelion	Taraxacum officinale
damiana, Mexican	Turnera aphrodisiaca
dogwood	Cornus florida
elder	Sambucus canadensis
elder, dwarf	Sambucus ebulus

elecampane	Inula helenium
ephedra	Ephedra sinica
eucalyptus	Eucalyptus globulus
eugenol	Caryophyllus aromaticus; Eugenia aromatica
European avens	Geum urbanum
European goldenrod	Solidago virgaurea
eyebright	Euphrasia officinalis
fennel	Foeniculum vulgare
feverfew	Chrysanthemum partheni- um
figwort	Scrophularia nodosa
flag, sweet	Acorus calamus
fringetree	Chionanthus viriginicus
garden thyme	Thymes vulgaris
German camomile	Matricaria chamomilla
ginkgo	Ginkgo biloba
goat's rue	Galega officinalis
goldenrod	Solidago virgaurea
gotu kola	Centella asiatica
ground pine	Lycopodium clavatum
ground seeds	Cucurbita maxima
guaiac	Guaiacum officinale; G. sanctum
guaiacum	Guaiacum officinale; G. sanctum
gum asafetida	Ferula assa-foetida
gum weed	Grindelia robusta
fennel	Foeniculum vulgare
flaxseed	Linum usitatissimum
fringetree	Chionanthus virginica
fumitory herb	Fumaria officinalis
goldenrod	Solidago odora
goldthread	Coptis trifolia
ground ivy	Glechoma hederacea
guaiac	Guaiacum officinale
gum Arabic	Acacia senegal
haircap moss	Polytrichum juniperum
hawthorn	Crataegus laevigata
hellebore	Veratrum viride
hemlock spruce	Tsuga canadensis; Pinus canadensis
henbane	Hyoscyamus niger
hoary plantain	Plantago media
horehound	Marrubium vulgare
horse nettle	Solanum carolinense
horse tail grass	Equisetum arvense; E. hyemale
hydrangea	Hydrangea arborescens
Iceland moss	Cetraria islandica
indian turnip	Arisaema triphyllum
Irish moss	Chondrus crispus

jack-in-the-pulpit	Arisaema triphyllum
jalap	Ipomoea purga; I. jalapa
John's bread	Ceratonia siliqua
jujube	Ziziphus jujuba; Z. vul- garis
knotgrass	Polygonum periscaria
kummell	Carum carvi
ladies bedstraw	Galium verum
ladies mantle	Alchemilla vulgaris
laurel	Laurus nobilis
lemon	Citrus limon
leptandra	Veronicastrum virginicum
lettuce, romaine	Lactuca sativa
lily of the valley	Convallaria majalis
linden	Tilia europaea
lippia	Lippia dulcis
liverwort	Anemone hepatica; Hepatica americana
loosestrife	Lythrum salicaria
ma-huang	ephedra species
maidenhair	Adiantum pedatum; A. capillus-veneris
manna	Fraxinus ornus
margoram	Origanum vulgare
margoram, sweet	Origanum majorana
meadowsweet	Filipendula ulmaria; Spiraea tomentosa
meliot	Melilotus alba
menthol	Mentha piperita
Mexican damiana	Turnera aphrodisiaca
mezereon bark	Daphne mezereum
mountain mahogany	Betula lenta
mugwort	Artemisia vulgaris
mustard	Brassica nigra; B. hirta
night bloom cereus	Selenicereus grandiflorus
nutmeg	Myristica fragrans
nux vomica	Strychnos nux vomica
oat straw	Avena sativa
olive	Olea Europaea
orange peel	Citrus aurantium; C. sinensis
oregano	Origanum vulgare
orris	Iris florentina
papaya	Carica papaya
peach	Prunus persica
pellitory-of-the-wall	Parietaria officinalis
pennyroyal, Amer.	Hedeoma pulegioides
pennyroyal, Europ.	Mentha pulegium
peony	Paeonia officinalis
pepper, water	Polygonum hydropiper- oides

persimmon	Diospyros virginiana
pile wort	Amaranthus hypochondriacus
Pimenta dioica	Pimento officinalis
pimento	Pimento officinalis
pine, white	Pinus strobus
pinus	Tsuga canadensis; Pinus canadensis
pipsissewa	Chimaphila umbellata
plantain, hoary	Plantago media
pleurisy root	Asclepias tuberosa
pond lily	Nymphaea odorata
poppy	Papaver somniferum
prince's feather	Amaranthus hypochondriacus
prince's pine	Chimaphila umbellata
quassia	Quassia amara; Picraena excelsa
queen of the meadow	Eupatorium purpureum; Filipendula ulmaria
queen's delight	Stillingia sylvatica
ragwort	Senecio jacobaea
red cock's amaranth	Amaranthus hypochondriacus
red poppy	Papaver somniferum
red root	Ceanothus americanus
red sage	Salvia colorata
rest harrow	Ononis spinosa
rock rose	Helianthemum canadense
romaine lettuce	Lactuca sativa
rose hips	Rosa species
rosemary	Rosmarinus officinalis
resin weed	Grindelia robusta
sacred bark	Rhamnus purshiana
saffron	Crocus sativus
sandalwood	Santalum album
saw palmetto	Serenoa repens
senega	Polygala senega
shavegrass	Equisetum arvense; E. hyemale
shepherd's purse	Capsella bursa-pastoris
silver weed	Potentilla anserina
skunk cabbage	Symplocarpus foetidus
snake root, Canada	Asarum canadense
sneezewort	Achillea ptarmica
socotrine aloes	Aloe perry
Spanish iris	Iris florentina
speedwell	Veronicastrum virginicum
spikenard	Aralia racemosa
squaw weed	Senecio jacobaea
steeplebush	Spiraea tomentosa
sticklewort	Agrimonia eupatoria
stillingia	Stillingia sylvatica
strawberry	Fragaria vesca
sunflower	Helianthus annuus
sweet almond	Prunus dulcis, var. dulcis
sweet birch	Betula lenta
sweet cicely	Osmorhiza longistylis
sweet flag	Acorus calamus
sweet majoram	Origanum majorana
thyme	Thymes vulgaris
tormentil	Potentilla erecta
tragacanth	Astragalus gummifer
turnip	Brassica rapa
twin leaf	Jeffersonia diphylla
unicorn root	Aletris farinosa
veronica	Veronica officinalis
vervain	Verbena officinalis
vervain, blue	Verbena hastata
violet	Viola odorata
Virginia creeper	Ampolopsis quinquefolia; Vitis hederacea
walnut	Juglans nigra
wake robin root	Trillium erectum; T. pendulum
water agrimony	Bidens tripartita
watercress	Nasturtium officinale
watermelon	Citrullus lanatus
water pepper	Polygonum hydropiperoides
water shamrock	Menyanthes trifoliata
white pine	Pinus strobus
wild geranium	Geranium maculatum
wild ginger	Asarum canadense
wild indigo	Baptisia tinctoria
wintergreen	Gaultheria procumbens
wood sanicle	Sanicula europaea
yellow bedstraw	Galium verum
yellow parilla	Menispermum canadense
yerba santa	Eriodictyon californicum
yucca	Yucca species

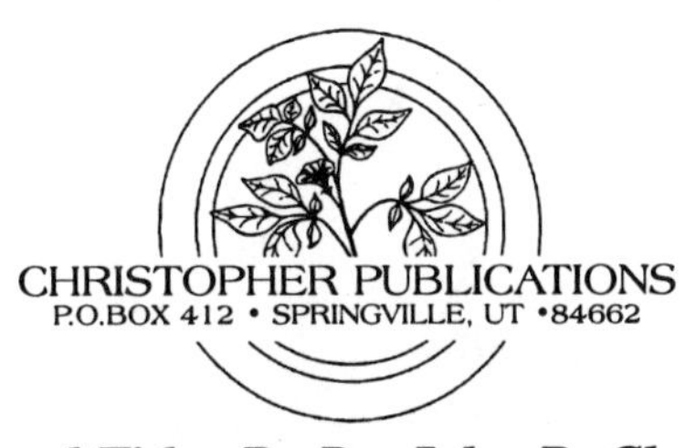

Additional Titles By Dr. John R. Christopher

DR. CHRISTOPHER'S HERBAL SEMINAR VIDEOS (VHS or PAL) • Witness America's premier natural healer sharing his knowledge and philosophies gained through years of experience. Enjoy over 16 hours of Dr. Christopher captured on video cassette at one of his last herbal seminars. • Complete Set • $395.00

DR. CHRISTOPHER'S NEW HERB LECTURES (10 audio cassettes - 1 hour ea.) • Listen and glean from the knowledge, wit and wisdom of Dr. Christopher teaching the benefits of herbs and natural healing techniques. Special Mind Trac Summaries at the end of each tape will aid the student to retain this valuable information. • (This set includes 2 bonus cassettes) • $69.95

HERBAL HOME HEALTH CARE • This volume from Dr. Christopher effectively deals with over 50 common ailments, listing them in convenient alphabetical order with concise definitions, symptom descriptions, causes, herbal aids, and other natural treatments. • 196 pages • $12.95

EVERY WOMAN'S HERBAL • The wisdom of Dr. Christopher and the practicality of Cathy Gileadi provides detailed information on herbal therapies for hormonal balance, proper menstruation, yeast control, pregnancy and more. For women of all ages. • 242 pages • $14.95

AN HERBAL LEGACY OF COURAGE • The first biography of Dr. Christopher. Read about his youth, his roots in herbalism, and his joys and struggles as he sought to heal and teach all who would hear. • 99 pages • $5.00

CAPSICUM • Dr. Christopher's research and case histories detailing the uses and healing powers of cayenne pepper. • 166 pages • $6.95

JUST WHAT IS THE WORD OF WISDOM? • Learn how the Word of Wisdom prompted Dr. Christopher toward a higher way of healthy living. • $1.75

REJUVENATION THROUGH ELIMINATION • Dr. Christopher discusses the necessity of cleansing and nourishing the bowel to obtain a disease free body. • $2.00

THE COLD SHEET TREATMENT • Dr. Christopher explains step by step his time tested treatment for colds, flu and any feverous or viral condition. • $1.75

THE INCURABLES • A natural treatment program for conditions deemed "incurable" by conventional methods of healing. Dr. Christopher shows that "there are no incurable diseases." • $2.00

DR. CHRISTOPHER'S NATURAL HEALING NEWSLETTERS • Over 6 volumes of back-issues available. 12 issues per volume • $25.00 • (issues are also sold separately)

A HEALTHIER YOU ~ AUDIO NEWSLETTER • A continuing series of newsletters in an audio cassette format. • 12 issue yearly subscription for $29.00

Christopher Publications carries over 100 titles! For a complete list, or to order any of the above titles, please call (800) 372-8255 or (801) 489-4254

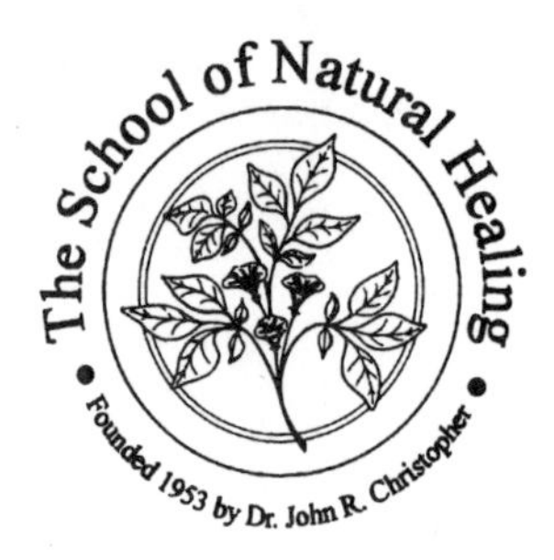

THE SCHOOL OF NATURAL HEALING

Because so many people are interested in Dr. Christopher's School of Natural Healing, we provide this overview of the training offered by the longest-running herbalist school in the United States.

The School of Natural Healing teaches the use of herbs within the framework of natural healing. We teach from the belief that the body has an inherent ability to self-correct. This discipline can be traced through written history beyond Hippocrates, who observed the body's needs and documented his use of herbal remedies and successful natural healing. Modernized by Dr. John R. Christopher, the principles of natural healing direct our up-to-date instruction on simple therapies and herbal usage to provide the body with the environment needed for vitality.

Herbalist Training

The herbalist training of The School of Natural Healing is organized for personal study of the herbs growing in your area. This is done through correspondence using regional materials. Study aid from qualified herbalists and instructors is available by phone (toll free in the United States). Regular classes, specialty courses, and upper-level certification seminars are also held either at our facilities or on satellite campuses. Training is organized in courses that begin with the basics and extend beyond Master Herbalist certification. The curriculum is arranged to accommodate those interested in increasing their understanding of certain areas of natural healing as well as those who want to receive certification. You can register for an individual course at any level of study or receive certification by completing any of the following study programs.

Be Your Own Doctor ~ Course Overview:

This first course introduces you to Herbology, the wonderful study of herbs and natural therapies. The texts, study guide, resource materials, and video and audio tapes of this course prepare you to effectively use Dr. Christopher's herbal formulas to cleanse, nourish, and build the body. You learn preventative medicine through your study of the cause of disease, therapy for the colon, and herbal cleansing for the entire system. Easy to follow natural therapies and health programs are discussed for over 50 common ailments. The recipes for some fundamental herbal formulas are also provided to get you started making your own remedies. Along with your study, you receive a biography of Dr. John Christopher.

Instruction:

- Fundamental principles of Herbology with David Christopher, M.H.
- Cleansing the body with herbs with David and Fawn Christopher.
- Simple, herbal therapies for over 50 common ailments with Dr. John Christopher.
- Correcting disease conditions of the bowel with Dr. John Christopher.

Completion:
After completing this course you will be skilled in your use of Dr. Christopher's commercial herbal combinations, some of the most widely-used herbal formulas in the world and the most accessible. You will also be able to implement the herbal cleansing routine developed by Dr. Christopher and improved by his son David Christopher. For over 50 years these herbs have been successfully used for many diseases.

The Vitalist Program ~ Overview:
This program will train you to become a Vitalist. What is a Vitalist? It is a person who understands the basic principles of natural healing and is able to help the body move towards wellness using wholesome herbs and simple therapies. The Vitalist Program includes the Be Your Own Doctor course and adds over 25 hours of dynamic instruction from master herbalists David Christopher and Dean Morris as well as other instructors from The School of Natural Healing. These video classes and workshops show you how to observe Nature for her answers to your health needs, and how to use herbs to reverse the cycle of disease. The Vitalist program teaches the basics in several areas providing an outline of the study required to become an effective natural healer. Conceptual instruction examines the cause of disease in the organism down to the cellular level. Therapeutic instruction provides specific herbs and therapies for individual organs and holistic programs for the entire system.

Instruction:
- History. The safety, and efficacy of herbalism since the earliest of times.
- Nutrition. Wholesome diet plans for increased energy, weight loss/gain, cancer, depression, cardiovascular disease, appendicitis, diabetes, allergies, and more.
- Science. Elementary study of botany and herb identification, therapeutic action of herbs, herb harvesting and preservation, plus the diagnostic art of iridology.
- Herbal Preparation. Step by step procedures for making herbal tea for shock, cleansing beverages for the liver, flaxseed poultices for congestion, herbal boluses (suppositories) for vaginal infection or hemorrhoids, hair conditioning vinegar extracts, earache oil extracts, first aid alcohol extracts, liniments for sore muscles, ointments for skin cancer, and more.
- Natural Therapy. Demonstrated techniques of massage for prolapsed organs, reflexology for the nervous system, hydrotherapy for arthritis, inflammation, colds, flu, fevers and more.

Completion:
A Vitalist certificate is awarded for completion of this study program.

The Herbalist Program ~ Overview:
The Herbalist program of The School of Natural Healing focuses on the School's mission of seeing a competent natural healer in every home. This program is designed to train you in the use of non-poisonous herbs and prepare you to be an effective teacher of the natural healing arts. Fortunately, Herbalists are not doctors and do not take responsibility for the health of others. Rather, an Herbalist teaches others to be responsible for their own health through natural, self-reliant means. The program begins with the basics of the Be Your Own Doctor and the Vitalist program courses, adding several more courses and completing your study with over 16 hours of instruction from Dr. John

Christopher himself. His eight Herbalist Seminar videos of the therapeutic categories of herbs and numerous case histories of successful, clinical application are yours to keep with this program.

Instruction:

- •Herbal History. Gain greater appreciation for herbs and the people who used them effectively as well as the politics and legalities of modern herbalism.
- •Herb Identification. Recognize the herbs which grow in your area using regional photographic field guides and illustrated identification keys and the botanical science of taxonomic classification.
- •Herbal Stewardship. Realize our dependence upon plants and our role as their caretakers through horticulture (growing of herbs), collection methodology, proper harvesting time and place, and the preservation and storage of herbs.
- •Herbal Usage. Develop proficiency in the application of herbs and natural therapies through the works of famous herbal practitioners such as; Jethro Kloss, Edward Shook, Mrs. M. Grieve, and of course, John Christopher.
- •Herbal Therapeutics. Become familiar with how herbs work through the categorization of their therapeutic actions.
- •Herbal Pharmacy. Acquire the skills to formulate and prepare your own herbal remedies with a significant study of the synergistic effects of combined herbs.

Completion:

Upon completion of this program you can earn the title of Herbalist and receive your Diploma from The School of Natural Healing.

The Master Herbalist Program ~ Overview:

This program is structured to prepare Herbalists to meet the demands of the professional market. As more and more people become interested in natural healing, the need for competent Herbalists continues to increase in a variety of health related areas. Through video and workbook presentation, you will receive training from the highest qualified botanists, herbal practitioners, herbal pharmacists and chemists in the field. You will then be qualified to attend a week's worth of the richest instruction from such notables as David Christopher, M.H., Christopher Hobbs, L. Ac., Richard Schulze, M.H., N.D., Steven Foster, Dianne Bjarnson, C.M. and Dean Morris, M.H. This six-day certification seminar is held at our facilities in the beautiful mountains outside of Springville, Utah.

Instruction:

Advanced studies in anatomy, botany, diagnostics, herbal chemistry, herbal pharmacognosy, jurisprudence, research, clinical applications, and commercial applications.

Completion:

Upon completion of this program you can earn the title of Master Herbalist and receive your Diploma from The School of Natural Healing.

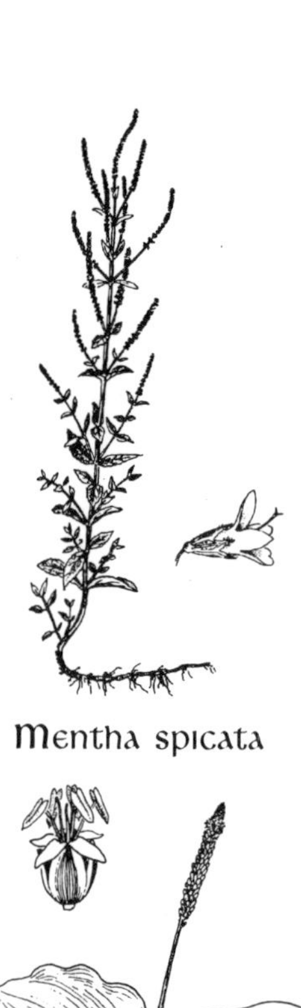

Mentha spicata

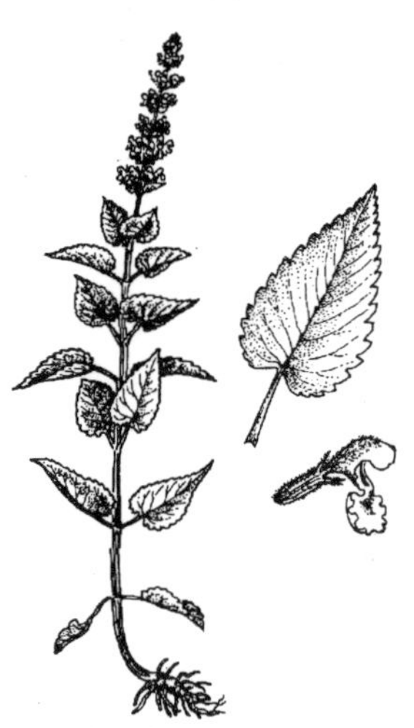

Nepeta cataria

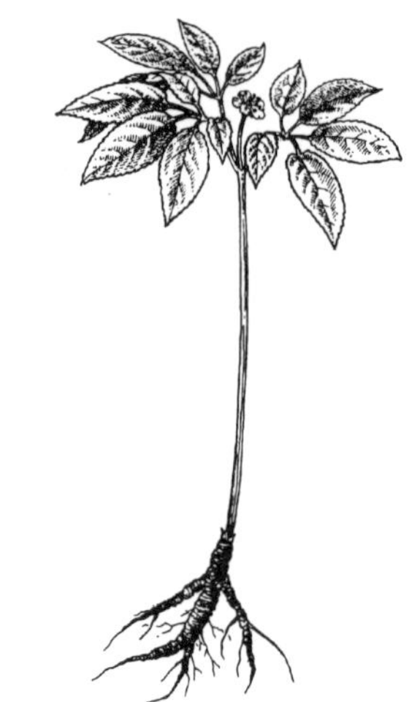

Panax quinquefolius

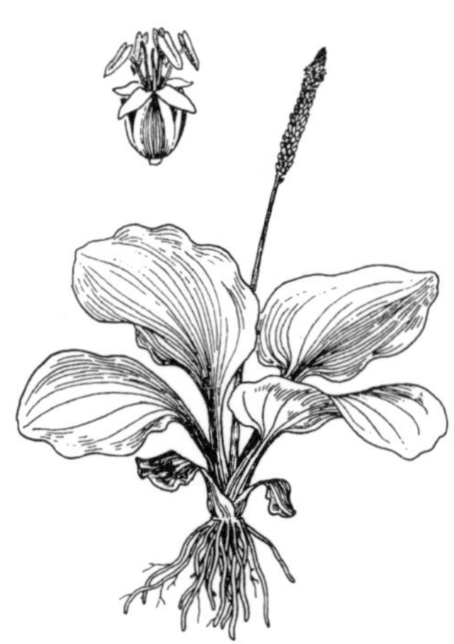

Plantago major

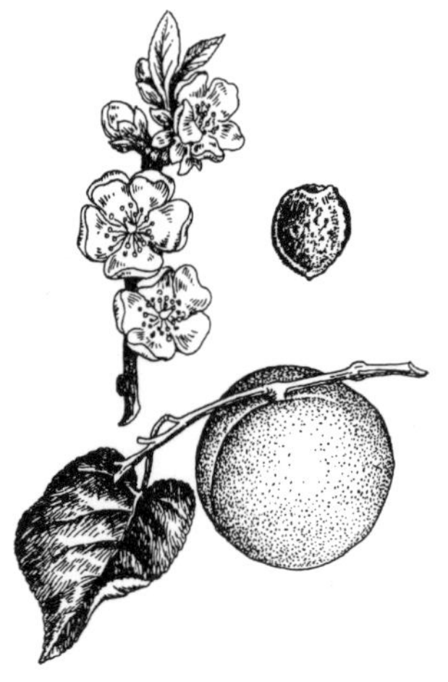

Prunus armeniaca

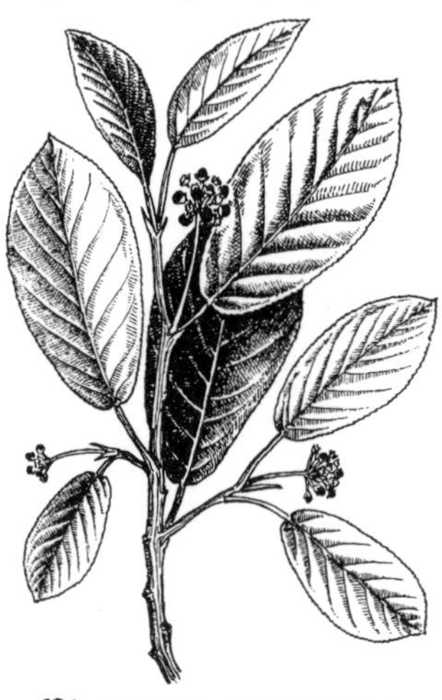

Rhamnus purshiana

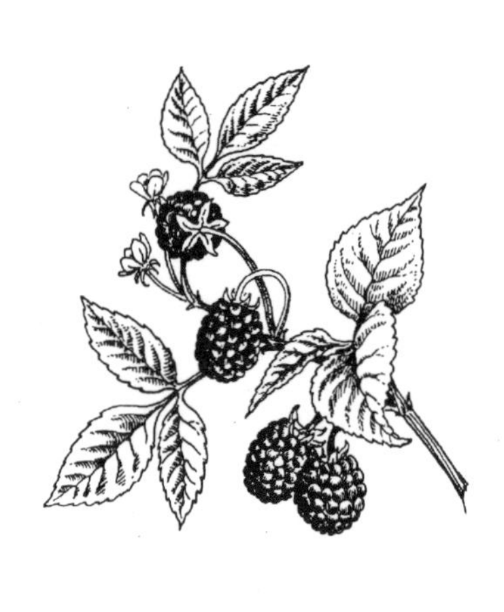

Rubus idaeus

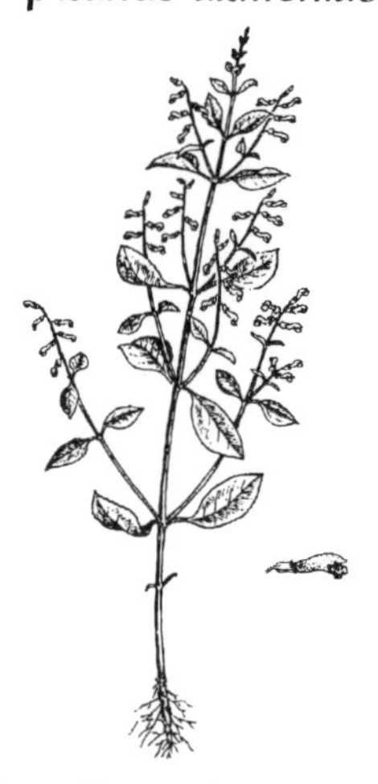

Scutellaria lateriflora

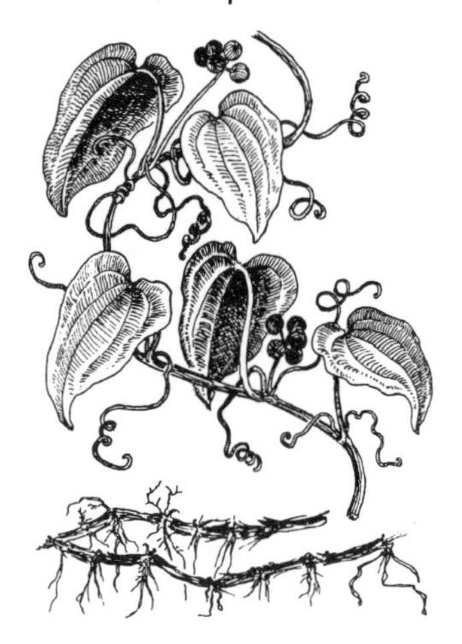

Smilax officinalis